T0210753

Lecture Notes in Computer Science 9005

Commenced Publication in 1973
Founding and Former Series Editors:
Gerhard Goos, Juris Hartmanis, and Jan van Leeuwen

More information about this series at http://www.springer.com/series/7412

Daniel Cremers · Ian Reid
Hideo Saito · Ming-Hsuan Yang (Eds.)

Computer Vision – ACCV 2014

12th Asian Conference on Computer Vision
Singapore, Singapore, November 1–5, 2014
Revised Selected Papers, Part III

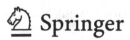
Springer

Editors

Daniel Cremers
Technische Universität München
Garching
Germany

Hideo Saito
Keio University
Yokohama, Kanagawa
Japan

Ian Reid
University of Adelaide
Adelaide, SA
Australia

Ming-Hsuan Yang
University of California at Merced
Merced, CA
USA

Videos to this book can be accessed at
http://www.springerimages.com/videos/978-3-319-16810-4

ISSN 0302-9743   ISSN 1611-3349   (electronic)
Lecture Notes in Computer Science
ISBN 978-3-319-16810-4   ISBN 978-3-319-16811-1   (eBook)
DOI 10.1007/978-3-319-16811-1

Library of Congress Control Number: 2015934895

LNCS Sublibrary: SL6 – Image Processing, Computer Vision, Pattern Recognition, and Graphics

Printed on acid-free paper

Springer International Publishing AG Switzerland is part of Springer Science+Business Media
(www.springer.com)

Preface

ACCV 2014 received a total of 814 submissions, a reflection of the growing strength of Computer Vision in Asia. We note, particularly, that a number of Area Chairs commented very positively on the overall quality of the submissions. The conference had submissions from all continents (except Antarctica, a challenge for the 2016 organizers perhaps) with 64 % from Asia, 20 % from Europe, and 10 % from North America.

The Program Chairs assembled a geographically diverse team of 36 Area Chairs who handled between 20 and 30 papers each. Area Chairs recommended reviewers for papers, and each paper received at least three reviews from the 638 reviewers who participated in the process. Paper decisions were finalized at an Area Chair meeting held in Singapore in September 2014. At this meeting, Area Chairs worked in triples to reach collective decisions about acceptance, and in panels of 12 to decide on the oral/poster distinction. The total number of papers accepted was 227, an overall acceptance rate of 28 %. Of these, 32 were selected for oral presentation.

We extend our immense gratitude to the Area Chairs and Reviewers for their generous participation in the process – the conference would not be possible if it were not for this huge voluntary investment of time and effort. We acknowledge particularly the contribution of 35 reviewers designated as "Outstanding Reviewers" (see page 14 in this booklet for a full list) who were nominated by Area Chairs and Program Chairs for having provided a large number of helpful, high-quality reviews.

The Program Chairs are also extremely grateful for the support, sage advice, and occasional good-natured prompting provided by the General Chairs. Each of them helped with matters that in other circumstances might have been left to the Program Chairs, so that it regularly felt as if we had a team of seven, not four Program Chairs. The PCs are very grateful for this.

Finally, we wish to thank the authors and delegates. Without their participation there would be no conference. The conference was graced with a uniformly high quality of presentations and posters, and we offer particular thanks to the three eminent keynote speakers, Stephane Mallat, Minoru Etoh, and Dieter Fox, who delivered outstanding talks.

Computer Vision in Asia is growing, and the quality of ACCV steadily climbing so that it is now, rightly, considered as one of the top conferences in the field. We look forward to future editions.

November 2014

Daniel Cremers
Ian Reid
Hideo Saito
Ming-Hsuan Yang

Organization

Organizing Committee

General Chairs

Michael S. Brown	National University of Singapore, Singapore
Tat-Jen Cham	Nanyang Technological University, Singapore
Yasuyuki Matsushita	Microsoft Research Asia, China

Program Chairs

Daniel Cremers	Technische Universität München, Germany
Ian Reid	University of Adelaide, Australia
Hideo Saito	Keio University, Japan
Ming-Hsuan Yang	University of California at Merced, USA

Organizing Chair

Teck Khim Ng	National University of Singapore, Singapore
Junsong Yuan	Nanyang Technological University, Singapore

Workshop Chairs

C.V. Jawahar	IIIT Hyderabad, India
Shiguang Shan	Institute of Computing Technology, Chinese Academy of Sciences, China

Demo Chairs

Bohyung Han	POSTECH, Korea
Koichi Kise	Osaka Prefecture University, Japan

Tutorial Chairs

Chu-Song Chen	Academia Sinica, Tawain
Brendan McCane	University of Otago, New Zealand

Publication Chairs

Terence Sim	National University of Singapore, Singapore
Jianxin Wu	Nanjing University, China

Industry Chairs

Hongcheng Wang	United Technologies Corporation, USA
Brian Price	Adobe, USA
Antonio Robles-Kelly	NITCA, Australia

Steering Committee

In-So Kweon	KAIST, Korea
Yasushi Yagi	Osaka University, Japan
Hongbin Zha	Peking University, China

Honorary Chair

Katsushi Ikeuchi	University of Tokyo, Japan

Area Chairs

Lourdes Agapito	Queen Mary University of London/University College London, UK
Thomas Brox	University of Freiburg, Germany
Tat-Jun Chin	University of Adelaide, Australia
Yung-Yu Chuang	National Taiwan University, Taiwan
Larry Davis	University of Maryland, USA
Yasutaka Furukawa	Washington University in St. Louis, USA
Bastian Goldluecke	University of Konstanz, Germany
Bohyung Han	POSTECH, Korea
Hiroshi Ishikawa	Waseda University, Japan
C.V. Jawahar	IIIT Hyderabad, India
Jana Kosecka	George Mason University, USA
David Kriegman	University of California, San Diego, USA
Shang-Hong Lai	National Tsing-Hua University, Taiwan
Ivan Laptev	Inria Rocquencourt, France
Kyoung Mu Lee	Seoul National University, Korea
Vincent Lepetit	École Polytechnique Fédérale de Lausanne, Switzerland
Jongwoo Lim	Hanyang University, Korea
Simon Lucey	CSIRO/University of Queensland, Australia
Ajmal Mian	University of Western Australia, Australia
Hajime Nagahara	Kyushu University, Japan
Ko Nishino	Drexel University, USA
Shmuel Peleg	The Hebrew University of Jerusalem, Israel
Imari Sato	National Institute of Informatics, Japan
Shin'ichi Satoh	National Institute of Informatics, Japan
Stefano Soatto	University of California, Los Angeles, USA
Jamie Shotton	Microsoft Research, UK
Ping Tan	Simon Fraser University, Canada
Lorenzo Torresani	Dartmouth College, USA
Manik Varma	Microsoft Research, India
Xiaogang Wang	Chinese University of Hong Kong, China
Shuicheng Yan	National University of Singapore, Singapore
Qing-Xiong Yang	City University of Hong Kong, Hong Kong
Jingyi Yu	University of Delaware, USA

Junsong Yuan   Nanyang Technological University, Singapore
Hongbin Zha   Peking University, China
Lei Zhang   Hong Kong Polytechnic University, Hong Kong,
                        China

Program Committee Members

Catherine Achard	Xun Cao	Jen-Hui Cheng
Hanno Ackermann	Gustavo Carneiro	Liang-Tien Chia
Haizhou Ai	Joao Carreira	Chen-Kuo Chiang
Emre Akbas	Umberto Castellani	Shao-Yi Chien
Naveed Akhtar	Carlos Castillo	Minsu Cho
Karteek Alahari	Turgay Celik	Nam Ik Cho
Mitsuru Ambai	Antoni Chan	Jonghyun Choi
Dragomir Anguelov	Kap Luk Chan	Wongun Choi
Yasuo Ariki	Kwok-Ping Chan	Mario Christoudias
Chetan Arora	Bhabatosh Chanda	Wen-Sheng Chu
Shai Avidan	Manmohan Chandraker	Albert C.S. Chung
Alper Ayvaci	Sharat Chandran	Pan Chunhong
Venkatesh Babu	Hong Chang	Arridhana Ciptadi
Xiang Bai	Kuang-Yu Chang	Javier Civera
Vineeth Balasubramanian	Che-Han Chang	Carlo Colombo
Jonathan Balzer	Vincent Charvillat	Yang Cong
Atsuhiko Banno	Santanu Chaudhury	Sanderson Conrad
Yufang Bao	Yi-Ling Chen	Olliver Cossairt
Adrian Barbu	Yi-Lei Chen	Marco Cristani
Nick Barnes	Jieying Chen	Beleznai Csaba
John Bastian	Yen-Lin Chen	Jinshi Cui
Abdessamad Ben Hamza	Kuan-Wen Chen	Fabio Cuzzolin
Chiraz BenAbdelkader	Chia-Ping Chen	Jeremiah D. Deng
Moshe Ben-Ezra	Yi-Ting Chen	Alessio Del Bue
AndrewTeoh Beng-Jin	Tsuhan Chen	Fatih Demirci
Benjamin Berkels	Xiangyu Chen	Xiaoming Deng
Jinbo Bi	Xiaowu Chen	Joachim Denzler
Alberto Del Bimbo	Haifeng Chen	Anthony Dick
Horst Bischof	Hwann-Tzong Chen	Julia Diebold
Konstantinos Blekas	Bing-Yu Chen	Thomas Diego
Adrian Bors	Chu-Song Chen	Csaba Domokos
Nizar Bouguila	Qiang Chen	Qiulei Dong
Edmond Boyer	Jie Chen	Gianfranco Doretto
Steve Branson	Jiun-Hung Chen	Ralf Dragon
Hilton Bristow	MingMing Cheng	Bruce Draper
Asad Butt	Hong Cheng	Tran Du
Ricardo Cabral	Shyi-Chyi Cheng	Lixin Duan
Cesar Cadena	Yuan Cheng	Kun Duan
Francesco Camastra	Wen-Huang Cheng	Fuqing Duan

Zoran Duric
Michael Eckmann
Hazim Ekenel
Naoko Enami
Jakob Engel
Anders Eriksson
Francisco Escolano
Virginia Estellers
Wen-Pinn Fang
Micha Feigin
Jiashi Feng
Francesc Ferri
Katerina Fragkiadaki
Chi-Wing Fu
Yun Fu
Chiou-Shann Fuh
Hironobu Fujiyoshi
Giorgio Fumera
Takuya Funatomi
Juergen Gall
Yongsheng Gao
Ravi Garg
Arkadiusz Gertych
Bernard Ghanem
Guy Godin
Roland Goecke
Vladimir Golkov
Yunchao Gong
Stephen Gould
Josechu Guerrero
Richard Guest
Yanwen Guo
Dong Guo
Huimin Guo
Vu Hai
Lin Hai-Ting
Peter Hall
Onur Hamsici
Tony Han
Hu Han
Zhou Hao
Kenji Hara
Tatsuya Harada
Mehrtash Harandi
Jean-Bernard Hayet
Ran He

Shengfeng He
Shinsaku Hiura
Jeffrey Ho
Christopher Hollitt
Hyunki Hong
Ki Sang Hong
Seunghoon Hong
Takahiro Horiuchi
Timothy Hospedales
Kazuhiro Hotta
Chiou-Ting Candy Hsu
Min-Chun Hu
Zhe Hu
Kai-Lung Hua
Gang Hua
Chunsheng Hua
Chun-Rong Huang
Fay Huang
Kaiqi Huang
Peter Huang
Jia-Bin Huang
Xinyu Huang
Yi-Ping Hung
Mohamed Hussein
Cong Phuoc Huynh
Du Huynh
Sung Ju Hwang
Naoyuki Ichimura
Ichiro Ide
Yoshihisa Ijiri
Sei Ikeda
Nazli Ikizler-Cinbis
Atsushi Imiya
Kohei Inoue
Yani Ioannou
Catalin Ionescu
Go Irie
Rui Ishiyama
Yoshio Iwai
Yumi Iwashita
Arpit Jain
Hueihan Jhuang
Yangqing Jia
Yunde Jia
Kui Jia
Yu-Gang Jiang

Shuqiang Jiang
Xiaoyi Jiang
Jun Jiang
Kang-Hyun Jo
Matjaz Jogan
Manjunath Joshi
Frederic Jurie
Ioannis Kakadiaris
Amit Kale
Prem Kalra
George Kamberov
Kenichi Kanatani
Atul Kanaujla
Mohan Kankanhalli
Abou-Moustafa Karim
Zoltan Kato
Harish Katti
Hiroshi Kawasaki
Christian Kerl
Sang Keun Lee
Aditya Khosla
Hansung Kim
Kyungnam Kim
Seon Joo Kim
Byungsoo Kim
Akisato Kimura
Koichi Kise
Yasuyo Kita
Itaru Kitahara
Reinhard Klette
Georges Koepfler
Iasonas Kokkinos
Kazuaki Kondo
Xiangfei Kong
Sotiris Kotsiantis
Junghyun Kown
Arjan Kuijper
Shiro Kumano
Kashino Kunio
Yoshinori Kuno
Cheng-hao Kuo
Suha Kwak
Iljung Kwak
Junseok Kwon
Alexander Ladikos
Hamid Laga

Antony Lam
Francois Lauze
Duy-Dinh Le
Guee Sang Lee
Jae-Ho Lee
Chan-Su Lee
Yong Jae Lee
Bocchi Leonardo
Marius Leordeanu
Matt Leotta
Wee-Kheng Leow
Bruno Lepri
Frederic Lerasle
Fuxin Li
Hongdong Li
Rui Li
Jia Li
Yufeng Li
Yongmin Li
Yung-Hui Li
Cheng Li
Xin Li
Peihua Li
Xirong Li
Annan Li
Xi Li
Chia-Kai Liang
Shu Liao
T. Warren Liao
Jenn-Jier Lien
Joseph Lim
Ser-Nam Lim
Huei-Yung Lin
Haiting Lin
Weiyao Lin
Wen-Chieh (Steve) Lin
Yen-Yu Lin
RueiSung Lin
Yuanqing Lin
Yen-Liang Lin
Haibin Ling
Hairong Liu
Cheng-Lin Liu
Qingzhong Liu
Miaomiao Liu
Jingchen Liu
Ligang Liu

Haowei Liu
Guangcan Liu
Feng Liu
Shuang Liu
Shuaicheng Liu
Xiaobai Liu
Si Liu
Lingqiao Liu
Chen Change Loy
Feng Lu
Tong Lu
Zhaojin Lu
Le Lu
Huchuan Lu
Ping Luo
Lui Luoqi
Ludovic Macaire
Arif Mahmood
Robert Maier
Yasushi Makihara
Koji Makita
Yoshitsugu Manabe
Rok Mandeljc
Al Mansur
Gian-Luca Marcialis
Stephen Marsland
Takeshi Masuda
Thomas Mauthner
Stephen Maybank
Chris McCool
Xing Mei
Jason Meltzer
David Michael
Anton Milan
Gregor Miller
Dongbo Min
Ikuhisa Mitsugami
Anurag Mittal
Daisuke Miyazaki
Henning Müller
Thomas Moellenhoff
Pascal Monasse
Greg Mori
Bryan Morse
Yadong Mu
Yasuhiro Mukaigawa
Jayanta Mukhopadhyay

Vittorio Murino
Atsushi Nakazawa
Myra Nam
Anoop Namboodiri
Liangliang Nan
Loris Nanni
P.J. Narayanan
Shawn Newsam
Thanh Ngo
Bingbing Ni
Jifeng Ning
Masashi Nishiyama
Mark Nixon
Shohei Nobuhara
Vincent Nozick
Tom O'Donnell
Takeshi Oishi
Takahiro Okabe
Ryuzo Okada
Takayuki Okatani
Gustavo Olague
Martin Oswald
Wanli Ouyang
Yuji Oyamada
Paul Sakrapee
Paisitkriangkrai
Kalman Palagyi
Hailang Pan
Gang Pan
Sharath Pankanti
Hsing-Kuo Pao
Hyun Soo Park
Jong-Il Park
Ioannis Patras
Nick Pears
Helio Pedrini
Pieter Peers
Yigang Peng
Bo Peng
David Penman
Janez Pers
Wong Ya Ping
Hamed Pirsiavash
Robert Pless
Dilip Prasad
Dipti Prasad Mukherjee
Andrea Prati

Vittal Premachandran
Brian Price
Oriol Pujol Pujol
Pulak Purkait
Zhen Qian
Xueyin Qin
Bogdan Raducanu
Luis Rafael Canali
Visvanathan Ramesh
Ananth Ranganathan
Nalini Ratha
Edel Garcia Reyes
Hamid Rezatofighi
Christian Riess
Antonio Robles-Kelly
Mikel Rodriguez
Olaf Ronneberger
Guy Rosman
Arun Ross
Amit Roy Chowdhury
Xiang Ruan
Raif Rustamov
Fereshteh Sadeghi
Satoshi Saga
Ryusuke Sagawa
Fumihiko Sakaue
Mathieu Salzmann
Jorge Sanchez
Nong Sang
Pramod Sankar
Angel Sappa
Michel Sarkis
Tomokazu Sato
Yoichi Sato
Jun Sato
Harpreet Sawhney
Walter Scheirer
Bernt Schiele
Frank Schmidt
Dirk Schnieders
William Schwartz
McCloskey Scott
Faisal Shafait
Shishir Shah
Shiguang Shan
Li Shen

Chunhua Shen
Xiaohui Shen
Shuhan Shen
Sanketh Shetty
Boxin Shi
YiChang Shih
Huang-Chia Shih
Atsushi Shimada
Nobutaka Shimada
Ilan Shimshoni
Koichi Shinoda
Abhinav Shrivastava
Xianbiao Shu
Gautam Singh
Sudipta Sinha
Eric Sommerlade
Andy Song
Li Song
Yibing Song
Mohamed Souiai
Richard Souvenir
Frank Steinbruecker
Ramanathan Subramanian
Yusuke Sugano
Akihiro Sugimoto
Yasushi Sumi
Yajie Sun
Weidong Sun
Xiaolu Sun
Deqing Sun
Min Sun
Ju Sun
Jian Sun
Ganesh Sundaramoorthi
Jinli Suo
Rahul Swaminathan
Yuichi Taguchi
Yu-Wing Tai
Taketomi Takafumi
Jun Takamatsu
Hugues Talbot
Toru Tamaki
Xiaoyang Tan
Robby Tan
Masayuki Tanaka
Jinhui Tang

Ming Tang
Kevin Tang
João Manuel R.S. Tavares
Mutsuhiro Terauchi
Ali Thabet
Eno Toeppe
Matt Toews
Yan Tong
Akihiko Torii
Yu-Po Tsai
Yi-Hsuan Tsai
Matt Turek
Seiichi Uchida
Hideaki Uchiyama
Toshio Ueshiba
Norimichi Ukita
Julien Valentin
Pascal Vasseur
Ashok Veeraraphavan
Matthias Vestner
Xiaoyu Wang
Dong Wang
Ruiping Wang
Sheng-Jyh Wang
Shenlong Wang
Lei Wang
Song Wang
Xianwang Wang
Yang Wang
Yunhong Wang
Yu-Chiang Frank Wang
Hanzi Wang
Hongcheng Wang
Chaohui Wang
Chen Wang
Cheng Wang
Changhu Wang
Li-Yi Wei
Longyin Wen
Gordon Wetzstein
Paul Wohlhart
Chee Sun Won
Kwan-Yee
    Kenneth Wong
John Wright
Jianxin Wu

Xiao Wu	Jimei Yang	Cha Zhang
Yi Wu	Chih-Yuan Yang	Hong Hui Zhang
Xiaomeng Wu	Bangpeng Yao	Hui Zhang
Rolf Wurtz	Jong Chul Ye	Guofeng Zhang
Tao Xiang	Mao Ye	Xiao-Wei Zhao
Yu Xiang	Sai Kit Yeung	Rui Zhao
Yang Xiao	Kwang Moo Yi	Gangqiang Zhao
Ning Xu	Alper Yilmaz	Shuai Zheng
Li Xu	Zhaozheng Yin	Yinqiang Zheng
Changsheng Xu	Xianghua Ying	Zhonglong Zheng
Jianru Xue	Ryo Yonetani	Weishi Zheng
Mei Xue	Ju Hong Yoon	Wenming Zheng
Yasushi Yagi	Kuk-Jin Yoon	Lu Zheng
Koichiro Yamaguchi	Lap Fai Yu	Baojiang Zhong
Kota Yamaguchi	Gang Yu	Lin Zhong
Osamu Yamaguchi	Xenophon Zabulis	Bolei Zhou
Toshihiko Yamasaki	John Zelek	Jun Zhou
Takayoshi Yamashita	Zheng-Jun Zha	Feng Zhou
Pingkun Yan	De-Chuan Zhan	Feng Zhu
Keiji Yanai	Kaihua Zhang	Ning Zhu
Jie Yang	Tianzhu Zhang	Pengfei Zhu
Ruigang Yang	Yu Zhang	Cai-Zhi Zhu
Ming Yang	Zhong Zhang	Zhigang Zhu
Hao Yang	Yinda Zhang	Andrew Ziegler
Meng Yang	Xiaoqin Zhang	Danping Zou
Xiaokang Yang	Liqing Zhang	Wangmeng Zuo
Yi Yang	Xiaobo Zhang	
Yongliang Yang	Changshui Zhang	

Best Paper Award Committee

James Rehg	Georgia Institute of Technology, USA
Horst Bischof	Graz University of Technology, Austria
Kyoung Mu Lee	Seoul National University, South Korea

Best Paper Awards

1. Saburo Tsuji Best Paper Award

A Message Passing Algorithm for MRF inference with Unknown Graphs and Its Applications
Zhenhua Wang (University of Adelaide), Zhiyi Zhang (Northwest A&F University), Geng Nan (Northwest A&F University)

2. Sang Uk Lee Best Student Paper Award [Sponsored by Nvidia]

Separation of Reflection Components by Sparse Non-negative Matrix Factorization
Yasuhiro Akashi (Tohoku University), Takayuki Okatani (Tohoku University)

3. Songde Ma Best Application Paper Award [Sponsored by NICTA]

Stereo Fusion using a Refractive Medium on a Binocular Base
Seung-Hwan Baek (KAIST), Min H. Kim (KAIST)

4. Best Paper Honorable Mention

Singly-Bordered Block-Diagonal Form for Minimal Problem Solvers
Zuzana Kukelova (Czech Technical University, Microsoft Research Cambridge),
Martin Bujnak (Capturing Reality), Jan Heller (Czech Technical University),
Tomas Pajdla (Czech Technical University)

5. Best Student Paper Honorable Mention [Sponsored by Nvidia]

On Multiple Image Group Cosegmentation
Fanman Meng (University of Electronic Science and Technology of China),
Jianfei Cai (Nanyang Technological University), Hongliang Li
(University of Electronic Science and Technology of China)

6. Best Application Paper Honorable Mention [Sponsored by NICTA]

Massive City-scale Surface Condition Analysis using Ground and Aerial Imagery
Ken Sakurada (Tohoku University), Takayuki Okatani (Tohoku Univervisty),
Kris Kitani (Carnegie Mellon University)

ACCV 2014 – Outstanding Reviewers

Emre Akbas	Catalin Ionescu	Bernt Schiele
Jonathan Balzer	Suha Kwak	Chunhua Shen
Steve Branson	Junseok Kwon	Sudipta Sinha
Sanderson Conrad	Fuxin Li	Deqing Sun
Marco Cristani	Chen-Change Loy	Yuichi Taguchi
Alessio Del Bue	Scott McCloskey	Toru Tamaki
Anthony Dick	Xing Mei	Dong Wang
Bruce Draper	Yasushi Makihara	Yu-Chiang Frank Wang
Katerina Fragkiadaki	Guy Rosman	Paul Wohlhart
Tatsuya Harada	Mathieu Salzmann	John Wright
Mehrtash Harandi	Pramod Sankar	Bangpeng Yao
Nazli Ikizler-Cinbis	Walter Scheirer	

ACCV 2014 Sponsors

Platnium	Singapore Tourism Board
Gold	Omron Nvidia Garena Samsung
Silver	Adobe ViSenze
Bronze	Lee Foundation Morpx Microsoft Research NICTA

Contents – Part III

Accurate Vessel Segmentation with Progressive Contrast Enhancement and Canny Refinement

Xin Yang[1,2(✉)], Kwang-Ting Tim Cheng[2], and Aichi Chien[3]

[1] Department of Electronics Information Engineering, HUST, Wuhan, China
xinyang@umail.ucsb.edu
[2] Department of Electrical Computer Engineering, UCSB, Santa Barbara, CA, USA
[3] Division of Interventional Neuroradiology, UCLA, Medical School,
Los Angeles, CA, USA

Abstract. Vessel segmentation is a key step for various medical applications, such as diagnosis assistance, quantification of vascular pathology, and treatment planning. This paper describes an automatic vessel segmentation framework which can achieve highly accurate segmentation even in regions of low contrast and signal-to-noise-ratios (SNRs) and at vessel boundaries with disturbance induced by adjacent non-vessel pixels. There are two key contributions of our framework. The first is a progressive contrast enhancement method which adaptively improves contrast of challenging pixels that were otherwise indistinguishable, and suppresses noises by weighting pixels according to their likelihood to be vessel pixels. The second contribution is a method called canny refinement which is based on a canny edge detection algorithm to effectively re-move false positives around boundaries of vessels. Experimental results on a public retinal dataset and our clinical cerebral data demonstrate that our approach outperforms state-of-the-art methods including the vesselness based method [1] and the optimally oriented flux (OOF) based method [2].

1 Introduction

The segmentation of vascular structures plays a significant role in diagnosis assistance, quantification of vascular pathologies, treatment and surgery planning. For instance, segmenting arteries and their bifurcations in the Circle of Willis, and quantifying their changes over a span of time can facilitate cerebral aneurysm detection and development analysis. In neurosurgical procedures, vessels, giving indication of where the blood supply of a lesion is drawn from and drained to, often serve as landmarks and guidelines to the lesion during surgery. The more accurate the vascular segmentation is, the more precise a computer-guided procedure can be made.

With growing streams of data generated by modern imaging modalities, such as computed tomography angiography (CTA) and magnetic resonance angiography (MRA), automatic vessel segmentation to minimize laborious and error-prone manual operations is in great demand. There have been numerous dedicated research efforts on this subject over years. Some of most successful ones apply

© Springer International Publishing Switzerland 2015
D. Cremers et al. (Eds.): ACCV 2014, Part III, LNCS 9005, pp. 1–16, 2015.
DOI: 10.1007/978-3-319-16811-1_1

filters (e.g. Hessian-based filters [1], optimally oriented flux (OOF) [2], steerable filters [19], and learned filters [3–8]) to individual pixels and classify a pixel as a part of a vessel or not based on its filter response. However, these filters mainly rely on image gradients or high-order derivatives, thus they can hardly provide accurate responses at regions with very low contrast and a poor signal-to-noises ratio (SNR). The top row of Figs. 1 (b) and (c) display a sub-region of a retinal vessel image of Fig. 1 (a) and a contrast-enhanced version, respectively. Due to low image contrast, several small vessels in Fig. 1 (b)-top can barely be distinguished. Applying contrast enhancement to this region could slightly improve the visibility of small vessels while greatly increase noises resulting in a low SNR (as shown in Fig. 1 (c)-top). As a result, most existing methods fail to achieve a high true-positive rate and a low false-positive rate in those regions (as shown in Fig. 1 (d)-top). Another limitation of existing methods is that vascular filters usually give similarly weak responses for pixels around vascular borders, either vessel or non-vessel pixels, resulting in inaccuracy in localizing the true boundary of a vessel tube. As shown in Fig. 1 (d)-bottom, most pixels in the neighborhood of vessel boundaries are incorrectly classified (as denoted in red) which could result in inaccurate quantification of vascular pathologies and diagnosis.

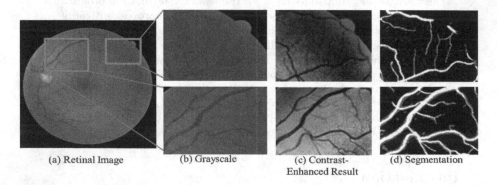

(a) Retinal Image   (b) Grayscale   (c) Contrast-Enhanced Result   (d) Segmentation

Fig. 1. Limitations of existing vessel segmentation methods. (a) An exemplar retinal image. (b) and (c) are grayscale images of two sub-regions and their contrast-enhanced results respectively. (d) Segmentation results for the contrast-enhanced images based on vesselness (i.e. the Frangi's method [1]), one of the most popular methods for vessel segmentation. White, green and red colors indicate true positives, false negatives and false positives, respectively. Two major limitations of the Frangi's method can be observed: (1) for regions with a low contrast and SNR, it fails to detect most of small vessels (green pixels in (d-top)) and incorrectly classifies many noises as vessels (red pixels in (d-top)); and (2) it fails to precisely localize boundaries of vessels (d-bottom). Although we use results of the Frangi's method for illustration, these two limitations are common for most existing methods (Color figure online).

In this paper, we present an automatic vessel segmentation framework, with the primary focus on achieving high accuracy in two challenging scenarios: in regions with low contrast and low SNR and at vessel boundaries. Specifically, there are two main contributions of the proposed framework:

1. We propose a progressive contrast enhancement method that iteratively excludes a subset of pixels, which have been identified as vessel pixels with high confidence in previous iterations, from contrast enhancement in the next iteration. Comparing to existing methods which process all pixels within a particular region, the proposed approach, adjusting the contrast only for the remaining pixels in each iteration, places more emphasis on challenging pixels which are difficult to be classified in previous iterations. As a result, our approach can better capture subtle vessel information in low contrast regions. To further suppress noises in low SNR regions, we weight the intensity of every pixel based on a function of shape responses to reduce the impact of noises in the contrast enhancement procedure. The idea behind this strategy is that the shape information is complementary to the intensity information and it is less likely that a non-vessel pixel with high noise could have both its shape response and its intensity value similar to those of a vessel pixel.

2. We propose a simple yet effective method, called canny refinement, for precisely localizing vessel pixels, particularly at vessel boundaries. Our method employs canny edge detection to identify pixels on the boundaries of vessels. Then a ro-bust and effective function is designed based on canny edges to determine whether a pixel is between two boundaries of a vessel or is outside a vessel. Based on the output of the function, the system method can refine the filtering results and minimize false positives which are outside a vessel. The rest of the paper is organized as follows. Section 2 reviews the related work. Section 3 presents details of the proposed method. In Sect. 4, we compare the performance of our method with two state-of-the-art methods. Section 5 concludes the paper.

2   Related Work

The broad application of vessel segmentation has stimulated the development of several categories of approaches, each of which has distinct strengths. Active contour within the level set framework [11–13], which is capable of handling topology changes and is adaptable to shapes of complex vessel structures, has proven to be effective for vessel segmentation. Several enhancements have been made for further performance improvement. Most recent efforts [9, 10] have been focusing on simplifying and automating the parameter settings to achieve optimized performance for a wide range of data content and quality.

Another category of approaches applies vessel enhancement filters to individual pixels and then classifies each pixel, as either a vessel or a non-vessel pixel, by thresholding the filtering score [1–3, 5–8, 20, 21]. Our framework belongs to this category. A number of vessel enhancement filters have been developed in recent years. Some of them utilize the second-order derivatives to distinguish specific tubular shape of vessels, which have a locally prominent low curvature orientation (i.e. the vessel direction) and have planes of a high intensity curvature (i.e. the cross-sectional planes) [1, 20–23]. The Hessian matrix is the most common tool to capture tubular structure information. Eigenvalues of the Hessian matrix can discriminate between plane-, blob- and tubular-like structures, and corresponding eigenvectors indicate the vessel orientations. A representative example of the Hessian-matrix based method is the vesselness filter proposed in Frangi et al. [1] which has been widely used in practice, owing to its intuitive geometric formulation. The Weingarten matrix is a less popular alternative to the Hessian matrix. Filters based on the Weingarten matrix include those proposed in [22,23].

Instead of analyzing the second-order derivatives, another category of methods exploit the local distribution of the gradient vectors. For instance, the method in [3] analyzes the eigenvalues of the gradient vectors' covariance matrix. Bauer and Bischof [24] leveraged a vector field obtained from the gradient vector flow (GVF) diffusion. Law and Chung proposed the use of optimally oriented flux (OOF) [2] which relies on the measure of gradient flux through the boundary of local spheres. Comparing to the Hessian-based filters, OOF could be more accurate and less sensitive to disturbances from adjacent structures.

It has been pointed out in recent literature [5–8] that real vascular structures, which do not necessarily conform to an ideal tubular shape model, can drastically impact the performance of methods relying on handcrafted shape filters. Several efforts have been made to learn filters to describe convoluted appearances and structures of vessels. For instance, Agam et al. [3] estimated the eigenvalue distribution of the gradient vectors' covariance matrix via Expectation Maximization. Support Vector Machines operating on the Hessian's eigenvalues have been used to discriminate between vascular and nonvascular pixels [4]. In [8], rotational features were computed at each pixel using steerable filters and fed to an SVM to classify pixels as vessel pixels or not. Inspired by [8], a series of improvements [5–7] were made which include more filters (i.e. vesselness [1] and OOF [2]), in addition to the steerable filters, and leverage more advanced machine learning techniques. A comprehensive survey of vessel segmentation methods can be found in [15,16]. The problem, however, is that both handcrafted and learned filters mainly rely on image gradients or high-order derivatives, thus their responses are sensitive to noises and often too weak to discriminate vascular and nonvascular pixels in low contrast regions. Today's angiograms inevitably contain noises and exhibit inhomogeneous contrast. The intensity of some vessels (particularly narrow vessels) could differ from the background by as little as four grey levels, yet the standard deviation of back-ground noise is around 2.3 grey levels. As a result, most, if not all, existing filters are ineffective in low contrast and/or low SNR regions. In addition, vascular filters usually produce weak responses around vascular borders, yielding difficulties in precisely localizing the exact boundary of a vessel tube. Imprecise boundary localization could consequently result in inaccurate quantification of pathologies and diagnosis. This paper focuses on addressing these two challenging problems. Specifically, we pro-posed two techniques: progressive contrast enhancement and canny refinement, which can be used together with existing filtering based methods and greatly boost their segmentation performance in low contrast, low SNR regions and at vascular boundaries.

3   Our Method

Figure 2 illustrates our vessel segmentation framework, which consists of three main components: vessel enhancement filtering (the orange block), canny refinement (the green block) and progressive contrast enhancement (the blue blocks). Given an input image, vessel enhancement filtering is first applied to every image pixel to obtain the likelihood of each pixel being a vessel pixel. In our implementation, we employ vesselness [1] and OOF filters [2], which are known as two of the best filters to date. Canny refinement is then applied to revise the filtering results: the filtering responses of those pixels classified to be outside a vessel by canny refinement are adjusted to zero (i.e. non-vessel pixel with the highest confidence). Based on the revised responses, pixels which can be classified with high confidence as either vessel or background pixels are added to the final segmentation results and removed from the image. The method adjusts the contrast of the remaining pixels by shape-weighted contrast enhancement and then restarts the above-mentioned procedure on the remaining pixels. Such procedure repeats until no more fine vessels can be detected or the number of iterations reaches a limit. In the following, we provide technical details and describe strengths of canny refinement and progressive contrast enhancement.

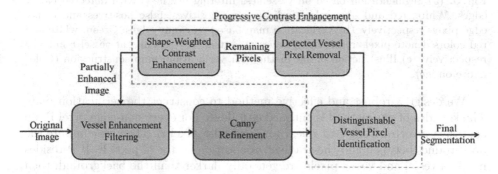

Fig. 2. Framework of vessel semgnetation with progressive contrast enhancement and canny refinement (Color figure online).

3.1   Canny Refinement

Canny [25] has been widely regarded as the best solution for robust edge detection and precise localization of edge pixels. Vascular boundaries which can be approx-imated as step edges should be accurately localized by canny. Figure 3 (a) displays the vessel segmentation based on vesselness filtering overlaid with detected canny edges (the blue pixels). Clearly, many canny edge pixels correctly locate at real vessel boundaries, forming "classification planes" which separate true positives (the white pixels) from false positives (the red pixels).

However, canny provides only the location of edges but could not determine whether a pixel adjacent to an edge is inside or outside of a vessel tube. Therefore, solely relying on the edge location cannot remove false positives. To address this problem, we construct a verification map based on canny edges. Each entry of the map is a value of quadruples 1, 0, -1, null (as shown in Fig. 3 (b)), i.e. 1 (green) and -1 (white) indicate pixels inside and outside a vessel tube, respectively. A 0 (red) de-notes a pixel at the boundary and null (back) indicate pixels far from any edges and thus are unnecessary to be examined in the current itera-tion. Based on the veri-fication map, the method can refine the filtering results, i.e. pixels with small filtering response values and are labeled as -1 in the verifi-cation map are re-classified as negatives.

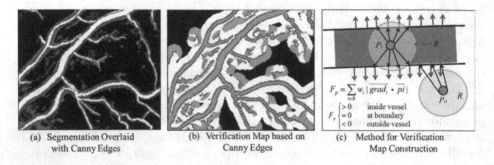

| (a) Segmentation Overlaid with Canny Edges | (b) Verification Map based on Canny Edges | (c) Method for Verification Map Construction |

Fig. 3. (a) Segmentation based on vesselness filtering overlaied with detected canny edges. White, red and blue colors indicate true positives, false positives and canny edge pixels respectively. (b) Verification map based on canny edges. Green, white and red colors denote pixels reside inside a vessel, outside a vessel and at vessel boundary respectively. (c) Illustruction of our method for verificatiom map construction (Color figure online).

We design a robust and effective method to construct the verification map. The key idea of our method is outlined as follows. For every non-edge pixel P, we construct a vector from P to a nearby canny edge pixel E. Then we compute the dot product between and the gradient orientation vector of pixel E. If P resides inside a vessel and vessel pixels are generally darker than the background, then the dot product is greater than zero; otherwise, the dot product is negative. Based on the sign of the dot product, we can determine whether a pixel is inside or outside a vessel. A verification map based on a single edge pixel is usually sensitive to noises. To improve the robustness, for every pixel P we consider a set of the canny edge pixels   near P and sum up the weighed dot product according to Eq. (1) (as illustrated in Fig. 3 (c)).

$$F_p = \sum_{E_i \in R} w_{E_i} \left| \overrightarrow{grad_{E_i}} \bullet \overrightarrow{PE_i} \right| \tag{1}$$

The weights w_{E_i} is sampled from a Gaussian distribution centered at P as Eq. (2), where (x_P, y_P), (x_{E_i}, y_{E_i}) are coordinates of pixels P and E_i, and σ is the standard deviation of the Gaussian distribution.

$$w_{E_i} = exp\left(\frac{(x_p - x_{E_i})^2 + (y_p - y_{E_i})^2}{2\sigma^2} \right) \tag{2}$$

Based on F_P we can construct a verification map V_p according to Eq. (3).

$$V_p = \begin{cases} 1, & F_p > 0 \text{ and } P \notin E \\ 0, & P \in E \\ -1, & F_p < 0 \text{ and } P \notin E \\ null, & R_p \cap E = \varnothing \end{cases} \tag{3}$$

3.2 Progressive Contrast Enhancement

In this section, we first briefly overview conventional contrast enhancement approaches and their limitations for vessel segmentation, followed by details of our progressive contrast enhancement method.

Histogram Equalization for Contrast Enhancement. Heterogeneous contrast, resulting from the contrast agent inhomogeneity, noises and image artifacts, is a common problem in many medical image modalities. Histogram equalization is a common tool to increase contrast by stretching out the overall inten-sity range of an image. More specifically, it maps one distribution (i.e. original histogram of a given image) to another distribution (i.e. a wider and more uniform distribu-tion of intensity values) based on a transformation function so that the intensity values can spread over the entire range. The transformation function is built based on the cumulative distribution function (CDF) defined as Eq. (4),

$$cdf_x(i) = \sum_{j=0}^{i} p_x(j), \qquad 0 \leq i \leq L \tag{4}$$

where $p_x(i)$ is the probability of an occurrence of gray level i in image x, L is the total number of gray levels in the image (typically 256). The desired image y should have a flat histogram with a linearized CDF across the entire range, for a constant K.

$$cdf_y(i) = iK \tag{5}$$

According to Eqs. (4) and (5), the intensity transformation function can be derived as

$$T(i) = round\left(\frac{cdf_x(i) - cdf_{x_{min}}}{(M \times N) - cdf_{x_{min}}} \times (L - 1) \right) \tag{6}$$

where $M \times N$ gives the total number of pixels in image x.

However, histogram equalization often fails to provide satisfactory results for medical images with inhomogeneous contrast. Regions that are much lighter or darker than the rest of the image cannot be sufficiently enhanced. In addition, it could over-amplify noises in relatively homogeneous regions. Figure 4 (c) displays the contrast-enhanced result for Fig. 4 (a) based on histogram equalization. Clearly, background noises are greatly amplified. Contrast Limited Adaptive Histogram Equalization (CLAHE) [15] is a popular solution to address these problems. It adjusts contrast locally by deriving a local transformation function from

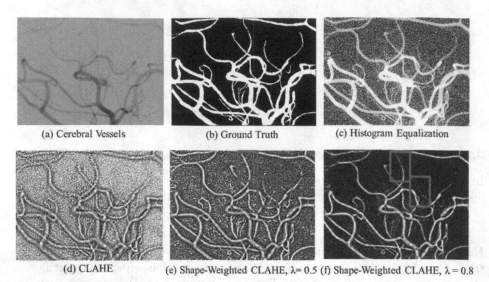

(a) Cerebral Vessels   (b) Ground Truth   (c) Histogram Equalization

(d) CLAHE   (e) Shape-Weighted CLAHE, λ= 0.5   (f) Shape-Weighted CLAHE, λ = 0.8

Fig. 4. Illustration of contrast enhancement results based on different methods. (a) Original image with cerebral vessels. (b) Ground truth obtained by manual label. (c) - (d) Contrast enhancement results based on histogram equalization and CLAHE with clip limit being 30, region size being 5050. (e) - (f) Contrast enhancement results based on shape-weighted CLAHE with λ being 0.5 and 0.8, respectively. Shape information is obtained by vesselness filtering.

a neighborhood region of each pixel, and clips the histogram at a predefined value before computing the CDF to prevent over-amplification of noises. However, for images with a very low SNR, CLAHE still cannot effectively suppress noises, resulting in a noisy background and rough vessel boundaries (as shown in Fig. 4 (d)). More importantly, although CLAHE performs equalization locally, it is inevitable that a local region contains both large vessels with good contrast to the background and fine vessels with low contrast (as shown in Fig. 1 (a)-top). For these regions, results are usually dominated by large vessels, resulting in insufficient enhancement for small vessels (as shown in Fig. 1 (b)-top). Our progressive contrast enhancement can more successfully suppress noises through weighting each pixel's intensity by its shape filtering response and focus mainly on enhancing contrast of challenging pixels (i.e. small vessel pixels) in each iteration.

Shape-Weighted Contrast Enhancement. CLAHE utilizes only the intensity of an image, thus is very sensitive to noises which have similar intensity values as vessels. The local geometric structure around each pixel is a discriminating feature useful for distinguishing vessel pixels from random noises. In addition, the local shape information is complementary to the intensity information, thus it is less likely that noise pixels have similar values of both shape responses and intensity as vessel pixels. Based on these observations, we propose to use local shape information $S(x)$ obtained from vessel enhancement filtering (i.e. vesselness or OOF) to weight the corresponding pixel intensities $I_{norm}(x)$

before per-forming CLAHE, as shown in Eq. (7). Intensities are normalized to the range of [0, 1] and for images in which vessel pixels are darker than the background, we reverse each pixel's intensity value by subtracting the original normalized intensity from 1. We set a parameter λ to adjust the impact of the weights. Larger results in greater impact of weighting and vice versa.

$$I_{new}(x) = \begin{cases} I_{norm}(x) \times (S(x))^\lambda, & vessel\ pixels\ are\ brighter\ than\ background \\ (1 - I_{norm}(x)) \times (S(x))^\lambda, & vessel\ pixels\ are\ darker\ than\ background \end{cases} \quad (7)$$

Figures 4 (e) and (f) show the enhanced results based on shape-weighted CLAHE with λ being 0.5 and 0.8, respectively. Pixels in homogeneous regions generally have small shape responses and thus most noises in those regions can be prevented from being amplified. Increasing λ from 0.5 to 0.8 can suppress more noises, while may also decrease the contrast for regions around small vessels (as indicated by red rectangles in Figs. 4 (e) and (f)), resulting from inaccurate shape responses due to low contrast at these regions. In our implementation, we set λ to 0.8 as the default value which produced the best empirical results.

Progressive Contrast Enhancement on Challenging Pixels. It's common that both large and fine vessels appear in the same regions (as illustrated by red rectangles in Fig. 5). Within such a region, large vessels have better contrast to the background (either darker or brighter) than small vessels. As a result, the intensity range is often dominated by large vessels, resulting in insufficient enhancement for small vessels in such a region. Reducing the region size of CLAHE could help limit the size differences in a region, but may also reduce the robustness of CLAHE.

To address this problem, we propose to progressively increase contrast for vessels of different sizes. In each iteration, we detect distinguishable vessel pixels that can be easily classified as vessels with high confidence and remove them from further consideration in future iterations. In each iteration, shape-weighted CLAHE is applied only to those remaining pixels, which usually contain smaller vessels which have not been detected in previous iterations. After the contrast enhancement to this subset of pixels in the image, more pixels in fine vessels can be detected and removed from consideration in future iterations. We repeat this iterative procedure until no more fine-vessel pixels can be detected or a limit on the iteration count is reached.

To classify vessel and background pixels with high confidence in each iteration, we set two strict thresholds. That is, pixels whose filtering responses are greater than a high threshold T_H or smaller than a low threshold T_L are classified as vessel and back-ground pixels respectively; the remaining pixels whose responses fall within the range of T_H and T_L are considered as unknown and their labeling will be done in future iterations. To guarantee that the true-positive and true-negative rates are both high for the classification, we exploited multiple settings of the parameters for running CLAHE to generate several enhanced results and performed vessel enhancement filtering and classification for every resulting image. Pixels which are classified as vessel pixels in all of the resulting images are considered as robust and distinguishable vessel pixels. They are then labeled as vessel pixels and excluded from consideration in future iterations.

Figure 5 compares the contrast enhancement results based on CLAHE and the 2nd round progressive contrast enhancement, respectively. We highlight a small region containing both small vessels and part of a larger vessel by a red rectangle and display the verification map of this region. Clearly, the result obtained by our progressive contrast enhancement provides better visibility of small vessels and contains fewer noises. As a result, the verification map is more accurate than that of CLAHE.

4   Experimental Results

In this section, we provide quantitative evaluation of our method using a public retinal dataset, DRIVE [18], and clinical cerebral data. We first describe our datasets and the evaluation metric, followed by the results and analysis.

4.1   Datasets

DRIVE [18] is a public-available dataset of 2D RGB retinal scans to enable comparative studies on segmentation of blood vessels in retinal images. Each image was captured using 8 bits per color plane at 768×584 pixels and was JPEG compressed. The entire dataset contains 40 images which are divided into a training set and a testing set, both containing 20 images. For each testing case, two ground truths obtained by manual segmentation are provided. We test

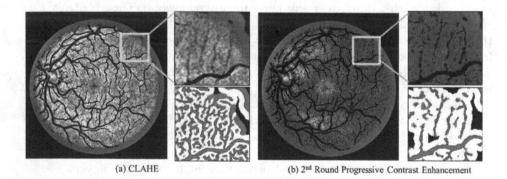

(a) CLAHE   (b) 2nd Round Progressive Contrast Enhancement

Fig. 5. Illustration of contrast enhancement results based on (a) CLAHE and (b) the 2nd round progressive contrast enhancement. A region including both challenging pixels (i.e. small vessels) and part of a larger vessel are highlighted by a red rectangle. Its enlarged version and the verification map are displayed on the right. Clearly, our progressive contrast enhancement can provide much fewer noises, better visibility of small vessels and hence a more accurate verification map for small vessels. The parameter settings for CLAHE are the same for both (a) and (b), i.e. clip limit = 30 and region size = 5050 (Color figure online).

our approach on the testing images of DRIVE. Figures 7 (a) and (b) show an exemplar image and one ground truth image from DRIVE.

We also evaluate our method on 2D clinical cerebral vessel data, approved by [re-moved for anonymous submission]. The image was obtained by digital subtraction angiography (DSA), represented using 8bits grayscale TIFF format, including 560 414 pixels. For quantitative evaluation, we asked two experts to manually label the image, yielding two ground truth images. Figures 8 (a) and (b) illustrate our cerebral vessel image and one of its ground truth images. The primary focus of this paper is to improve the segmentation performance in challenging scenarios. Thus, the ground truth data must be able to facilitate evaluation and performance comparison for the challenging cases. For this purpose, we further divide all pixels in each ground truth image into two parts: vessel pixels which can be correctly classified by all baseline methods we have implemented are labeled as easy pixels and pixels which are incorrectly labeled by at least one baseline method are marked as challenging pixels. Specifically, we implemented two baseline methods: vesselness based method and OOF based method (details about baselines can be Sec. 4.3). The threshold for binary classification is adjusted so that the precision is above 95 %. Figures 7 (c) and (d), and Figs. 8 (c) and (d) illustrate the easy and challenging vessel pixels in the ground truth images, respectively. Obviously, challenging pixels are mainly located around vessel boundaries and at small vessels which have very low contrast to its surrounding background.

4.2 Evaluation Metric

We use recall and precision to evaluate the segmentation performance. Recall is de-fined as the number of true positives which are identified as vessel pixels in both ground truth and segmented image divided by the total number of vessel pixels in the ground truth. Precision is defined as the number of true positives divided by the total number of pixels that are identified as vessel pixels in segmented images. As mentioned in Sect. 4.1, we focus our evaluation on challenging pixels, thus we exclude easy vessel pixels from the precision-recall calculation, as shown in Eqs. (8) and (9),

$$Recall = \frac{TP - TP_{easy}}{challenging\ vessel\ pixels\ in\ ground\ truth} \tag{8}$$

$$Precision = \frac{TP - TP_{easy}}{challenging\ vessel\ pixels\ in\ segmented\ image} \tag{9}$$

We plot the Recall-Precision curve to demonstrate the overall segmentation performance when varying the threshold parameter for binary classification. The larger is the area under the curve, the better the performance of the method.

4.3 Experimental Setup

Any existing vessel enhancement filter can be used in the first step of our segmentation framework (the orange block of Fig. 2). In this work, we experimented with two filters: multi-scale vesselness and multi-scale OOF, due to their widely-acknowledged good performance for delineating tubular structures. We utilized the ITK implementation for multi-scale vesselness filtering and relied on [17] for the implementation of OOF. For each filter, we manually adjusted parameters to obtain the best performance and used the same parameter settings throughout the entire evaluation process. For both filters, we used identical parameters for multi-scale processing - the minimum and maximum standard deviations for Gaussian are set to 0.5 and 5, respectively, and the total number of scales is set to 10.

In our experiments, we compared six methods: vesselness, OOF, vesselness with canny refinement (i.e. vesselness+CR), OOF with canny refinement (OOF+CR), vesselness with the two proposed techniques (Pro-vesselness+CR), and OOF with the two proposed techniques (Pro-OOF+CR).

4.4 Results

Figures 6 (a) and (b) show the comparison results on the retinal and cerebral data respec-tively. First, we evaluate the effectiveness of canny refinement. We compare the performance of vesselness and vesselness+CR, as shown by red and light green curves in Figs. 6 (a) and (b). When the recall is relatively small (e.g. below 75 % in (a) and below 70 % in (b)), canny refinement can greatly improve the precision by removing false positives arising from random noises and the disturbing objects adjacent to vessel boundaries. However, when the recall is greater than a certain value, canny refinement could adversely decrease the precision. This is mainly because canny edge detection may incur errors, e.g. missing true edges of vessels and mistakenly detecting edges on noises, especially in regions with poor contrast and a low SNR. Incorrect canny edges may lead to errors in the verification map, yielding incorrect removal of true vessel pixels.

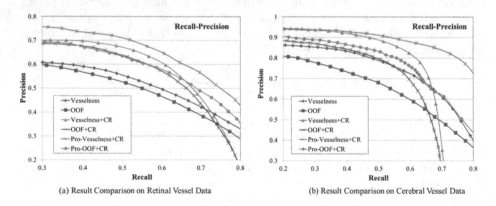

(a) Result Comparison on Retinal Vessel Data   (b) Result Comparison on Cerebral Vessel Data

Fig. 6. Recall-Precision curves obtained for (a) the retinal vessel data and (b) the cerebral vessel data. Our method with canny refinement and progressive contrast enhancement outperforms vesselness and OOF over the entire range (Color figure online).

As a result, reducing the threshold cannot improve the recall any more while reduce the precision. Similar results can be observed by comparing the results of OOF (blue curves) and OOF+CR (purple curves) for both datasets.

Next, we examine the effectiveness of progressive contrast enhancement. We compare the performance of vesselness (the red curves), vesselness+CR (the light green curves) and Pro-vesselness+CR (the light blue curves). Clearly, Pro-vesselness+CR outperforms the other two methods over the entire range. In particular, for large recall (i.e. greater than 70 %) progressive contrast enhancement can help greatly boost the performance of vesselness+CR and maintain superior performance to vesselness. This result demonstrates that progressive contrast enhancement can effectively improve the contrast and SNR in low quality regions, and in turn increase the detection rate of vessels in those regions. Similar results can be also observed for methods based on OOF filters.

The second row of Figs. 7 and 8 illustrate the segmentation results for a retinal and a cerebral image respectively. We omit the results for OOF+CR and Pro-OOF+CR since their results are similar to those of vesselness+CR and Pro-vesselness+CR. For the first three methods ((e)-(g)), i.e. vesselness, OOF and vesselness+CR, we manually tune the threshold so that the recalls for all the three methods are similar (57 % 58 %). We then compare their precisions (as shown under the segmentation results). For the retinal image, vesselness+CR achieves 10 % and 5 % greater precision than vesselness and OOF respectively. For the cerebral image, it is 10 % and 22.7 % higher than those of vesselness and OOF respectively. We further applied progressive contrast enhancement to the results of vesselness+CR (as shown in (h)), which improves the recall by another 10 % 15 % while maintaining the precision.

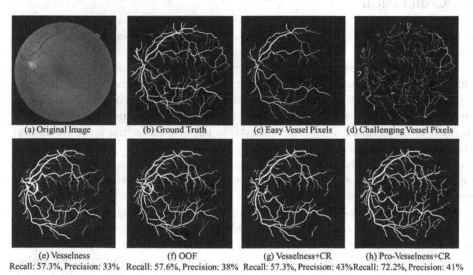

(a) Original Image   (b) Ground Truth   (c) Easy Vessel Pixels   (d) Challenging Vessel Pixels

(e) Vesselness   (f) OOF   (g) Vesselness+CR   (h) Pro-Vesselness+CR
Recall: 57.3%, Precision: 33%   Recall: 57.6%, Precision: 38%   Recall: 57.3%, Precision: 43%   Recall: 72.2%, Precision: 41%

Fig. 7. Illsutration of segmentation results on an exemplar retinal image. (a) Original image. (b) A ground truth image. (c) and (d) indicate easy and challenging vessel pixels on the ground truth image. (e) - (h) show the segmentation results of four methods. Pro-vesselness+CR achieves the best performance.

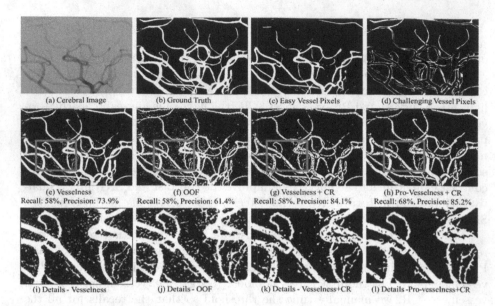

Fig. 8. Illsutration of segmentation results on a cerebral image. (a) Original image. (b) A ground truth image. (c) and (d) indicate easy and challenging vessel pixels on the ground truth image. (e) - (h) display the segmentation results of four methods. (i)-(l) show segmentation details of a region. Pro-vesselness+CR achieves the best performance.

5 Conclusion

In this paper, we present a framework for accurate vessel segmentation in two challenging scenarios: in regions with poor contrast and a low SNR, and at vessel boundaries. We propose and validate two techniques: progressive contrast enhancement and canny refinement. Progressive contrast enhancement involves an iterative procedure where each iteration emphasizes only on challenging pixels (usually pixels of small vessels) which were not distinguishable in previous iterations. Experimental results demonstrate that by excluding large vessel pixels detected in previous iterations from contrast enhancement, small vessel pixels can be better highlighted by CLAHE. In addition, progressive contrast enhancement can effectively suppress noises spread in a homogeneous background by weighting pixels according to their shape responses.

This paper also demonstrates that canny refinement which constructs a verification map based on canny edges can successfully minimize false positives around boundaries of vessels. Experimental results on a retinal dataset and a cerebral data demonstrate that the two proposed techniques can greatly improve the performance of state-of-the-art filtering-based segmentation methods, such as vesselness and OOF.

Acknowledgement. This work was supported in part by the Society of Interventional Radiology (SIR) Foundation Dr. Ernest J. Ring Academic Development Grant, The Aneurysm and AVM Foundation (TAAF) Cerebrovascular Research Grant, and a UCLA Radiology Exploratory Research Grant.

References

1. Frangi, A.F., Niessen, W.J., Vincken, K.L., Viergever, M.A.: Multiscale vessel enhancement filtering. In: Wells, W.M., Colchester, A.C.F., Delp, S.L. (eds.) MICCAI 1998. LNCS, vol. 1496, pp. 130–137. Springer, Heidelberg (1998)
2. Law, M., Chung, A.: Three dimensional curvilinear structure detection using optimally oriented flux. In: Forsyth, D., Torr, P., Zisserman, A. (eds.) Computer Vision–ECCV 2008. LNCS, vol. 5305, pp. 368–382. Springer, Berlin (2008)
3. Agam, G., Wu, C.: Probabilistic modeling-based vessel enhancement in thoracic CT scans. In: Proceedings of CVPR (2005)
4. Santamaría-Pang, A., Colbert, C.M., Saggau, P., Kakadiaris, I.: Automatic centerline extraction of irregular tubular structures using probability volumes from multiphoton imaging. In: Ayache, N., Ourselin, S., Maeder, A. (eds.) Medical Image Computing and Computer-Assisted Intervention – MICCAI 2007. LNCS, vol. 4792, pp. 486–494. Springer, Berlin (2007)
5. Rigamonti, R., Lepetit, V.: Accurate and efficient linear structure segmentation by leveraging ad hoc deatures with learned filters. In: Ayache, N., Delingette, H., Golland, P., Mori, K. (eds.) Medical Image Computing and Computer-Assisted Intervention – MICCAI 2012. LNCS, vol. 7510, pp. 189–197. Springer, Berlin (2012)
6. Becker, C., Rigamonti, R., Lepetit, V., Fua, P.: Supervised feature learning for curvilinear structure segmentation. In: Mori, K., Sakuma, I., Sato, Y., Barillot, C., Navab, N. (eds.) MICCAI 2013, Part I. LNCS, vol. 8149, pp. 526–533. Springer, Heidelberg (2013)
7. Rigamonti, R., Sironi, A., Lepetit, V., Fua, P.: Learning separable filters. In: Proceedings of CVPR (2013)
8. Gonzalez, G., Fleuret, F., Fua, P.: Learning rotational features for filament detection. In: Proceedings of CVPR (2009)
9. Yang, X., Cheng, K.-T., Chien, A.-C.: Geodesic Active Contour with Adaptive Configuration for Cerebral Vessel and Aneurysm Segmentation. In: Proceedings of ICPR (2014)
10. Yushkevich, P.A., Piven, J., Hazlett, H.C., Smith, R.G., Ho, S., Gee, J.C., Gerig, G.: User-guided 3D Active Contour Segmentation of Anatomical Structures: Significantly improved efficiency and reliability. Neuroimage $31(3)$, 1116–1128 (2006)
11. Nain, D., Yezzi, A.J., Turk, G.: Vessel segmentation using a shape driven flow. In: Barillot, C., Haynor, D.R., Hellier, P. (eds.) MICCAI 2004. LNCS, vol. 3216, pp. 51–59. Springer, Heidelberg (2004)
12. Caselles, V., Kimmel, R., Sapiro, G.: Geodesic Active Contours. Int. J. Comput. Vis. 22, 61–79 (1997)
13. Zhu, S.C., Yullie, A.: Region Competition: Unifying Snakes, Region Growing, and Bayes/MDL for Multiband Image Segmentation. IEEE Trans. Pattern Anal. Mach. Intell. $18(9)$, 884–900 (1996)
14. Lesage, D., Angelini, E.D., Bloch, I., Funka-Lea, G.: A Review of 3D Vessel Lumen Segmentation Techniques: Models, Features and Extraction Schemes. Med. Image Anal. 13, 819–845 (2009)

15. Zuiderveld, K.: Contrast limit adaptive histogram equalization. Graphics Gems IV, pp. 474–485. Academic Press, Boston (1994)
16. Kirbas, C., Quek, F.: A Review of Vessel Extraction Techniques and Algorithms. J. ACM Comput. Surv. **36**(2), 81–121 (2004)
17. Optimally Oriented Flux implementation. https://github.com/fethallah/ITK-TubularGeodesics
18. Staal, J.J., Abramoff, M.D., Niemeijer, M., Viergever, M.A., van Ginneken, B.: Ridge based Vessel Segmentation in Color Images of the Retina. IEEE Trans. Med. Imaging **23**, 501–509 (2004)
19. Freeman, W.T., Adelson, E.H.: The Design and Use of Steerable Filters. IEEE Trans. Pattern Anal. Mach. Intell. **13**, 891–906 (1991)
20. Shikata, H., Hoffman, E.A., Sonka, M.: Automated Segmentation of Pulmonary Vascular Tree from 3D CT Images. Proc. SPIE Med. Imaging **5369**, 107–116 (2004)
21. Lin, Q.: Enhancement, Detection, and Visualization of 3D Volume Data. Ph.D. Thesis, Dept. EE, Linkoping University, SE-581 83 Linkoping, Sweden, Dissertations No. 824, May 2003
22. Armande, N., Montesinos, P., Monga, O.: A 3D thin nets extraction method for medical imaging. In Proceedings of ICPR, p. 642 (1996)
23. Prinet, V., Monaga, O., Ge, C., Xie, S.L., Ma, S.D.: Thin network extraction in 3D images: application to medical angiograms. In Proceedings of ICPR, pp. 386–390 (1996)
24. Bauer, C., Bischof, H.: A novel approach for detection of tubular objects and its application to medical image analysis. In: Rigoll, G. (ed.) DAGM 2008. LNCS, vol. 5096, pp. 163–172. Springer, Heidelberg (2008)
25. Canny, J.: A Computational Approach To Edge Detection. IEEE Trans. Pattern Anal. Mach. Intell. **8**(6), 679–698 (1986)

Eigen-PEP for Video Face Recognition

Haoxiang Li[1]($\boxtimes$), Gang Hua[1], Xiaohui Shen[2], Zhe Lin[2], and Jonathan Brandt[2]

[1] Stevens Institute of Technology, Hoboken, USA
hli18@stevens.edu
[2] Adobe Systems Inc., San Jose, USA

Abstract. To effectively solve the problem of large scale video face recognition, we argue for a comprehensive, compact, and yet flexible representation of a face subject. It shall comprehensively integrate the visual information from all relevant video frames of the subject in a compact form. It shall also be flexible to be incrementally updated, incorporating new or retiring obsolete observations. In search for such a representation, we present the Eigen-PEP that is built upon the recent success of the probabilistic elastic part (PEP) model. It first integrates the information from relevant video sources by a part-based average pooling through the PEP model, which produces an intermediate high dimensional, part-based, and pose-invariant representation. We then compress the intermediate representation through principal component analysis, and only a number of principal eigen dimensions are kept (as small as 100). We evaluate the Eigen-PEP representation both for video-based face verification and identification on the YouTube Faces Dataset and a new Celebrity-1000 video face dataset, respectively. On YouTube Faces, we further improve the state-of-the-art recognition accuracy. On Celebrity-1000, we lead the competing baselines by a significant margin while offering a scalable solution that is linear with respect to the number of subjects.

1 Introduction

With the proliferation of videos accumulated in online social multimedia, *e.g.*, hundreds of hours videos are uploaded to YouTube every minute, the problem of video face recognition in the wild has caught more and more attention in recent years. Compared with image-based face recognition, face recognition from videos not only presents new challenges, but also offers new opportunities. As shown in Fig. 1, faces in the videos are generally in lower quality, present more pose variations, and often suffer from motion blur. These factors can induce more visual variations of the faces and negatively influence the recognition accuracy. On the other hand, a video clip of a face usually contains hundreds of frames which present varied appearance of the same subject. This obviously offers additional opportunities to better model the visual variations for more robust face recognition by integrating the information from all the frames.

A naive approach to video face recognition would be applying existing image based face recognition algorithms [1], such as those top performers on the Labeled

© Springer International Publishing Switzerland 2015
D. Cremers et al. (Eds.): ACCV 2014, Part III, LNCS 9005, pp. 17–33, 2015.
DOI: 10.1007/978-3-319-16811-1_2

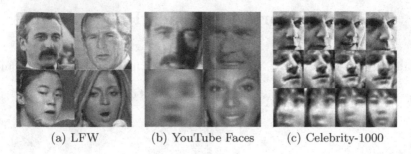

|(a) LFW|(b) YouTube Faces|(c) Celebrity-1000|

Fig. 1. Sample images in three unconstrained face recognition datasets: the image-based Labeled Faces in the Wild (LFW), video-based YouTube Faces Database, and video-based Celebrity-1000 dataset.

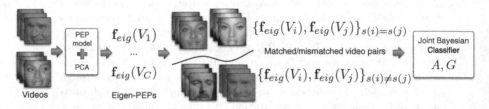

Fig. 2. The high-level training work-flow of our method.

Faces in the Wild (LFW) [2–7], to conduct frame-to-frame matching and then fusing the matching results across all the frame pairs together when comparing two video faces. This is obviously not a scalable solution as the complexity of a single match is already $O(n^2)$ with respect to the number of frames n each video possesses.

Previous work on the video face recognition includes methods representing the video data by linear combination of the training data [8,9], utilizing probabilistic methods to exploit the intrinsic manifolds [10–12], etc. We refer readers to Zhao *et al.* [13] for a more comprehensive survey of earlier literatures. Notwithstanding the demonstrated efficacy of these methods, the computational expense is a hurdle when applied to large-scale video face recognition.

We argue that, to effectively solve the problem of large scale video face recognition, we need a comprehensive, compact, and yet flexible representation of a face subject. By comprehensive, we mean that it shall integrate the visual information from all relevant video frames (even those from multiple videos) of a subject to better model the visual variations. By compact, we mean that it is scalable both in terms of computing and storage. By flexible, we mean that it can be incrementally updated, either incorporating new observations, or retiring obsolete observations, without the need to revisit all the video frames used to build the original representation.

To address these requirements, we propose a new video face representation named Eigen-PEP for video face recognition in the wild. The Eigen-PEP representation is built upon the recent success of the probabilistic elastic part (PEP) model proposed by Li *et al.* [14,15] The Eigen-PEP integrates information from all the video frames by a part-based average pooling through the PEP model, which produces an intermediate high dimensional, part-based, pose-invariant representation. It then compacts the high dimensional intermediate representation by principal component analysis (PCA), after which only a small number (as small as 100) of principal eigen dimensions is retained. This compact video representation maintains the flexibility from the nature of average pooling to incorporate or exclude frames incrementally. We then adopt the joint Bayesian classifier [16] to implement face recognition based on the Eigen-PEP representation. The high-level work-flow of the video face recognition system based on Eigen-PEP is summarized in Fig. 2. We utilize the PEP model [14,15] and PCA to construct the Eigen-PEPs for videos (Sect. 3.2). In the training stage, the joint Bayesian classifier [16] is trained from a set of matched and mismatched video pairs (Sect. 3.3) represented in the Eigen-PEPs. The classifier is then applied to compare two face videos in the testing stage for either video face verification or identification. In practice, the storage size of an Eigen-PEP produced from one video or multiple videos of a subject can be less than 400 bytes. Hence a system based on Eigen-PEP is highly scalable and the matching process can be very efficient.

In particular, without resorting to more advanced indexing scheme, a video face identification system based on the proposed Eigen-PEP representation would have a run-time that is linear to the number of subjects presented in the gallery database. This is achieved by generating one Eigen-PEP representation per subject, from all videos associated with that subject. Another advantage of the proposed Eigen-PEP representation is that its size is invariant to the length of the input video. Hence, the Eigen-PEP representation can be readily used with more advanced indexing methods, such as tree-based indexing, to further reduce the run-time complexity for identification to be $O(log(n))$, which we defer to our future work.

We evaluate our method on two large-scale video face recognition databases, and an image face recognition dataset, both for face verification and identification. We also participated the recent Point-and-Shoot Face Recognition Challenge (PaSC)[1] and our method significantly outperforms other competitors under the video-to-video face recognition setting [17]. Note the proposed method can be applied to image face recognition naturally by processing an image as a one-frame video. We can also flip the image horizontally to generate a two-frame video, from which we built the Eigen-PEP representation. Therefore, our research contributes to video face recognition in the following aspects:

- We propose a comprehensive, compact, and flexible Eigen-PEP video face representation with superb recognition accuracy.
- We present a highly scalable video face recognition system based on the Eigen-PEP representation.

---

[1] http://www.cs.colostate.edu/~vision/pasc/ijcb2014/.

– We outperform the state-of-the-art recognition accuracy over three challenging face recognition datasets.

2   Review of the PEP Model

As we have mentioned, the proposed Eigen-PEP representation is built upon the PEP representation proposed by Li *et al.* [14,15]. The PEP representation can deal with a single face or a face set. The PEP representation itself has been shown to be robust to pose variations. When it is applied to video face recognition, a PEP model selects a set of image patches out of all video frames and concatenates the descriptors of the selected image patches into a single vector as the PEP representation.

Although the PEP model presents great potential in modeling human faces, there are several issues when applying it to more practical and large-scale video face recognition. First, the PEP representation is high dimensional (*e.g.*, 1024×128 dimensional using SIFT) which is memory demanding. Second, Li *et al.* [14] used a kernel Support Vector Machine (SVM) to match two PEP representations for recognition, which is not scalable (Sect. 4.2).

Third, for modeling video faces, the PEP representation may lose valuable information from appearance variations presented in the video, since it keeps only a small portion of feature descriptors by a part-based probabilistic max pooling. Because of this, although the PEP representation can be incrementally updated to incorporate new observations, it cannot be incrementally updated to remove obsolete observations.

Compared to the PEP representation, the Eigen-PEP representation is more compact, flexible, and comprehensive. We integrate the information from all video frames (even those from multiple videos) by introducing a part-based average pooling to the PEP model. Since we build PEP representation for every frame, the appearance variations under different poses, expressions, and illuminations etc., are integrated.

Because the PEP representations are part-based and robust to pose variations, the corresponded selected descriptors consistently come from the same facial part. Intuitively, the mean of the descriptors from each part can naturally suppress the appearance variations, leading to a robust representation. To address the high-dimensionality problem, we apply PCA over all video-level PEP representations and only retain a small number of principal eigen dimensions.

Since an Eigen-PEP integrates the appearance of different poses and expressions, it is very suitable to represent a subject in a large-scale video face identification system by building a single representation from all videos associated with that subject. Once each gallery person has a single vector representation to incorporate all available videos of him/her, even the brute-force complexity in the testing stage will be linear to the number of gallery identities, instead of the number of gallery videos.

In addition to its compactness and comprehensiveness, the Eigen-PEP benefits from the nature of the average pooling to be flexible for incremental modifications (Sect. 3.2). For example, we can update the Eigen-PEP incrementally to incorporate new video frames of the same subject, or to remove obsolete video frames, without the need to access all the other video frames used to build the initial representation.

3   The Eigen-PEP Representation

3.1   The PEP Representation

The PEP representation has been shown to be effective in modeling human faces [14,15]. We refer the readers to Li *et al.* [14] for the details. To build the PEP representation for a video, all the video frames are firstly processed into a set of descriptors $\{\mathbf{f}\} = \{[\mathbf{a}_i\ \mathbf{l}_i]\}_{i=1}^{M}$, where $[\mathbf{a}_i\ \mathbf{l}_i]$ denotes one spatial-appearance descriptor; $\mathbf{a}$ is the appearance part and $\mathbf{l}$ is the spatial part.

The training stage builds a PEP model (or Universal Background Model in [14]) parameterized by Θ over training descriptors with the Expectation-Maximization (EM) algorithm. The PEP model is a Gaussian mixture model with K spherical Gaussian components,

$$P([\mathbf{a}\ \mathbf{l}]|\Theta) = \sum_{k=1}^{K} \omega_k \mathcal{G}([\mathbf{a}\ \mathbf{l}]|\boldsymbol{\mu}_k, \sigma_k^2 \mathbf{I}), \tag{1}$$

where $\Theta = (\omega_1, \boldsymbol{\mu}_1, \sigma_1, \ldots, \omega_K, \boldsymbol{\mu}_K, \sigma_K)$; $\mathbf{I}$ is an identity matrix; ω_k is the mixture weight of the k-th Gaussian component; $\mathcal{G}(\boldsymbol{\mu}_k, \sigma_k^2 \mathbf{I})$ is a spherical Gaussian with mean $\boldsymbol{\mu}_k$ and variance $\sigma_k^2 \mathbf{I}$. Each one of the K Gaussian components commits one descriptor with the highest generative probability and the PEP representation of $\{\mathbf{f}\}$ is the concatenation of the appearance part of the K selected descriptors, i.e.,

$$\mathcal{F} = [\mathbf{a}_{g_1}\ \mathbf{a}_{g_2}\ \ldots\ \mathbf{a}_{g_K}], \quad g_k = \arg\max_i \omega_k \mathcal{G}([\mathbf{a}_i\ \mathbf{l}_i]|\boldsymbol{\mu}_k, \sigma_k^2 \mathbf{I}). \tag{2}$$

3.2   The Eigen-PEP Extension

Given a video of multiple frames, we process each single video frame into its PEP representation. Because the PEP representation is part-based and pose-invariant, the PEP representations from the video frames are aligned facial part descriptors. Since the PEP representation is concatenated local descriptors of facial parts, the mean of the corresponding descriptors naturally suppresses the appearance variations across all video frames. Hence the mean of the PEP representations over all the frames is an intermediate high-dimensional part-based video-level representation.

To reduce its dimensionality, we apply Principle Component Analysis (PCA) and keep d principal eigen dimensions. The PCA is trained over all the video-level intermediate PEP representations from the training data. We hence name the video-level representation after PCA the Eigen-PEP.

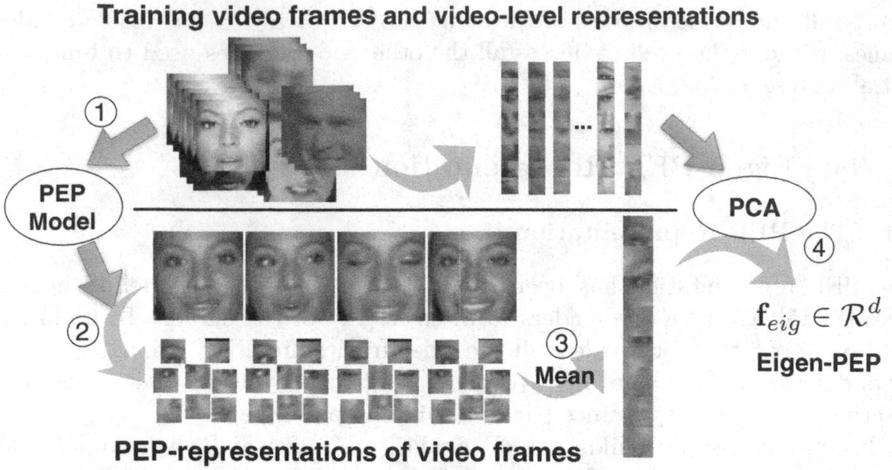

Training video frames and video-level representations

Fig. 3. Workflow for building the Eigen-PEP of a video: (1) the PEP model is learned from training video frames; (2) for each frame in the testing video, the PEP representation is partially visualized as the selected image patches of which the patches at the same location are consistent in semantics but varied in appearance across the video frames; (3) visualization of the intermediate video level representation as the pixel-level mean; (4) apply PCA to project the intermediate video level representation into a low-dimensional space to build the Eigen-PEP; the PCA is trained over all video level intermediate representations.

The workflow for building the Eigen-PEP is shown in Fig. 3. Formally, let $\mathcal{F}_1, \mathcal{F}_2, \ldots, \mathcal{F}_N$ denote the PEP representations for video V with N frames; and P denotes the PCA projection. The Eigen-PEP for the video V is

$$f_{eig}(V) = P^T \frac{1}{N} \sum_{n=1}^{N} \mathcal{F}_n. \tag{3}$$

Compared with the PEP representation, the Eigen-PEP is more comprehensive and compact. In building the intermediate video level representation of the video V, each Gaussian component of the PEP model actually commits N descriptors (one from each video frame), and therefore encodes more appearance variations. The intermediate representation is then built by average pooling per Gaussian component over the N descriptors it selected.

Besides that, benefiting from the nature of this part-based average pooling, the intermediate representation is flexible to incremental modification. Furthermore, the linear nature of the PCA allows the Eigen-PEP to maintain this flexibility. Specifically, with a new video frame $\mathcal{F}_{N+1}$, the Eigen-PEP can be updated incrementally without the need of accessing other video frames, *i.e.*,

$$f_{eig}(V) \leftarrow \frac{N}{N+1} f_{eig}(V) + \frac{1}{N+1} P^T \mathcal{F}_{N+1}. \tag{4}$$

Similarly, to retire the n-th frame it can be deducted from the representation without accessing the other video frames by

$$f_{eig}(V) \leftarrow \frac{N}{N-1} f_{eig}(V) - \frac{1}{N-1} P^T \mathcal{F}_n. \tag{5}$$

3.3   Joint Bayesian Classifier

Chen *et al.* [16] propose the joint Bayesian classifier to explicitly model the intra-person and extra-person variations as zero-mean Gaussians with covariance matrices Σ_I and Σ_E respectively. The similarity of a face pair (x_1, x_2) is then measured by the likelihood ratio

$$r(x_1, x_2) = log \frac{P(x_1, x_2|H_I)}{P(x_1, x_2|H_E)} = x_1^T A x_1 + x_2^T A x_2 - 2x_1^T G x_2, \tag{6}$$

where

$$\begin{pmatrix} F & G \\ G & F \end{pmatrix} = \Sigma_I^{-1}, \quad \begin{pmatrix} A & 0 \\ 0 & A \end{pmatrix} = \Sigma_E^{-1} - \begin{pmatrix} F & 0 \\ 0 & F \end{pmatrix}. \tag{7}$$

H_I and H_E denote the intra-person and extra-person hypothesis parameterized by the covariance matrices Σ_I and Σ_E respectively.

Chen *et al.* [16] utilizes an EM algorithm relying on identity information to estimate the matrices A and G. In practice, when the identity information is not available, we can estimate Σ_I and Σ_E from matched and mismatched face pairs directly i.e.,

$$\Sigma_I = cov(X_I, X_I), \quad \Sigma_E = cov(X_E, X_E), \tag{8}$$

where X_I and X_E are the sets of concatenated Eigen-PEP pairs of the matched and mismatched face pairs respectively.

In face verification, we use the joint Bayesian classifier without EM to bypass the necessity of identity information. In face identification, since the identity information is available, we follow the one with EM for better recognition accuracy. Note that only the training time complexity is different in these two cases, the run-time efficiency is the same.

4   Experiments

We perform extensive experiments to evaluate the effectiveness of the proposed representation under different scenarios including video face verification on the YouTube Faces Database [1], large-scale video based face identification on the Celebrity-1000 dataset [18][2], and image face verification on the Labeled Face in the Wild (LFW) dataset [19]. Over all three datasets, our method achieves superior performance compared to the state-of-the-art algorithms.

---

[2] http://www.lv-nus.org/facedb/.

4.1   Video Face Verification on YouTube Faces Database

In video face verification, the training data is given in the form of matched and mismatched video face pairs. We follow Eqs. 7 and 8 to learn the matrices A and G.

In the testing stage, the input is a pair of videos V_1 and V_2. After processing the video face pair into Eigen-PEPs $f_{eig}(V_1)$ and $f_{eig}(V_2)$, the joint Bayesian classifier is applied following Eq. 6 to assign the similarity score to this video pair, i.e.,

$$r(f_{eig}(V_1), f_{eig}(V_2)) = f_{eig}(V_1)^T A f_{eig}(V_1) + f_{eig}(V_2)^T A f_{eig}(V_2)$$
$$- 2 f_{eig}(V_1)^T G f_{eig}(V_2).$$

We evaluate our method on the YouTube Faces Dataset (YTFaces) published by Wolf *et al.* [1], and compare the result with the state-of-the-art. This dataset contains 3,425 videos of 1,595 different people. Each video consists of 181.3 frames on average. Faces are detected by the Viola-Jones detector and aligned by fixing the coordinates of automatically detected facial feature points [1]. We follow the standard protocol to report the average accuracy over 10-folds evaluation.

In our experiments, video frames are center cropped to 100×100 before feature extraction. To leverage the left-right facial symmetry in the Eigen-PEP, we flip the original video frames horizontally as additional new video frames. We report the recognition accuracy with and without the flipped frames separately.

For the parameters in our system, the SIFT descriptors are extracted over a 3-scale Gaussian image pyramid with scaling factor 0.9, densely from a 8×8 sliding window with 2-pixel spacing. The PEP model consists of 1024 Gaussian components and we keep top 100 eigen vectors in the PCA. Hence the dimensionality of Eigen-PEPs is 100. The storage size of Eigen-PEP for a single video is hence only 400 bytes (100 float values).

Table 1. Performance comparison over YouTube Faces

Algorithm	Accuracy $\pm$ Error (%)
MBGS [1]	76.4 ± 1.8
MBGS+SVM- [22]	78.9 ± 1.9
STFRD+PMML [23]	79.5 ± 2.5
VSOF+OSS(Adaboost) [24]	79.7 ± 1.8
APEM (fusion) [14]	79.1 ± 1.5
VF^2 [20]	84.7 ± 1.4
DDML (combined) [25]	82.3 ± 1.5
Our method	82.40 ± 1.7
Our method (with flipped frames)	$\mathbf{84.80 \pm 1.4}$
Our method (with flipped frames, corrected labels)	$\mathbf{85.04 \pm 1.49}$

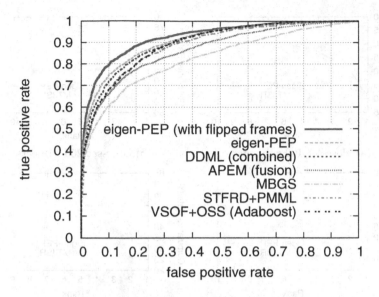

Fig. 4. Performance comparison over YouTube Faces.

As shown in Table 1 and Fig. 4, our method outperforms the state-of-the-art algorithms on the YouTube Faces Database under the restricted protocol. Although the Parkhi *et al.* [20] achieves comparable performance to our method, their method relies on large amount of training data in the discriminative dimensionality reduction. As a result, under the restricted protocol, their method produces very high dimensional video representations. Note that on the same dataset, Taigman *et al.* [21] pushed the accuracy as high as $91.4 \pm 1.1\%$. However they leveraged massive outside training data (4 million) while we only use the provided 4,500 pairs of face tracks for training. Note that there is a list of label errors uploaded to the YouTube Faces webpage recently [21], we also report our result with the corrected labels.

4.2 Video face identification on Celebrity-1000

In terms of video face identification on Celebrity-1000 dataset, there are two categories of protocols: the open-set face identification and the close-set face identification. In both protocols, the task is to identify the identity of the probe face video given a set of gallery face videos. In the open-set protocol, the gallery face videos are not in the training data.

In the training stage, we use the training data to learn the PEP model and PCA projections for the Eigen-PEP representation. After that, for each gallery subject, we build one Eigen-PEP from all his/her videos as the representation of the subject. Since the identity information is available, instead of following Eq. 8, we follow Chen *et al.* [16] to train the joint Bayesian classifier.

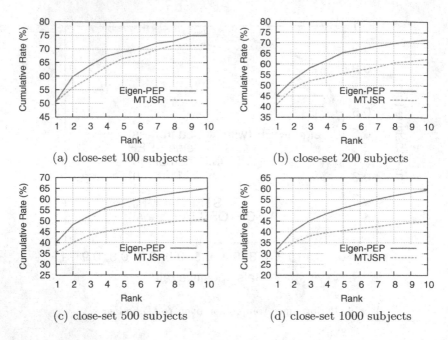

Fig. 5. Performance comparison over Celebrity-1000 dataset (close-set): the curve describes the rank K recognition accuracy.

In the testing stage, the probe face video is firstly processed into Eigen-PEP. Then the similarity between the probe face and each gallery face is measured by the joint Bayesian classifier. The performance of the identification is measured by the cumulative match characteristic curve (CMC) [26] which reports the top k recognition accuracy with varying k.

Liu *et al.* [18] published the Celebrity-1000 dataset to study the large-scale unconstrained video-based face identification problem. This dataset contains 159,726 video sequences of 1,000 human subjects. Faces are detected by the OMRON face detector. We evaluate our method under both the open-set and close-set protocols.

In the open-set protocol, 200 subjects are used for training. In the testing stage, videos are provided as the gallery set and probe set. There are 4 different experimental settings with different number of probe and gallery subjects: 100, 200, 400 and 800. In the close-set protocol, dataset is divided into training (gallery) subset and testing (probe) subset. Similarly, there are 4 settings for close-set: 100, 200, 500 and 1000 subjects.

Considering the relatively low-resolution of the video frames (80×64) in Celebrity-1000, we extract SIFT descriptors in a 8×8 sliding windows with 1-pixel spacing. The PEP model consists of 200 components. In the PCA, we keep 90 % accumulated eigen values. We use a maximum of 20, 000 training videos in the PCA. As a result, the dimensionality of Eigen-PEPs varies from 100 to 400 for different settings. For the open-set protocol, the Eigen-PEP dimension is set

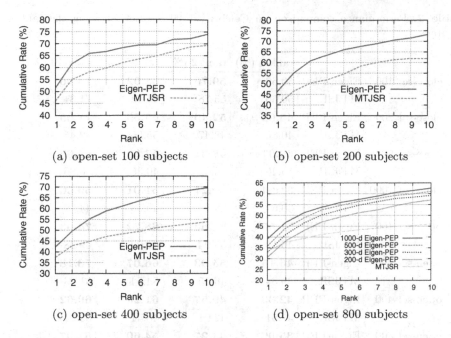

(a) open-set 100 subjects   (b) open-set 200 subjects

(c) open-set 400 subjects   (d) open-set 800 subjects

Fig. 6. Performance comparison over Celebrity-1000 dataset (open-set): the curve describes the rank K recognition accuracy.

to 500. Hence, the storage size of Eigen-PEP for a single gallery subject is no more than 2 kbytes.

We compare our method with the Multi-task Joint Sparse Representation (MTJSR) [8] which is the current state-of-the-art on Celebrity-1000 [18][3]. As shown in Figs. 5 and 6, and Table 2, our method outperforms the MTJSR algorithm under both the open-set and close-set protocols.

In addition to the superior accuracy, our system is more efficient than the MTJSR. In the testing stage of MTJSR, it solves an optimization problem to represent every frame of the probe video sequence as a sparse linear combination of video sequences of a gallery subject. The classification is then based on the accumulated reconstruction error.

Denote the number of gallery subjects as M, the number of frames of the probe video is N; the number of matching times of MTJSR is generally $N \times M$. Moreover, each matching needs to solve an optimization problem of a sparse representation which by itself is a complex computation. Given the same probe video, the number of matching times in our system, after processing the probe video into Eigen-PEP, is only M. Besides, each matching operation in our system is exactly three times of vector-matrix multiplications and two times of add operations of scalar values. Considering the typical dimension of Eigen-PEP is only a few hundred, our matching operation is far faster.

---

[3] We thank the authors for sharing theirs results.

Table 2. Performance comparison on Celebrity-1000 dataset: showing the rank-K accuracy.

		rank-1 (%)	rank-2 (%)	rank-5 (%)	rank-10 (%)
close-set 100	Eigen-PEP	50.60	**59.76**	**68.92**	**74.90**
	MTJSR	50.60	55.78	66.53	71.31
close-set 200	Eigen-PEP	**45.02**	**52.49**	**65.33**	**71.65**
	MTJSR	40.80	48.47	55.56	62.45
close-set 500	Eigen-PEP	**39.97**	**48.21**	**57.85**	**65.09**
	MTJSR	35.46	40.05	46.35	50.86
close-set 1000	Eigen-PEP	**31.94**	**40.27**	**51.01**	**59.50**
	MTJSR	30.04	34.88	40.58	44.77
open-set 100	Eigen-PEP	**51.55**	**61.63**	**68.22**	**74.03**
	MTJSR	46.12	55.04	62.02	69.38
open-set 200	Eigen-PEP	**46.15**	**55.03**	**66.07**	**73.18**
	MTJSR	39.84	46.55	54.64	61.93
open-set 400	Eigen-PEP	**42.33**	**49.57**	**61.23**	**69.62**
	MTJSR	37.51	42.91	48.41	53.91
open-set 800	Eigen-PEP	**35.90**	**44.27**	**54.60**	**61.07**
	MTJSR	33.50	37.71	42.41	46.03

Specifically, in the close-set protocol with 1000 gallery subjects, the run-time of evaluating one probe video in our system is about 2 s, most of which is for building the Eigen-PEP, and the matching time is only 0.05 s. In comparison, the evaluation time of MTJSR for one test sequence, as reported by [18], is 1.6×10^3 s. Besides, our experiment is conducted on a single machine with 12 CPU cores (2.4 GHz) while Liu *et al.* [18] used a cluster with 14 workstations each of which has 8 CPU cores (3 GHz). On average, their run-time is roughly 6 orders of magnitude greater than ours.

We also evaluate the performance of using SVM with the PEP-representations as described in Li *et al.* [14] which takes 41 s (matching time) for one query in the 1000 gallery subjects face identification task. Hence in terms of the matching time, our system is 800 times faster than theirs and our video representations are far more storage-efficient.

To further explore how the number of dimensions influence the effectiveness of the Eigen-PEP. We perform an experiment on the open-set 800 subjects setting to evaluate the identification accuracy with Eigen-PEPs of differing dimensions, *i.e.*, 200, 300, 500 and 1000. As shown in Fig. 7, except for the rank-1 accuracy when Eigen-PEP is of only 200 or 300 dimensions, all Eigen-PEPs outperforms the MTJSR by a significant margin. This observation also suggests that the dimension of the Eigen-PEP can be a trade-off parameter to balance the accuracy and efficiency.

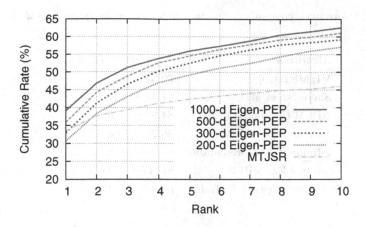

Fig. 7. Performance of different dimensional Eigen-PEPs over Celebrity-1000 dataset.

We present an example result in Fig. 9. As observed, different video sequences of the same gallery subject present varied appearance. Nevertheless by representing a subject as one Eigen-PEP representation our system can successfully identify the probe video. This observation demonstrates the Eigen-PEP as a comprehensive video representation.

4.3   Image Face Verification

Although we propose the compact PEP representation for video-based face recognition, it naturally applies to the image-based setting by processing the image as a one-frame video. Furthermore, we can actually generate a two-frame video by horizontally flipping the face image to better leverage the facial symmetry in the Eigen-PEP representation. The Labeled Faces in the Wild (LFW) [19] dataset is designed to address the unconstrained image-based face verification problem. This challenging dataset contains more than 13,000 images from 5,749 people.

We follow the *image-restricted, no outside data* protocol of LFW [27] using the faces roughly aligned with the funneling method [28]. Besides that we do not leverage any external data for strong face alignment, feature extraction or recognition model training.

Similarly, we extract SIFT descriptors in 8×8 sliding window with 2-pixel spacing in the center cropped 150×150 images. The PEP model is of 1024 components and the PCA reduces the dimensionality to 100.

As shown in Table 3 and Fig. 8, our method outperforms the state-of-the-art algorithms on LFW. We also evaluate the performance of combining the joint Bayesian classifier with the PEP representation. Since it is not practical to apply joint Bayesian classifier over the high-dimensional PEP representation directly due to the large size of covariance matrices, we apply PCA to reduce the dimensionality of PEP representation to be 100 as well. To be fair, the PCA is trained separately over training PEP representations.

Table 3. Performance comparison on the LFW, under *image-restricted, no outside data* protocol

Algorithm	Accuracy ± Error (%)
V1/MKL [29]	79.35 ± 0.55
Simonyan et al. [30]	87.47 ± 1.49
APEM (Fusion) [14]	84.08 ± 1.20
1-frame Eigen-PEP	86.27 ± 1.06
2-frame PEP representation	87.37 ± 0.66
2-frame Eigen-PEP	**88.47 ± 0.91**
2-frame Eigen-PEP (fusion)	**88.97 ± 1.32**

In a single frame case, our method is equivalent to applying the joint Bayesian classifier for the PEP representation after PCA. Compared with the results from APEM by Li *et al.* [14], which is essentially the PEP representation with a kernel SVM on the absolute difference of the PEP representations for verification with an additional step of Bayesian adaptation, it clearly shows the advantage of adopting the joint Bayesian classifier. We believe that taking the absolute difference of two PEP representations resulted in loss of important discriminative information.

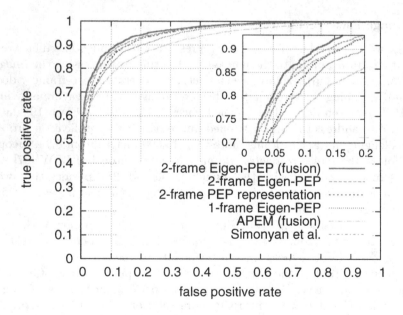

Fig. 8. Performance comparison on the LFW, under *image-restricted, no outside data* protocol

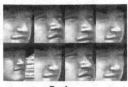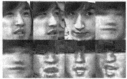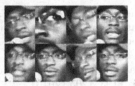

| Probe | Rank 1 | Rank 2 |

Fig. 9. Qualitative result on Celebrity-1000: shows a successful query and the top 2 candidates ranked by our system; 8 frames of the probe video are shown; 8 frames of the gallery subjects are selected from 8 video sequences chosen randomly.

We also compare with the 2-frame PEP representation setting, in which a single PEP representation is built for the two images. Similarly, PCA is applied to the PEP representation and the joint Bayesian classifier is adopted for classification. As observed, the Eigen-PEP consistently outperforms the PEP representation in all the cases.

Following similar process in Li *et al.* [14], by fusing the additional result using Local Binary Pattern (LBP) [31] descriptors with a linear SVM, we observe further improvement on LFW.

5 Conclusion

In this paper, we propose the Eigen-PEP video face representation. We combine the Eigen-PEP with the joint Bayesian classifier for video face recognition. The Eigen-PEP naturally integrates information from all video frames and is flexible to dynamical modification. The small footprint of the proposed Eigen-PEP makes the overall video face recognition framework to be scalable and be suitable for large-scale video face identification. Extensive experiments are conducted over three challenging real-world face recognition datasets to evaluate the proposed method in video face verification, video face identification and image face verification. The proposed method outperforms the existing state-of-the-art algorithms under all three tasks.

Acknowledgement. Research reported in this publication was partly supported by the National Institute Of Nursing Research of the National Institutes of Health under Award Number R01NR015371. The content is solely the responsibility of the authors and does not necessarily represent the official views of the National Institutes of Health. This work is also partly supported by US National Science Foundation Grant IIS 1350763, China National Natural Science Foundation Grant 61228303, GH's start-up funds form Stevens Institute of Technology, a Google Research Faculty Award, a gift grant from Microsoft Research, and a gift grant from NEC Labs America.

References

1. Wolf, L., Hassner, T., Maoz, I.: Face recognition in unconstrained videos with matched background similarity. In: CVPR (2011)

2. Chen, D., Cao, X., Wen, F., Sun, J.: Blessing of dimensionality: high dimensional feature and its efficient compression for face verification. In: CVPR (2013)
3. Cao, X., Wipf, D., Wen, F., Duan, G.: A practical transfer learning algorithm for face verification. In: ICCV (2013)
4. Liao, S., Jain, A., Li, S.: Partial face recognition: alignment-free approach. T-PAMI **35**, 1193–1205 (2013)
5. Barkan, O., Weill, Y., Wolf, L., Aronowitz., H.: Fast high dimensional vector multiplication based face recognition. In: ICCV (2013)
6. Lei, Z., Pietikainen, M., Li, S.Z.: Learning discriminant face descriptor. T-PAMI **36**, 289–302 (2014)
7. Cao, Q., Ying, Y., Li, P.: Similarity metric learning for face recognition. In: ICCV (2013)
8. Yuan, X.T., Liu, X., Yan, S.: Visual classification with multitask joint sparse representation. IEEE Trans. Image Process. **21**, 4349–4360 (2012)
9. Chen, Y.C., Patel, V., Shekhar, S., Chellappa, R., Phillips, P.: Video-based face recognition via joint sparse representation. In: 2013 10th IEEE International Conference and Workshops on Automatic Face and Gesture Recognition (FG) (2013)
10. Zhou, S., Krueger, V., Chellappa, R.: Probabilistic recognition of human faces from video. Comput. Vis. Image Underst. **91**, 214–245 (2003)
11. Lee, K.C., Ho, J., Yang, M.H., Kriegman, D.: Video-based face recognition using probabilistic appearance manifolds. In: Proceedings of 2003 IEEE Computer Society Conference on Computer Vision and Pattern Recognition (2003)
12. Zhang, Y., Martnez, A.M.: A weighted probabilistic approach to face recognition from multiple images and video sequences. Image Vis. Comput. **24**, 626–638 (2006)
13. Zhao, W., Chellappa, R., Rosenfeld, A., Phillips, P.J.: Face recognition: a literature survey. ACM Comput. Surv. **35**, 399–458 (2003)
14. Li, H., Hua, G., Lin, Z., Brandt, J., Yang, J.: Probabilistic elastic matching for pose variant face verification. In: CVPR (2013)
15. Li, H., Hua, G., Lin, Z., Brandt, J., Yang, J.: Probabilistic elastic part model for unsupervised face detector adaptation. In: ICCV (2013)
16. Chen, D., Cao, X., Wang, L., Wen, F., Sun, J.: Bayesian face revisited: a joint formulation. In: Fitzgibbon, A., Lazebnik, S., Perona, P., Sato, Y., Schmid, C. (eds.) ECCV 2012, Part III. LNCS, vol. 7574, pp. 566–579. Springer, Heidelberg (2012)
17. Beveridge, J.R., et al.: The IJCB 2014 pasc video face and person recognition competition. In: IJCB (2014)
18. Liu, L., Zhang, L., Liu, H., Lao, S., Yan, S.: Towards large-population face identification in unconstrained videos. In: CSVT (2013)
19. Huang, G.B., Mattar, M., Berg, T., Learned-Miller, E.: Labeled faces in the wild: a database for studying face recognition in unconstrained environments. In: Faces in Real-Life Images Workshop in ECCV (2008)
20. Parkhi, O.M., Simonyan, K., Vedaldi, A., Zisserman, A.: A compact and discriminative face track descriptor. In: CVPR (2014)
21. Taigman, Y., Yang, M., Ranzato, M., Wolf, L.: DeepFace: closing the gap to human-level performance in face verification. In: CVPR (2014)
22. Wolf, L., Levy, N.: The SVM-minus similarity score for video face recognition. In: CVPR (2013)
23. Cui, Z., Li, W., Xu, D., Shan, S., Chen, X.: Fusing robust face region descriptors via multiple metric learning for face recognition in the wild. In: CVPR (2013)
24. Mendez-Vazquez, H., Martinez-Diaz, Y., Chai, Z.: Volume structured ordinal features with background similarity measure for video face recognition. In: ICB (2013)

25. Hu, J., Lu, J., Tan, Y.P.: Discriminative deep metric learning for face verification in the wild. In: CVPR (2014)
26. Moon, H., Phillips, P.J.: Computational and performance aspects of pca-based facerecognition algorithms. Perception **30**, 303–321 (2001)
27. Huang, G.B., Learned-Miller, E.: Labeled faces in the wild: updates and new reporting procedures. Technical report UM-CS-2014-003, UMass Amherst (2014)
28. Huang, G., Jain, V., Learned-Miller, E.: Unsupervised joint alignment of complex images. In: ICCV (2007)
29. Pinto, N., DiCarlo, J.J., Cox, D.D.: How far can you get with a modern face recognition test set using only simple features? In: CVPR (2009)
30. Simonyan, K., Parkhi, O.M., Vedaldi, A., Zisserman, A.: Fisher vector faces in the wild. In: BMVC (2013)
31. Ahonen, T., Hadid, A., Pietikäinen, M.: Face recognition with local binary patterns. In: Pajdla, T., Matas, J.G. (eds.) ECCV 2004. LNCS, vol. 3021, pp. 469–481. Springer, Heidelberg (2004)

Local Generic Representation for Face Recognition with Single Sample per Person

Pengfei Zhu[1], Meng Yang[2], Lei Zhang[1]([✉]), and Il-Yong Lee[3,4]

[1] Department of Computing, The Hong Kong Polytechnic University,
Hong Kong, China
`cslzhang@comp.polyu.edu.hk`
[2] Computer Vision Institute, School of Computer Science and Software Engineering,
Shenzhen University, Shenzhen, China
[3] LG Electronics Institute of Technology, Seoul, Korea
[4] Department of Computer Science, Yonsei University, Seoul, Korea

Abstract. Face recognition with single sample per person (SSPP) is a very challenging task because in such a scenario it is difficult to predict the facial variations of a query sample by the gallery samples. Considering the fact that different parts of human faces have different importance to face recognition, and the fact that the intra-class facial variations can be shared across different subjects, we propose a local generic representation (LGR) based framework for face recognition with SSPP. A local gallery dictionary is built by extracting the neighboring patches from the gallery dataset, while an intra-class variation dictionary is built by using an external generic dataset to predict the possible facial variations (e.g., illuminations, pose, expressions and disguises). LGR minimizes the total representation residual of the query sample over the local gallery dictionary and the generic variation dictionary, and it uses correntropy to measure the representation residual of each patch. Half-quadratic analysis is adopted to solve the optimization problem. LGR takes the advantages of patch based local representation and generic variation representation, showing leading performance in face recognition with SSPP.

1 Introduction

Face recognition (FR) is a very active topic in computer vision research because of its wide range of applications, including access control, video surveillance, social network, photo management, criminal investigation, etc. [1]. Though FR has been studied for many years, it is still a challenging task due to the many types of large face variations, e.g., pose, expressions, illuminations, corruption, occlusion and disguises. Furthermore, in applications such as smart cards, law enforcement, etc., we may have only one template sample of each subject, resulting in the single sample per person (SSPP) problem [2]. SSPP makes FR much more difficult because we have little information from the gallery set to predict the variations in the query face image [3].

Since the intra-class variations cannot be well estimated in the SSPP problem, the traditional discriminative subspace learning based FR methods can fail

© Springer International Publishing Switzerland 2015
D. Cremers et al. (Eds.): ACCV 2014, Part III, LNCS 9005, pp. 34–50, 2015.
DOI: 10.1007/978-3-319-16811-1_3

to work. In addition, since the number of samples per class is so small, the robustness of extracted features and the generalization ability of learned classifiers can be much reduced. To alleviate these difficulties of FR with SSPP, researchers have proposed to generate virtual samples of each subject, extract more discriminative features, and learn the facial variations from external data, etc. Generally speaking, the existing FR methods for SSPP can be categorized into three groups: virtual sample generation, generic learning and patch/block based methods.

Virtual sample generation aims to estimate the intra-class face variations by simulating extra samples for each subject. Virtual samples can be generated by perturbation-based approaches [4], geometric transform and photometric changes [5], SVD decomposition [6] and 3D methods [7], etc. With the virtual samples, intra-class scatter can be calculated to make Fisher linear discriminant analysis feasible in the scenario of SSPP [4–6]. Although virtual samples are helpful to FR with SSPP, they are highly correlated with the original face images and cannot be considered as independent samples for feature extraction. Therefore, there may exist much redundancy in the learned discriminative feature subspace [4,8].

Considering the similarity of face images across subjects, a generic training set can be used to compensate for the shortage of samples in FR. On one hand, the face variation information in the generic training set can be used to learn a projection matrix to extract discriminative features [9–12]. In [9] and [12], discriminative pose-invariant and expression-invariant projection matrices are learned by using a collected generic training set for pose-invariant and expression-invariant FR tasks, respectively. On the other hand, the abundant intra-class variations in the generic training set are very useful to more accurately represent a query face with unknown variations [3,13,14]. The sparse representation based classification (SRC) [15] represents a query face as a sparse linear combination of training samples from all classes. SRC shows interesting FR results; however, its performance will deteriorate significantly when the number of training samples of each class is very small because in such cases the variation space of each subject cannot be well spanned. The extended SRC (ESRC) [13] constructs an intra-class variation dictionary to represent the changes between the gallery and query images. In the case of SSPP, Yang et al. [3] learned a sparse variation dictionary by taking the relationship between the gallery set and the external generic set into account. The so-called sparse variation dictionary learning (SVDL) scheme shows state-of-the-art performance in FR with SSPP. However, SVDL ignores the distinctiveness of different parts of human faces.

Patch/block based methods [8,16–19] partition each face image into several patches/blocks, and then perform feature extraction and classification on them. First, patches can be viewed as independent samples for feature extraction [8,16]. In [16], the patches of each subject are considered as the samples of this class and then the within-class scatter matrix can be computed. In [8], the patches of each subject are considered to form a manifold and a projection matrix is learned by maximizing the manifold margin. Second, a weak classifier can be obtained from each patch, and then the classifiers on all patches can be combined to output the final decision (i.e., a strong classifier) [17,18]. In [17], the nearest neighbor classifier (NNC) is used for classification on each patch, and a kernel plurality method is proposed to combine the decisions on all patches. In [18], the collaborative representation based classifier (CRC) [20] is applied to each patch, and the majority voting is used for decision combination. Although the patch based methods in [17] and [18] significantly improve the FR performance compared with the original NNC and CRC classifiers, respectively, they do not solve the problem of lacking facial variations in the gallery set.

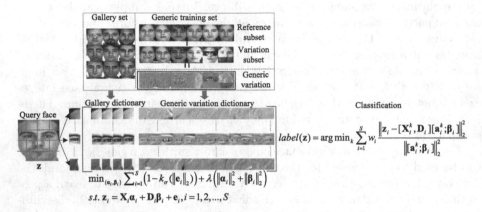

Fig. 1. Framework of local generic representation based classification. Gallery set is composed of the training face images. Generic training set includes reference subset and variation subset, while reference subset is composed of the neutral face images or the mean faces of each subject, and variation subset is composed of face images with different facial variations.

In this paper, we propose a local generic representation (LGR) based scheme for FR with SSPP, whose framework is illustrated in Fig. 1. The training samples in the gallery set are used to build a gallery dictionary. To introduce the face intra-class variation information that is lacked in the gallery set, a generic training set, which contains a reference subset and several variation subsets, is collected. A generic variation dictionary is then constructed as the difference between the reference subset and the variation subsets. Considering the different importance of different facial parts in FR, we adopt a local representation approach, i.e., each patch of the query sample is represented by the patch gallery dictionary and patch variation dictionary at the corresponding location. LGR aims to minimize the total representation residual of all patches. Since the residuals are non-Gaussian distributed, we use correntropy to measure the loss in minimization. The half-quadratic optimization technique is used to solve the optimization problem. Finally, the classification is performed based on the overall representation residual of the query sample by each class. The experimental results on benchmark face databases, including Extended Yale B [21], CMU Multi-PIE [22], AR [23] and LFW [24], show that LGR outperforms many state-of-the art methods for FR with SSPP.

2   Local Generic Representation

2.1   Generic Representation

In FR with SSPP, we have a gallery set $X = [x_1, ..., x_k, ..., x_K] \in \mathbb{R}^{d \times K}$, where $x_k \in \mathbb{R}^d$ is the only single gallery sample of class k, $k = 1, 2, ..., K$. Given a query sample $z \in \mathbb{R}^d$, representation based classifiers such as SRC [15] represent it over the gallery set X as:

$$z = X\alpha + e \tag{1}$$

If the gallery set has many training samples for each subject, most of the facial variations in the query sample can be synthesized by the multiple samples from the same class, and consequently correct classification can be made via comparing the representation residual of each class. For FR with SSPP, unfortunately, there is only one training sample per subject, and the variations (e.g., illumination, pose, expression, etc.) in z cannot be well represented by the single same-class sample in X. Thus, the representation residual of z can be big, and z can be wrongly represented by samples from other classes, leading to misclassification of z. Figure 2(a) shows an example. The query image has some illumination change compared with the single gallery sample of its class. We use the SRC model to solve the representation in Eq. (1), i.e., $\min_{\alpha} \|z - X\alpha\|_2^2 + \lambda\|\alpha\|_1$. One can see from Fig. 2(a) that the synthesized image $X\alpha$ does not overcome the problem of illumination change, and the illumination change is put forward into the representation residual e. Such a representation will cause trouble in the classification stage.

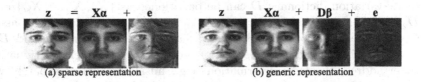

(a) sparse representation   (b) generic representation

Fig. 2. Sparse representation versus generic representation.

Considering that the intra-class facial variations caused by illumination, pose, and expression changes and disguise can be shared across subjects, an external generic training set which consists of enough face images with various types of variations can be adopted to construct an intra-class variation dictionary [3,13]. Suppose that we have collected a generic training set $G = [G^r, G^v]$, where G^r and G^v are the reference subset and variation subset, respectively. The reference subset $G^r \in \mathbb{R}^{d \times n}$ is composed of neutral face images or the mean faces of each subject. The variation subset G^v involves M possible facial variations: $G^v = [G_1^v, ..., G_m^v, ..., G_M^v]$, where G_m^v is the subset of the mth variation, $m = 1, 2, ..., M$. In [3], a sparse variation dictionary is learned from G. In our work, we simply construct an intra-class variation dictionary, denoted by D, by using the difference between G^r and G^v:

$$D = [G_1^v - G^r, ..., G_m^v - G^r, ..., G_M^v - G^r] \in \mathbb{R}^{d \times nM} \tag{2}$$

We then propose to represent the query sample z over the gallery set X and the generic variation dictionary D simultaneously:

$$z = X\alpha + D\beta + e \tag{3}$$

where α and β are the representation vectors of z over X and D, respectively, and e is the representation residual. We call the representation in Eq. (3) generic representation, which uses a generic intra-class variation dictionary D to account for the variations in the query sample. Figure 2(b) shows the generic representation of the query sample in Fig. 2(a). We use the following model to solve Eq. (3): $\min_{\{\alpha,\beta\}} \|z - X\alpha - D\beta\|_2^2 + \lambda(\|\alpha\|_1 + \|\beta\|_1)$. One can clearly see that the illumination change in the query sample is well encoded by the generic variation dictionary D, and the residual e has much lower energy ($\|e\|_2^2 = 0.0049$) than the residual in Fig. 2(a) ($\|e\|_2^2 = 0.0502$).

2.2 Patch Based Local Generic Representation

Different parts (e.g., eye, mouth, nose, cheek) of human faces exhibit distinct structures, and they have different importance in identifying the identity of a face. Taking this fact into account, we propose to localize the representation model in Eq. (3) and present a patch based local generic representation scheme.

We partition the query sample z into S (overlapped) patches and denote these patches as $\{z_1, z_2, ..., z_S\}$. Correspondingly, the gallery dictionary X and the generic variation dictionary D can be partitioned as $\{X_1, X_2, ..., X_S\}$ and $\{D_1, D_2, ..., D_S\}$, respectively. For each local patch $z_i, i = 1, 2, .., S$, its associated local gallery dictionary and local variation dictionary are X_i and D_i, respectively. To increase the representation power of local gallery dictionaries and better address the local deformation (e.g., misalignment) of a patch, we extract the neighborhood patches at location i from each gallery sample, and add them to X_i. Such a sample expansion of local gallery dictionaries can improve much the stability and robustness of local representation [18]. In our implementation, the 8 closet neighboring patches to the underlying patch at location i are extracted. With X_i and D_i, we can represent each local patch z_i as:

$$z_i = X_i\alpha_i + D_i\beta_i + e_i, i = 1, 2, ..., S \tag{4}$$

where α_i and β_i are the representation vectors of z_i over X_i and D_i, respectively, and e_i is the representation residual.

Clearly, in order to find meaningful solutions of vectors α_i and β_i, appropriate loss function should be defined on the representation residual e_i and appropriate regularization can be imposed on α_i and β_i. Denote by $l(\|e_i\|_2)$ the loss function defined on the l_2-norm of e_i and denote by $R(\alpha_i, \beta_i)$ some regularizer imposed on the representation coefficients. We consider the following optimization problem to solve $\{\alpha_i, \beta_i\}$:

$$\min_{\{\alpha_i, \beta_i\}} \sum_{i=1}^{S} l(\|e_i\|_2) + \lambda R(\alpha_i, \beta_i)$$
$$s.t. \ z_i = X_i a_i + D_i \beta_i + e_i, \ i = 1, 2, ..., S \tag{5}$$

The problem now turns to how to define the loss function $l(\|e_i\|_2)$ and regularizer $R(\alpha_i, \beta_i)$.

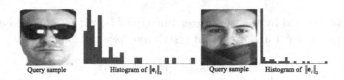

Query sample   Histogram of $\|e_i\|_2$ Query sample   Histogram of $\|e_i\|_2$

Fig. 3. The histogram of $\|e_i\|_2, i = 1, 2, ..., S$, for two query samples.

Let $e_i = \|e_i\|_2$. Due to the special structure of human face, the different patches will have very different representation residuals e_i. We solve $\{\hat{\alpha}_i, \hat{\beta}_i\} = \min_{\{\alpha_i, \beta_i\}} \|z_i - X\alpha_i + D_i\beta_i\|_2^2 + \lambda(\|\alpha_i\|_2^2 + \|\beta_i\|_2^2)$ and then calculate $e_i = \left\|z_i - X\hat{\alpha}_i + D_i\hat{\beta}_i\right\|_2$. Figure 3 illustrates the distribution for e_i for two query face images. One can see that the distribution of e_i is highly non-Gaussian. The widely used l_2-norm loss function relies highly on the Gaussianity assumption of the data [25] and hence it is not suitable to measure such non-Gaussian distributed residual. In [26], the concept of correntropy is proposed to measure the loss of non-Gaussian data. A correntropy induced metric (CIM) for residual e_i is defined as [26]:

$$\text{CIM}(e_i) = (k_\sigma(0) - k_\sigma(e_i))^{1/2} \tag{6}$$

where $k_\sigma(\cdot)$ is a kernel function. The Gaussian kernel function $k_\sigma(x) = \exp(-x^2/2\sigma^2)$ is widely used with good performance [25,26]. The robustness of CIM to non-Gaussian residual/noise has been verified in signal processing [27], feature selection [28], and FR [29]. Hence, we adopt correntropy to model the representation residual of different patches.

For the regularizer $R(\alpha_i, \beta_i)$, we define it as the l_2-norm of α_i and β_i. It has been shown that the l_2-norm regularization on representation coefficients can lead to similar classification performance to l_1-norm regularization but with much less computational cost [20]. Finally, the proposed local generic representation (LGR) model becomes:

$$\min_{\{\alpha_i, \beta_i\}} \sum_{i=1}^{S} (1 - k_\sigma(\|e_i\|_2)) + \lambda \left(\|\alpha_i\|_2^2 + \|\beta_i\|_2^2\right)$$
$$s.t. z_i = X_i\alpha_i + D_i\beta_i + e_i, i = 1, 2, ..., S \tag{7}$$

3 Optimization and Classification

3.1 Half-Quadratic Optimization

The minimization problem in Eq. (7) can be solved by half-quadratic optimization [27]. If a function $\phi(x)$ satisfies the following conditions [27]: (a) $x \to \phi(x)$

is convex on $\mathbb{R}$; (b) $x \to \phi(\sqrt{x})$ is concave on $\mathbb{R}_+$; (c) $\phi(x) = \phi(-x), x \in \mathbb{R}$; (d) $x \to \phi(x)$ is C^1 on $\mathbb{R}$; (e) $\phi''(0^+) > 0$; (f) $\lim_{x \to \infty} \phi(x)/\|x\|_2^2 = 0$, there exists a dual function φ such that

$$\phi(x) = \inf_{w \in \mathbb{R}} \left\{ \frac{1}{2}wx^2 + \varphi(w) \right\} \tag{8}$$

where w is determined by the minimizer function $\delta(\cdot)$ with respect to $\phi(\cdot)$. $\delta(\cdot)$ admits an explicit form under certain restrictive assumptions [27]:

$$w = \begin{cases} \delta(t) = \phi''(0^+), & \text{if } t = 0 \\ \phi''(t)/t, & \text{if } t \neq 0 \end{cases} \tag{9}$$

Obviously, $\phi_\sigma(x) = 1 - k_\sigma(x) = 1 - \exp(-x^2/2\sigma^2)$ satisfies all the conditions from (a) to (f). Then the problem in Eq. (7) can be equivalently written as the following augmented minimization problem:

$$\min_{A,w} \sum_{i=1}^S \left(\frac{1}{2}w_i \|z_i - X_i\alpha_i - D_i\beta_i\|_2^2 + \varphi(w_i) \right) + \lambda \|A\|_2^2 \tag{10}$$

where $A = [a_1, a_2, ..., a_S]$ with $a_i = [\alpha_i; \beta_i]$, and $w = [w_1, w_2, ..., w_S]$.

According to the half-quadratic analysis [27], Eq. (10) can be easily minimized by updating A and w alternatively, and there is no need to have an explicit form of the dual function $\varphi(w_i)$. When w is fixed, A can be solved by

$$\hat{A} = \arg\min_A \sum_{i=1}^S \left(w_i \|z_i - X_i\alpha_i - D_i\beta_i\|_2^2 \right) + \lambda \|A\|_F^2 \tag{11}$$

Clearly, the above minimization is a least square regression problem, and we have the closed-form solution of each $\{\alpha_i, \beta_i\}$:

$$[\hat{\alpha}_i; \hat{\beta}_i] = w_i(w_i[X_i, D_i]^T[X_i, D_i] + \lambda I)^{-1}[X_i, D_i]^T z_i \tag{12}$$

When A is fixed, the weights w can be updated as

$$\hat{w}_i = \frac{1}{\sigma^2} \exp(-\|z_i - X_i\alpha_i - D_i\beta_i\|_2^2/2\sigma^2) \tag{13}$$

The weight w_i corresponds to the ith patch, and it is used to control the portion of $\|e_i\|_2$ in the whole energy of Eq. (10). If the representation residual of a patch is big (e.g., caused by sunglasses, scarf and/or other large variations), the corresponding weight w_i will become small, and consequently the effect of this patch in the overall representation will be suppressed.

3.2 LGR Based Classification

After the optimal solutions of A and w are resolved by the half-quadratic optimization in Sect. 3.1, an LGR based classification scheme can be proposed to determine the class label of query face z. Let $X_i = [X_i^1, ..., X_i^k, ..., X_i^K]$, where X_i^k is sub-gallery dictionary associated with class k. Accordingly, the representation vector α_i can be written as $\alpha_i = [\alpha_i^1; ...; \alpha_i^k; ...; \alpha_i^K]$, where α_i^k is the coefficients vector associated with class k. By using the class-specific sub-gallery dictionary X_i^k and the generic variation dictionary D_i, we can calculate the representation residual of each patch z_i by each class k. Then the sum of the weighted residual (by w_i) over all patches can be calculated. Our classification principle is to check which class can lead to the minimal residual over all patches. Specifically, the classification rule of query face z is as follows:

$$label(z) = \arg\min_k \sum_{i=1}^{S} w_i \left\| z_i - [X_i^k, D_i][\alpha_i^k; \beta_i] \right\|_2^2 / \left\| [\alpha_i^k; \beta_i] \right\|_2^2 \qquad (14)$$

Note that in Eq. (14), we also use the l_2-norm of $[\alpha_i^k; \beta_i]$ to adjust the residual of patch i by class k. $1/ \left\| [\alpha_i^k; \beta_i] \right\|_2^2$ can be considered as a "class weight". If class k has a larger $\left\| [\alpha_i^k; \beta_i] \right\|_2^2$, it means that the query patch is more similar to the gallery patch of class k, and thus a smaller weight should be assigned to weaken the representation residual by this class. The query sample z is classified to the class which has the minimal weighted representation residual over all patches. The algorithm of LGR based classification is summarized in Table 1.

Table 1. The algorithm of local generic representation (LGR) based classification.

Input: The query sample z, gallery set X, reference subset G^r,   variation subset G^v and regularization parameter λ.   Output: The class label of z
1: Initialize $w = [1, 1, ..., 1]$;   2: Caculate $D = [G_1^v - G^r, G_2^v - G^r, ..., G_m^v - G^r]$.   3: Partition z, X and D into patches.   4: While convergence   5:   Update A by Eq. (11);   6:   Update w by Eq. (13);   7: End   8: Output the class label of sample z by Eq.(14).

3.3 Convergence and Complexity

According to half-quadratic optimization [27], the objective function in Eq. (10) is non-increasing under the update rules in Eq. (11) and Eq. (13). Therefore, our algorithm is guaranteed to converge based on the theory of half-quadratic optimization [27]. In Fig. 4, the convergence curve of LGR on the AR database [23] is shown (please refer to Sect. 4.4 for the details of experiment setting). We can see that the LGR algorithm converges after 5 iterations.

The main computational cost of LGR is spent on solving the least square regression problem in Eq. (11), whose time complexity is $O(S(n_d^3 + n_d^2 d_p))$, where S is the number of patches, n_d is the total number of patches in $[X_i, D_i]$ and d_p is the feature dimension of patches. Denote by T the total number of iteration in our algorithm, the time complexity of LGR is $O(TS(n_d^3 + n_d^2 d_p))$.

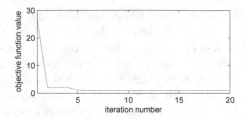

Fig. 4. The convergence curve of LGR on the AR database.

4   Experimental Analysis

We test the performance of LGR on four benchmark face databases, including three face databases in controlled environment, i.e., Extended Yale B [21], large-scale CMU Multi-PIE [22], and AR [23], and one face database in uncontrolled environment, i.e., Labeled Faces in the Wild (LFW) database [24]. Extended Yale B database contains illumination variations; AR database contains illumination and expression variations and disguises; Multi-PIE database contains pose, illumination and expression variations; LFW reflects the variations in real-world applications. We compare the proposed LGR method with the following eleven methods:

- Baseline methods: Nearest neighbor classifier (NNC) [30], support vector machines (SVM) [31], sparse representation based classifiers (SRC) [15] and collaborative representation based classifiers (CRC) [20];
- Generic learning methods: Adaptive generic learning (AGL) [32], extended SRC (ESRC) [13] and sparse variation dictionary learning (SVDL) [3];
- Patch/block based methods: Block linear discriminative analysis (BlockLDA) [16], patch based NN (PNN) [17], patch based CRC (PCRC) [18], and discriminative multi-manifold analysis (DMMA) [8].

Note that the generic learning method SVDL learns a sparse variation dictionary from the generic training set. The proposed LGR also belongs to the generic learning methods; however, we use the raw face difference images as the dictionary rather than learning a dictionary with some objective function. Among the competing methods, we implement NN and DMMA; the code of SVM is from [33]; and the codes of all the other methods are obtained from the original authors.

4.1   Parameter Setting

In all the experiments, the face images are resized to 80×80 (using the Matlab function "resize.m"). For patch/block based methods including BlockLDA, PNN, PCRC, DMMA, and the proposed LGR, the patch size is fixed as 20×20 and the overlap between neighboring patches is 10 pixels. That is, the query sample is partitioned into $S = 49$ patches.

Apart from the setting of patch size and patch number, there are only two parameters to set in the proposed LGR. The first is the regularization parameter λ in Eq. (6). We fix it as $\lambda = 0.001$ in all our experiments. Another is the scale parameter σ of the kernel function $k_\sigma(x)$. Based on our experimental experience, if the representation residual is big, a large value of σ could be set to make the representation more robust. Therefore, we adaptively set σ as the average representation residual after solving the coefficients α_i and β_i in the first iteration of our algorithm; that is, $\sigma = \sqrt{\frac{1}{2S} \sum_{i=1}^{S} \|z_i - X_i \alpha_i - D_i \beta_i\|_2^2}$.

For the competing algorithms, we tune their parameters for the best results. In particular, for SVDL we follow the parameter setting in [3]. The three parameters λ_1, λ_2, λ_3 are set as 0.001, 0.01, 0.0001, respectively, and the number of dictionary atoms is set as 400 in the initialization. For SRC, CRC and PCRC, the optimal regularization parameter λ is chosen from $\{0.0005, 0.001, 0.005, 0.01\}$. As BlockLDA and AGL are sensitive to the feature dimension, the best result of different feature dimensions is reported.

4.2 Extended Yale B Database

The Extended Yale B face database [21] contains 38 human subjects and 2,414 face images with 64 illumination conditions. The frontal faces with light source directions at 0 degree azimuth (A + 000) and at 0 degree elevation (E + 00) are used as the gallery set, and the face images under other illumination conditions are used as the query set. We use the face images of the first 30 subjects to form the gallery and query sets, and use the face images of the other 8 subjects as the generic set.

Table 2 lists the recognition rates by different methods. By combining the decisions of different patches, the PCRC method achieves much higher recognition rate than the baseline methods. The generic learning based method SVDL achieves the second highest recognition rate by learning a dictionary that consists of different illumination variations. By exploiting the advantages of both patch based local representation and generic variation information, the proposed LGR method achieves the highest recognition accuracy.

4.3 CMU Multi-PIE Database

The Multi-PIE database [22] contains a total of more than 750,000 images from 337 individuals, captured under 15 viewpoints and 19 illumination conditions

Table 2. Recognition rate (%) on Extended Yale B database.

Method	NNC [30]	SVM [31]	SRC [15]	CRC [20]	BlockLDA [16]	AGL [32]
Accuracy	46.5	41.4	49.2	51.2	49.2	59.5
Method	DMMA [8]	PNN [17]	PCRC [18]	ESRC [13]	SVDL [3]	LGR
Accuracy	61.7	67.5	77.8	67.9	85.0	**86.6**

Table 3. Recognition accuracy (%) on Multi-PIE with illumination variations.

Method	Session 2	Session 3	Session 4
NNC [30]	44.3	40	43.8
SVM [31]	43.6	40.5	40.1
SRC [15]	51.9	46.5	50.6
CRC [20]	52.8	47.4	50.5
BlockLDA [16]	68.2	60.4	65.1
AGL [32]	84.5	79.6	78.5
DMMA [8]	64.1	56.6	60.1
PNN [17]	65.1	55.6	60.8
PCRC [18]	83.7	72.7	77.7
ESRC [13]	92.6	84.6	87.6
SVDL [3]	94.2	87.5	90.4
LGR	**96.9**	**90.5**	**94.4**

in four recording sessions. The face images of the first 100 subjects in session 1 are used for the gallery set and the other 149 subjects are used as generic set. Following the experiment setting in [3], in the generic training set, the frontal images with illumination 7 and neutral expression are used as the reference subset and the face images with different variations in Session 1 are used as the variation subset.

Illumination Variations. In this experiment, we test the performance of LGR under different illuminations. The frontal face images with neutral expression from session 2, session 3 and session 4 are used as the query set, respectively. The recognition rates on Multi-PIE with illumination variations are listed in Table 3. LGR shows superior performance to all the other competing methods. Compared with SVDL, which achieves the second highest accuracy, the recognition rate is improved by 2.7%, 3.0% and 4.0% on session 2, session 3 and session 4, respectively. Compared with PCRC, the recognition rate is improved by about 15%. The performance of SRC and CRC is very poor because with only one gallery face image per person, the query image cannot be well represented.

Expression and Illumination Variations. We then test the robustness of the proposed LGR method to face images with both expression and illumination variations. The query set includes the frontal face images with smile expression in session 1 (Smile-S1), smile expression in session 3 (Smile-S3) and surprise expression (Surprise-S2). Table 4 presents the recognition results in this experiment. Clearly, LGR outperforms all the other methods. SVDL still works the second best, but it lags behind LGR by 1.8%, 5.6% and 21.7% for Smile-S1, Smile-S3 and Surprise-S2, respectively.

Table 4. Recognition accuracy (%) on Multi-PIE with expression and illumination variations.

Method	Smile-S1	Smile-S3	Surprise-S2
NNC [30]	46.8	29.1	18.3
SVM [31]	46.8	29.1	18.3
SRC [15]	50.1	28.1	21.1
CRC [20]	50	29.7	22.4
BlockLDA [16]	49.5	30	26.2
AGL [32]	85.2	39.5	31.5
DMMA [8]	58.5	33.4	23
PNN [17]	53.1	31.1	31.4
PCRC [18]	74.9	44.1	44.9
ESRC [13]	82	50.8	49.9
SVDL [3]	88.9	59.6	52.8
LGR	**90.7**	**65.2**	**74.5**

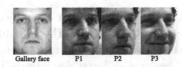

Gallery face   P1   P2   P3

Fig. 5. Images of Multi-PIE database with pose, expression and illumination variations.

Pose, Expression and Illumination Variations. In this experiment, there are pose, expression and illumination variations in the query set simultaneously. We select the face images with pose 05_0 in Session 2 (P1), pose 04_1 in Session 3 (P2), and pose 04_1 and smile expression in Session 3 (P3) as the query set. Some face images from the gallery and query set are illustrated in Fig. 5.

Table 5 lists the recognition rate of all methods. LGR achieves the highest accuracy on all the three query sets. Because of the large variations caused by pose, expression and illumination variations, the FR rates in this experiment are relatively lower than the experimental results in Tables 3 and 4. The patch based methods such as PCRC do not work well because they are sensitive to pose variation. The generic learning methods, including AGL, ESRC, SVDL and the proposed LGR, outperform the other methods since they can exploit the variation information from the external generic training set. LGR consistently exhibits better results than SVDL, which still works the second best.

4.4 AR Face Database

The AR face database [23] contains about 4,000 color face images of 126 people, which consists of the frontal faces with different facial expressions, illuminations and disguises. There are two sessions and each session has 13 face images per subject. Following the SSPP experiment setting in [13], a subset with face images

Table 5. Recognition accuracy (%) on Multi-PIE with pose, expression and illumination variations.

Method	P1	P2	P3
NNC [30]	25.7	8.8	11.9
SVM [31]	25.7	8.8	11.9
SRC [15]	23.9	6.1	10.1
CRC [20]	24.9	5.4	9.0
BlockLDA [16]	29.5	13.2	15.8
AGL [32]	66.4	25.5	24.0
DMMA [8]	28.2	5.5	12.1
PNN [17]	35.3	11.8	13.5
PCRC [18]	37.3	8.0	10.2
ESRC [13]	63.8	31.9	27.0
SVDL [3]	76.0	37.9	33.5
LGR	**79.1**	**39.5**	**36.3**

of 50 males and 50 females is selected. The first 80 subjects from sessions 1 are used for the gallery and query set while the other 20 subjects are used as the generic training set. We also use the face images from session 2 as the query set to test the FR performance. There are different variations, including illumination, expression, and disguise (scarf and sunglass) in this experiment.

The experimental results on session 1 and session 2 are shown in Tables 6 and 7, respectively. LGR exhibits significantly better performance than all the other methods on both sessions. In particular, on session 2 LGR outperforms SVDL by 16.4 %, 10.8 %, 32.5 % and 34.7 % under different variations. Note that in this experiment the performance of patch based methods such as PCRC is very competitive. This is because the disguises (i.e., scarf and sunglass) can be well dealt with by patch/block based methods. Therefore, PCRC can achieve higher recognition rate than the global representation based SVDL though it does not learn any variation information from a generic dataset. The proposed LGR utilizes both local presentation and generic information, leading to very promising performance for the task of FR with SSPP.

4.5   LFW Database

The LFW database [24] contains images of 5,749 different individuals in unconstrained environment. LFW-a is a version of LFW after alignment using commercial face alignment software [34]. Following the experiment setting in [18] and [3], a subset of 158 subjects with more than 10 images per person is collected. Each face image is cropped to 120×120 and then resized to 80×80. One can see that although face alignment has been conducted, the variations in this database is still very large compared with the face databases in the controlled environment. Face images of the first 50 subjects are selected to form the gallery

Table 6. Recognition accuracy (%) on AR face database (session1).

Method	Illumination	Expression	Disguise	Illumination + Disguise
NNC [30]	70	79.2	39.4	23.5
SVM [31]	55.8	90.4	43.1	29.4
SRC [15]	80.8	85.4	55.6	25.3
CRC [20]	80.5	80.4	58.1	23.8
BlockLDA [16]	75.3	81.4	65.4	53.5
AGL [32]	93.3	77.9	70.0	53.8
DMMA [8]	92.1	81.4	46.9	30.9
PNN [17]	84.6	86.7	90.0	72.5
PCRC [18]	95.0	86.7	95.6	81.3
ESRC [13]	99.6	85.0	83.1	68.6
SVDL [3]	98.3	86.3	86.3	79.4
LGR	**100**	**97.9**	**98.8**	**96.3**

Table 7. Recognition accuracy (%) on AR face database (session2).

Method	Illumination	Expression	Disguise	Illumination + Disguise
NNC [30]	41.7	58.8	26.3	12.8
SVM [31]	40.0	58.8	26.9	14.4
SRC [15]	55.8	68.8	29.4	12.8
CRC [20]	55.8	69.6	35.0	13.5
BlockLDA [16]	54.7	61.2	31.9	21.0
AGL [32]	70.8	55.8	40.6	30.7
DMMA [8]	77.9	61.7	28.1	21.9
PNN [17]	77.5	73.8	71.9	52.8
PCRC [18]	88.8	71.7	81.8	63.1
ESRC [13]	87.9	70.4	59.4	45.0
SVDL [3]	87.1	74.2	61.3	54.1
LGR	**97.5**	**85.0**	**93.8**	**88.8**

and query sets, while the face images of the remaining subjects are used to build the generic training set. Since there are no frontal neutral face images in this database, the mean face of each person is used to form the reference subset in the generic set.

The face recognition rates of different methods are listed in Table 8. Because of the challenging face variations in uncontrolled environment, no method achieves very high accuracy in this experiment. Nonetheless, LGR still works the best among all competing methods. The patch based method PCRC works better than the global representation based CRC, which is similar to what we observed

Table 8. Recognition accuracy (%) on LFW database.

Method	NNC [30]	SVM [31]	SRC [15]	CRC [20]	BlockLDA [16]	AGL [32]
Accuracy	12.2	11.6	20.4	19.8	16.4	19.2
Method	DMMA [8]	PNN [17]	PCRC [18]	ESRC [13]	SVDL [3]	LGR
Accuracy	17.8	17.6	24.2	27.3	28.6	**30.4**

in the experiments of previous sections. SVDL again achieves the second highest recognition rate, demonstrating that the face variation information learned from other subjects is indeed helpful to improve the robustness of FR with SSPP, no matter in controlled or uncontrolled environment.

5   Conclusions

We proposed a local generic representation (LGR) based approach for the challenging task of face recognition with single sample per person (SSPP). LGR utilizes the advantages of both patch based local representation and generic learning. A generic intra-class variation dictionary was constructed from a generic dataset, and it can well compensate for the face variations lacked in the SSPP gallery set. A patch gallery dictionary was built by using the gallery samples, which can more accurately represent the different parts of face images. Considering that the distribution of representation residual of different patches is highly non-Gaussian, a correntropy based metric was adopted to measure the loss of each patch so that the importance of different patches in face recognition can be more robustly evaluated. As a result, LGR can adaptively suppress the role of patches with large variations. The extensive experimental results on four benchmark face databases showed that LGR always achieves higher face recognition rate than the state-of-the-art SSPP methods used in competition.

Acknowledgement. This work was (partially) supported by LG Electronics Co., Ltd.

References

1. Jain, A.K., Li, S.Z.: Handbook of Face Recognition. Springer, London (2005)
2. Tan, X., Chen, S., Zhou, Z.H., Zhang, F.: Face recognition from a single image per person: a survey. Pattern Recogn. **39**, 1725–1745 (2006)
3. Yang, M., Gool, L.V., Zhang, L.: Sparse variation dictionary learning for face recognition with a single training sample per person. In: Proceedings of the 14th IEEE International Conference on Computer Vision (ICCV) (2013) (in press)
4. Martínez, A.M.: Recognizing imprecisely localized, partially occluded, and expression variant faces from a single sample per class. IEEE Trans. Pattern Anal. Mach. Intell. **24**, 748–763 (2002)
5. Shan, S., Cao, B., Gao, W., Zhao, D.: Extended fisherface for face recognition from a single example image per person. In: IEEE International Symposium on Circuits and Systems, ISCAS 2002, vol. 2., pp. II–81. IEEE (2002)

6. Gao, Q.X., Zhang, L., Zhang, D.: Face recognition using FLDA with single training image per person. Appl. Math. Comput. **205**, 726–734 (2008)
7. Vetter, T.: Synthesis of novel views from a single face image. Int. J. Comput. Vis. **28**, 103–116 (1998)
8. Lu, J., Tan, Y.P., Wang, G.: Discriminative multimanifold analysis for face recognition from a single training sample per person. IEEE Trans. Pattern Anal. Mach. Intell. **35**, 39–51 (2013)
9. Kim, T.K., Kittler, J.: Locally linear discriminant analysis for multimodally distributed classes for face recognition with a single model image. IEEE Trans. Pattern Anal. Mach. Intell. **27**, 318–327 (2005)
10. Wang, J., Plataniotis, K.N., Lu, J., Venetsanopoulos, A.N.: On solving the face recognition problem with one training sample per subject. Pattern Recogn. **39**, 1746–1762 (2006)
11. Kan, M., Shan, S., Su, Y., Xu, D., Chen, X.: Adaptive discriminant learning for face recognition. Pattern Recogn. **46**, 2497–2509 (2013)
12. Mohammadzade, H., Hatzinakos, D.: Projection into expression subspaces for face recognition from single sample per person. IEEE Trans. Affect. Comput. **4**, 69–82 (2013)
13. Deng, W., Hu, J., Guo, J.: Extended SRC: undersampled face recognition via intraclass variant dictionary. IEEE Trans. Pattern Anal. Mach. Intell. **34**, 1864–1870 (2012)
14. Huang, D.A., Wang, Y.C.F.: With one look: robust face recognition using single sample per person. In: Proceedings of the 21st ACM International Conference on Multimedia, pp. 601–604. ACM (2013)
15. Wright, J., Yang, A., Ganesh, A., Sastry, S., Ma, Y.: Robust face recognition via sparse representation. IEEE Trans. Pattern Anal. Mach. Intell. **31**, 210–227 (2009)
16. Chen, S., Liu, J., Zhou, Z.: Making FLDA applicable to face recognition with one sample per person. Pattern Recogn. **37**, 1553–1555 (2004)
17. Kumar, R., Banerjee, A., Vemuri, B.C., Pfister, H.: Maximizing all margins: pushing face recognition with kernel plurality. In: 2011 IEEE International Conference on Computer Vision (ICCV), pp. 2375–2382 (2011)
18. Zhu, P., Zhang, L., Hu, Q., Shiu, S.C.K.: Multi-scale patch based collaborative representation for face recognition with margin distribution optimization. In: Fitzgibbon, A., Lazebnik, S., Perona, P., Sato, Y., Schmid, C. (eds.) ECCV 2012, Part I. LNCS, vol. 7572, pp. 822–835. Springer, Heidelberg (2012)
19. Kumar, R., Banerjee, A., Vemuri, B.C.: Volterrafaces: discriminant analysis using volterra kernels. In: IEEE Conference on Computer Vision and Pattern Recognition, CVPR 2009, pp. 150–155. IEEE (2009)
20. Zhang, L., Yang, M., Feng, X.: Sparse representation or collaborative representation: which helps face recognition? In: International Conference on Computer Vision (2011)
21. Georghiades, A., Belhumeur, P., Kriegman, D.: From few to many: illumination cone models for face recognition under variable lighting and pose. IEEE Trans. Pattern Anal. Mach. Intell. **23**, 643–660 (2001)
22. Gross, R., Matthews, I., Cohn, J., Kanade, T., Baker, S.: Multi-pie. Image Vis. Comput. **28**, 807–813 (2010)
23. Martinez, A.: The ar face database. CVC Technical Report 24 (1998)
24. Huang, G.B., Ramesh, M., Berg, T., Learned-Miller, E.: Labeled faces in the wild: a database for studying face recognition in unconstrained environments. Technical Report 07–49, University of Massachusetts, Amherst (2007)

25. Lu, C., Tang, J., Lin, M., Lin, L., Yan, S., Lin, Z.: Correntropy induced l2 graph for robust subspace clustering. In: Proceedings of 14th IEEE International Conference on Computer Vision (ICCV) (2013) (in press)
26. Liu, W., Pokharel, P.P., Príncipe, J.C.: Correntropy: properties and applications in non-gaussian signal processing. IEEE Trans. Sig. Process. **55**, 5286–5298 (2007)
27. Nikolova, M., Ng, M.K.: Analysis of half-quadratic minimization methods for signal and image recovery. SIAM J. Sci. Comput. **27**, 937–966 (2005)
28. He, R., Tan, T., Wang, L., Zheng, W.S.: $l_{2,1}$-regularized correntropy for robust feature selection. In: 2012 IEEE Conference on Computer Vision and Pattern Recognition (CVPR), pp. 2504–2511. IEEE (2012)
29. He, R., Zheng, W.S., Tan, T., Sun, Z.: Half-quadratic-based iterative minimization for robust sparse representation. IEEE Trans. Pattern Anal. Mach. Intell. **36**, 261–275 (2014)
30. Cover, T., Hart, P.: Nearest neighbor pattern classification. IEEE Trans. Inf. Theory **13**, 21–27 (1967)
31. Cortes, C., Vapnik, V.: Support vector machine. Mach. Learn. **20**, 273–297 (1995)
32. Su, Y., Shan, S., Chen, X., Gao, W.: Adaptive generic learning for face recognition from a single sample per person. In: 2010 IEEE Conference on Computer Vision and Pattern Recognition (CVPR), pp. 2699–2706. IEEE (2010)
33. Chang, C.C., Lin, C.J.: LIBSVM: a library for support vector machines. ACM Trans. Intell. Syst. Technol. (TIST) **2**, 27 (2011)
34. Wolf, L., Hassner, T., Taigman, Y.: Similarity scores based on background samples. In: Zha, H., Taniguchi, R., Maybank, S. (eds.) ACCV 2009, Part II. LNCS, vol. 5995, pp. 88–97. Springer, Heidelberg (2010)

Unsupervised Image Co-segmentation Based on Cooperative Game

Bo-Chen Lin, Ding-Jie Chen$^{(\boxtimes)}$, and Long-Wen Chang

Department of Computer Science, National Tsing Hua University, Hsinchu, Taiwan
dj_chen_tw@yahoo.com.tw

Abstract. In computer vision, co-segmentation is defined as the task of jointly segmenting the common objects in a given set of images. Most proposed co-segmentation algorithms have the assumptions that the common objects are singletons or with the similar size. In addition, they might assume that the background features are simple or discriminative. This paper presents a cooperative co-segmentation without these assumptions. In the proposed cooperative co-segmentation algorithm, each image is treated as a player. By using the cooperative game, heat diffusion, and image saliency, we design a constrained utility function for each player. This constrained utility function push all players, with the instinct to maximize their self-utility, to cooperatively define the common-object labels. We then use cooperative cut to segment the common objects according to the common-object labels. Experimental results demonstrate that the proposed method outperforms the state-of-the-art co-segmentation methods in the segmentation accuracy of the common objects in the images.

1 Introduction

Image segmentation is a fundamental problem in computer vision. Segmentation partitions an image into several regions that each region shares certain similar appearances. The goal of segmentation is to simplify the representation of an image for locating the objects. An important issue of image segmentation is that the regions found by a typical image segmentation algorithm usually tend to be fragmented or lack semantic meanings. That is, it is difficult to locate the objects from a single image. Therefore, Rother et al. [1] proposed the idea of co-segmentation that one additional image is provided to segment both images together to increase the accuracy of the object segmentation.

Recently, co-segmentation has been widely studied in computer vision. The goal of image co-segmentation refers to segment the similar regions from two or more images. Although the authors [1–9] proposed some methods to solve this problem, there are still some restrictions as follows:

(1) Some algorithms are supervised.
(2) The given images have only one instance of the common object.
(3) The backgrounds of the given images are discriminative.

© Springer International Publishing Switzerland 2015
D. Cremers et al. (Eds.): ACCV 2014, Part III, LNCS 9005, pp. 51–63, 2015.
DOI: 10.1007/978-3-319-16811-1_4

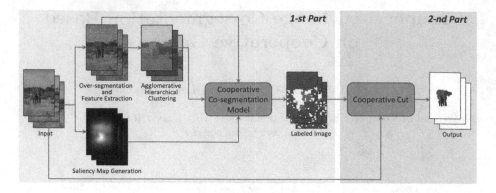

Fig. 1. The block diagram of the proposed image co-segmentation method.

Heat diffusion framework [9–11] is a successful technique in image processing and computer vision. It can be applied in image segmentation [10], and optical flow estimation [11]. Here we adopt the heat-gain of this framework to measure the segmentation confidence [9]. In order to deal with images with similar back-ground, we use the saliency map [12] in our algorithm to provide an initial guess about the object positions. Game theory [13] has been widely used as a powerful method to solve problems in social science, biology, economics, computer science [14,15], etc. It is the study of the rational choice of strategies by interacting agents called players. In this paper, we model the labeling problem as a cooperative game to constrain the labeling procedure.

The co-segmentation problem implies cooperative feasibility for jointly segmenting the common objects among the images. In this paper, we base on the cooperative game, heat diffusion, and image saliency to propose a cooperative co-segmentation framework (see Fig. 1) for overcoming the aforementioned restrictions. In the proposed method, each image is treated as a player in the heat diffusion system, and her heat gain is treated as her utility. In the first part, the superpixels with very low saliency value are labeled as background. Next, all players cooperatively define the common-object superpixels with their constrained utility function. The remaining unlabeled superpixels are treated as neutral. In the second part, we apply the cooperative cut [16] with the aid of the labeled superpixels and thus generate the pixel-level segmentation.

There are three advantages of the proposed cooperative co-segmentation method. First, the proposed method can discover multiple instances of the common objects. Secondly, our method is capable of handling images whose backgrounds are similar. Thirdly, we can segment the common objects with different scales and achieve higher accuracy than other methods [6,9].

1.1 Related Work

Existing image co-segmentation works [1,5,7,8] formulated the co-segmentation problem as a binary labeling problem. Their objectives are minimization of an energy function with a histogram difference term which derived from the input

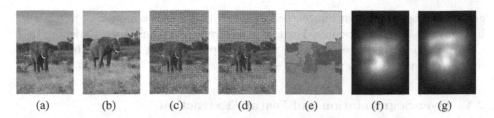

Fig. 2. (a) and (b) are Elephants-safari from the CMU-Cornell iCoseg dataset [2]. (c) the over-segmentation of (a). (d) the representative superpixels set of (c). (e) The yellow sky region corresponding to the yellow representative superpixel of (d). (f) and (g) are the corresponding saliency maps of (a) and (b) (Color figure online).

image pairs. The histogram difference term penalizes the difference between the foreground histograms calculated from the input images. Since the histogram difference term is computed between any two images, the energy function is computationally intractable as the number of the input images increase. In addition, these methods implicitly assume that only one object appears in each image.

Joulin et al. [6] proposed a discriminative clustering based image co-segmentation. The main idea in this method is to train a supervised classifier for maximal separation of the foreground and the background. Although it can solve the co-segmentation problem for up to dozens of images, the segmentation results are not satisfactory for the number of the input images less than a certain number. Kim et al. [9] proposed the distributed co-segmentation algorithm based on temperature maximization on anisotropic heat diffusion. The approach can deal with a large number of input images. Chu et al. [4] proposed a method that has the ability to segment multiple objects that repeatedly appear among input images. It incorporates a common pattern discovery algorithm, that using the SIFT descriptor, with an energy function. The method can achieve high accuracy of segmentation when the common objects have high texture complexity.

However, the above unsupervised co-segmentation methods [1,4–9] require the testing dataset to be chosen carefully, because their methods would fail for images with similar background. For example, in Fig. 2(a) and (b), the backgrounds of images are so similar that the common objects cannot be cut out via unsupervised co-segmentation methods. Due to this problem, some interactive co-segmentation techniques were proposed [2,3], which allow users to decide where the foreground or background is, and then users can guide the output of the co-segmentation algorithm toward it via scribbles.

2   Cooperative Image Co-segmentation

Given a set of input images, the co-segmentation goal is to segment the common objects among these images. The block diagram of our method is given in Fig. 1, which is divided into two parts. The first part consists of four stages, namely *over-segmentation and feature extraction*, *agglomerative hierarchical clustering*, *saliency map generation*, and *cooperative co-segmentation model*. In this part, the goal is to label each input image. We label the images with common-object-label, background-label, and neutral-label. The neutral-label is just used to denote the unsure regions. In the second part, we use cooperative cut [16] with the labeled image-regions to obtain the final result.

2.1   Over-Segmentation and Feature Extraction

In order to reduce the computational loading in the following heat diffusion system, we represent each image as a set of superpixels. We adopt the over-segmentation method [17] to obtain the regular-size superpixels. Figure 2(c) shows an example of the over-segmentation [17] that applied on Fig. 2(a).

After over-segmentation, we need some descriptors to describe each superpixel. Color and texture descriptors are commonly used in computer vision. The color of a superpixel can be represented in terms of average color or color histogram. Texture descriptor is used to describe the superpixel in terms of its texture property. Here we simply represent each superpixel as a 3-dimensional average color vector.

2.2   Agglomerative Hierarchical Clustering

To select the representative superpixels as the candidate heat sources in the following heat diffusion system, we apply the agglomerative hierarchical clustering [9] to find out some representative superpixels. Precisely, a set of superpixels with the similar features will be represented as one representative superpixel. Figure 2(c) is the superpixel representation of Fig. 2(a). A region, for example, the sky in Fig. 2(e), consists of a set of superpixels of similar features and represented with the yellow representative superpixel in Fig. 2(d).

2.3   Saliency Map Generation

We assume that the objects in the foreground usually have higher saliency value than those in background. The saliency detection methods usually focus on identifying the fixation points that human viewer would focus on at the first glance. Harel et al. [12] proposed a method of computing bottom-up saliency maps which shows a remarkable consistency with the deployment of attention of human subjects.

For an input image, the method [12] extracts three kinds of features of each pixel, thus generate three kinds of feature maps. For each kind of feature map, the method obtains corresponding activation map by computing Markov chains. Finally, the method normalizes and averages the three kinds of activation maps to generate the saliency map. The saliency maps of Fig. 2(a)–(b) are shown as Fig. 2(f)–(g).

2.4   Cooperative Co-segmentation Model

With a heat diffusion system, each image can evaluate the segmentation confidence of each region with the value of heat gain [9]. In addition, the heat gain is proportional to this segmentation confidence in a heat diffusion system.

The image co-segmentation goal is to segment the common object region. Intuitively, the common object region should has as high segmentation confidence, i.e., heat gain, as possible. However, we observed that a representative superpixel with high heat gain could be the foreground or the background. In order to label the representative superpixels right on the foreground as the common object, here we consider the image saliency.

In image co-segmentation scenario, a superpixel is considered as the common object candidate if it has similar appearance with the superpixels from other images. This means that an image should selects its superpixels as the common object with considering what are the selected superpixels of other images. This kind of consideration is like the scenario in game theory, that is, each player choose her best strategy according to the strategies chosen by other players.

In game theory [13], one assumption is that each player is rational. Namely, each player maximizes her utility, given the adopted strategies of other players. In cooperative game, each player still need to maximize her utility. However, the designed utility functions also trigger them to maximize the coalition utility. In this paper, we design a utility function constrained on the other players' strategies, self heat gain, and self image saliency. To begin with labeling, the superpixels with very low saliency value are regarded as background. Then, all players cooperatively define the common-object-label via maximizing their constrained utility functions. The remaining unlabeled superpixels are assigned the neutral-label. Finally, we use the cooperative cut [16] with the label information to finely segment the images.

Heat Diffusion System. Each image corresponds to a heat diffusion system while the images correspond to those systems are coupled together. In each system, there are K_i heat sources, i.e., representative superpixels.

Given an input image set I. For each input image $I_i \in I$ ($i = 1, ..., N$) consider a graph $\mathcal{G}_i = (\mathcal{V}_i, \mathcal{E}_i)$ where the node set $\mathcal{V}_i$ is the set of superpixels of I_i, and the edge set $\mathcal{E}_i$ connect all pairs of adjacent superpixels in $\mathcal{V}_i$. The heat diffusion system [9] has the following definitions:

(1) Each input image I_i is an insulated heat diffusion system T_i. A heat diffusion system T_i contains: (i). a temperature function u_i. (ii). an environment node g_i with zero temperate, denoted by $u_i(g_i) = 0$. (iii). a heat source node h_i with constant temperate, denoted by $u_i(h_i) = 1$.
(2) Each node v_x in T_i diffuses heat to its neighbors and is connected to an environment node with constant diffusivity of z_{v_x}. The diffusivity between any two nodes $v_x, v_y \in \mathcal{V}_i$ are defined by their Gaussian similarity:

$$d_{v_x,v_y} = \begin{cases} \exp(-\gamma \| f^c(v_x) - f^c(v_y) \|^2), & \text{if } (v_x, v_y) \in \mathcal{E}_i \\ 0, & \text{otherwise} \end{cases}, \qquad (1)$$

where $f^c(v_x)$ is the average color of the pixels in v_x, γ is a constant parameter.
(3) The diffusion equation for $v_x \in \mathcal{V}_i$ is defined as follows:

$$u_i(v_x) = \frac{1}{a_{v_x}} \sum_{(v_x,v_y) \in \mathcal{E}_i} d_{v_y v_x} u_i(v_y), \qquad (2)$$

where $a_{v_x} = \Sigma_{(v_x, v_y) \in \mathcal{E}_i} d_{v_y v_x} + z_{v_x}$ is a normalization factor.

(4) Assume that the system temperature is zero before putting the heat source h_i on v_x. Once putting a heat source h_i on v_x, the corresponding heat gain δ_i is computed by

$$\delta_i(v_x) = \sum_{(v_x, v_y) \in \mathcal{E}_i} u_i(v_y). \tag{3}$$

Cooperative Label Generation Model. We propose a cooperative game model to assign the common-object-label to each image, which is configured as follows:

Players: Given an input image set I, each image I_i $(i = 1, ..., N)$ is regarded as a player in the game. The superpixels of I_i are separated into K_i clusters with the aforementioned agglomerative hierarchical clustering. The collection of these representative superpixels of I_i are denoted by R_i.

Strategies: The strategy set of each player I_i is $R_i = \{v_{i_1}, v_{i_2}, ..., v_{i_{K_i}}\}$. Each player choose one strategy $v_i \in R_i$ to put her heat source in one diffusion process. We denote the strategy profile $\mathbf{v}$ of all players as $(v_1, v_2, ..., v_N) \in R_1 \times R_2 \times ... \times R_N$.

Preference: We treat the image set I with the common objects as a coalition. In a cooperative game, each player should takes the strategy with considering what are the adopted strategies of other players. Thus we define the preference of each player I_i is represented by the constrained utility function U_i as follows:

$$U_i(v_i | \mathbf{v}) = \pi(v_i | \mathbf{v}) \delta_i(v_i) \left(\frac{1}{|N-1|} \sum_{j \in -i} \psi(v_i, v_j) \right), \tag{4}$$

where $-i$ denotes all players except i. Precisely, the similarity function ψ of any two representative superpixels $v_i \in R_i, v_j \in R_j$ is defined as the Gaussian similarity:

$$\psi(v_i, v_j) = \exp(-\gamma \| f^c(v_i) - f^c(v_j) \|^2), \tag{5}$$

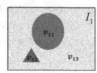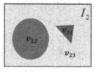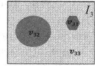

Fig. 3. An example to explain the cooperative behavior conditioned on function π. Each image I_i has three different regions, and each region can be represented as the corresponding representative superpixels v_{i_1}, v_{i_2}, and v_{i_3}. Since the objects usually have higher saliency value than background, the strategies $v_{11}, v_{12}, v_{21}, v_{22}, v_{31}, v_{32}$ can pass the saliency function ϕ in π. Since any pair from the two strategy sets $\{v_{11}, v_{22}, v_{32}\}$ and $\{v_{12}, v_{21}, v_{31}\}$ have similar color features, the pairs from these two sets can obtain high values of the similarity function ψ. Thus, the strategy profiles which can pass the π function will belong to $\{v_{11}, v_{12}\} \times \{v_{21}, v_{22}\} \times \{v_{31}, v_{32}\}$. However, the optimal strategy profile is (v_{11}, v_{22}, v_{32}) because it has the largest sum of the pairwise feature similarities according to the constrained utility function.

where $f^c(v_i)$ is the average color of the superpixels v_i, and γ is a constant parameter. Considering with the image saliency, the candidate strategy s_i of player I_i obeys the following function:

$$\pi(v_i|\mathbf{v}) = \begin{cases} 1, \text{ if } \psi(v_i, v_{-i}) > \alpha \text{ and } \phi(v_i) > \beta \\ 0, \text{ otherwise} \end{cases}, \tag{6}$$

where α and β are threshold parameters, $\phi(v_i)$ is the average saliency value of all pixels in v_i. Equation (6) shows that we only concern the superpixel v_i with high saliency value and with feature similar to other players' strategies. Figure 3 shows a simple example to explain the cooperative behavior conditioned on function π.

The goal of the cooperative model is to find the optimal strategy profile $\mathbf{v}^*$ that maximizes the coalition utility. That is,

$$\mathbf{v}^* = \underset{\mathbf{v}}{\operatorname{argmax}}(\sum_{i=1}^{N} U_i(v_i|\mathbf{v})), \tag{7}$$

where $\mathbf{v} = (v_1, v_2, ..., v_N) \in R_1 \times R_2 \times ... \times R_N$. In the designed utility function, the best response of each player I_i is conditioned on not only the heat gain δ of herself but also the feature similarity ψ comparing with other players' strategies. It is hard to calculate the exact optimal strategy profile $\mathbf{v}^* \in R_1 \times R_2 \times ... \times R_N$. In practice, we use loopy belief propagation (LBP) [18] to approximate the optimal strategy profile.

Algorithm 1. Label Generation

Input: N players: image set $\{I_1, I_2, \cdots, I_N\}$; Strategy set: each I_i has strategy set $R_i = \{v_{i_1}, v_{i_2}, \cdots, v_{i_{K_i}}\}$; Parameter set: $\{\alpha, \beta\}$.
Output: Background-label set: $\mathbf{V}_B$; Common-object-label set: $\mathbf{V}_C$; Neutral-label set: $\mathbf{V}_N$;
1: $\mathbf{V}_B = \emptyset; \mathbf{V}_C = \emptyset; \mathbf{V}_N = \emptyset$;
2: For all $v_i \in R_i$, if $\phi(v_i) < \beta$ then remove v_i from R_i and $\mathbf{V}_B = \mathbf{V}_B \cup v_i$;
3: Construct graph G with node $\{R_1, R_2, \cdots, R_N\}$ and edge $\{(v_i, v_j)|v_i \in R_i, v_j \in R_{-i}\}$;
4: **for all** $v_i \in R_i, v_j \in R_{-i}$ **do**
5:    **if** $\psi(v_i, v_{-i}) > \alpha$ **then**
6:       define edge weight $w(v_i, v_j) = \frac{\delta_i(v_i)\psi(v_i, v_j)}{|N-1|}$;
7:    **else**
8:       define edge weight $w(v_i, v_j) = 0$;
9:    **end if**
10: **end for**
11: Iteration $t = 1$;
12: **while** each R_i is non-empty **do**
13:    $\mathbf{v}^*_t \leftarrow LBP(G)$; /* state set of image I_i is R_i */
14:    **for all** R_i **do**
15:       for all $v_i \in R_i$, if $v_i \in \mathbf{v}^*_t$ then remove v_i from R_i;
16:    **end for**
17:    $\mathbf{V}_C = \mathbf{V}_C \cup \mathbf{v}^*_t; t = t + 1$;
18:    reconstruct graph G with updated R_i as line 3 to line 10;
19: **end while**
20: **return** $\mathbf{V}_B, \mathbf{V}_C, \mathbf{V}_N = \{R_i|i = 1, ..., N\}$; /* $\mathbf{V}_N$: the remaining unlabeled strategies */

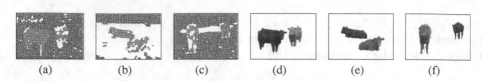

| (a) | (b) | (c) | (d) | (e) | (f) |

Fig. 4. The co-segmentation result of the proposed method. Figure 5(a)–(c) are the input images. (a)–(c) show the labeled results generated by the proposed cooperative game. The red parts are the common object labels, the blue parts are the background labels, and the white parts are the neutral labels. (d)–(f) show the segmentation results after the cooperative cut (Color figure online).

The common objects usually represented as several representative superpixels (see Fig. 2(d)). That is, we need to find more than one optimal strategy profiles $\mathbf{v}^*$ as the common-object-label. We summarize the complete label generation as Algorithm 1 which based on the greedy method and LBP. In algorithm 1, before assigning the common-object-label, the background-label is assigned to the representative superpixels which have very low saliency values. After assigning the common-object-label, the neutral-label is assigned to the remaining unlabeled representative superpixels. Notice that, once a representative superpixel v_i is labeled, all the superpixel represented by it will get the same label.

2.5   Cooperative Cut

For the input images, the proposed cooperative co-segmentation generate the corresponding labeled images such as Fig. 4(a)–(c). The remaining problem is to label the neutral-label regions as the common-object or the background, and thus yielding the final segmentation results such as Fig. 4(d)–(f). Given some labeled image regions, a cut-algorithm [16,19–21] is used to label the remaining unlabeled image regions. In practice, graph cuts [19–21] is known to shortcut elongated boundaries, especially in low contrast or shaded region. Thus, Jegelka et al. proposed the cooperative cut [16] to utilize edge cooperation to selectively reward global features of true boundaries in the image. It has ability to segment fine structured objects and objects with shading variation.

In our experiments, we use the cooperative cut [16] with the given common-object regions and background regions to label the neutral-label regions in the pixel-level. The parameter setting is the same as [16].

3   Experimental Results

We discuss the experimental results on several image sets for evaluating the performance of the proposed cooperative co-segmentation method. The test images are collected from various database such as CMU-Cornell iCoseg dataset [2], MSRC dataset [22], and ImageNet [23]. We present qualitative and quantitative results of our algorithm. The segmentation accuracy of a given image is measured by the intersection-over-union metric. The metric defined as $Acc_i = \frac{GT_i \cap S_i}{GT_i \cup S_i}$, where GT is the ground truth segment, S is the segment obtained by the co-segmentation algorithm.

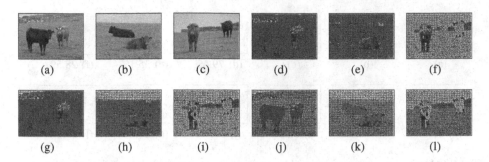

Fig. 5. Effect of the constrained utility function. (a)–(c) are the input images. (d)–(f) represent the labeled results of noncooperative behavior. (g)–(i) show the labeled results for cooperative players without considering the saliency maps. (j)–(l) show the labeled results with considering the saliency maps.

3.1 Cooperative Behavior

In the proposed cooperative co-segmentation, we designed the constrained utility function. The effects of the constrained utility function are shown in Fig. 5. Figure 5(a)–(c) are the input images. Figure 5(d)–(f) show the common-object-label results of noncooperative behavior. That is, the utility function only consider the heat gain and all edges have the same weight. We can find that each player just chooses the strategy to maximize his own heat gain. Figure 5(g)–(i) shows the common-object-label results of the constrained utility function without considering the saliency maps. Figure 5(j)–(l) shows the common-object-label results of the constrained utility function with considering the saliency maps.

3.2 Comparison

The parameter α and β, which represent the similarity and saliency threshold respectively, are the only two free parameters in our method. We usually set $\alpha = 0.5$, $\beta = 0.25$ in general condition, and $\alpha = 0.8$, $\beta = 0.5$ for high-variability images. Note that we use the default parameters to generate the results of [6] and [9]. Precisely, we use the sixth output image, i.e. the output of function $disp\_draw\_imgs\_clust\_cut$ of [9] for comparison.

Figures 6, 7, 8, and 9 illustrate some results obtained by the proposed method on a set of images in different conditions. (1). The images with multiple common objects. (2). The images with similar backgrounds. (3). The common objects for different scales. (4). The images with complex backgrounds.

We first evaluated the proposed method on multiple common objects. The result is shown in Fig. 6. In Fig. 7, these sets of images (iCoseg dataset) are particularly difficult to segment due to the high similarity on the image background. Thanks to the saliency map, our result performs much better than [6,9]. Figure 8 shows comparative results on MSRC dataset. Our method outperforms state-of-the-art co-segmentation methods [6,9]. When the objects among images are with different scales. We can observe that even if there is enormous size differences

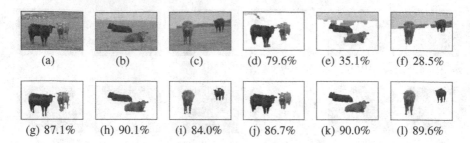

(a)   (b)   (c)   (d) 79.6%   (e) 35.1%   (f) 28.5%

(g) 87.1%   (h) 90.1%   (i) 84.0%   (j) 86.7%   (k) 90.0%   (l) 89.6%

Fig. 6. Multiple common objects. The percentage under each image denotes the segmentation accuracy. (a)–(c) are the input images. (d)–(f) show the co-segmentation of [6]. (g)–(i) show the co-segmentation of [9]. (j)–(l) show the proposed cooperative co-segmentation.

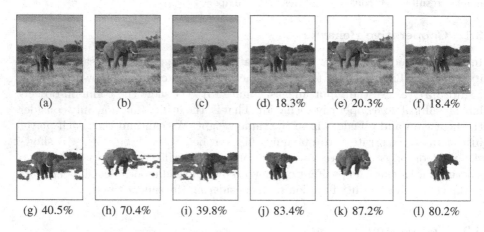

(a)   (b)   (c)   (d) 18.3%   (e) 20.3%   (f) 18.4%

(g) 40.5%   (h) 70.4%   (i) 39.8%   (j) 83.4%   (k) 87.2%   (l) 80.2%

Fig. 7. Images with similar backgrounds. The percentage under each image denotes the segmentation accuracy. (a)–(c) are the input images. (d)–(f) show the co-segmentation of [6]. (g)–(i) show the co-segmentation of [9]. (j)–(l) show the proposed cooperative co-segmentation.

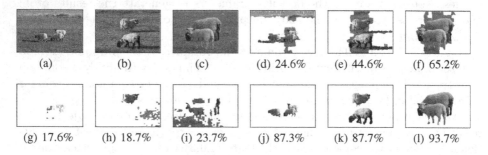

(a)   (b)   (c)   (d) 24.6%   (e) 44.6%   (f) 65.2%

(g) 17.6%   (h) 18.7%   (i) 23.7%   (j) 87.3%   (k) 87.7%   (l) 93.7%

Fig. 8. Different-scale common objects. The percentage under each image denotes the segmentation accuracy. (a)–(c) are the input images. (d)–(f) show the co-segmentation of [6]. (g)–(i) show the co-segmentation of [9]. (j)–(l) show the proposed cooperative co-segmentation.

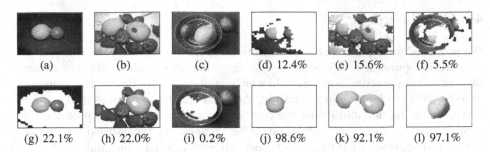

<table>

(a)   (b)   (c)   (d) 12.4%   (e) 15.6%   (f) 5.5%

(g) 22.1%   (h) 22.0%   (i) 0.2%   (j) 98.6%   (k) 92.1%   (l) 97.1%
</table>

Fig. 9. Common objects with complicated backgrounds. The percentage under each image denotes the segmentation accuracy. (a)–(c) are the input images. (d)–(f) show the co-segmentation of [6]. (g)–(i) show the co-segmentation of [9]. (j)–(l) show the proposed cooperative co-segmentation.

Table 1. Co-segmentation results on the iCoseg dataset

iCoseg dataset	Ours	Joulin [6]	Kim [9]
Elephants	83.6	19.0	50.2
Kite	75.0	29.2	47.1
Kite panda	85.0	37.9	46.1
Gymnastics1	90.9	47.0	41.5
Gymnastics2	83.9	39.2	41.6
Gymnastics3	86.4	51.8	59.0
Taj Mahal	76.0	30.4	28.4
Stonehenge	70.4	71.9	40.5
Liberty Statue	79.2	45.5	64.5
Skating	86.8	12.6	23.9
Livepool FC	78.2	40.7	36.5
Helicopter	79.6	55.1	6.2
Mean accuracy	81.3	40.0	40.5

among objects, the proposed method still achieve high accuracy up to 93.7 %. Another difficult problem of co-segmentation is shown in Fig. 9. There is only one common object (i.e. the yellow lemon) among images but backgrounds are complicated. As shown in the figure, both [6,9] cannot recognize the common object, lead to extremely low accuracy. On the contrary, our method produces the satisfactory results with more than 96 % averaged segmentation accuracy in these images. For more general comparisons, Table 1 shows the comparative results on the iCoseg dataset. Since the dataset contains images with similar background, our method can reach higher average accuracy than [6,9].

4 Conclusion

We proposed a cooperative co-segmentation algorithm by using the concepts of cooperative game, heat diffusion, and image saliency. Our method takes advantage of a cooperative game model, which enables us to detect the common objects unsupervisedly and accurately. We treat images as players in the cooperative game model, and define the constrained utility function to promote the cooperation on the label estimation. After generating the labeled image, we apply the cooperative cut to precisely segment each labeled image independently. Compared to other co-segmentation methods, our method can solve those co-segmentation problems for images with similar or complex background, or images with objects of different scales or numbers. Experimental results demonstrate that our method outperforms the state-of-the-art co-segmentation algorithms.

References

1. Rother, C., Minka, T.P., Blake, A., Kolmogorov, V.: Cosegmentation of image pairs by histogram matching - incorporating a global constraint into MRFs. In: CVPR, vol. 1, pp. 993–1000 (2006)
2. Batra, D., Kowdle, A., Parikh, D., Luo, J., Chen, T.: iCoseg: interactive co-segmentation with intelligent scribble guidance. In: CVPR, pp. 3169–3176 (2010)
3. Batra, D., Kowdle, A., Parikh, D., Luo, J., Chen, T.: Interactively co-segmentating topically related images with intelligent scribble guidance. Int. J. Comput. Vis. **93**, 273–292 (2011)
4. Chu, W.-S., Chen, C.-P., Chen, C.-S.: MOMI-cosegmentation: simultaneous segmentation of multiple objects among multiple images. In: Kimmel, R., Klette, R., Sugimoto, A. (eds.) ACCV 2010, Part I. LNCS, vol. 6492, pp. 355–368. Springer, Heidelberg (2011)
5. Hochbaum, D.S., Singh, V.: An efficient algorithm for co-segmentation. In: ICCV, pp. 269–276 (2009)
6. Joulin, A., Bach, F.R., Ponce, J.: Discriminative clustering for image co-segmentation. In: CVPR, pp. 1943–1950 (2010)
7. Mukherjee, L., Singh, V., Dyer, C.R.: Half-integrality based algorithms for coseg-mentation of images. In: CVPR, pp. 2028–2035 (2009)
8. Vicente, S., Kolmogorov, V., Rother, C.: Cosegmentation revisited: models and optimization. In: Daniilidis, K., Maragos, P., Paragios, N. (eds.) ECCV 2010, Part II. LNCS, vol. 6312, pp. 465–479. Springer, Heidelberg (2010)
9. Kim, G., Xing, E.P., Li, F.F., Kanade, T.: Distributed cosegmentation via sub-modular optimization on anisotropic diffusion. In: ICCV, pp. 169–176 (2011)
10. Zhang, J., Zheng, J., Cai, J.: A diffusion approach to seeded image segmentation. In: CVPR, pp. 2125–2132 (2010)
11. Bruhn, A., Weickert, J., Schnörr, C.: Lucas/kanade meets horn/schunck: combining local and global optic flow methods. Int. J. Comput. Vis. **61**, 211–231 (2005)
12. Harel, J., Koch, C., Perona, P.: Graph-based visual saliency. In: NIPS, pp. 545–552 (2006)
13. Osborne, M.: An Introduction to Game Theory. Oxford University Press, Oxford (2004)

14. Chen, Y., Wang, B., Lin, W.S., Wu, Y., Liu, K.J.R.: Cooperative peer-to-peer streaming: an evolutionary game-theoretic approach. IEEE Trans. Circ. Syst. Video Techn. **20**, 1346–1357 (2010)
15. Hsiao, P.C., Chang, L.W.: Image denoising with dominant sets by a coalitional game approach. IEEE Trans. Image Process. **22**, 724–738 (2013)
16. Jegelka, S., Bilmes, J.: Submodularity beyond submodular energies: coupling edges in graph cuts. In: CVPR, pp. 1897–1904 (2011)
17. Levinshtein, A., Stere, A., Kutulakos, K.N., Fleet, D.J., Dickinson, S.J., Siddiqi, K.: Turbopixels: fast superpixels using geometric flows. IEEE Trans. Pattern Anal. Mach. Intell. **31**, 2290–2297 (2009)
18. Murphy, K.P., Weiss, Y., Jordan, M.I.: Loopy belief propagation for approximate inference: an empirical study. In: UAI, pp. 467–475 (1999)
19. Rother, C., Kolmogorov, V., Blake, A.: "grabcut": interactive foreground extraction using iterated graph cuts. ACM Trans. Graph. **23**, 309–314 (2004)
20. Vicente, S., Kolmogorov, V., Rother, C.: Graph cut based image segmentation with connectivity priors. In: CVPR (2008)
21. Boykov, Y., Jolly, M.P.: Interactive graph cuts for optimal boundary and region segmentation of objects in n-d images. In: ICCV, pp. 105–112 (2001)
22. Winn, J.M., Criminisi, A., Minka, T.P.: Object categorization by learned universal visual dictionary. In: ICCV, pp. 1800–1807 (2005)
23. Deng, J., Dong, W., Socher, R., Li, L.J., Li, K., Li, F.F.: Imagenet: a large-scale hierarchical image database. In: CVPR, pp. 248–255 (2009)

A High Performance CRF Model
for Clothes Parsing

Edgar Simo-Serra[1]([✉]), Sanja Fidler[2], Francesc Moreno-Noguer[1],
and Raquel Urtasun[2]

[1] IRI (CSIC-UPC), Barcelona, Spain
esimo@iri.upc.edu
[2] University of Toronto, Toronto, Canada

Abstract. In this paper we tackle the problem of clothing parsing: Our
goal is to segment and classify different garments a person is wearing. We
frame the problem as the one of inference in a pose-aware Conditional
Random Field (CRF) which exploits appearance, figure/ground segmentation, shape and location priors for each garment as well as similarities
between segments, and symmetries between different human body parts.
We demonstrate the effectiveness of our approach on the Fashionista
dataset [1] and show that we can obtain a significant improvement over
the state-of-the-art.

1 Introduction

The impact of fashion and clothing is tremendous in our society. According to
the Forbes magazine [2], excluding auctions, US online retail sales are expected
to reach 262 billion dollars this year, 13 % higher than the total in 2012. The
situation is similar in Europe, with the expectation being that it will reach 128
billion euros. This is reflected in the growing interest in recognizing clothing
from images [3–10], as this can enable a wide variety of applications such as
trying on virtual garments in online shopping. Being able to automatically parse
clothing is also key in order to conduct large-scale sociological studies related to
family income or urban groups. For instance, several researches have attempted
to estimate sociological patterns from clothing inferred from images, predicting
for example occupation [11] or urban tribes [12].

In the context of fashion, Yamaguchi et al. [1], created *Fashionista*, a dataset
of images and clothing segmentation labels. Great performance was obtained
when the system was given information about which garment classes, but not
their location, are present for each test image. Unfortunately, the performance of
the state-of-the-art methods [1,8] is rather poor when this kind of information is
not provided at test time. This has been very recently partially addressed in [13]

Electronic supplementary material The online version of this chapter (doi:10.
1007/978-3-319-16811-1_5) contains supplementary material, which is available to
authorized users.

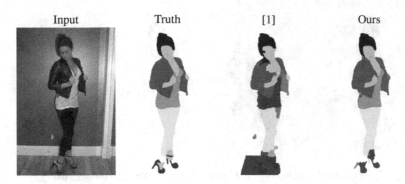

Fig. 1. Example of our result in a scenario where no a priori knowledge of which garments are worn is provided. We compare against state-of-the-art. Despite some mistakes, our result looks visually much more natural than the competing method.

by utilizing over 300,000 weakly labeled images, where the weak annotations are in the form of image-level tags. In this paper, we show an approach which outperforms the state-of-the-art significantly without requiring these additional annotations, by exploiting the specific domain of the task: clothing a person. An example of our result can be seen in Fig. 1.

The complexity of the task of human semantic segmentation comes from the inherent variability of pose and cloth appearances, the presence of self-occlusions as well as the potentially large number of classes. Consider for example Fig. 2: an autonomous system needs to distinguish between blazers and cardigans, stockings and tights, and heels, wedges and shoes, where the intra-class variability is fundamentally much larger than the inter-class variability. This fine-grained categorization is difficult to resolve even for humans who are not familiar with the fashion industry. The problem is further aggravated by the power law distribution of classes, as certain categories have very few examples. Thus, extra-care has to be taken into account to not over-predict the classes that are very likely to appear in each image, e.g., skin, hair.

In this paper we address some of these challenges and formulate the problem as the one of inference in a Conditional Random Field (CRF), which takes into account the complex dependencies between clothing and human pose. Specifically, we develop a rich set of potentials which encode the person's global appearance and shape to perform figure/ground segmentation, shape and location likelihoods for each garment, which we call *clothelets*, and long-range similarity between segments to encourage, for example, T-Shirt pixels on the body to agree with the T-shirt pixels on the person's arm. We further exploit the fact the people are symmetric and dress as such as well by introducing symmetry-based potentials between different limbs. We also use a variety of different local features encoding cloth appearance as well as local shape of the person's parts. We demonstrate the effectiveness of our approach of the Fashionista dataset [1] and show that our approach significantly outperforms the existing state-of-the-art.

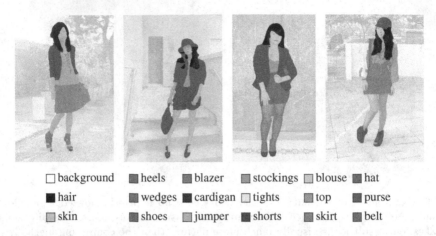

☐ background   ■ heels   ■ blazer   ■ stockings   ☐ blouse   ■ hat

■ hair   ■ wedges   ■ cardigan   ☐ tights   ☐ top   ■ purse

☐ skin   ■ shoes   ☐ jumper   ■ shorts   ☐ skirt   ■ belt

Fig. 2. Examples of fine-grained annotations in Fashionista [1]. Many of the different classes are very difficult to distinguish even for humans. Observe the subtle differences between some classes such as footwear (heels, wedges, and shoes), blazer and cardigan, or stockings and tights. We also point out that this dataset has been annotated via super-pixels, and thus the ground truth contains errors when superpixels do not align with the actual garments. We have not modified the ground truth segmentation in any way (Color figure online).

2   Related Work

There has been a growing interest in recognizing outfits and clothing from still images. One of the first approaches on the subject was Chen et al. [14], which manually built a composite clothing model, that was then matched to input images. This has led to more recent applications for learning semantic clothing attributes [5], which are in turn used for describing and recognizing the identity of individuals [4,6], their style [3], and performing sociological studies such as predicting the occupation [11] or urban tribes [12]. Other tasks like outfit recommendations [15] have also been investigated. However, in general, these approaches do not perform accurate segmentation of clothing, which is the goal of our approach. Instead, they rely on more coarse features such as bounding boxes and focus on producing generic outputs based on the presence/absence of a specific type of outfit. It is likely that the performance of such systems would improve if accurate clothing segmentation would be possible.

Recent advances in 2D pose estimation [16,17] have enabled a more advanced segmentation of humans [18]. However, most approaches have focused on figure/ground labeling [19,20]. Additionally, pose information has been used as a feature in clothing related tasks such as finding similar worn outfits in the context of online shopping [9].

Segmentation and classification of garments has been addressed in the restrictive case in which the labels are known beforehand [1]. The original paper tackled this problem in the context of fashion photographs which depicted one person typically in an upright pose. This scenario also been extended to the case where more than one individual can be present in the image [8]. In order to perform the segmentation, conditional random fields are used with potentials linking clothing and pose. However, the performance of these approaches drops significantly when no information about the outfit is known a priori (i.e., no tags are provided at test time). The paper doll approach [13] uses over 300,000 weakly labeled training images and a small set of fully labeled examples in order to enrich the model of [1] with a prior over image labels. As we will show in the experimental evaluation, our method can handle this scenario without having to resort to additional training images. Furthermore, it consistently outperforms [1,13].

CRFs have been very successful in semantic segmentation tasks. Most approaches combine detection and segmentation by using detectors as additional image evidence [21,22]. Co-occurrence potentials have been employed to enforce consistency among region labels [23]. Part-based detectors have also been aligned to image contours to aid in object segmentation [24]. All these strategies have been applied to generic segmentation problems, where one is interested in segmenting classes such as car, sky or trees. Pixel-wise labeling of clothing is, however, a much more concrete task, where strong domain specific information, such as 2D body pose, can be used to reduce ambiguities.

3   Clothing a Person

We pose the clothing parsing problem as one of inference in a Conditional Random Field (CRF), which takes into account complex dependencies that exist between garments and human pose. We obtain pose by employing a 2D articulated model by Yang et al. [17] which predicts the main keypoints such as head, shoulders, knees, etc. As [1], we will exploit these keypoints to bias the clothing labeling in a plausible way (e.g., a hat is typically on the head and not the feet). To manage the complexity of the segmentation problem we represent each input image with a small number of superpixels [25]. Our CRF contains a variable encoding the garment class (including background) for each superpixel. We also add limb variables which encode the garment associated with a limb in the human body and correspond to edges in the 2D articulated model. We use the limb variables to propagate information while being computationally efficient.

Our CRF contains a rich set of potentials which exploit the domain of the task. We use the person's global appearance and shape to perform figure/ground segmentation in order to narrow down the scope of cloth labeling. We further use shape and location likelihoods for each garment, which we call *clothelets*. We exploit the fact that people are symmetric and typically dress as such by forming long-range consistency potentials between detected symmetric keypoints of the human pose. We finally also use a variety of different features that encode appearance as well as local shape of superpixels.

3.1   Pose-Aware Model

Given an input image represented with superpixels, our goal is to assign a clothing label (or background) to each of them. More formally, let $y_i \in \{1, \cdots, C\}$ be

Table 1. Overview of the different types of potentials used in the proposed CRF model.

Type	Name	Description
unary	Simple features ($\phi_{i,j}^{simple}(y_i)$)	Assortment of simple features [1]
unary	Object mask ($\phi_{i,j}^{obj}(y_i)$)	Figure/ground segmentation ask
unary	Clothelets ($\phi_{i,j}^{cloth}(y_i)$)	Pose-conditioned garment likelihood masks
unary	Ranking ($\phi_{i,j}^{o2p}(y_i)$)	Rich set of region ranking features
unary	Bias ($\phi_j^{bias}(y_i)$ and $\phi_{p,j}^{bias}(l_p)$)	Class biases
pairwise	Similarity ($\phi_{m,n}^{simil}(y_m, y_n)$)	Similarity between superpixels
pairwise	Compatibility ($\phi_{i,p}^{comp}(y_i, l_p)$)	Edges between limb segments and superpixels

the class associated with the i-th superpixel, and let l_p be the p-th limb segment defined by the edges in the articulated body model. Each limb l_p is assumed to belong to one class, $l_p \in \{1, \cdots, C\}$. To encode body symmetries in an efficient manner, we share limb variables between the left and right part of the human body, e.g., the left and the right leg share the same limb variables. We propose several domain inspired potentials, the overview of which is presented in Table 1. We emphasize that the weights associated with each potential in our CRF will be learned using structure prediction. We now explain each potential in more detail.

Simple Features: Following [1], we concatenate a diverse set of simple local features and train a logistic regression classifier for each class. In particular, we use color features, normalized histograms of RGB and CIE L*a*b* color; texture features, Gabor filter responses; and location features: both normalized 2D image coordinates and pose-relative coordinates. The output of the logistic functions are then used as unary features in the CRF. This results in a unary potential with as many dimensions as classes:

$$\phi_{i,j}^{simple}(y_i) = \begin{cases} \sigma_j^{simple}(f_i), & \text{if } y_i = j \\ 0, & \text{otherwise} \end{cases} \tag{1}$$

where $\sigma_j^{simple}(f_i)$ is the score of the classifier for class j, and f_i is the concatenation of all the features for superpixel i. Notice we have used C different unary potentials, one for each class. By doing this, we allow the weights of a variety of potentials and classes be jointly learned within the model.

Figure/Ground Segmentation: To facilitate clothing parsing we additionally compute how likely each superpixel belongs to a person. We do this by computing a set of bottom-up region proposals using the CPMC approach [26]. We take top K (we set $K = 100$) regions per image and use O2P [27] to score each region into figure/ground (person-vs-background). Since we know that there is a person in each image, we take at least the top scoring segment per image, no matter its score. For images with multiple high scoring segments, we take the union of

Image   Person Mask   Limbs   Image   Person Mask   Limbs

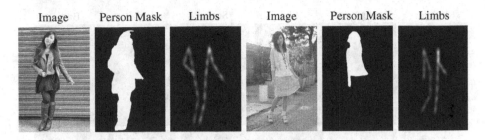

Fig. 3. Visualization of CPMC object segments [26] and limbs (obtained via [17]). Note that CPMC typically generates high quality results, e.g. the one in the left image, but can also completely miss large parts of the body as shown in the image on the right.

all segments with scores higher than a learned threshold [27]. We define a unary potential to encourage the superpixels that lie inside the foreground mask to take any of the clothing labels (and not background):

$$\phi_{i,j}^{obj}(y_i) = \begin{cases} \sigma^{cpmc} \cdot |\neg M_{fg} \cap S_i|/|S_i|, & \text{if } y_i = 1 \\ \sigma^{cpmc} \cdot |M_{fg} \cap S_i|/|S_i|, & \text{otherwise} \end{cases} \quad (2)$$

where $y_i = 1$ encodes the background class, o^{cpmc} is the score of the foreground region, S_i, M_{fg} are binary masks defining the superpixel and foreground, respectively, and $\neg M_{fg}$ is a mask of all pixels not in foreground. Figure 3 shows examples of masks obtained by [27]. Note that while in some cases it produces very accurate results, in others, it performs poorly. These inaccurate masks are compensated by other potentials.

Clothelets: Our next potential exploits the statistical dependency between the location on the human body and garment type. Its goal is to make use of the fact that e.g. jeans typically cover the legs and not the head. We compute a likelihood of each garment appearing in a particular relative location of the human pose. In particular, for each training example we take a region around the location of each joint (and limb), the size of which corresponds to the size of the joint part template encoded in [17]. We average the GT segmentation masks for each class across the training examples. In order to capture garment classes that stray away from the pose, we use boxes that are larger than the part templates in [17]. At test time, the masks for each class are overlaid relative to the inferred pose and normalized by the number of non-zero elements. Areas with no information are assigned to the background class. The potential is then defined as

$$\phi_{i,j}^{cloth}(y_i) = \begin{cases} (\text{clothelet}_i^j \cdot S_i)/|S_i|, & \text{if } y_i = j \\ 0, & \text{otherwise} \end{cases} \quad (3)$$

where clothelet_i^j is the clothelet for the j-th class, and $\cdot$ is the dot product. Figure 4 depicts clothelets for a few sample classes.

Shape Features: This potential uses a set of rich features that exploit both the shape and local appearance of garments. In particular, we use eSIFT and

Image	Background	Skin	Socks	Jacket	Bag

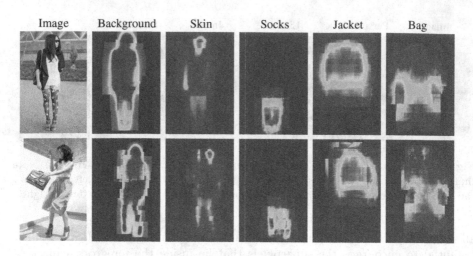

Fig. 4. Visualization of different clothelets for two different input images.

eMSIFT proposed by [27] for region description. Given a region, both descriptors extract SIFT inside the region and enrich it with the relative location and scale within the region. Second-order pooling is used to define the final region descriptor. eSIFT and eMSIFT differ slightly in how the descriptors are pooled, eSIFT pools over both the region and background of the region, while eMSIFT pools over the region alone. While [27] defines the features over full object proposals, here we compute them over each superpixel. As such, they capture more local shape of the part/limb and local appearance of the garment. We train a logistic classifier for each type of feature and class and use the output as our potential:

$$\phi_{i,j}^{o2p}(y_i) = \begin{cases} \sigma_j^{o2p}(r_i), & \text{if } y_i = j \\ 0, & \text{otherwise} \end{cases} \quad (4)$$

with $\sigma_j^{o2p}(r_i)$ the classifier score for class j, and r_i the feature vector for superpixel i.

Bias: We use a simple bias for the background to encode the fact that it is the class that appears more frequently. Learning a weight for this bias is equivalent to learning a threshold for the foreground, however within the full model. Thus:

$$\phi^{bias}(y_i) = \begin{cases} 1, & \text{if } y_i = 1 \\ 0, & \text{otherwise} \end{cases} \quad (5)$$

Similarity: In CRFs, neighboring superpixels are typically connected via a (contrast-sensitive) Potts model encouraging smoothness of the labels. For clothing parsing, we want these connections to act on a longer range. That is, a jacket is typically split in multiple disconnected segments due to a T-shirt, tie, and/or a bag. Our goal is to encourage superpixels that are similar in appearance to agree on the label, even though they may not be neighbors in the image.

We follow [28] and use size similarity, fit similarity that measures how well two superpixels fit each other; and color and texture similarity, with the total of 12 similarity features between each pair of superpixels. We then train a logistic regression to predict if two superpixels should have the same label or not. In order to avoid setting connections on the background, we only connect superpixels that overlap with the bounding box of the 2D pose detection. Note that connecting all pairs of similar superpixels would slow down inference considerably. To alleviate this problem, we compute the minimum spanning tree using the similarity matrix and use the top 10 edges to connect 10 pairs of superpixels in each image. We form a pairwise potential between each connected pair:

$$\phi_{m,n}^{simil}(y_m, y_n) = \begin{cases} \sigma_{m,n}^{simil}, & \text{if } y_m = y_n \\ 0, & \text{otherwise} \end{cases} \tag{6}$$

where $\sigma_{m,n}^{simil}$ is the output of the similarity classifier.

Limb Segment Bias: We use a per-class bias on each limb segment to capture a location specific bias, e.g., hat only appears in the head:

$$\phi_{p,j}^{bias}(l_p) = \begin{cases} 1, & \text{if } l_p = j \\ 0, & \text{otherwise} \end{cases} \tag{7}$$

These potentials allow us to compute which classes are more frequent in each limb.

Compatibility Segmentation-Limbs: We define potentials connecting limb segments with nearby superpixels encouraging them to agree in their labels. Towards this goal, we first define a Gaussian mask centered between two joints. More formally, for two consecutive joints with coordinates $J_a = (u_a, v_a)$ and $J_b = (u_b, v_b)$, we define the mask based on the following Normal distribution:

$$M(J_a, J_b) = \mathcal{N}\left(\frac{J_a + J_b}{2}, \quad R\begin{pmatrix} q_1\|J_a - J_b\| & 0 \\ 0 & q_2 \end{pmatrix} R^{\mathrm{T}}\right) \tag{8}$$

where R is a 2D rotation matrix with an angle $\arctan(\frac{u_a - u_b}{v_a - v_b})$, and q_1 and q_2 are two hyperparameters controlling the spread of the mask longitudinally and transversely, respectively. The strength of the connection is based on the overlap between the superpixels and the Gaussian mask:

$$\phi_{i,p}^{comp}(y_i, l_p) = \begin{cases} M(J_a, J_b) \cdot S_i, & \text{if } y_i \neq 1 \text{ and } y_i = k_p \\ 0, & \text{otherwise} \end{cases} \tag{9}$$

For computational efficiency, edges with connection strengths below a threshold are not set in the model. Some examples of the limb segment masks are shown in Fig. 3. We can see the masks fit the body tightly to avoid overlapping with background superpixels.

Full Model: We define the energy of the full model to be the sum of three types of energies encoding unary and pairwise potentials that depend on the superpixel labeling, as well as an energy term linking the limb segments and the superpixels:

$$E(\mathbf{y}, \mathbf{l}) = E_{unary}(\mathbf{y}) + E_{similarity}(\mathbf{y}) + E_{limbs}(\mathbf{y}, \mathbf{l}) \tag{10}$$

This energy is maximized during inference. The unary terms are formed by the concatenation of appearance features, figure/ground segmentation, clothelets, shape features and background bias for a total of $K = (1 + 5C)$ features

$$E_{unary}(\mathbf{y}) = \sum_{i=1}^{N} \sum_{j=1}^{K} \mathbf{w}_j^{unaries} \phi_{i,j}^{unary}(y_i) \tag{11}$$

where N is the number of superpixels. The pairwise features encode the similarity between different pairs of superpixels as we describe above

$$E_{similarity}(\mathbf{y}) = \sum_{(m,n) \in \text{pairs}} w^{simil} \phi_{m,n}^{simil}(y_m, y_n) \tag{12}$$

The limb-superpixel compatibility term is defined as

$$E_{limbs}(\mathbf{y}, \mathbf{l}) = \sum_{p=1}^{M} \left(\sum_{j=1}^{C} \left(w_j^{bias} \phi_{p,j}^{bias}(l_p) + \sum_{i=1}^{N} w_{j,p}^{comp} \phi^{comp}(y_i, l_p) \right) \right) \tag{13}$$

for a total of $(M + C)$ features, with M the number of limb segments.

3.2 Learning and Inference

Our model is a multi-label CRF which contains cycles and thus inference is NP-hard. We use a message passing algorithm, distributed convex belief propagation [29] to perform inference. It belongs to the set of LP-relaxation approaches, and has convergence guarantees. This is not the case in other message passing algorithms such as loopy-BP.

To learn the weights, we use the primal-dual method of [30] (we use the implementation of [31]), shown to be more efficient than other structure prediction learning algorithms. As loss-function, we use the semantic similarity between the different classes in order to penalize mistakes between unrelated classes more than similar ones. We do this via Wordnet [32], which is a large lexical database in which sets of cognitive synonyms (synsets) are interlinked by means of semantic and lexical relationships. We can unambiguously identify each of the classes with a single synset, and then proceed to calculate similarity scores between these synsets that represent the semantic similarity between the classes, in order to penalize mistakes with dissimilar classes more.

In particular, we choose the corpus-independent Leacock-Chodorow Similarity score. This score takes into account the shortest path length p between both synsets and the maximum depth of the taxonomy d at which they occur. It is defined as the relationship $-\log(p/2d)$. A visualization of the dissimilarity

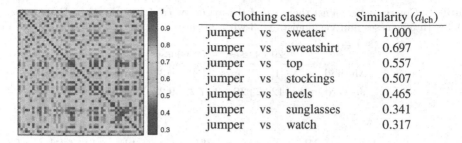

Clothing classes			Similarity (d_{lch})
jumper	vs	sweater	1.000
jumper	vs	sweatshirt	0.697
jumper	vs	top	0.557
jumper	vs	stockings	0.507
jumper	vs	heels	0.465
jumper	vs	sunglasses	0.341
jumper	vs	watch	0.317

Fig. 5. Inverse of the Leacock-Chodorow Similarity between the classes in the Fashionista dataset. We display the similarity matrix between all the classes on the left. Some individual values of the similarity between the jumper class and several other classes can be seen on the right.

between all the classes in the dataset can be seen in Fig. 5. We therefore define the loss-function as:

$$\Delta^y(y_i, y_i^*) = \begin{cases} 0, & \text{if } y_i = y_i^* \\ d_{\text{lch}}(y_i, y_i^*), & \text{otherwise} \end{cases} \qquad (14)$$

with $d_{\text{lch}}(\cdot, \cdot)$ being the inverse Leacock-Chodorow Similarity score between both classes. For the limb segments we use a 0-1 loss:

$$\Delta^k(k_i, k_i^*) = \begin{cases} 0, & \text{if } k_i = k_i^* \\ 1, & \text{otherwise} \end{cases} \qquad (15)$$

4 Experimental Evaluation

We evaluate our approach on both a the Fashionista dataset v0.3 [1], and the setting of [13] with the Fashionista dataset v0.2. Both datasets are taken from http://www.chictopia.com in which a single person appears wearing a diverse set of garments. The dataset provides both annotated superpixels as well as 2D pose annotations. A set of evaluation metrics and the full source code of approaches [1,13] are provided. Version 0.2 has 685 images and v0.3 has 700 images. Note that v0.3 is not a superset of v0.2.

We have modified the Fashionista v0.3 dataset in two ways. First we have compressed the original 54 classes into 29. This is due to the fact that many classes that appear have very few occurrences. In fact, in the original dataset, 13 classes have 10 or fewer examples and 6 classes have 3 or fewer instances. This means that when performing a random split of the samples into training and test subsets, there is a high probability that some classes will only appear in one of the subsets. We therefore compress the classes by considering both semantic similarity and the number of instances. The final classes in this setting can be seen in the supplemental material of this paper.

For evaluation on Fashionista v0.3 we consider a random 50-50 train-test split. As previously stated, we do not have information about which classes

Table 2. Comparison against the state-of-the-art on two different datasets: Fashionista v0.2 with 56 classes and Fashionista v0.3 with 29 classes.

	29 Classes		56 Classes		
Method	[1]	Ours	[1]	[13]	Ours
Jaccard index	12.32	**20.52**	7.22	9.22	**12.28**

are present in the scene. We employ the publicly available code of [1] as the baseline. We evaluate on Fashionista v0.2 according to the methodology in [13]. This consists of a split with 456 images for training and 229 images for testing. Note that [13] uses 339,797 additional weakly labeled images from the Paper doll dataset for training, which we do not use.

Following PASCAL VOC, we report the average class intersection over union (Jaccard index). This metric is the most similar to human perception as it considers all true positives, true negatives and false positives. It is nowadays a standard measure to evaluate segmentation and detection [33–35].

Comparison to State-of-the-Art: We compare our approach against [1,13]. The approach of [1] uses a CRF with very simple features. We adapt the code to run in the setting in which the labels that appear in the image are not known a priori. Note also that [13] uses a look-up approach on a separate dataset to parse the query images. The results of the comparison can be seen in Table 2. Note that our approach consistently outperforms both competing methods on both datasets, even though [13] uses 339,797 additional images for training. We roughly obtain a 60 % relative improvement on Jaccard index metric with respect to [1] and a 30 % improvement over [13]. The full confusion matrix of our method can be seen in Fig. 6. We can identify several classes that have large appearance variation and similar positions that get easily confused, such as Footwear with Shoes and Jeans with Pants.

Foreground Segmentation: We also evaluate person-background segmentation results. Note that the binary segmentation in our model is obtained by putting all foreground garment classes to the person class. In Table 3, we show results for both pixel accuracy considering all the different classes, and the two class case of foreground/background segmentation accuracy. We see that the best results are obtained by the approaches reasoning jointly about the person and clothing. Our approach outperforms the baseline CPMC [27] by 12 %, and achieves a 4 % over [1] and 2 % over [13].

Table 3. Evaluation on foreground segmentation task on the Fashionista v0.2 dataset.

Method	CPMC [27]	[1]	Clothelets	[13]	Ours
Pixel Accuracy	-	77.98	77.09	84.68	**84.88**
Person/Bck. Accuracy	85.39	93.79	94.77	95.79	**97.37**

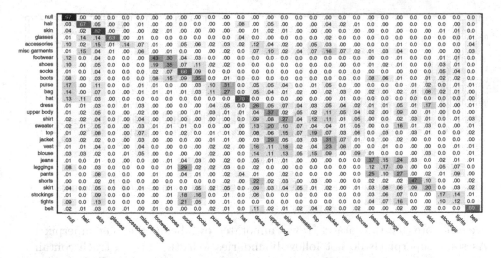

Fig. 6. Confusion matrix for our approach on the Fashionista v0.3 dataset.

Pose Influence: We next investigate the importance of having an accurate pose estimate. Towards this goal, we analyze three different scenarios. In the first one, the pose is estimated by [17]. The second case uses the ground-truth pose, while the last one does not use pose information at all. As shown in Table 4, the poses in this dataset are not very complex as performance does not increase greatly when using ground truth instead of estimated pose. However, without pose information, performance drops 20 %. This shows that our model is truly pose-aware. A breakdown of the effect of pose on all the classes is shown in Fig. 7. Some classes like hat, belt or boots benefit greatly from pose information while others like shorts, tights or skin do not really change.

Oracle Performance: Unlike [1], we do not use the fine level superpixels, but instead use coarser superpixels to speed up learning and inference. Table 5 shows that using coarser superpixels lowers the maximum achievable performance. However, by having larger areas, the local features become more discriminative.

Table 4. Influence of pose. We compare against the state-of-the-art in three different scenarios: estimated 2D pose, ground truth 2D pose and no pose information at all.

Method		29 Classes	56 Classes
[1]	Estimated	12.32	7.22
	GT Pose	12.39	7.41
	No Pose	10.54	5.22
Ours	Estimated	20.52	12.28
	GT Pose	21.01	12.46
	No Pose	16.56	9.64

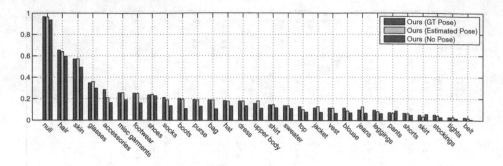

Fig. 7. Per class results for our model using Jaccard index metric on Fashionista v0.3.

We also note that the dataset [1] was annotated by labeling the finer superpixels. As some superpixels do not follow boundaries well, the ground truth contains a large number of errors. We did not correct those, and stuck with the original annotations.

Table 5. Oracle performance for different of superpixels for the Fashionista v0.3 dataset.

Threshold	0.16	0.10	0.05
Mean superpixels/image	50	120	290
Jaccard index	69.44	83.07	100

Importance of the Features: We also evaluate the influence of every potential in our model in Table 6. The eSIFT features obtain the best results under the Jaccard index metric. The high performance of eSIFT can be explained by the fact that it also takes into account the super pixel's background, thus capturing local context of garments. This feature alone surpasses the simple features from [1] despite that it does not use pose information. By combining all the features we are able to improve the results greatly. We show some qualitative examples of the different feature activations in Fig. 8. We also evaluate the model in a leave-one-out fashion. That is, for each unary we evaluate the rest of the unaries in the model without it. Results are shown in Table 7.

Qualitative Results: We show qualitative results for both our approach and the current state-of-the-art in Fig. 9. We can see a visible improvement over [1],

Table 6. Different results using only unary potentials in our model.

Method	Simple features [1]	Clothelets	eSIFT [27]	eMSIFT [27]
29 Classes	13.80	8.91	16.65	13.65
56 Classes	7.93	3.02	9.29	7.80

Input	Truth	Person Mask [27]	eSIFT	Similarity	Features [1]	Full Model

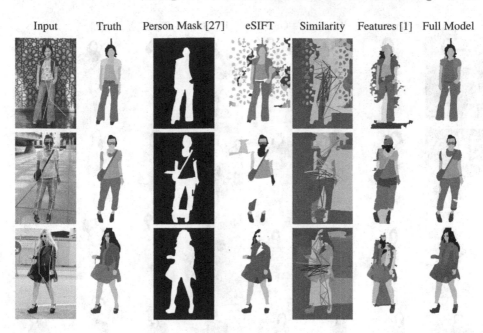

Fig. 8. We show various feature activations for example images. For similarity we display the connections between the superpixels. While both the features from [1] and eSIFT provide decent segmentation results, they have poorly defined boundaries. These are corrected via person masks [27] and clothelets. Further corrections are obtained by pairwise potentials such as symmetry and similarity. These results highlight the importance of combining complementary features. For class colors we refer to Fig. 9 (Color figure online).

especially on person/bckgr classification due to the strength of the proposed clothelets and person masks which in combination give strong cues on person segmentation. There are also several failure cases of our algorithm. One

Table 7. Importance of the different potentials in our model in the 56 class setting.

Method	Jaccard index
Full Model	12.28
No similarity ($\phi_{m,n}^{simil}(y_m, y_n)$)	11.64
No limb segments ($\phi_{i,p}^{comp}(y_i, l_p)$)	12.24
No simple features ($\phi_{i,j}^{simple}(y_i)$)	10.07
No clothelets ($\phi_{i,j}^{cloth}(y_i)$)	11.94
No object mask ($\phi_{i,j}^{obj}(y_i)$)	10.02
No eSIFT ($\phi_{i,j}^{o2p(eSIFT)}(y_i)$)	10.70
No eMSIFT ($\phi_{i,j}^{o2p(eMSIFT)}(y_i)$)	12.25

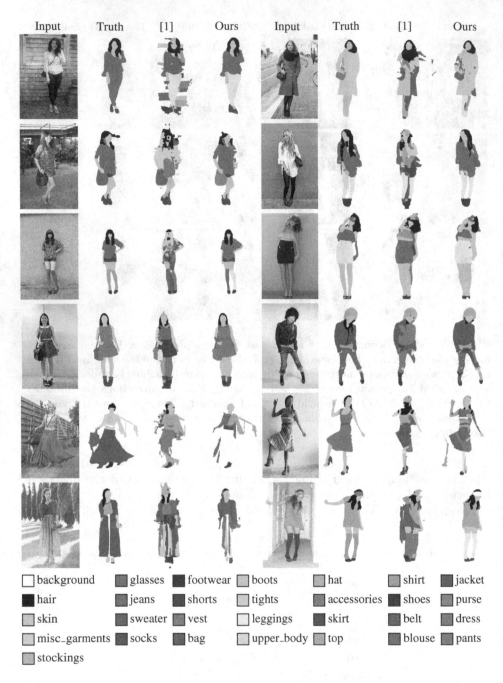

Fig. 9. Results on Fashionista v0.2 with 29 classes, comparing our approach with the state-of-the-art. In the top four rows we show good results obtained by our model. In the bottom two rows we show failure cases that are in general caused by 2D pose estimation failure, superpixel failures or chain failures of too many potentials (Color figure online).

of the main failure cases is a breakdown of the superpixels caused by clothing texture. An excess of texture leads to an oversegmentation where the individual superpixels are no longer discriminative enough to individually identify (Fig. 9-bottom-left), while too much similarity with the background leads to very large superpixels that mix foreground and background. Additionally it can be seen that failures in pose detection can lead to missed limbs (Fig. 9-bottom-right).

Computation Time: Our full model takes several hours to train and roughly 20 min to evaluate on the full test set (excluding feature computation), on a single machine. On the same machine [1] takes more than twice the time for inference. Additionally, [1] uses grid-search for training, which does not scale to a large amount of weights, that as we have shown, are able to provide an increase in performance. Even with only 2 weights, [1] is several times slower to train than our model. Furthermore, [13] reports a training time of several days in a distributed environment.

5   Conclusions

We have tackled the challenging problem of clothing parsing. We have shown that our approach is able to obtain a large improvement over the state-of-the-art in the challenging Fashionista dataset by exploiting appearance, figure/ground segmentation, shape and location priors for each garment as well as similarity between segments and symmetries between different human body parts. Despite these promising results, we believe much can still be done to improve. For example, one of the most occurring mistakes are missing glasses or other small garments. We believe a multi-resolution approach is needed to handle the diversity of garment classes. Additionally, we believe that using 3D pose instead of 2D, e.g [36], would be beneficial to handle self-occlusions better.

Acknowledgements. This work has been partially funded by Spanish Ministry of Economy and Competitiveness under projects PAU+ DPI2011-27510 and ERA-Net Chistera project ViSen PCIN-2013-047.

References

1. Yamaguchi, K., Kiapour, M.H., Ortiz, L.E., Berg, T.L.: Parsing clothing in fashion photographs. In: CVPR. (2012)
2. Forbes Magazine: US online retail sales to reach $370B By 2017; €191B in Europe (2013). http://www.forbes.com. Accessed 14 March 2013
3. Bossard, L., Dantone, M., Leistner, C., Wengert, C., Quack, T., Gool, L.V.: Apparel classifcation with style. In: ACCV (2012)
4. Bourdev, L., Maji, S., Malik, J.: Describing people: a poselet-based approach to attribute classification. In: ICCV (2011)
5. Chen, H., Gallagher, A., Girod, B.: Describing clothing by semantic attributes. In: Fitzgibbon, A., Lazebnik, S., Perona, P., Sato, Y., Schmid, C. (eds.) ECCV 2012, Part III. LNCS, vol. 7574, pp. 609–623. Springer, Heidelberg (2012)

6. Gallagher, A.C., Chen, T.: Clothing cosegmentation for recognizing people. In: CVPR (2008)

7. Hasan, B., Hogg, D.: Segmentation using deformable spatial priors with application to clothing. In: BMVC (2010)

8. Jammalamadaka, N., Minocha, A., Singh, D., Jawahar, C.: Parsing clothes in unrestricted images. In: BMVC (2013)

9. Liu, S., Song, Z., Liu, G., Xu, C., Lu, H., Yan, S.: Street-toshop: Cross-scenario clothing retrieval via parts alignment and auxiliary set. In: CVPR (2012)

10. Wang, N., Ai, H.: Who blocks who: simultaneous clothing segmentation for grouping images. In: ICCV (2011)

11. Song, Z., Wang, M., s. Hua, X., Yan, S.: Predicting occupation via human clothing and contexts. In: ICCV (2011)

12. Murillo, A.C., Kwak, I.S., Bourdev, L., Kriegman, D., Belongie, S.: Urban tribes: analyzing group photos from a social perspective. In: CVPR Workshops (2012)

13. Yamaguchi, K., Kiapour, M.H., Berg, T.L.: Paper doll parsing: retrieving similar styles to parse clothing items. In: ICCV (2013)

14. Chen, H., Xu, Z.J., Liu, Z.Q., Zhu, S.C.: Composite templates for cloth modeling and sketching. In: CVPR (2006)

15. Liu, S., Feng, J., Song, Z., Zhang, T., Lu, H., Changsheng, X., Yan, S.: Hi, magic closet, tell me what to wear! In: Proceedings of the 20th ACM International Conference on Multimedia (2012)

16. Bourdev, L., Malik, J.: Poselets: body part detectors trained using 3d human pose annotations. In: ICCV (2009)

17. Yang, Y., Ramanan, D.: Articulated pose estimation using flexible mixtures of parts. In: CVPR (2011)

18. Dong, J., Chen, Q., Xia, W., Huang, Z., Yan, S.: A deformable mixture parsing model with parselets. In: ICCV (2013)

19. Ladicky, L., Torr, P.H.S., Zisserman, A.: Human pose estimation using a joint pixel-wise and part-wise formulation. In: CVPR (2013)

20. Wang, H., Koller, D.: Multi-level inference by relaxed dual decomposition for human pose segmentation. In: CVPR (2011)

21. Yao, Y., Fidler, S., Urtasun, R.: Describing the scene as a whole: Joint object detection, scene classification and semantic segmentation. In: CVPR (2012)

22. Fidler, S., Sharma, A., Urtasun, R.: A sentence is worth a thousand pixels. In: CVPR (2013)

23. Ladicky, L., Russell, C., Kohli, P., Torr, P.H.S.: Graph cut based inference with co-occurrence statistics. In: Daniilidis, K., Maragos, P., Paragios, N. (eds.) ECCV 2010, Part V. LNCS, vol. 6315, pp. 239–253. Springer, Heidelberg (2010)

24. Brox, T., Bourdev, L., Maji, S., Malik, J.: Object segmentation by alignment of poselet activations to image contours. In: CVPR (2011)

25. Arbelaez, P., Maire, M., Fowlkes, C., Malik, J.: Contour detection and hierarchical image segmentation. In: PAMI (2011)

26. Carreira, J., Sminchisescu, C.: CPMC: automatic object segmentation using constrained parametric min-cuts. TPAMI 34, 1312–1328 (2012)

27. Carreira, J., Caseiro, R., Batista, J., Sminchisescu, C.: Semantic segmentation with second-order pooling. In: Fitzgibbon, A., Lazebnik, S., Perona, P., Sato, Y., Schmid, C. (eds.) ECCV 2012, Part VII. LNCS, vol. 7578, pp. 430–443. Springer, Heidelberg (2012)

28. Uijlings, J.R.R., van de Sande, K.E.A., Gevers, T., Smeulders, A.W.M.: Selective search for object recognition. IJCV 104, 154–171 (2013)

29. Schwing, A., Hazan, T., Pollefeys, M., Urtasun, R.: Distributed message passing for large scale graphical models. In: CVPR (2011)
30. Hazan, T., Urtasun, R.: A primal-dual message-passing algorithm for approximated large scale structured prediction. In: NIPS (2010)
31. Schwing, A.G., Hazan, T., Pollefeys, M., Urtasun, R.: Efficient structured prediction with latent variables for general graphical models. In: ICML (2012)
32. Miller, G.A.: Wordnet: a lexical database for english. Commun. ACM **38**, 39–41 (1995)
33. Everingham, M., Van Gool, L., Williams, C.K.I., Winn, J., Zisserman, A.: The pascal visual object classes (voc) challenge. Int. J. Comput. Vis. **88**, 303–338 (2010)
34. Geiger, A., Lenz, P., Stiller, C., Urtasun, R.: Vision meets robotics: the kitti dataset. Int. J. Robot. Res. (IJRR) **32**, 1231–1237 (2013)
35. Deng, J., Dong, W., Socher, R., jia Li, L., Li, K., Fei-fei, L.: Imagenet: a large-scale hierarchical image database. In: CVPR (2009)
36. Simo-Serra, E., Quattoni, A., Torras, C., Moreno-Noguer, F.: A joint model for 2D and 3D pose estimation from a single image. In: CVPR (2013)

Real-Time Head Orientation from a Monocular Camera Using Deep Neural Network

Byungtae Ahn, Jaesik Park, and In So Kweon$^{(\boxtimes)}$

KAIST, Daejeon, Republic of Korea
{btahn,jspark}@rcv.kaist.ac.kr, iskweon77@kaist.ac.kr

Abstract. We propose an efficient and accurate head orientation estimation algorithm using a monocular camera. Our approach is leveraged by deep neural network and we exploit the architecture in a data regression manner to learn the mapping function between visual appearance and three dimensional head orientation angles. Therefore, in contrast to classification based approaches, our system outputs continuous head orientation. The algorithm uses convolutional filters trained with a large number of augmented head appearances, thus it is user independent and covers large pose variations. Our key observation is that an input image having 32×32 resolution is enough to achieve about 3 degrees of mean square error, which can be used for efficient head orientation applications. Therefore, our architecture takes only 1 ms on roughly localized head positions with the aid of GPU. We also propose particle filter based post-processing to enhance stability of the estimation further in video sequences. We compare the performance with the state-of-the-art algorithm which utilizes depth sensor and we validate our head orientation estimator on Internet photos and video.

1 Introduction

Head pose estimation is crucial for face related applications such as face recognition, facial expression recognition, driver state monitoring, gaze estimation, etc. Accordingly, a variety of methods have been proposed for more than two decades [1]. In the context of computer vision, head pose estimation infer the position and orientation (roll, pitch, and yaw) of head from a face image.

Existing approaches can be categorized into two methods: appearance based methods and model based methods. Appearance based methods [2–12] use visual feature of the whole face appearance with machine learning techniques. The methods are relatively robust to large head pose variation and low image resolution. However, most of them utilize discrete head poses for training and treat the head pose estimation as a classification problem. As a result, the estimates are quantized (typically more than $10°$) as well. Model based methods [13–18] use geometric cues or non-rigid facial models. Model based methods have advantages that the outputs are continuous values; not discrete. Also they can obtain not only head pose but also facial feature locations for various applications. However, since their performance heavily rely on facial feature localization, the

© Springer International Publishing Switzerland 2015
D. Cremers et al. (Eds.): ACCV 2014, Part III, LNCS 9005, pp. 82–96, 2015.
DOI: 10.1007/978-3-319-16811-1_6

model based methods are sensitive to large variation of head pose, facial expression, and low resolution of input image.

The objective of this paper is to do head orientation estimation that is accurate, continuous, operating beyond real time, and robust to large variation of head pose and low resolution. We achieve this by exploiting deep neural network as a data regression manner. We demonstrate that the proposed estimator outperforms previous literatures. Our approach is adequate for real time applications such as driver drowsiness detection, gaze estimation, and face verification.

2   Related Works

Appearance Based Methods. These methods seek relationship between 3D face pose and its appearance on 2D image. Balasubramanian *et al.* [9] and Foytik and Asari [2] presented manifold embedding frameworks which maps the high-dimensional space of face appearance to low-dimensional manifolds. The latter paper introduces a framework composed of two steps, in which head pose is estimated in a coarse-to-fine manner. Gruji *et al.* [8] utilized image retrieval which compares an input image of head to a set of large exemplars. The initially estimated head orientation is refined using the candidate images in the database. The reported test error of [2,8] on Pointing'04 dataset [19] is larger than 13°. Huang *et al.* [5] used Gabor feature based random forests as the discrete label classifier. They combined the random forest with linear discriminative analysis (LDA) to improve the discriminative power. Zhu and Ramanan [3] proposed a unified model for face detection, head pose estimation, and facial landmark localization. They use a mixture of tree-structured part models to find topological changes due to rotation along yaw axis. Though it conducts unified task, it classifies just a few discrete yaw angles of head poses, and the computation takes a few seconds per VGA resolution image.

Compared to those discrete labeling approaches, BenAbdelkader [6] and Ji *et al.* [4] treated head pose estimation as a nonlinear regression problem which computes continuous 3D pose. Other approaches [10–12] exploited depth information for continuous head pose estimation. Breitenstein *et al.* [10] aligned a range image with reference poses. Their GPU implementation operates in 10 fps. Fanelli *et al.* [12] introduced a random forest based voting framework for real-time and continuous head pose estimation. They also extended it to 3D facial feature localization. They provide an head pose database containing tuples of color, depth and ground truth head pose. The use of depth data has some advantages that it can be available even at night and can generate 3D face model, but a specific device is required. Also the device cannot be used in outdoors because of its sensing mechanism.

Model Based Methods. In contrast to most of appearance based methods, model based methods output continuous head pose. Hu *et al.* [13] roughly estimated face pose by using asymmetric distribution of facial components. The pose is refined with 3D-to-2D geometrical model. Active shape models (ASM) [15] and active appearance models (AAM) [16] are very popular statistical models of face. They were proposed for facial landmark localization first, but have been extended for estimating head pose [17]. Morency *et al.* [18] presented generalized adaptive view-based appearance model (GAVAM) for stable head pose estimation, which takes some benefits of automatic initialization, user-independence, and key frame tracking. These methods generally depend on some specific facial landmarks, so they are sensitive to initialization, large variation of head pose or facial expression, occlusions, and resolution of input image.

Deep Convolutional Neural Network. As graphic processing unit (GPU) has been developed, and accessibility to big data has become easy, deep learning techniques has been actively studied. Among those deep learning methods, convolutional neural network (CNN) [20] has been successfully applied to computer vision tasks such as image classification [21], pedestrian detection [22], and image denoising [23]. Recently, deep convolutional neural network (DNN) are widely utilized for face related applications and body pose estimation as well. Sun *et al.* [24] and Zhou *et al.* [25] introduced DNN into coarse-to-fine facial feature localization. The former paper proposed three-level cascaded structure composed of one DNN and two shallow neural networks. They also analyzed on effects of some schemes such as absolute value rectification and local weight sharing on facial feature localization. Toshev and Szegedy [26] applied DNN to human body pose estimation, namely DeepPose. They designed DNN architecture composed of regressor and refiner. The architecture is used for every body joint individually, and the outputs are linked to each other for building the body pose. They report state-of-the art performance.

Inspired by recent success of DNN based approaches, we design a DNN architecture for estimating head orientation. We found that DNN architecture is appropriate for head orientation estimation. In our experiment, we observe that it outperforms previous approach which exploits depth data while we use only gray scale images. Especially, we analyze the effects of input image size, the number of layers, and the number of feature maps. We suggest a novel head orientation estimator showing remarkable accuracy in 1 ms.

3 Preliminaries: Representation of Head Pose

Before introducing our approach, we provide preliminary discussion for describing and displaying head pose. Compared to 6D description of object's pose which is general, the head pose in image coordinate can be described as $(x_h, y_h, \psi, \theta, \phi)$. $\mathbf{x}_h = (x_h, y_h)$ is head position in image coordinate and a triplet (ψ, θ, ϕ) stands for the rotation angles of roll, pitch, and yaw. They are all bounded in $[-\frac{\pi}{2}, \frac{\pi}{2}]$ and [0,0,0] denotes frontal view of the head. We use the conventional definition of (ψ, θ, ϕ) in right-handed Cartesian coordinates as shown in Fig. 1. According to the definition, ψ and θ correspond to clockwise rotation angles about x-axis and y-axis. ϕ corresponds to counter clockwise rotation angle about z-axis. The 3D head orientation matrix $R_{head} = R_\psi R_\theta R_\phi$ is then determined as

$$R_\psi = \begin{bmatrix} 1 & 0 & 0 \\ 0 & \cos\psi & \sin\psi \\ 0 & -\sin\psi & \cos\psi \end{bmatrix}, R_\theta = \begin{bmatrix} \cos\theta & 0 & -\sin\theta \\ 0 & 1 & 0 \\ \sin\theta & 0 & \cos\theta \end{bmatrix}, R_\phi = \begin{bmatrix} \cos\phi & -\sin\phi & 0 \\ \sin\phi & \cos\phi & 0 \\ 0 & 0 & 1 \end{bmatrix}.$$

(1)

As a counter conversion, unique (ψ, θ, ϕ) is determined from R_{head} as

$$(\psi, \theta, \phi) = \left(\arctan(\frac{R_{32}}{R_{33}}), \arctan(\frac{-R_{31}}{\sqrt{R_{32}^2 + R_{33}^2}}), \arctan(\frac{R_{21}}{R_{11}}) \right),$$

(2)

where R_{ij} is the element of R_{head} at i-th row and j-th column.

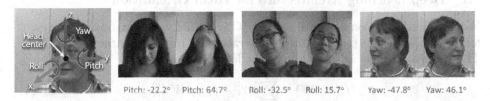

Pitch: -22.2°   Pitch: 64.7°   Roll: -32.5°   Roll: 15.7°   Yaw: -47.8°   Yaw: 46.1°

Fig. 1. Representation of head orientation. We use conventional definition of roll, pitch and yaw rotation directions shown in the left figure. Some examples of rotation angles and their corresponding head images are shown in the right side. The dataset is provided by Fanelli *et al.* [12].

The head pose $(x_h, y_h, \psi, \theta, \phi)$, can be visualized by means of the 3D axis and a circle on yz plane around the head as shown in Fig. 6. To do so, we transform (ψ, θ, ϕ) into R_{head} and we project the axes and the circle onto the input image by using an orthographic projection matrix:

$$P = \begin{bmatrix} R_{11} & R_{12} & R_{13} & x_h \\ R_{21} & R_{22} & R_{23} & y_h \\ 0 & 0 & 0 & 1 \end{bmatrix},$$

(3)

where P is defined in homogeneous coordinate.

4   Proposed Method

In this section, our head pose estimation approach is introduced. We assume that we have head position and its corresponding scale. In our implementation, we utilize robust head detection algorithm by Zhu *et al.* [3] which uses tree structured part model for elastic deformation.

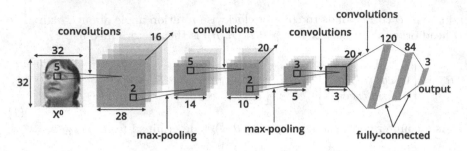

Fig. 2. Proposed structure of deep neural network (referred as N2 in Table 1) for head orientation estimation. It uses 32×32 pixels gray scale image as an input. The output is head orientation (ψ, θ, ϕ).

4.1 Deep Learning Architecture for Head Orientation

We review convolutional neural network (CNN) briefly and introduce our design for head orientation task. Figure 2 illustrates the proposed structure of DNN. The trained filters in DNN minimize the following loss error:

$$E(X_i; W) = \sum_i ||Y_i - f(X_i; W)||_2^2, \tag{4}$$

where i indicates an index of training samples, W is a set of weight values in convolution filters, X is estimated angles (ψ, θ, ϕ), and Y denotes the target (ground truth) of head orientation. Training CNN consists of two phases: prediction and update. Prediction means feed forward through the network. Update means evolving weights and biases between layers by error back-propagation. In the prediction phase, one convolutional layer accompanies three steps. First, convolution operation is performed on the input image with trained filters. Second, the outputs of the convolutions are passed through an activation function. Third, they are downscaled (sub-sampling) for introducing small translation invariance and improving generalization. Sub-sampling step can be disregarded according to applications. In update phase, loss errors are calculated at the end node (the output of the network). Based on the errors, the weights and biases of the network are updated from the last layer to the first layer by stochastic gradient descent (SGD). This is called backward propagation of errors (or back-propagation). Hyperbolic tangent, sigmoid, and rectified linear unit (ReLU) [21] functions are commonly used as the activation function. The sigmoid function $f(x) = (1 + e^{-\beta x})^{-1}$ maps $[-\infty, +\infty] \rightarrow [0, 1]$, while hyperbolic tangent function $f(x) = \tanh(x)$ maps $[-\infty, +\infty] \rightarrow [-1, +1]$. Thus, the outputs from the sigmoid function are typically not close to zero on average, while average of the outputs from hyperbolic tangent function is close to zero. In this aspect, with a normalized dataset whose mean and variance are 0 and 1 respectively, the hyperbolic tangent function is recommendable due to convergence during gradient descent [27]. ReLU tends to train faster than other activation functions [21].

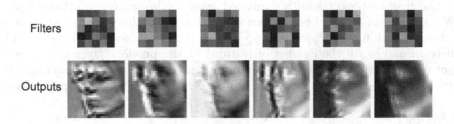

Fig. 3. Some trained filters and their outputs of an input image in the first convolutional layer. The sizes of filters and the outputs are 5×5 and 28×28 pixels respectively.

Now, we introduce our DNN design for head orientation estimation. Our DNN structure follows a principle introduced by Coates *et al.* [28]. According to the literature, since our dataset may not cover head appearances of every people, we use small filter size (5×5 which is smallest in convention) and smallest convolutional stride (1 pixel). Regarding the number of layers, we follow insights from [24], which states that performance improves as the number of layers increases (more than 3 at least). The number of filters is also an important factor on accuracy. Our design is composed of 4 convolutional layers having 16, 20, 20, and 120 filters respectively, which produces an acceptable trade-off between the performance and computational speed.

Our architecture takes an input image of 32×32 pixels which is relatively small compared to other DNN architectures for other face applications [3,24,25,29]. We normalize intensities of an input image, so that the mean and variance are 0 and 1 respectively. This allows us to use hyper-tangent as the activation function. Max-pooling is performed after convolutional layers. The outputs of the first convolutional layer followed by max-pooling is the input of the second convolutional layer. They are convolved with 20 filters of 5×5 pixels. In the same manner, third and forth convolutional layers take the outputs of the previous layers as input, and convolve it with 20 and 120 filters of 5×5 and 3×3 pixels respectively. The max-pooling is not conducted in the third and fourth convolutional layer. The l-th convolutional layer is defined as

$$X_v^{l+1} = \tanh \left(\sum_{u=1}^{I} W_{uv}^l \otimes X_u^l + b_v^l \right), \tag{5}$$

where W_{uv}^l and X_u^l are the trained filter and the image patch, and u and v indicate the index of input and output channels respectively. For example, in the first convolutional layer, $u = 1$ and $v \in \{1, \cdots, 16\}$. Therefore, X_v^{l+1} is the output from v-th channel which is the input to the $(l+1)$-th layer. b_v means the bias vectors, and $\otimes$ denotes convolution operator. Figure 3 shows some of the trained filters in the first convolutional layer. Note that the features are not correlated, and edges and some important parts for estimating head orientation (e.g. eye, nose, and chin) are enhanced in their output.

The first and second fully connected layers following convolutional layers are composed of 120 and 84 neurons respectively. The fully connected layer is performed with function $y_j = \tanh\left(\sum_{i=0}^{m-1} x_i \cdot w_{i,j} + b_j\right)$, for $j \in \{0, \cdots, n-1\}$, where m and n are the number of neurons at the previous layer and current layer respectively. Equation (4) is non-linear due to the activation function. We solve it by back-propagation method using stochastic gradient descent (SGD) as in [21].

4.2   Temporally Stable Head Pose Estimation

Given an input video, if we handle input frames independently, the estimated head orientation may be temporally unstable since the head appearance often changes abruptly due to shadows or occlusions. In order to obtain stable head orientation in the time domain, we apply Bayesian sequential estimation which uses the past observation to update the posterior distribution and to predict the current state. The distribution required for filtering procedure can be effectively approximated by sequential Monte Carlo estimation, or known as particle filter [30]. We empirically choose particle filter instead of linear filter such as Kalman due to high non-linearity of state changes. We operate two particle filters, which are for head orientation and head position due to the multi-modality and weak correlation between the two states. For propagating particles, we use a first-order dynamic model which regards constant angular or positional displacements over the period $[t-1, t]$. In this manner, head orientation state $\mathbf{o} = (\mathbf{s}, \mathbf{d})$ is updated as:

$$\mathbf{s}_t = \mathbf{s}_{t-1} + \mathbf{d}_{t-1}\Delta t + \epsilon_\mathbf{s}, \tag{6}$$

$$\mathbf{d}_t = \mathbf{d}_{t-1} + \epsilon_\mathbf{d}, \tag{7}$$

where $\mathbf{s} := (\psi, \theta, \phi)$ represents head orientation state, $\mathbf{d} := (d_\psi, d_\theta, d_\phi)$ is angular displacement, subscript t notes time stamp at t, and $\epsilon_{\mathbf{s},\mathbf{d}}$ are process noise come from zero-mean Gaussian distribution. We exploit the *bootstrap filter* where the density of state transition is used for estimating the probability function [31]. The importance weight $w_{t,ang}^i$ for i-th particle $\mathbf{o}_t^i$ is described by:

$$w_{t,ang}^i \propto w_{t-1,ang}^i \times p(\mathbf{o}_{t,obs}|\mathbf{o}_t^i), \tag{8}$$

where $\mathbf{o}_{t,obs} = (\mathbf{s}_{t,obs}, \mathbf{d}_{t,obs})$ is a new observation at t and $\mathbf{o}_t^i$ is the propagated particles. $w_{t-1,ang}$ can be regarded as constant since resampling is performed on fixed number of particles. We define $w_{t,ang}^i$ as:

$$w_{t,ang}^i = \exp\left(\frac{\|\mathbf{o}_{t,obs} - \mathbf{o}_t^i\|^2}{\sigma_{ang}^2}\right), \tag{9}$$

Note that we have another state $\mathbf{h} = (x, y, v_x, v_y)$ which represents head position and its velocity in image domain. For this state, the importance weight $w_{t,pos}$ for particle $\mathbf{h}^i$ is defined as:

$$w_{t,pos}^i = \exp\left(\frac{f(x^i, y^i)^2}{\sigma_{pos}^2}\right), \tag{10}$$

where $f(\cdot)$ is 2D confidence map built up by head detector. Since $\mathbf{h}$ also uses constant velocity model, it is similarly updated as Eqs. (6) and (7).

5 Experimental Result

In this section, we provide experimental results in various aspects. First, we evaluate networks while altering parameters of the networks such as the number of feature maps and size of input image with the depth of networks. We will also discuss the effect of particle filter as a post processing. Finally, the proposed method will be compared with the state-of-the-art method [12].

5.1 Dataset for Evaluation

We evaluate our method using Biwi Kinect Head Pose Database [12]. The dataset contains 15,678 upper body images of 20 people (4 people were recorded twice but they appear different hair style and clothing), and ground truth head pose information from user-specific 3D template based head tracker [32]. It provides 3D rotation matrix for head orientation. By using Eq. (2), we convert the rotation matrix into (ψ, θ, ϕ). The triplet is used for training described in Sect. 4. The head orientation covers about $\pm75°$ for yaw, $\pm60°$ for pitch, and $\pm50°$ for roll. The dataset provides depth to facial center as well. From the perspective camera model without lens distortion, the size of head image patch is determined as $\frac{fR}{Z}$ where f is focal length, R is radius of head, Z is metric depth to head center. We use $R = 120\,\text{mm}$ and fix it over the evaluation. The extracted head images are resized to 100×100 pixels.

Among 15,678 patches, we randomly selected a subset of 2,178 patches as our validation set, and remaining 13,500 patches were used for training. For the training samples, we first did data augmentation on the extracted patches to avoid over-fitting. We did this by randomly cropping the extracted patches. The size of smaller patch varies from 86×86 to 100×100 pixels. Then, the augmented patches are resized to 32×32 pixels for the proposed DNN. At test time, five patches of 86×86 pixels are extracted from each 100×100 pixels of input patch (four from each corner patch and one from center). The five patches are also resized to 32×32 pixels. Note that the size of input patch can be 64×64 pixels as well, which will be discussed in Sect. 5.2. All training and test patches are gray-scaled and their intensity values are modified by histogram normalization. We used GPU accelerated implementation, and training continues until convergence.

5.2 Analysis on Various Network Structures

In order to find most efficient and effective network, we design various types of DNN structures with different parameters (the number of feature maps, and the size of an input image, and the number of convolutional layers) on estimating head orientation. Note that the image size decreases when it passes each layer. Therefore, the number of layer and size of input have dependency. Our selected configurations are summarized in Table 1. N2 containing four convolutional layers is the proposed DNN structure illustrated in Fig. 2. The networks N1–N4 include four convolutional layers, and perform with the input images of 32 × 32 pixels. The networks N5–N8 contain five convolutional layers, with the input images of 64 × 64 pixels. Figure 4 and Table 2 show the performance of the networks in Table 1.

Table 1. Summary of DNN structures. $I(s, s)$ denotes a square input image of s pixels on a side. $C(k, n)$ means convolutional layer with square filters of k pixels on a side, where n is the number of filters. Pooling layer is denoted by $P(p)$, where p is the size of the square pooling regions. $F(e)$ indicates fully connected layer, where e is the number of neurons.

	L0	L1	L2	L3	L4	L5	L6	L7	L8	L9	L10
N1	I(32,32)	C(5,30)	P(2)	C(5,30)	P(2)	C(3,30)	C(3,120)	F(84)	F(3)		
N2	**I(32,32)**	**C(5,16)**	**P(2)**	**C(5,20)**	**P(2)**	**C(3,20)**	**C(3,120)**	**F(84)**	**F(3)**		
N3	I(32,32)	C(5,10)	P(2)	C(5,20)	P(2)	C(3,20)	C(3,120)	F(84)	F(3)		
N4	I(32,32)	C(5,10)	P(2)	C(5,10)	P(2)	C(3,10)	C(3,120)	F(84)	F(3)		
N5	I(64,64)	C(5,30)	P(2)	C(5,30)	P(2)	C(4,30)	P(2)	C(3,30)	C(3,120)	F(84)	F(3)
N6	I(64,64)	C(5,16)	P(2)	C(5,20)	P(2)	C(4,20)	P(2)	C(3,20)	C(3,120)	F(84)	F(3)
N7	I(64,64)	C(5,10)	P(2)	C(5,20)	P(2)	C(4,20)	P(2)	C(3,20)	C(3,120)	F(84)	F(3)
N8	I(64,64)	C(5,10)	P(2)	C(5,10)	P(2)	C(4,10)	P(2)	C(3,10)	C(3,120)	F(84)	F(3)

Figure 4 shows the comparison results on mean and standard deviation of the errors. Processing time shown in Fig. 4 over the eight DNN structures are tested on Nvidia^{TM} GTX Titan Black 6 GB GPU. Results show that the performance can be slightly improved when the networks have more than four convolutional layers and use high quality input images of 64 × 64 pixels. However, in these networks, processing is much slower. It seems that four convolutional layers with low quality images of 32 × 32 pixels are satisfied for accurate head orientation estimation. 32 × 32 resolution is approximately two times smaller than [29] which is designed for recovering canonical view with important parts of face images.

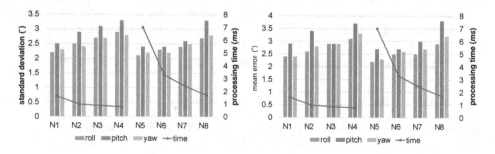

Fig. 4. Mean and standard deviation of the errors, and processing speed of various networks defined in Table 1.

Table 2. Mean and standard deviation of the errors, and processing time of various networks. N1-N4 structures are composed of four convolutional layers, and N5-N8 structures consists of five convolutional layers.

	Mean error ± standard deviation (°)			Time (ms)
	Roll	Pitch	Yaw	
N1	2.4 ± 2.2	2.9 ± 2.5	2.4 ± 2.3	1.60
N2	**2.6 ± 2.5**	**3.4 ± 2.9**	**2.8 ± 2.4**	**0.98**
N3	2.9 ± 2.7	2.9 ± 3.1	2.9 ± 2.7	0.87
N4	3.1 ± 2.9	3.7 ± 3.3	3.3 ± 2.8	0.78
N5	2.2 ± 2.1	2.7 ± 2.4	2.3 ± 2.2	7.00
N6	2.5 ± 2.3	2.7 ± 2.4	2.6 ± 2.2	3.30
N7	2.5 ± 2.4	3.0 ± 2.6	2.7 ± 2.5	2.41
N8	2.9 ± 2.7	3.8 ± 3.3	3.2 ± 2.8	1.71

In face orientation problem, we believe relative location of the chin, nose and eyes regardless of the individual person still works as a useful cue in 32×32 resolution, even though they are not shown obviously. In addition, due to the reduced dimensions, we could achieved impressive computational time. When comparing the networks having the same depth, as the number of feature maps increases, the result tends to be improved. However, since the processing time is increased as well, deciding the number of feature maps depends on its applications (Table 3).

5.3 Temporally Stable Head Orientation Estimation

We validate our particle filter based module described in Sect. 4.2 on the Robe-Safe [33] dataset. The video contains the driver who moves his/her head smoothly during driving. Note that the driver data is not used for training in our pipeline. Figure 5 shows estimated head orientation over some periods. The estimated head orientation however, shows inconsistent orientation over adjacent time due to abrupt change of the appearance and occlusion (around 15th frame in the Fig. 5) not by the physical head movement.

5.4 Comparison with Fanelli et al. [12]

We compare with the state-of-the-art approach for real time head pose estimation, which uses random forest regression with depth sensor, Kinect. They provide and use the same dataset in our experiments. Table 2 shows comparison results on mean and standard deviation of the errors, and processing time of both [12] and ours. Note that all the results on accuracy and precision from the networks we design (Table 2) significantly outperform those of the state-of-the-art approach. While the method in [12] compares internal depth values from extracted random patches for voting head poses, our DNN based approach uses

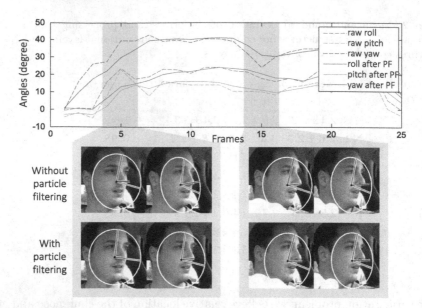

Fig. 5. Validation on RobeSafe driver monitoring dataset [33]. The method in Sect. 4.2 stabilizes abrupt changes of head orientation which is occurred by shadow and occlusion not by physical movement of the head. The comparison of the head orientations without and with particle filtering is displayed.

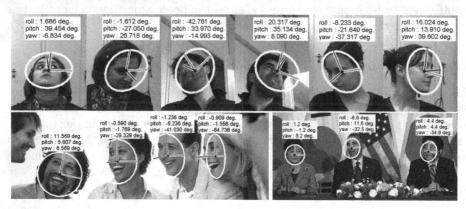

Fig. 6. Our head orientation estimation on validation set [12](first row) and the web photos (second row).

filters automatically learned from many training images without handcraft low level features (intensity difference, edge etc.). Our approach results in implicitly extracting important high level information (relative position of eyes, nose, chin etc.). In addition, the approach using depth values from the Kinect sensor may be affected by noise and low-resolution of depth maps. In contrast, the level of noise in grey scale image is lesser than that of depth map, which is another

Table 3. Comparison with Fanelli *et al.* [12] on mean and standard deviation of the errors, and processing time. The test environment used in [12] is a 2.67 GHz Intel Core i7 CPU, and ours is the same level of CPU with Nvidia^{TM} GTX Titan Black 6 GB GPU. Our time is only for estimating head orientation whereas [12] includes time for abrupt face detection using depth map.

	Mean error $\pm$ standard deviation ($^\circ$)			Time (ms)
	Roll	Pitch	Yaw	
Fanelli stride 5	5.4±6.0	3.5±5.8	3.8±6.5	44.7
Fanelli stride 10	5.5±6.2	3.6±6.0	4.0±7.1	17.8
Fanelli stride 15	5.5±6.2	3.8±6.4	4.2±7.8	10.7
Ours N2	**2.6±2.5**	**3.4±2.9**	**2.8±2.4**	**0.98**

benefit. Some examples of the estimation are shown in Fig. 6, where the center of the white circle with radius 120 mm is on the head center. It demonstrates that our method is reasonable even though the person has various facial expressions and poses. We believe that it is a result from training a large database which consists of various facial expressions and poses. Given roughly localized head position, our approach requires less than 1 ms to estimate head orientation. For comparing computational time, we analyze with the reported time in [12], although [12] performs face detection and head orientation simultaneously. Since [12] finds the head region abruptly by thresholding depth values, their reported time is mainly for processing depth values for head orientation.

Figure 7 illustrates the normalized success rates of the estimations on the validation set for each 15 × 15 degrees. Angular error below 15° is regarded as a success, and the background color of the the heat map reflects the number of images present in each region. In almost all regions, the estimates show the

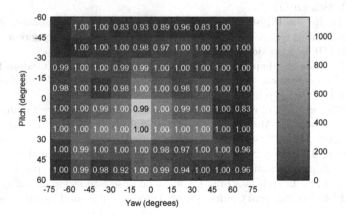

Fig. 7. Normalized success rates. Angular error below 15° is regraded as success. The background color represents the number of images in each bin, as illustrated by the side bar (Color figure online).

results of 100 % or close to 100 % success rates, which outperform the equivalent plot in [12]. Also, it shows that the algorithm works well over large variations of head orientations.

6 Conclusion

In this work, we introduce an efficient and accurate method for estimating head orientation. Inspired by the remarkable success of deep neural network which automatically learns desirable features, we design network structure which achieves notable performance and speed comparable to the state-of-the-art algorithm. We tested our algorithm on various types of video and photos. Possible application scenarios include measuring driver's attention, robust face recognition and saliency estimation. Our future work is designing a general-purpose head detection algorithm as well to make a comprehensive deep neural network for 5D head pose estimation. We expect that the complete system will boost up the accuracy and usefulness in practice.

Acknowledgement. We appreciate constructive comments from anonymous reviewers. This work was supported by the National Research Foundation of Korea(NRF) grant funded by the Korea government(MSIP) (No. 2010-0028680).

References

1. Murphy-Chutorian, E., Trivedi, M.M.: Head pose estimation in computer vision: a survey. IEEE Trans. Pattern Anal. Mach. Intell. (TPAMI) **31**, 607–626 (2009)
2. Foytik, J., Asari, V.K.: A two-layer framework for piecewise linear manifold-based head pose estimation. Int. J. Comput. Vis. (IJCV) **101**, 270–287 (2013)
3. Zhu, X., Ramanan, D.: Face detection, pose estimation and landmark localization in the wild. In: Proceedings of Computer Vision and Pattern Recognition (CVPR), pp. 2879–2886 (2012)
4. Ji, H., Liu, R., Su, F., Su, Z., Tian, Y.: Robust head pose estimation via convex regularized sparse regression. In: Proceedings of International Conference on Image Processing (ICIP), pp. 3617–3620 (2011)
5. Huang, C., Ding, X., Fang, C.: Head pose estimation based on random forests for multiclass classification. In: Proceedings of International Conference on Pattern Recognition (ICPR), pp. 934–937 (2010)
6. BenAbdelkader, C.: Robust head pose estimation using supervised manifold learning. In: Daniilidis, K., Maragos, P., Paragios, N. (eds.) ECCV 2010, Part VI. LNCS, vol. 6316, pp. 518–531. Springer, Heidelberg (2010)
7. Aghajanian, J., Prince, S.J.: Face pose estimation in uncontrolled environments. In: Proceedings of British Machine Vision Conference (BMVC), pp. 1–11 (2009)
8. Gruji, N., Ili, S., Lepetit, V., Fua, P.: 3d facial pose estimation by image retrieval. In: 8th IEEE International Conference on Automatic Face and Gesture Recognition (2008)
9. Balasubramanian, V.N., Ye, J., Panchanathan, S.: Biased manifold embedding: a framework for person-independent head pose estimation. In: Proceedings of Computer Vision and Pattern Recognition (CVPR), pp. 1–7 (2007)

10. Breitenstein, M.D., Kuettel, D., Weise, T., van Gool, L.: Real-time face pose estimation from single range images. In: Proceedings of Computer Vision and Pattern Recognition (CVPR), pp. 1–8 (2008)
11. Padeleris, P., Zabulis, X., Argyros, A.A.: Head pose estimation on depth data based on particle swarm optimization. In: IEEE Computer Society Conference on Computer Vision and Pattern Recognition Workshops (CVPRW), pp. 42–49 (2012)
12. Fanelli, G., Dantone, M., Gall, J., Fossati, A., Gool, L.V.: Random forests for real time 3d face analysis. Int. J. Comput. Vis. (IJCV) **101**, 437–458 (2013)
13. Hug, Y., Chen, L., Zhoug, Y., Zhang, H.: Estimating face pose by facial asymmetry and geometry. In: 6th IEEE International Conference on Automatic Face and Gesture Recognition, FG 2004, pp. 651–656 (2004)
14. Pathangay, V., Das, S., Greiner, T.: Symmetry-based face pose estimation from a single uncalibrated view. In: 8th IEEE International Conference on Automatic Face and Gesture Recognition, FG 2008, pp. 1–8 (2008)
15. Cootes, T.F., Taylor, C.J., Cooper, D.H., Graham, J.: Active shape models-their training and application. Comput. Vis. Image Underst. (CVIU) **61**, 38–59 (1995)
16. Cootes, T.F., Edwards, G., Taylor, C.: Active appearance models. IEEE Trans. Pattern Anal. Mach. Intell. (TPAMI) **23**, 681–685 (2001)
17. Martins, P., Batista, J.: Accurate single view model-based head pose estimation. In: 8th IEEE International Conference on Automatic Face and Gesture Recognition, FG 2008, pp. 1–6 (2008)
18. Morency, L.P., Whitehill, J., Movellan, J.: Monocular head pose estimation using generalized adaptive view-based appearance model. Image Vis. Comput. **28**, 754–761 (2009)
19. Gourier, N., Hall, D., Crowley, J.L.: Estimating face orientation from robust detection of salient facial features. In: Proceedings of Pointing 2004, ICPR, International Workshop on Visual Observation of Deictic Gestures (2004)
20. Lecun, Y., Boser, B., Denker, J., Henderson, D., Howard, R., Hubbard, W., Jackel, L.: Backpropagation applied to handwritten zip code recognition. Neural Comput. **1**, 541–551 (1989)
21. Krizhevsky, A., Sutskever, I., Hinton, G.E.: Imagenet classification with deep convolutional neural networks. In: Advances in Neural Information Processing Systems (NIPS) (2012)
22. Sermanet, P., Kavukcuoglu, K., Chintala, S., LeCun, Y.: Pedestrian detection with unsupervised multi-stage feature learning. In: Proceedings of Computer Vision and Pattern Recognition (CVPR), pp. 3626–3633 (2013)
23. Burger, H.C., Schuler, C.J., Harmeling, S.: Image denoising: can plain neural networks compete with bm3d? In: Proceedings of Computer Vision and Pattern Recognition (CVPR) (2012)
24. Sun, Y., Wang, X., Tang, X.: Deep convolutional network cascade for facial point detection. In: Proceedings of Computer Vision and Pattern Recognition (CVPR), pp. 3476–3483 (2013)
25. Zhou, E., Fan, H., Cao, Z., Jiang, Y., Yin, Q.: Extensive facial landmark localization with coarse-to-fine convolutional network cascade. In: IEEE International Conference on Computer Vision Workshops (ICCVW), pp. 386–391 (2013)
26. Toshev, A., Szegedy, C.: Deeppose: human pose estimation via deep neural networks. In: Proceedings of Computer Vision and Pattern Recognition (CVPR) (2014)
27. Lecun, Y., Bottou, L., Bengio, Y., Haffner, P.: Gradient-based learning applied to document recognition. Proc. IEEE **86**, 2278–2324 (1998)

28. Coates, A., Lee, H., Ng, A.Y.: An analysis of single-layer networks in unsupervised feature learning. In: International Conference on Artificial Intelligence and Statistics (AISTATS), pp. 215–233 (2011)
29. Zhu, Z., Luo, P., Wang, X., Tang, X.: Recover canonical-view faces in the wild with deep neural networks. Computing Research Repository (CoRR), arXiv (2014)
30. Doucet, A., Freitas, N.D., Gorden, N.: Sequential Monte Carlo Methods in Practice. Springer, New York (2001)
31. Gordon, N., Salmond, D., Smith, A.: Novel approach to nonlinear/nongaussian Bayesian state estimation. IEE Proc. Radar Sig. Process. **140**, 107–113 (1993)
32. Weise, T., Bouaziz, S., Li, H., Pauly, M.: Realtime performance-based facial animation. In: Proceedings of SIGGRAPH (2011)
33. Nuevo, J., Bergasa, L.M., Jiménez, P.: Rsmat: Robust simultaneous modeling and tracking. Pattern Recogn. Lett. **31**, 2455–2463 (2010)

Jointly Learning Dictionaries and Subspace Structure for Video-Based Face Recognition

Guangxiao Zhang[1]([⊠]), Ran He[2], and Larry S. Davis[2]

[1] Institute for Advanced Computer Studies, University of Maryland,
College Park, MD 20742, USA
gxzhang@umiacs.umd.edu
[2] Institute of Automation, Chinese Academy of Sciences,
95 Zhongguancun East Road, P.O. Box 2728, Beijing 100190, China
rhe@nlpr.ia.ac.cn, lsd@umiacs.umd.edu

Abstract. In video-sharing websites and surveillance scenarios, there are often a large amount of face videos. This paper proposes a joint dictionary learning and subspace segmentation method for video-based face recognition (VFR). We assume that the face images from one subject video lie in a union of multiple linear subspaces, and there exists a global dictionary to represent these images and segment them to their corresponding subspaces. This assumption results in a "chicken and egg" problem, where subspace clustering and dictionary learning are mutually dependent. To solve thiss problem, we propose a joint optimization model that includes three parts. The first part seeks a low-rank representation for subspace segmentation; the second part encourages the dictionary to accurately represent the data while tolerating frame-wise corruption or outliers; and the third part is a regularization on the dictionary. An alternating minimization method is employed as an efficient solution to the proposed joint formulation. In each iteration, it alternately learns the subspace structure and the dictionary by improving the learning results. Experiments on three video-based face databases show that our approach consistently outperforms the state-of-the-art methods.

1 Introduction

Video-based face recognition (VFR) has become an active research topic in recent years in the computer vision community [1–7]. Compared to still-image face recognition, the task in video-to-video recognition is to efficiently exploit multiple frames, and to build a model robust against variations of the same subject appearing in different videos. This is challenging because faces detected from videos are usually acquired under non-ideal acquisition conditions in which illumination, pose, and facial expression variations dominate. Moreover, the cropped face images are often of low resolution, which makes many local feature methods inapplicable.

Electronic supplementary material The online version of this chapter (doi:10.1007/978-3-319-16811-1_7) contains supplementary material, which is available to authorized users.

© Springer International Publishing Switzerland 2015
D. Cremers et al. (Eds.): ACCV 2014, Part III, LNCS 9005, pp. 97–111, 2015.
DOI: 10.1007/978-3-319-16811-1_7

To solve the video-based face recognition problem, researchers have proposed numerous methods. Early frame-based attempts include fusing frame-based recognition results by voting [8], finding the minimal distance between two frames across videos [9], and matching the key frames with exemplars in the gallery [10]. Most of the recent approaches are based on either temporal models or image sets. Some researchers extract spatial-temporal representations from videos to enhance face recognition [11,12]. Others discard the temporal information and treat the videos as image sets [1–3,13–16]. The problem of VFR then becomes a more general image-set matching or classification problem. To solve this problem, many statistical models were proposed to describe the image sets as linear subspaces or manifolds. Under the linear subspace assumptions, methods such as [13,14] (DCC) measure the distance or similarity between two subspaces by computing the angles between the principle components. Hu et al. [1] (SANP) find the minimal distance of the two nearest points, which can be sparsely approximated from the samples of their respective subspaces. Under the nonlinear manifold assumptions, [17] defines the distance between subspaces over Grassmann manifold, and then constructs the Sparse Approximated Nearest Subspaces (SANS) adaptively from the samples of the query image set. It approaches the nearest point to the reference point by minimizing the joint sparse representation error. Wang et al. [15] proposed Manifold-to-Manifold Distance learning (MMD), which partitions a manifold into several local linear models and integrates the pair-wise distances. They also extended MMD to a supervised version called Manifold Discriminant Analysis(MDA) [16]. Moreover, Wang et al. [2] represent image sets with their covariance matrices, and compute the distance between manifolds by mapping the covariance matrix from the Riemannian manifold to a Euclidean space (Cov+PLS). While those methods have received great success, Cui et al. [3] raised an uncertainty issue that commonly arises when partitioning a nonlinear manifold into local linear subspaces. They argue that face images with similar appearance can be clustered to different subspaces or clusters in different video sequences, making the distance between two manifolds ill-defined. They proposed to align the gallery set and the query set with respect to a pre-defined reference sequence [3] (ImgSetAlign). This image set alignment issue is also addressed in [18]. Given a well-aligned, high quality gallery, they combine three tasks in a unified framework: aligning faces geometrically, performing recognition, and selecting good quality frames (CAR). Another image set method proposed by Lu et. al [19] computes the holistic multiple order statistics features of the image sets, and performs multi-kernel metric learning. These methods have achieved the state of the art on several public face databases.

Most recently, sparse representation for videos has attracted attention. Although the advantage of dictionary learning for robust face recognition in still images has been widely recognized [20], dictionary learning for VFR is relatively new. Chen et al. [4,5] proposed a joint sparse representation method under a minimal reconstruction error criterion. It divides a video sequence into K partitions in order to capture different poses or illumination conditions. Next, partition-level sub-dictionaries are learned by minimizing the total reconstruction error within the partition. Experiments have demonstrated that the dictionary-based method also achieved the state of the art (Fig. 1).

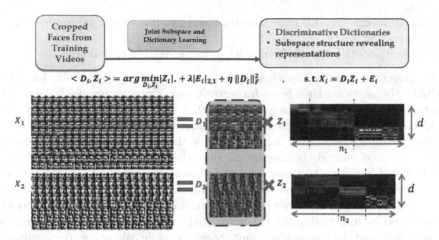

Fig. 1. An overview of our method. Sequences of cropped faces detected from videos are sent as inputs to our Jointly Learning Dictionary and Subspace Structure (JLDSS) algorithm. It learns class-specific dictionaries and the corresponding low-rank representations simultaneously. Examples of face sequences X_1, X_2, our dictionaries D_1, D_2, and the low-rank matrices Z_1, Z_2 are shown in the figure. The low-rank matrices can also be employed for video segmentation. Such examples are shown by the red dashed lines on Z_1 and Z_2.

The dictionary-based method falls into the category of image-set methods. The basic assumption can be summarized as follows: all face images from one subject video lie in a union of multiple linear subspaces. In each of those subspaces, there exists a sub-dictionary that can represent the data well. However, as in other manifold-partitioning-to-multiple-linear-subspaces methods, the clustering uncertainty issue recognized in [3] also exists here. Subspace clustering and dictionary learning are mutually beneficial and dependent on one another. To learn the sub-dictionaries, or perform any within subspace operations in general, subspace clustering, or equivalently "sequence partitioning" in [4] and [5], needs to be performed first. Yet it is impossible to define an "optimal" clustering result until the final reconstruction error is obtained. In other words, one needs to have the dictionaries in advance for reconstruction to make an appropriate choice of subspace clustering that captures the true characteristics of the video.

To address the above issue, we propose a joint learning framework that simultaneously learns a global dictionary and reveals the intrinsic subspace structure of the video. We assume that faces from one subject video lie in multiple linear subspaces, and there exists a global dictionary that can represent all the faces and reflects the subspace structure of the image set. The objective function of our model includes three parts. The first part forces the data to lie in multiple linear subspaces, in each of which one point can be represented by a set of bases called a dictionary that spans the same linear subspace; the second part encourages the dictionary to represent the data well with tolerance to outliers; the third part regularizes the learned dictionary. An alternating minimization method is employed as an efficient solution to the joint formulation. In each iteration, it alternately learns the subspace structure and the dictionary by improving the learning results.

The main contributions of our work are summarized as follows:

- We present a joint subspace and dictionary learning framework for VFR. Unlike the partition-then-learn framework, our approach implicitly learns the subspace segmentation along with a global dictionary simultaneously. The video-dictionaries are compact and compliant to the subspace structure of the data, meaning the more dynamic videos with larger variation are automatically assigned more dictionary atoms than the more static videos.
- Our model is robust to variation and frame-wise corruption. Since we model the same face under various poses and illumination as data points lying in multiple subspaces, it allows our model to handle data with large variation. Moreover, by minimizing the $l_{2,1}$ norm of the reconstruction error matrix, we essentially fuse the frame-wise results together while tolerating corruption and outliers, making our model robust.
- Experiments shows that our method not only achieves the best recognition performances on three standard databases, but also yields interpretable low-rank representations and more natural dictionaries.

1.1 Related Work

There are a couple of recent works focusing on subspace recovery [21–24]. One of the related models to our work is [21]. Liu et al. proposed a low-rank minimization framework to recover the subspace structures in the presence of noise, outliers, and corruption. The main interest of those works, however, is to analyze the subspace structures of a given set of observation points without considering how it generalizes to unseen data. For that reason, [21] first constructs a dictionary, and keeps it unchanged throughout the process. On the contrary, our model is designed for classification purpose and therefore the generative power is important. We *learn* a set of dictionaries that best represent the observation points. The recovery of the subspace structures in our model facilitates the dictionary learning and enhances the representation.

2 Preliminaries

2.1 Subspace Learning via Low-Rank Minimization

Suppose we have a set of corrupted data points (in columns), $X = [x_1, x_2, \ldots, x_n]$, drawn from a union of multiple subspaces $\mathcal{S}_1, \ldots, \mathcal{S}_k$. We wish to decompose the data matrix as the sum of a clean, self-expressive, and low-rank matrix plus a matrix of noise or outliers. This can be achieved by solving:

$$Z^* = \arg\min_Z \operatorname{rank}(Z) + \gamma \|E\|_l, \quad \text{s.t. } X = DZ + E \tag{1}$$

where D is a pre-defined dictionary that linearly spans the entire data space, and Z is the representation with respect to D. The optimal solution is then used for estimating the lowest-rank recovery of the corrupted data DZ^{*1}. With replacement of the rank function with the nuclear norm, the problem becomes a convex optimization and can be solved by the Augmented Lagrange Multiplier (ALM) algorithm, also known as an alternating direction method:

$$Z^* = \arg \min_Z \ \|Z\|_* + \gamma \|E\|_l, \quad \text{s.t. } X = DZ + E \tag{2}$$

Depending on the error types in different applications, one can choose:

- $l = 0$ to model element-wise sparse error. As minimizing the l_0 norm is NP hard, the l_1 norm is often employed as a good relaxation, which is defined by $\|E\|_1 := \sum_{i,j} |[E]_{i,j}|$.
- $l = 2$ to model Gaussian noise (white noise). $\|E\|_2 := \sqrt{\sum_{i,j} |E_{i,j}|^2}$.
- $l = 2, 1$ to model sample-wise sparse error. This is suitable when outliers and corruption exist. $\|E\|_{2,1} := \sum_i \|[E]_{:,i}\|_2$.

In most of the literature, the dictionary D in (2) is pre-defined. In particular, by setting $D = X$, one essentially assumes that any data point (column of X) can be represented by a linear combination (with the coefficients given by columns of Z) of all the other points in the same subspace. Columns of Z thereby are considered as new representations of the original points [21].

Low-rank minimization and subspace structure recovery have been successfully used in applications such as data clustering, image denoising, saliency detection, and recognition and classification. In particular, for recognition and classification where the dataset contains multiple subjects, samples of one subject are considered to be drawn from the same linear subspace, while samples of different subjects are drawn from different linear subspaces. However, for video-based face recognition, it is beneficial to consider a nonlinear subspace or multiple linear subspaces for one subject because of large appearance variations [4,5,14,15].

2.2 Dictionary Learning for Sparse Representation

Suppose we have the original training data $X = [X_1, X_2, \ldots, X_c]$, where X_i is the data from the ith class. We wish to learn a set of bases D_i, called "dictionaries", such that the projection of X_i to the bases is "sparse", i.e.

$$\min_{D_i, Z_i} \|X_i - D_i Z_i\|_F^2, \quad \text{s.t. } \|z_j\| \leq T_0, \forall j = 1, \ldots, n_i \tag{3}$$

where $Z_i = [z_1, z_2, \ldots, z_{n_i}]$ is the sparse representation of the original data X_i with respect to D_i. T_0 is the sparsity constant which specifies the maximum number of nonzero elements.

The standard solution to (3) alternates between sparse coding and dictionary learning. There are many off-the-shelf algorithms to find the sparse codes

---

[1] Here and for the rest of the paper, a variable with a superscript * denotes the optimal solution. One should not confuse the notation with the symbol of Hermitian transpose.

for a given dictionary, such as Orthogonal Matching Pursuit (OMP), coordinate descent, first-order/proximal methods, etc. Conversely, given the sparse representation, one can derive the optimal dictionary by finding the least-square-based closed form solution, or adopt the popular K-SVD algorithm [25] for its computational efficiency.

3   Joint Discriminative Dictionary Learning and Subspace Structure Recovery for Videos

3.1   Problem Formulation

Suppose we have a set of cropped faces from the training videos (gallery) for N people. Denote the face sequence of person i as $X_i = [x_1^{[i]}, \ldots, x_{n_i}^{[i]}]$, where $x_j^{[i]}$ is a column feature vector that describes the jth face in the sequence for person i. Due to facial expression, pose, and illumination changes, we assume that $x_j^{[i]}, j = 1, \ldots, n_i$ are noisy data points drawn from a union of an unknown number of subspaces. The objective is to learn a dictionary D_i that: (1) is good for reconstruction; (2) yields a new representation Z_i, which has low rank and reveals the multiple subspace structure of the "clean" data. This can be formulated as the following optimization problem:

$$< D_i, Z_i > = \arg \min_{D_i, Z_i} \|Z_i\|_* + \lambda \|E_i\|_{2,1} + \eta \|D_i\|_F^2,$$

$$\text{s.t. } X_i = D_i Z_i + E_i, \quad \text{for all } i. \tag{4}$$

The first term is the low-rank requirement. The second one, which is the $l_{2,1}$ norm of the reconstruction error, encourages accurate reconstruction while tolerating sample-specific corruption such as occlusion and outliers. The choice of the trade-off parameter λ depends on the nature of the data. For example, if the person's face in a video appears to be fairly still (with small changes in pose and expression) and switches to another still pose very quickly, then that means that the data points are lying in the subspaces with few outliers, therefore the low-rank constraint should be relaxed and the dictionary should aim to achieve better reconstruction. Conversely, if the person's facial expression or pose changes gradually over time with no obvious cutoff, then the low-rank constraint should be emphasized more so it allows the dictionary to capture key features. The third term is the regularization.

3.2   Optimization

For the rest of this section, the class index i is dropped for convenience. Following the standard procedures of the Augmented Lagrangian Multiplier method, we introduce auxiliary variables J, Y_1, Y_2 and μ. The optimization problem above becomes:

$$\min_{D, Z, E, J} \|J\|_* + \lambda \|E\|_{2,1} + \eta \|D\|_F^2, \text{s.t.} X = DZ + E, Z = J \tag{5}$$

Algorithm 1. Video-based face recognition by JLDSS

Input: $X_1, X_2, \ldots, X_C$, Y, λ, and η
Output: Recognition p
Initialization:
    Initialize D_i by finding the first d principle components on columns of X_i.
Training:
for i=1:C **do**
    Learn D_i and Z_i by Algorithm 2 (JLDSS), given X_i, D_i, λ, and η.
end for
    $D = [D_1|D_2|\ldots|D_C]$
Testing:
    Find Z_y in (12) by Algorithm 2 without updating D, given Y, D, and λ.
    Recognize p given by equation (13).

---

with the Lagrangian function given by

$$\mathcal{L}(D, Z, J, E, Y_1, Y_2, \mu) = \|J\|_* + \lambda\|E\|_{2,1} + \eta\|D\|_F^2$$
$$+ \langle Y_1, X - DZ - E \rangle + \langle Y_2, Z - J \rangle$$
$$+ \frac{\mu}{2} \left(\|X - DZ - E\|_F^2 + \|Z - J\|_F^2 \right) \qquad (6)$$

where $\langle A, B \rangle = trace(A^T B)$. This problem can be optimized in an alternating way described as follows. In each iteration, it first solves for Z with D fixed, and then solves for D with Z fixed. Repeat until the convergence is achieved.

Solve for Z. With D fixed, (5) becomes a typical low-rank minimization problem with auxiliary variable J:

$$\min_{Z,J,E} \|J\|_* + \lambda\|E\|_{2,1}, \text{s.t.} X = DZ + E, Z = J \qquad (7)$$

with solutions given by,

$$J^* = \arg\min_J \frac{1}{\mu}\|J\|_* + \frac{1}{2}\|J - (Z + Y_2/\mu)\|_F^2 \qquad (8)$$

$$Z^* = (I + D^T D)^{-1} \left(D^T(X - E) + J + (D^T Y_1 - Y_2)/\mu \right) \qquad (9)$$

$$E^* = \arg\min \frac{\lambda}{\mu}\|E\|_{2,1} + \frac{1}{2}\|E - (X - DZ + Y_1/\mu)\|_F^2 \qquad (10)$$

Details of derivation are provided in the supplemented material.

Solve for D. Once we have updated Z, J, and E, the Lagrangian function (6) becomes a quadratic function of D. Finding the solution to $\nabla_D \mathcal{L}(D; Z, J, E, Y_1, Y_2, \mu) = 0$ is equivalent to:

$$\min_D \left\{ \eta\|D_i\|_F^2 + \langle Y_1, X - DZ - E \rangle + \frac{\mu}{2}\|X - DZ - E\|_F^2 \right\} \qquad (11)$$

which has a closed form solution: $(D^*)^T = \left(\frac{2\eta}{\mu}I + ZZ^T \right)^{-1} Z \left((X - E) + \frac{Y_1}{\mu} \right)^T$.
See the supplemented material for derivation.

The advantage of our method is that for each class, it seeks a solution for D and Z simultaneously without conducting explicit subspace clustering. Yet if one wants to, one can easily find the subspace structure by performing spectral clustering on Z [21]. The typical matrices are displayed in Fig. 2(d) and (e). It clearly shows that the video contains 3 distinct poses or illumination conditions.

We describe the complete algorithm in Algorithm 1.

Algorithm 2. JLDSS: Jointly Learning Dictionary and Subspace Structure

---

Input: X, D_0, λ, and η
Output: D and Z
Initialization:
$Z = J = 0, D = D_0, E = 0, Y_1 = 0, Y_2 = 0, \mu = 10^{-6}, \mu_{max} = 10^6, \rho = 1.1$, and $tol = 10^{-6}$
while not converge **do**
Update $J \leftarrow J^*$, where

$$J^* = \arg\min_J \frac{1}{\mu}\|J\|_* + \frac{1}{2}\|J - (Z + Y_2/\mu)\|_F^2$$

Update $Z \leftarrow Z^*$, where

$$Z^* = (I + D^T D)^{-1}\left(D^T(X - E) + J + (D^T Y_1 - Y_2)/\mu\right)$$

Update $E \leftarrow E^*$, where

$$E^* = \arg\min \frac{\lambda}{\mu}\|E\|_{2,1} + \frac{1}{2}\|E - (X - DZ + Y_1/\mu)\|_F^2$$

(For recognition, skip this step) Update the dictionary $D \leftarrow D^*$, where

$$(D^*)^T = \left(\frac{2\eta}{\mu}I + ZZ^T\right)^{-1} Z\left((X - E) + \frac{Y_1}{\mu}\right)^T$$

Update the parameter $\mu \leftarrow \min(\rho\mu, \mu_{max})$
Update the multipliers

$$Y_1 \leftarrow Y_1 + \mu(X - DZ - E), \quad Y_2 \leftarrow Y_2 + \mu(Z - J)$$

Check the convergence conditions: $\|X - DZ - E\|_\infty < tol$ and $\|Z - J\|_\infty < tol$.
end while

3.3 Recognition

Once we obtain the class-specific dictionaries $D_1, D_2, \ldots, D_C$, the global dictionary is the concatenation, i.e. $D = [D_1|D_2|\ldots|D_C]$. Denote the test sequence (query) of a face as Y. We assume all the faces belong to a single subject to be recognized. The low-rank representation is given by:

$$Z_y = \arg\min_{Z_y} \|Z\|_* + \lambda\|E_y\|_{2,1}, \quad \text{s.t. } Y = DZ_y + E_y \tag{12}$$

Suppose we have d dictionary atoms for each class-specific dictionary. The first d rows of Z_y correspond to the dictionary of the 1st class; the second d rows, or the $(d+1)$-th to the $2d$-th rows, of Z_y correspond to the dictionary of the 2nd class; and so on. Denote the k-th d rows of Z_y as $Z_{y,k}$. Choose the subject $p*$ with the best reconstruction given by D_k and $Z_{y,k}$ as our recognition decision:

$$p* = \arg \min_{k \in 1,\ldots,C} \|Y - D_k Z_{y,k}\|_{2,1} \tag{13}$$

4   Experiments

We evaluated the proposed method on three data sets for video-based face recognition: Honda/UCSD video database [12], the CMU Motion of Body (MoBo) database [26], and the more challenging YouTube Celebrities Face Tracking and Recognition dataset [11].

4.1   Comparison Methods

The methods we compare ours against include:

- A linear subspace method: discriminative canonical correlations (DCC) [14];
- A nonlinear manifold method: manifold discriminant analysis (MDA) [15];
- An affine subspace method: sparse approximated nearest point (SANP) [1];
- A covariance-on-manifold method: covariance discriminative learning (Cov+ PLS) [2];
- A manifold alignment method: image sets alignment (ImgSetsAlign) [3];
- A dictionary based method: sparse representation for video (SRV) and its kernelized version KSRV [5]. The higher recognition rates between the two versions are adopted for comparison, which we denote as (K)SRV.

We compare our method especially to the dictionary-based method (K)SRV to show the effect of learning subspace structure with the dictionary without performing video partitioning. The recognition rates for other competing methods are cited directly from their papers, except for (K)SRV in Honda/UCSD, because [5] had a slightly different setting.

4.2   Experimental Set-Up

For all experiments, we extracted face sequences by a cascaded face detector [27], and resized them to 20*20 gray images (30*30 for YouTube Celebrities database). The feature vectors are simply the vectorized faces with histogram equalization for reducing lighting effects. We also doubled the size of the gallery by adding the mirror-symmetric faces. This avoids the tendency of assigning unknown profile faces to the one with similar poses in the gallery.

Honda/UCSD Database. There are 59 videos for 20 people in a wide range of different poses in Honda/UCSD database. Each person has at least 2 videos.

We randomly selected 1 video as training and tested on the rest, and repeated for 10 times. To follow the procedures in [1], we tested four cases of maximum set length: 50, 100, and full length. Note that for 50/100 maximum length, we tested on the first 50/100 frame as an standard setting, as well as on randomly selected 50/100 frames as in [5] for fair comparison. With the randomly chosen frames, we achieved 100 % accuracy for both 50 frames case and 100 frames case. The average recognition rates over 10 trials under the standard setting are reported in Table 1. Our rates are obtained by setting the dictionary size $d = 10$. Performance is not sensitive to the choices of λ and η. We outperform all other methods in all settings.

CMU MoBo Database. The CMU MoBo contains 96 sequences of 24 subjects, each of which has 4 sequences (roughly 300 frames each) captured in different walking situations. We performed 10-fold cross validation where 1 video was randomly chosen as training and the remaining 3 for testing. The average recognition rate is shown in Table 1. For our method, we set $d = 20, \lambda = 0.1,$ and $\eta = 0.01$. For (K)SRV, we set the number of partitions $K = 3$. The dictionary size for each subject is $d = 7 * 3$ (7 for each partition), which is comparable to 20 in our method. Again we achieved the best performance among all.

YouTube Celebrities. The YouTube Celebrities contains 1910 video clips of 47 human subjects from YouTube. Roughly 41 clips were segmented from 3 unique videos for each person. This dataset is challenging because it contains a lot of noise and facial variations (see Fig. 2(a)). Following the standard setup, we selected 3 training clips, 1 from each unique video, and 6 test clips, 2 from each unique video, per person. The performance of all methods is summarized in Table 1. Our rates are obtained by setting $d = 30, \lambda = 0.1,$ and $\eta = 0.001$.

To the best of our knowledge, the top performance levels on this dataset are reported as 80.75 % in [7], 78.9 % in [6], and 74.6 % in [3]. However, their experiments employed different protocols from the standard one. [7] not only benefits from its own tracker, which gives 92 % success rate versus 80 % using the standard tracker, but also takes advantage of sophisticated features including LBP, HOG and Gabor wavelets. Other methods only use 30*30 vectorized faces as features. [6] only tested on the videos of the first 29 celebrities out of 47, which makes the task easier than the standard one. Recognition rates are of course higher when a smaller number of subjects are included. In addition to the 3 training clips for each subject in the gallery, [3] uses one more sequence from any subject as a reference for alignment. This gives their method an advantage of seeing more faces in the gallery. We also noticed that [3] reported higher recognition rates than the literature for the competing methods that we also used for comparison: DCC: 0.673 in [3] vs 0.648 in [2], and MDA: 0.676 [3] vs 0.653 [16], suggesting a systematic bias might exist. Under the standard settings, our performance is the best, and it could be further improved with better tracking and advanced features.

4.3   Analysis and Discussions

As seen in Table 1, we consistently outperformed other competing methods in all datasets under all settings, especially compared with the other dictionary-based

Table 1. Recognition rates on three databases. We cited the recognition rates of the competing methods from the literature except for (K)SRV. The highest rate in each experiment is highlighted in bold font. In the last row, the number with the superscript * was achieved by employing a different protocol than the standard one.

Dataset		DCC [14]	MDA [16]	SANP [1]	Cov+ PLS [2]	ImgSets Align [3]	(K)SRV [5]	Our method
Honda/ UCSD [12]	50 frames	0.769	0.744	0.846	-	-	0.846±0.02	**0.872±0.01**
	100 frames	0.846	0.949	0.923	-	-	0.964±0.02	**0.974±0.01**
	full length	0.949	0.974	**1.000**	**1.000**	0.989	0.974±0.01	**1.000**
	Average	0.856	0.889	0.923	-	-	0.931±0.01	**0.949±0.01**
CMU MoBo [26]		0.903	0.947	0.900	0.941	0.950	0.952±0.03	**0.968±0.02**
YouTube [11]		0.648	0.653	0.684	0.701	**0.746***	0.684±0.03	0.723±0.03

method [5]. We take the video clips for one subject from YouTube Celebrities as an example to further demonstrate the benefit of jointly learning a dictionary and subspace structure.

The Effect of λ. The comparison between Fig. 2(b) and (c) shows the effect of the choice of λ, which is the trade-off between low-rank and reconstruction accuracy. When λ is small, we assume the data is more uniform, thus the dictionary atoms from the same subspace look very similar to each other in Fig. 2(b).The faces which look different from the dictionary atoms are considered as outliers. When λ is large, we assume the data contains large variations and therefore put more emphasis on the reconstruction accuracy. As a result, the dictionary contains faces with more variety as shown in Fig. 2(c). The corresponding low-rank representations also reflect the impact of choosing different λ, where the columns of the matrix in Fig. 2(d) look quite similar to each other while the columns in Fig. 2(e) are much more diverse. However, the subspace segmentation results are the same.

Low-rank Matrix Interpretation. Figure 2(d) and (e) show a typical low-rank representation of original faces from training videos constructed by our method, which has a block diagonal structure indicating the subspace structure of the data. The brightness indicates the value of each entry, where the darkest entries are zeros. Looking at the columns, one can easily construct a similarity matrix and apply spectral clustering to it if explicit segmentation is desired. Furthermore, since each row of the matrix corresponds to the coefficients of a particular dictionary atom, the row structure also reflects the structure of the dictionary. A skinny and tall block in the low-rank matrix suggests a relatively short clip with large variation, so that it requires many dictionary atoms to represent it, whereas a fat and short block indicates a long clip with little variation so that only a small number of dictionary atoms are needed.

Dictionary Comparison. Figure 2(a) shows the sequence of cropped faces from our training clips, where the red line shows the true partition of the

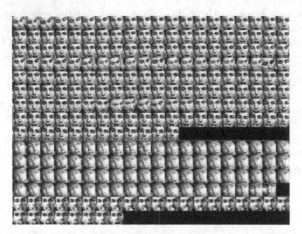

(a) A sequence of cropped faces from 3 training videos

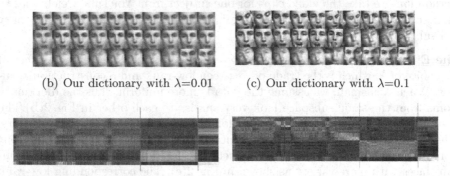

(b) Our dictionary with λ=0.01   (c) Our dictionary with λ=0.1

(d) The low-rank matrix with λ=0.01   (e) The low-rank matrix with λ=0.1

Fig. 2. An example of the training faces from YouTube Celebrities database (a), the dictionaries (b) (c), and the low-rank representations (d) (e).

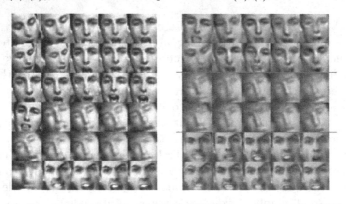

(a) Our dictionary with λ=0.1 (b) Dictionary learned by SRV

Fig. 3. Dictionary comparison of our method and SRV [5] using the true video partitions. The red dashed lines separate the partition-level sub-dictionaries (Color figure online).

sequence that is used in our implementation of [5]. The dictionaries learned by both methods with $d = 30$ are shown in Fig. 3. It clearly shows the limitations of the partition-level dictionaries. First, [5] assigns the same number of dictionary atoms regardless of the length and variation present in each clip. The first clip obviously contains much larger variation than the second clip. As a result, the first 10 dictionary faces learned by SRV [5] are blurry, indicating the dictionary is not big enough to capture the variation, while the second 10 dictionary faces are more or less uniform, indicating 10 atoms are more than necessary. Increasing the size of dictionary or the number of partitions might help, but with bigger dictionaries the computational cost will increase dramatically, especially in the testing stage when partition-level decisions need to be made. In addition, SRV suffers from the unknown length of each partition. In such situations where the shortest partition contains fewer frames than the size of sub-dictionary, artificial frames need to be inserted to obtain an augmented partition. In contrast, our method enjoys the flexibility of no explicit partitioning, so that the dictionary reflects the distribution of the training data.

5   Conclusion and Future Work

We introduced a novel joint learning framework for video-based face recognition. We modeled the set of faces as a union of multiple subspaces, and attempted to find a global dictionary that reveals the subspace structure. To achieve this goal, we proposed an objective function that encourages low-rank representation and reduces reconstruction error. We explained how our optimization problem can be solved with an alternating minimization algorithm. Finally, we conducted experiments on three data sets which resulted in the state-of-the-art performance. Future work to achieve better VFR includes running the face tracker and identifying the faces online, incorporate alignment with recognition, and developing a more effective down-sampling method that resizes the tracked face images to smaller size but preserves discriminative information.

Acknowledgement. This work was supported by the Army Research Office MURI Grant W911NF-09-1-0383. We also thank Dr. Ruiping Wang for sharing the processed data.

References

1. Hu, Y., Mian, A., Owens, R.: Sparse approximated nearest points for image classification. In: Proceedings of IEEE Conference on Computer Vision and Pattern Recognition (2011)
2. Wang, R., Guo, H., Davis, L., Dai, Q.: Covariance discriminative learning: a natural and efficient approach to image set classification. In: Proceedings of IEEE Conference on Computer Vision and Pattern Recognition (2012)
3. Cui, Z., Zhang, H., Lao, S., Chen, X.: Image sets alignment for video-based face recognition. In: Proceedings of IEEE Conference on Computer Vision and Pattern Recognition (2012)

4. Chen, Y.C., Patel, V., Phillips, P., Chellappa, R.: Dictionary-based face recognition from video. In: Proceedings of European Conference of Computer Vision (2012)
5. Chen, Y.C., Patel, V., Shekhar, S., Chellappa, R., Phillips, P.: Video-based face recognition via joint sparse representation. In: Proceedings of IEEE Conference on Automatic Face and Gesture Recognition (2013)
6. Yang, M., Zhu, P., Zhang, L.: Face recognition based on regularized points between image sets. In: Proceedings of IEEE Conference on Automatic Face and Gesture Recognition (2013)
7. Ortiz, E., Wright, A., Shah, M.: Face recognition in movie trailers via mean sequence spars representation-based classification. In: Proceedings of IEEE Conference on Computer Vision and Pattern Recognition (2013)
8. Shakhnarovich, G., Fisher, J., Darrell, T.: Face recognition from long-term observations. In: Proceedings of European Conference on Computer Vision (2002)
9. Satoh, S.: Conparative evaluation on face sequence matching for content-based video access. In: Proceedings of IEEE Automatic Face and Gesture Recognition (2000)
10. Krüger, V., Zhou, S.: Exemplar-based face recognition from video. In: Heyden, A., Sparr, G., Nielsen, M., Johansen, P. (eds.) ECCV 2002, Part IV. LNCS, vol. 2353, pp. 732–746. Springer, Heidelberg (2002)
11. Kim, M., Kumar, S., Pavlovic, V., Rowley, H.: Face tracking and recognition with visual constraints in real-world videos. In: Proceedings of IEEE Conference on Computer Vision and Pattern Recognition (2008)
12. Lee, K., Ho, J., Yang, M., Kriegman, D.: Visual tracking and recognition using probabilistic appearance manifolds. In: Proceedings of Computer Vision and Image Understanding (2005)
13. Cevikalp, H., Triggs, B.: Face recognition based on image sets. In: Proceedings of IEEE Conference on Computer Vision and Pattern Recognition (2010)
14. Kim, T., Arandjelovic, O., Cipolla, R.: Discriminative learning and recognition of image set classes using canonical correlations. IEEE Trans. Pattern Anal. Mach. Intell. 29, 1005–1018 (2007)
15. Wang, R., Shan, S., Chen, X., Gao, W.: Manifold-manifold distance with application to face recognition based on image set. In: Proceedings of IEEE Conference on Computer Vision and Pattern Recognition (2008)
16. Wang, R., Chen, X.: Manifold discrimininant analysis. In: Proceedings of IEEE Conference on Computer Vision and Pattern Recognition (2009)
17. Chen, S., Sanderson, C., Harandi, M.T., Lovell, B.: Improved image set classification via joint sparse approximated nearest subspaces. In: Proceedings of IEEE Conference on Computer Vision and Pattern Recognition (2013)
18. Huang, Z., Shan, S., Wang, R., Chen, X.: Coupling alignments with recognition for still-to-video face recognition. In: IEEE International Conference on Computer Vision (2013)
19. Lu, J., Wang, G., Moulin, P.: Image set classification using holistic multiple order statistics features and localized multi-kernel metric learning. In: IEEE International Conference on Computer Vision (2013)
20. Wright, J., Yang, A., Ganesh, A., Sastry, S., Ma, Y.: Robust face recognition via sparse representation. IEEE Trans. Pattern Anal. Mach. Intell. 31, 210–227 (2009)
21. Liu, G., Lin, Z., Yu, Y.: Robust subspace segmentation by low-rank representation. In: International Conference on Machine Learning (2010)
22. Elhamifar, E., Vidal, R.: Sparse subspace clustering: algorithm, theory, and applications. IEEE Trans. Pattern Anal. Mach. Intell. 35, 2765–2781 (2013)

23. Favaro, P., Vidal, R., Ravichandran, A.: A closed form solution to robust subspace estimation and clustering. In: Proceedings of IEEE Conference on Computer Vision and Pattern Recognition (2011)
24. He, R., Sun, Z., Tan, T., Zheng, W.S.: Recovery of corrupted low-rank matrices via half-quadratic based non convex minimization. In: Proceedings of IEEE Conference on Computer Vision and Pattern Recognition (2011)
25. Aharon, M., Elad, M., Bruckstein, A.: K-svd: an algorithm for designing over-complete dictionaries for sparse representation. IEEE Trans. Signal Process. **54**, 4311–4322 (2006)
26. Gross, R., Shi, J.: The cmu motion of body (mobo) database. Technical Report CMU-RI-TR-01-18, Robotics Institute, Pittsburgh, PA (2001)
27. Viola, P., Jones, M.: Robust real-time face detection. Int. J. Comput. Vision **57**, 137–154 (2004)

Visual Salience Learning via Low Rank Matrix Recovery

Junxia Li, Jundi Ding, and Jian Yang[✉]

School of Computer Science and Engineering,
Nanjing University of Science and Technology, Nanjing, China
csjyang@njust.edu.cn

Abstract. Detection of salient object regions is useful for many vision tasks. Recently, a variety of saliency detection models have been proposed. They often behave differently over an individual image, and these saliency detection results often complement each other. To make full use of the advantages of the existing saliency detection methods, in this paper, we propose a salience learning model which combines various saliency detection methods such that the aggregation result outperforms each individual one. In our model, we first obtain several saliency maps by different saliency detection methods. The background regions of each saliency map usually lie in a low-dimensional subspace as most of them tend to have lower salience values, while the object regions that deviating from this subspace can be considered as sparse noises. So, an individual saliency map can be represented as a low rank matrix plus a sparse matrix. We aim at learning a unified sparse matrix that represents the salient regions using these obtained individual saliency maps. The sparse matrix can be inferred by conducting low rank matrix recovery using the robust principal component analysis technique. Experiments show that our model consistently outperforms each individual saliency detection approach and state-of-the-art methods.

1 Introduction

Humans have a remarkable ability to effortlessly judge the importance of image pixels or regions in real time, and pay more attention to those important and informative parts. Detection of such salient pixels or regions of an image automatically is an active research area in recent decades. There are two major research directions of visual attention modeling, including eye fixation prediction and salient object detection. The former is to identify a few human fixation locations on natural images, which is helpful for many high-level vision tasks. The later focuses on uniformly highlighting entire salient object regions, thus benefiting wide applications in computer vision like: salient object segmentation [1–3], object based image retrieval [4], content-aware image resizing [5], automatic image cropping [6], and adaptive image compression [7]. In this paper, we focus on the salient object detection.

Although a rich literature has been appeared on image saliency analysis [8–19], a few commonly noticeable and critically influencing issues still endure. They

© Springer International Publishing Switzerland 2015
D. Cremers et al. (Eds.): ACCV 2014, Part III, LNCS 9005, pp. 112–127, 2015.
DOI: 10.1007/978-3-319-16811-1_8

are related to complexity of patterns and behave differently in natural images, since different saliency models are based on variety of theories and techniques. The saliency maps obtained by different methods vary remarkably from each other. Each of them has its advantages and disadvantages. Figure 1 shows a few results from several previous representative salient object detection methods. We can clearly see that each method just works well for some parts of an image. As shown in Fig. 1(b-c), some objects boundaries are well-defined, but most of the salient regions do not stand out. Differently, the detection results shown in Fig. 1(d-f) well highlight most of the object regions, but some background regions are also detected as salient regions shown in white. As shown in the 'Board' image of Fig. 1(d), the trees around the board also stand out simultaneously with the salient board regions. More interestingly, it is observed that these results can complement each other in general. This is mainly because each saliency detection method often captures some aspects of the visual information from different perspectives (*e.g.* local/ global contrast, sparsity or spatial distribution). *This motivates us to combine different saliency maps to get better results. Specifically, for a given image, we can first obtain several saliency maps by different saliency detection methods, and then try to find a way to utilize the advantages of these methods and meanwhile suppress the disadvantages of them, aiming to effectively combine these saliency maps.*

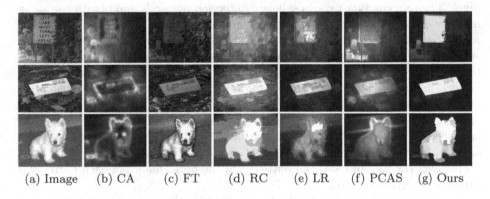

(a) Image   (b) CA   (c) FT   (d) RC   (e) LR   (f) PCAS   (g) Ours

Fig. 1. Visual salience learning. Individual salience maps, such as CA [10], FT [9], RC [11], LR [14], PCAS [19] often complement each other. Visual salience learning can effectively combine their results and perform better than each of them.

Although there are several approaches attempting to integrate different saliency maps to detect saliency [12,13], they might not make use of the advantages and disadvantages of these saliency maps for each input image. A. Borji et al. [12] presented a simple combination model for saliency detection using pre-defined functions. It takes each individual model all equal in the integration process. However, this strategy may not fully capture the advantages of each individual saliency detection method. L. Mai et al. [13] proposed an approach for saliency aggregation using a conditional random field framework. Sometimes, this method can better determine the contribution for each input saliency map in the aggregation, as it considers the performance gaps among different saliency analysis methods. Unfortunately, the cross-information among individual saliency maps is not well utilized in the aggregation process. It is often difficult for such models that are use linear or nonlinear fusion strategy to produce reliable results.

For the saliency maps obtained by various saliency detection methods, if we first segment the original image into many homogeneous sub-regions, the background regions of each saliency map usually lie in a low-dimensional subspace since most of them tend to have the lower salience values shown in black, while the object regions that deviating from this subspace can be represented by a sparse matrix. Inspired by this, we are dedicated to learning a unified sparse matrix that represents the salient regions using these obtained individual saliency maps. And our saliency detection can be cast as a sparse matrix pursuit problem. Our idea differs from the previous saliency detection models which also based on the theory of low-rank-sparsity matrix decomposition [14,20,21] in its motivation. In [14,20,21], the saliency map is inferred by integrating multiple types of features of the given image. However, in their models, for many complex natural images, the assumptions that the background matrix has a low rank and the salient regions correspond to a sparse matrix may not hold.

In our method, we first decompose a given image into many homogeneous sub-regions by an image segmentation technology, each of which is called a super-pixel. Then we conduct various saliency detection methods and obtain the same number of saliency maps. Each saliency map is represented by a vector, where each element of the vector corresponds to the mean of the saliency value of that super-pixel. Arranging these vectors forms a combinational matrix representation of these saliency maps. The sparse matrix indicating the salient regions can be well inferred by conducting low-rank matrix recovery using the robust principal component analysis (RPCA) technique [22]. Since the cross-information among individual saliency maps has been well considered, such a sparsity pursuit scheme can produce more accurate and reliable results than the saliency aggregation models of using simple linear or nonlinear fusing strategy with fixed coefficients [12,13], and also can outperform the performance of each individual saliency detection method.

Compared with existing methods, the contributions of our method mainly include:

- Our proposed approach considers the cross-information among individual saliency detection methods, it performs better than these methods which combine saliency maps through weighted averaging.
- In our proposed approach, the contribution of each saliency map is not equally constant, but learned adaptive to each image.
- Our proposed approach treats the saliency detection as a sparsity pursuit problem based on the theory of low rank matrix recovery. It provides an interesting perspective for visual saliency learning framework.

2   Related Work

To serve as the baseline of our approach, a set of saliency detection methods need to be chosen to produce individual saliency maps. Today, there are many saliency analysis methods based on variety of techniques with interesting performance. In the following we give a review of saliency detection methods that are related to our approach.

The major difference among these saliency detection approaches is the strategy for measure saliency. In recent years, a growing number of saliency detection methods have been proposed. Here, we classify existing saliency object detection models into three categories: contrast based methods, spatial distribution based methods and sparsity based methods. Note that, these three kinds of methods are not completely disjoint, they are interspersed with each other to some extent.

As a pioneer, Itti et al. [23] use center-surround differences across multi-scale image features to detect image saliency. Hereafter, many contrast based models have been proposed to extend this approach, including the fuzzy growth model (MZ) by Ma and Zhang [24], and graph based visual saliency model (GB) by Harel et al. [25]. Later, a method presented by Achanta et al. (AC) [8] which determine salient regions using low level features of color and luminance. Achanta et al. [9] implemented a frequency-tuned method (FT) to define pixel saliency based on the color difference from the average color of entire image. Recently, Margolin et al. [19] use PCA (PCAS) to represent the set of patches of an image and use this representation to determine patch distinctness. Cheng et al. [11] consider the global region contrast differences with respect to the whole image and spatial coherence across the regions to define saliency map (RC). However, since spatial distribution among patches is not formulated, RC cannot well handle images with cluttered and textured backgrounds. To deal with the images which contain small-scale structures, Yan et al. [16] presented a hierarchical saliency model (HS) that infers saliency values from multiple image layers. These contrast based methods have their difficulty in distinguishing among similar saliency cues (e.g. color, structure) in both foreground and background regions. Besides, they generally fail when the images are with large-scale objects.

Spatial distribution based methods are generally built on two common priors which come from the basic rule of photographic composition. The first one is the object prior which considers that salient regions are likely to appear at the center of an image. The second one is the background prior which assumes that the image boundary is mostly background. Based on these two priors there are many saliency detection models have been presented, e.g., graph-based manifold ranking model [32], absorbing markov chain model [17] and dense and sparse reconstruction model [15]. Spatial distribution based models have achieved success in many images, but still have certain limitations. Typically, if the assumption of the object prior or background prior is not hold, it nevertheless provides useful visual information which can be utilized to guide the salience detection.

Sparsity based models are performed under the assumption that in a certain feature space the salient region is sparse compared with the background regions. SR [26] proposed by Hou and Zhang is a typical sparsity based model which measures saliency via spectral residual in the frequency domain. Later, several low-rank-sparsity matrix decomposition theory based models have been proposed, which infer saliency map by integrating multiple types of features of the given image [14,18,20,21].

Although still each year many new saliency models are introduced, there is a large gap between models and human performance in detecting salient object regions in free-viewing of natural scenes. It is nice to see that these models often vary over an individual image and complement each other. In our model, we choose newly published methods HS [16], PCAS [19], GC [31], DS [15], AMC [17], GBMR [32] and SLR [18] to produce individual saliency maps for our saliency aggregation. Note that as more and more saliency detection models have been developed recently, more existing and forthcoming saliency models can also used in our individual initial saliency maps production.

It should be noted that the idea of employing the low-rank matrix recovery for saliency detection is not new [14,21]. In [21], an image is partitioned into non-overlapping patches of size $p \times q$ pixels, each of which is represented by a feature vector. These feature vectors are then arranged to form a multiple-feature matrix for low rank matrix recovery. However, when the object of the image is not small enough, the noises expected to indicate saliency will no longer be sparse. This violates the underlying assumption of the model. Different from this method, the approach proposed in [14] represents the image in another way. It incorporated image segmentation into the saliency detection and partitioned an image into many small regions after multi-scale feature extraction. To ensure the validity of the low rank recovery model, they modulated the image features with a learnt transform matrix. However, the learnt transform matrix is somewhat biased toward the training data set, it suffers from limited adaptability.

Differing from these approaches, we select various saliency maps to form a matrix for low rank matrix recovery. After the over-segmentation, the input image is divided into many regions. Thus, for each saliency map, the corresponding background regions can be represented by a low rank matrix, and the salient regions can be indicated by a sparse matrix. We use the matrix combined by various saliency maps to conduct the low rank recovery. By this way, our model can adaptively make use of the advantages of individual saliency maps and yield a satisfactory result even without higher-level prior.

3   Salience Learning by Low Rank Affinity Pursuit

Our method starts from running a set of d saliency detection methods on a given image $\mathbf{I}$, and produces d saliency maps, $\{S_k || 1 \leq k \leq d\}$, one for each method. Each element $S_k(p)$ in a saliency map is the salience value of the pixel p. In each saliency map, the values of pixels are represented in gray and normalized in the range $[0, 1]$. Our goal is to take these d salience maps as original input and learn a final salience map S. In this section, we describe details of our learning model of salience maps aggregation.

3.1   Problem Formulation

In this subsection, we will describe the formulation of our problem in detail. And Fig. 2 gives an illustration for easy understanding of our procedure.

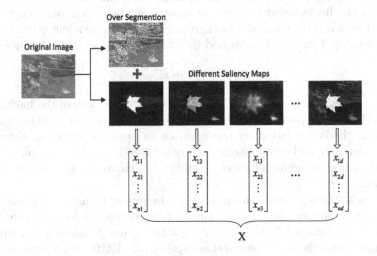

Fig. 2. Illustration of our problem formulation.

In order to get an effective representation for a saliency map, we use super-pixels other than image pixels or patches with the same size as basic image elements. We choose mean-shift clustering [27] to produce our required image segmentation. Each sub-region is called a super-pixel. With suitable parameters selection, the image background also contains multiple super-pixels even if it is visually homogeneous. See the first row of Fig. 2 for an example, the original is divided into a set of super-pixels $\{P_i\}_{i=1,\ldots,n}$, where n is the number of super-pixels. Combining the over-segmentation result, saliency map S_k can be represented by a n-dimensional vector $X_k = [x_{1k}, x_{2k}, \ldots, x_{nk}]^T$, the $i-th$ element of the vector corresponds to the mean of the saliency values of super-pixel P_i. By arranging these vectors into a matrix, we get the combinational matrix representation of all the saliency maps $\mathbf{X} = [X_1, X_2, \ldots, X_d]$. $\mathbf{X} \in R^{n \times d}$, where each X_i corresponds to the $i-th$ saliency map, d denotes the number of saliency maps. Then, our goal is to find an assignment function $S(P_i) \in [0, 1]$. Function $S(P_i)$ is referred to as the final saliency map, where the value of $S(P_i)$ represents the probability of super-pixel P_i belonging to the salient objects.

3.2   Saliency Aggregation Using Robust PCA

Our task described by the above formulation is to find a criterion for measuring and detecting the final saliency which can effectively utilize the advantages of individual saliency methods and meanwhile suppress the disadvantages of them.

For the previous saliency detection methods, the term "sparsity" is an important perspective for detecting salient objects. It is in essence similar to the contrast (another point of view for saliency), since the pixels or regions different from their surroundings usually receive higher response on contrast-based features (*e.g.*, color or texture). From this perspective, the salient regions are different from the background regions are mostly sparse. Then, an image can be considered as a combination of a background part with a salient part. In other words, the image $\mathbf{I}$ can be decomposed into two parts in a certain feature space:

$$\emptyset(\mathbf{I}) = \mathbf{A} + \mathbf{E}, \tag{1}$$

where $\emptyset$ is a feature transformation, $\mathbf{A}$ and $\mathbf{E}$ denote matrices of the background part and the salient part, respectively. Although most of the existing saliency detection methods are based on the contrast or sparsity criterion, they often perform differently and complement each other (see Fig. 1 for example). Therefore, we design a 'powerful alliances' strategy to achieve a satisfactory saliency aggregation.

Since each saliency detection method is a nonlinear transformation from the given image to the saliency map, then $\mathbf{X}$ can be treated as a feature representation of the image $\mathbf{I}$ in the saliency feature space (to distinguish this new feature space from the traditional feature space, *e.g.*, RGB color space, we called the feature space composed by various saliency maps as saliency feature space). Naturally, Eq. 1 can be rewritten as:

$$\mathbf{X} = \mathbf{A} + \mathbf{E}, \tag{2}$$

Equation 2 is a severely under-constrained problem. Theoretically speaking, it is almost impossible to find $\mathbf{A}$ and $\mathbf{E}$ without any restrictions information. In other words, without imposing any restrictions to Eq. 2, there are an infinite number of solutions with regard to $\mathbf{A}$ and $\mathbf{E}$. To seek a suitable solution that is benefit for our saliency detection, some criteria for characterizing matrices $\mathbf{A}$ and $\mathbf{E}$ are needed. To this end, we here consider two basic principles. On the one hand, the background regions usually lie in a low dimensional subspace so that they can be represented as a low rank matrix. This suggests that matrix $\mathbf{A}$ may have the property of low rankness. On the other hand, in a saliency map, only a small portion of superpixels are salient regions even when the object size is large, since salient objects usually have characteristic and spatial coherence. So, we can regard the salient regions that are deviate from the low dimensional subspace as noises or errors, *i.e.*, matrix $\mathbf{E}$ is sparse. The relation between low-rank-sparsity and saliency is consistent with the fact that only the distinctive sensory information is selected for further processing in a human vision system. In summary, we incorporate two criteria to solve the Eq. 2, *i.e.*, the low rank constraint for the background regions and the sparsity constraint for the salient regions. Therefore, the saliency detection can be cast as a sparse matrix recovery problem. Fortunately, the recently established robust principle component analysis (RPCA) technique [22] may fit well to the saliency detection problem. For matrix $\mathbf{X} = [X_1, X_2, \ldots, X_d]$ with each column representing a corresponding saliency detection method, RPCA is appropriate to efficiently and exactly recover the sparse matrix $\mathbf{E}$ by solving a tractable optimization problem:

$$\min_{\mathbf{A},\mathbf{E}} ||\mathbf{A}||_* + \lambda ||\mathbf{E}||_1$$

$$s.t. \mathbf{X} = \mathbf{A} + \mathbf{E} \tag{3}$$

where $||\cdot||_*$ denotes the nuclear norm (sum of the singular values of a matrix), $||\cdot||_1$ is the ℓ_1-norm and parameter $\lambda > 0$ balances the effects between rank and sparsity. In our implementation, we set $\lambda = 0.06$. Note that, problem (3) is a convex optimization problem. Recent theoretic analysis indicates that there are various algorithms can be used to recover the sparse matrix $\mathbf{E}$ in high probability [22, 28]. Here, we apply the exact ALM method [28] to extract the sparse matrix $\mathbf{E}$.

As the minimization of the ℓ_1-norm encourages the columns of $\mathbf{E}$ to be zero, *i.e.*, the columns of $\mathbf{E}$ are sparse, it fits well to our visual saliency learning problem. Naturally, the sparse matrix $\mathbf{E}$ measures the contribution of each individual saliency method and detects satisfactory visual saliency. For a row corresponding to the $i - th$ super-pixel, larger element implies that the corresponding saliency detection method made a greater contribution in terms of aggregation. That is, in the saliency aggregation process, our model learned a set of combinational coefficents for each super-pixel rather than simply combining the saliency responses through weighted averaging.

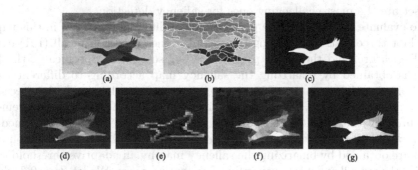

Fig. 3. Illustration on our saliency learning. (a) input image, (b) over-segmentation result by mean-shift, (c) ground truth, (d) saliency aggregation result using predefined function [12], (e) sparse coding result [20], which only highlights some edges, (f) detected saliency by LR [14] without high-level prior interaction, better than (e), but has some high saliency values in the background, (g) saliency by our model, which is better than others.

Let $\mathbf{E}^*$ be the optimal solution (with respect to $\mathbf{E}$) to optimization problem (3). To obtain a saliency value for the super-pixel P_i, we only need a following step to quantify the response of the obtained sparse matrix $\mathbf{E}^*$:

$$S(P_i) = ||\mathbf{E}^*(i,:)||_1 = \sum_{j=1}^{d} |\mathbf{E}^*(i,j)| \tag{4}$$

Here, $\|\mathbf{E}^*(i,:)\|_1$ is the ℓ_1-norm of the $i-th$ row of $\mathbf{E}^*$. Larger (smaller) magnitude of $S(P_i)$ implies that the super-pixel P_i is more salient (non-salient), then we assign a higher (lower) value to it. In this way, the final saliency map is accordingly generated. Figure 3(g) presents our saliency aggregation result and shows that our model outperforms others.

4   Experiments

4.1   Experimental Setup

Data Sets and Evaluation Metrics. In order to comprehensively evaluate the performance of our proposed method, we conducted extensive experiments on four benchmark datasets. The first one is ASD dataset provided by Achanta et al. [9], which contains 1000 images with accurate human-marked labels for salient objects. The second one is the SED1 dataset [29] with 100 images of a single salient object. The third one is the SED2 dataset [29] which contains 100 images of two salient objects. Both SED1 and SED2 are with ground truths labeled by three different users. The SOD dataset [30] contains 300 images, which is based on Berkeley segmentation dataset. The fifth one is the PASCAL-1500 dataset [18] in which many images contain multiple objects with various locations and scales, and highly cluttered background. This dataset is first used for image segmentation evaluation [33]. Both SOD dataset and PASCAL-1500 dataset are the most challenging ones for saliency detection.

To evaluate the quantitative performance of different methods, in this paper we adopt three metrics including two popular ones precision recall (PR) curve and F-measure, and the newly presented VOC score [34]. Specifically, the PR curve is obtained by binarizing the saliency map according to different fixed thresholds ranging from 0 to 255. At each value of the threshold, the precision and recall are computed. The F-measure is the overall performance measurement computed by the weighted harmonic of precision and recall, which defined as $F = ((\beta^2 + 1)P * R)/(\beta^2 P + R)$ (P = precision, R = recall). Here, precision and recall are obtained by binarizing the saliency map by an adaptive threshold that is twice the overall mean saliency value of the entire image. We set $\beta^2 = 0.3$ which is the same as in [9,11,14]. The VOC score is defined as $VOC = (S \cap G)/(S \cup G)$, where S is the object segmentation result obtained by binarizing the saliency map using the same adaptive threshold as in the computation of F-measure, and G is the ground-truth.

4.2   Quantitative Evaluations

We first compared the performance of our method with seven used individual saliency detection methods, i.e., DS [15], AMC [17], GBMR [32], SLR [18], HS [16], PCAS [19] and GC [31]. In addition, we also compared our method with other five classical approaches, including FT [9], HC [11], LC [35] RC [11] and SR [26]. Most of them were presented recently or have a high citation rate. Note that,

SLR is the extension of the LR [14] which also uses idea of employing the low-rank matrix recovery for saliency detection, so here we are no longer report the results of LR. And, theoretically, a comparison with the related approach, namely the saliency aggregation method proposed by L. Mai et al. [13] is necessary. However, we could not find the authors' implementation.

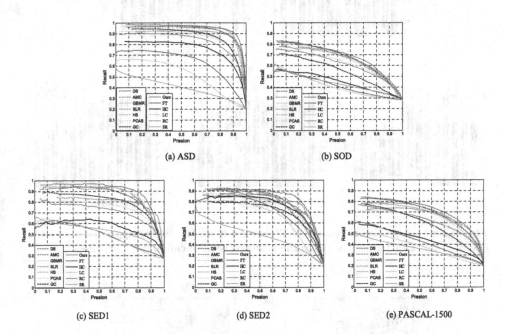

(a) ASD   (b) SOD

(c) SED1   (d) SED2   (e) PASCAL-1500

Fig. 4. Precision recall curves of all the twelve methods on the five datasets. Clearly, our approach obtains a better PR performance than the other approaches.

Figure 4 shows the PR carves with fixed thresholds of all the above methods on the five datasets, which demonstrate that our method achieves the consistent and favorable performance against the other competing approaches. From the Fig. 5, it is observed that our proposed approach achieves the best F-measure performance. Further, Fig. 6 presents the corresponding VOC scores of all the twelve approaches. It can be seen from the bar graphs, our model obtains the highest VOC scores over the five datasets. Overall, our approach consistency outperforms each individual saliency detection approach and state-of-the-art methods.

4.3 Visual Comparison

Figure 7 presents some results of our method with the seven selected individual saliency detection methods. All of these images are from the four datasets ASD, SOD, SED1, SED2. Visually, these images are simple, however, most of them are with cluttered object or background. In the individual saliency maps, some

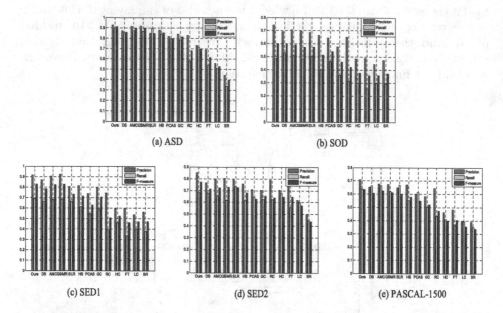

Fig. 5. Average precision, recall and F-measure of all the twelve approaches over the five datasets. Our method achieves the best precision, recall and F-measure.

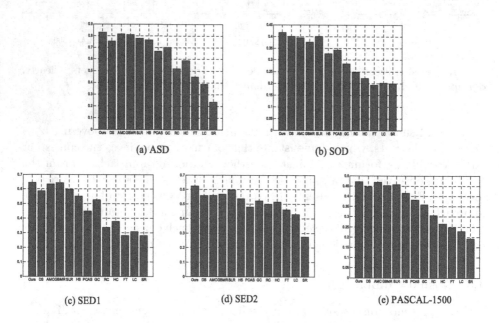

Fig. 6. Quantitative VOC performance of all the twelve methods on the five datasets. Our approach achieves the highest VOC scores over the five datasets.

salient regions are not pop not from the background, especially for the images which come from the SED2 dataset. And, the results shown in Fig. 7(h), some parts of background pixels or regions also stand out simultaneously with the object regions. Compared with the ground truth shown in Fig. 7(j), we can clearly see that our approach consistently outperforms each individual saliency detection method. This confirms that our model can effectively integrate the results of these methods. More comparison results on the PASCAL-1500 dataset are shown in Fig. 8.

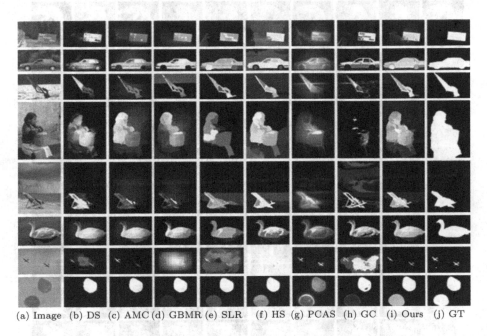

(a) Image (b) DS   (c) AMC (d) GBMR (e) SLR   (f) HS (g) PCAS (h) GC   (i) Ours   (j) GT

Fig. 7. Examples of saliency learning on the four datasets: ASD (rows 1–2), SOD (rows 3–4), SED1 (rows 5–6), and SED2 (rows 7–8). Given an input image (a), we conduct some saliency detection methods and obtain corresponding individual saliency maps (b)-(h), (i) shows the saliency map produced by our model. Compared with the ground truth (j), our model achieved best performance visually.

In addition, some saliency maps of the evaluated methods are shown in Fig. 9. We note that the proposed method can uniformly highlight the salient regions and preserve object boundaries well than the other approaches.

4.4 Limitations

Up until now, we have evaluated the effectiveness of our model which can consistently improve the performance of each individual saliency detection method. However, some difficult images are still challenging for our model as well as other

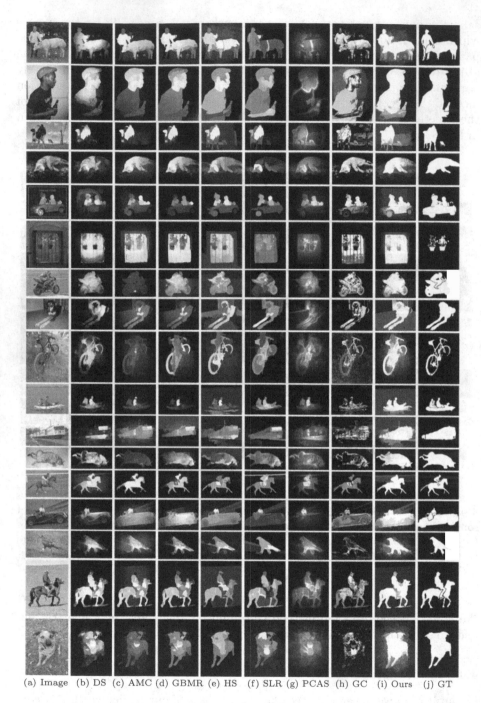

(a) Image   (b) DS   (c) AMC   (d) GBMR   (e) HS   (f) SLR   (g) PCAS   (h) GC   (i) Ours   (j) GT

Fig. 8. More comparison results on the PASCAL-1500 dataset. Compared with the ground truth (j), our model achieved best performance visually.

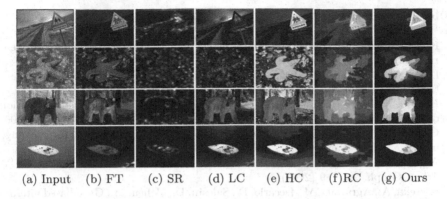

(a) Input   (b) FT   (c) SR   (d) LC   (e) HC   (f)RC   (g) Ours

Fig. 9. Visual comparisons between five classical methods and our proposed approach.

state-of-the-art saliency models. As shown in Fig. 10, most of the saliency models fail to identify the salient regions for an image. In this case, the advantages of some saliency maps are not learned into the low rank matrix recovery based framework to help the final saliency combination.

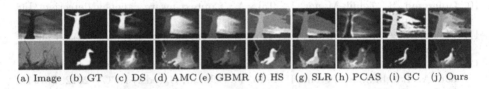

(a) Image   (b) GT   (c) DS   (d) AMC (e) GBMR   (f) HS   (g) SLR (h) PCAS   (i) GC   (j) Ours

Fig. 10. Failure cases. The advantages of some saliency maps are not learned into our framework to help the final saliency combination.

5   Conclusions and Future Work

In this paper, we propose a saliency learning model for saliency aggregation that integrates saliency maps produced by multiple saliency detection methods. Specifically, we cast the saliency detection as a sparsity pursuit problem. Our method provides a robust way to combine individual saliency detection methods into a more powerful one. Experimental results prove that our proposed approach performs better than the individual saliency detection methods and outperforms the state-of-the-art approaches.

With the development of saliency detection technology, we believe that our method can benefit from the forthcoming saliency methods. In the future, we plan to investigate a strategy to learn which method can improve the performance of our aggregation model. Furthermore, we will focus on how to overcome the failure of our method and how to improve its speed.

References

1. Ko, B.C., Nam, J.Y.: Object-of-interest image segmentation based on human attention and semantic region clustering. JOptSoc Am. **23**, 2462–2470 (2006)
2. Li, J., Ma, R., Ding, J.: Saliency-seeded region merging: automatic object segmentation. In: ACPR, pp. 691–695 (2011)
3. Han, J., Ngan, K., Li, M., Zhang, H.: Unsupervised extraction of visual attention objects in color images. IEEE Trans. Circ. Syst. Video. Technol. **16**, 141–145 (2006)
4. Chen, T., Cheng, M., Tan, P., Shamir, A., Hu, S.: Sketch2photo: internet image montage. ACM Trans. Graph. **28**, 1–10 (2009)
5. Avidan, S., Shamir, A.: Seam carving for content-aware image resizing. ACM Trans. Graph. **26**, 1–9 (2007)
6. Santella, A., Agrawala, M., Decarlo, D., Salesin, D., Cohen, M.: Gaze-based interaction for semi-automatic photo cropping. In: Proceedings of the Conference Human Factors in Computing Systems pp. 771–780 (2006)
7. Christopoulos, C., Skodras, A., Ebrahimi, T.: The JPEG2000 still image coding system: an overview. IEEE Trans. Consum. Elec. **46**, 1103–1127 (2002)
8. Achanta, R., Estrada, F.J., Wils, P., Süsstrunk, S.: Salient region detection and segmentation. In: Gasteratos, A., Vincze, M., Tsotsos, J.K. (eds.) ICVS 2008. LNCS, vol. 5008, pp. 66–75. Springer, Heidelberg (2008)
9. Achanta, R., Hemami, S.,Estrada, F.J., Susstrunk., S.: Frequency-tuned salient region detection. In: CVPR, pp. 1597–1604 (2009)
10. Goferman, S., Zelnik-Manor, L., Tal., A.: Context-aware saliency detection. In: CVPR, pp. 2376–2383 (2010)
11. Cheng, M., Zhang, G., Mitra, N.J., Huang, X., Hu, S.: Global contrast based salient region detection. In: CVPR, pp. 409–416 (2010)
12. Borji, A., Sihite, D.N., Itti, L.: Salient object detection: a benchmark. In: Fitzgibbon, A., Lazebnik, S., Perona, P., Sato, Y., Schmid, C. (eds.) ECCV 2012, Part II. LNCS, vol. 7573, pp. 414–429. Springer, Heidelberg (2012)
13. Mai, L., Niu, Y., Liu, F.: Saliency aggregation: a data-driven approach. In: CVPR, pp. 4321–4328 (2013)
14. Shen, X., Wu, Y.: A unified approach to salient object detection via low rank matrix recovery. In: CVPR, pp. 853–860 (2012)
15. Li, X., Lu, H., Zhang, L., Ruan, X., Yang, M.: Saliency detection via dense and sparse reconstruction. In: ICCV, pp. 2976–2983 (2013)
16. Yan, Q., Xu, L., Shi, J., Jia, J.: Hierarchical saliency detection. In: CVPR, pp. 1155–116 (2013)
17. Jiang, B., Zhang, L., Lu, H., Yang, M.: Saliency detection via absorbing markov chain. In: ICCV, pp. 1665–1672 (2013)
18. Zou, W., Kpalma, K., Liu, Z., Ronsin, J.: Segmentation driven low-rank matrix recovery for saliency detection. In: BMVC, pp. 1–13 (2013)
19. Margolin, R., Tal, A., Manor, L.: What makes a patch distinct? In: CVPR, pp. 1139–1146 (2013)
20. Yan, J., Zhu, M., Liu, H., Liu, Y.: Visual saliency detection via sparsity pursuit. IEEE Sig. Process. Lett. **17**, 739–742 (2010)
21. Lang, C., Liu, G., Yu, J., Yan, S.: Saliency detection by multitask sparsity pursuit. IEEE Trans. Image Process. **21**, 1327–1338 (2012)
22. Wright, J., Ganesh, A., Rao, S., Peng, Y., Ma, Y.: Robust principal component analysis: exact recovery of corrupted low-rank matrices via convex optimization. In: NIPS (2009)

23. Itti, L., Koch, C., Niebur, E.: A model of saliency-based visual attention for rapid scene analysis. IEEE TPAMI **20**, 1254–1259 (1998)
24. Ma, Y., Zhang, H.: Contrast-based image attention analysis by using fuzzy growing. In: ACM Multimedia, pp. 374–381 (2003)
25. Harel, J., Koch, C., Perona, P.: Graph-based visual saliency. In: NIPS, pp. 545–552 (2006)
26. Hou, X., Zhang, L.: Saliency detection: a spectral residual approach. In: CVPR, pp. 1–8 (2007)
27. Comaniciu, D., Meer, P.: Mean shift: a robust approach toward feature space analysis. J. Foo **24**, 603–619 (2002)
28. Lin, Z., Chen, M., Wu, L., Ma, Y.: The augmented lagrange multiplier method for extract recovery of corrupted low rank matrices UIUC. Technical report, UILU-ENG-09-2215 (2009)
29. Alpert, S., Galun, M., Basri, R., Brandt, A.: Image segmentation by probabilistic bottom-up aggregation and cue integration. In: CVPR, pp. 1–8 (2007)
30. Movahedi, V., Elder, J.: Design and perceptual validation of performance measures for salient object segmentation. In: CVPRW, pp. 49–56 (2010)
31. Cheng, M., Warrell, J., Lin, W., Zheng, S., Vineet, V., Crook, N.: Efficient salient region detection with soft image abstraction. In: ICCV, pp. 1529–1536 (2013)
32. Yang, C., Zhang, L., Lu, H., Ruan, X., Yang, M. : Saliency detection via graph-based manifold ranking. In: CVPR, pp. 3166–3173 (2013)
33. Everingham, M., Van Gool, L., Williams, C.K.I., Winn, J., Zisserman, A.: The pascal visual object classes (VOC) challenge. IJCV **88**, 303–338 (2010)
34. Rosenfeld, A., Weinshall, D.: Extracting foreground masks towards object recognition. In: ICCV, pp. 1371–1378 (2011)
35. Zhai, Y., Shah, M.: Visual attentation detection in video sequences using spatiotemporal cues. In: ACM Multimedia, pp. 815–824 (2006)

A New Framework for Multiclass Classification Using Multiview Assisted Adaptive Boosting

Avisek Lahiri$^{(\boxtimes)}$ and Prabir Kumar Biswas

Indian Institute of Technology, Kharagpur, India
avisek@ece.iitkgp.ernet.in

Abstract. Multiview representation of data is common in disciplines such as computer vision, bio-informatics, etc. Traditional fusion methods train independent classifiers on each view and finally conglomerate them using weighted summation. Such approaches are void from interview communications and thus do not guarantee to yield the best possible ensemble classifier on the given sample-view space. This paper proposes a new algorithm for multiclass classification using multi-view assisted supervised learning (MA-AdaBoost). MA-AdaBoost uses adaptive boosting for initially training baseline classifiers on each view. After each boosting round, the classifiers share their classification performances. Based on this communication, weight of an example is ascertained by its classification difficulties across all views. Two versions of MA-AdaBoost are proposed based on the nature of final output of baseline classifiers. Finally, decisions of baseline classifiers are agglomerated based on a novel algorithm of reward assignment. The paper then presents classification comparisons on benchmark UCI datasets and eye samples collected from FERET database. Kappa-error diversity diagrams are also studied. In majority instances, MA-AdaBoost outperforms traditional AdaBoost, variants of AdaBoost, and recent works on supervised collaborative learning with respect to convergence rate of training set and generalization errors. The error-diversity results are also encouraging.

1 Introduction

Adaptive Boosting [1,2] yields a strong classifier by combination of several feeble rules of thumb. After each boosting round, AdaBoost updates a weight distribution based on difficulty of the sample space at that round. The final classifier is a weighted combination of individual trained classifiers. Though initially formulated for supervised learning, AdaBoost has been used extensively in semi supervised learning under multi view setting. In applications such as computer vision, biomedical signal processing, bioinformatics, data is acquired from different view points (feature spaces) [3,4]. Each view has its own discriminative property which is absent in other views. Usually statistical methods [5,6] are applied for extracting the best discriminative feature from each view. By dimensionality reduction, such methods yield a compact representation of data. But these methods tend to ignore the localized subtle features in each view which are usually beneficial for classification in presence of data perturbation.

© Springer International Publishing Switzerland 2015
D. Cremers et al. (Eds.): ACCV 2014, Part III, LNCS 9005, pp. 128–143, 2015.
DOI: 10.1007/978-3-319-16811-1_9

Multiview learning in semi supervised learning tries to minimize manual labeling effort by iteratively learning on labeled and unlabeled instance spaces. The pioneering work of Query-by-Committee (QBC) algorithm [7] required that the views be independent of each other. The work was closely followed by Co-training [8] which still preserved the restrictive assumption of QBC. Since then there has been plethora of research on multiview semi supervised learning [9–14]. Recently, Co-Training-by-Committee [15] eliminates the requirement that the representative views be mutually orthogonal.

There is dearth of literature on collaborative multiview learning for multiclass classification in supervised learning. This is the primary motivation of the paper. In the era of Big Data we need a scalable learning framework to learn from different information sources. Previous works have focused on combining classifiers learnt on different views by fusion methods. Early fusion manifests data in a macro environment by combining discriminating features from the available views and then trains a single classifier. Late fusion trains separate classifiers on each view and ultimately combines them by plurality voting. Empirical studies performed on multimedia domain reveals that late fusion tends to perform better than early fusion [16]. But neither of the two methods encompasses assistive learning communications across views. Some recent works have focused on multiview learning in supervised learning arena. Liu et al. proposed Co-AdaBoost [17,18] for classification of software document based on Co-training algorithm. Koco et al. proposed an algorithm (Mumbo) [19,20] for multiclass classification with multiview collaborative learning. Recent attempts to model frameworks for assisted multiview learning in supervised learning is the primary invigoration of this paper.

2 Contributions of Proposed Work

The paper proposes a new supervised learning framework(MA-AdaBoost) for multiclass classification where a sample space is represented by multiple views. The paper places no restrictions on orthogonality of the feature spaces. The proposed work differs from Co-AdaBoost in the following aspects:

1. Co-AdaBoost mandates the views be disjoint for effective learning. The proposed MA-AdaBoost does not place any such restrictions on the views.
2. Co-AdaBoost is limited to binary classification with maximum two view representations. MA-AdaBoost is designed for multiclass classification and can be scaled for any finite cardinality view sets.
3. Co-AdaBoost conglomerates the boosted classifiers by simple weighted majority voting but MA-AdaBoost formulates a novel reward function for mixing ensemble learners.

Some of the key differences between Mumbo and MA-AdaBoost are:

1. For each view Mumbo maintains a cost matrix M(i, j) which denotes cost of assigning label j to training example x_i. For a V view problem, the storage requirement is $\mathcal{O}(V*m*K)$, where m and K are cardinality of instance

space and label space respectively. Such space requirements are debatable in many real life problems. MA-AdaBoost calculates mislabeling cost on global basis after each round of assisted communication and hence need not store misclasification costs over local views.

2. Mumbo assumes the presence of a major view which is assisted by several minor views. The minor views intervene only if the average error on major view exceeds than that of random guessing. But selection of such major view from real life data is tedious and undermines the fundamental purpose of multiview learning. MA-AdaBoost adaptively rewards the views based on classification performances on each boosting round and thus the user is free from tediously selecting the best possible view.

At a particular boosting round (t), both Co-AdaBoost and Mumbo considers a sample-view space to be boostable if

$$\sum_{i:h_{t,v}(x_i)\neq y_i} W_{t,v}(i) \leq 0.5 \tag{1}$$

whereas MA-AdaBoost deems a space boostable if

$$\prod_{v=1}^{V}\left[\sum_{i:h_{t,v}(x_i)\neq y_i} W_{t,v}(i)\right] \leq 0.5 \tag{2}$$

where $W_{t,v}$ is weight distribution over view v and $h_{t,v}(x)$ is a local trained hypothesis on view v. Naturally MA-AdaBoost imposes less rigid restrictions on local hypotheses compared to Mumbo and Co-AdaBoost.

3 MA-AdaBoost Algorithm

This section formally introduces the MA-AdaBoost algorithm in the context of supervised learning for multiview assisted multiclass classification.

3.1 Initial Parameters

MA-AdaBoost initializes with learning space $X = \{(x_1,y_1), (x_2,y_2),..(x_m, y_m)\}$, label space $L = \{1,2,.K\}$ and view space $VS = \{v_1,v_2,.v_V\}$. Each $y_i \in L$. An uniform weight $W_1(i) = 1/m$ is initiated over all x_i and v_i. A single learning algorithm such as ANN, SVM, C4.5, etc. is selected as local hypothesis over each view.

3.2 Inter View Communication and Group Learing

Misclassification cost of a local hypothesis $h_{t,v}(x)$ over a view v on t^{th} boosting round is given by

$$P_{W_t}(h_{t,v}(x_i)) \neq y_i \tag{3}$$

After each boosting round, the local hypotheses communicate their classification performances and the overall misclassification cost of the entire learning group is assigned as:

$$\chi_t = \prod_{v_1}^{v_V} P_{W_t}(h_{t,v}(x_i) \neq y_i) \tag{4}$$

Such a cost function obviates the strict restrictions of Eq. 1. MA-AdaBoost then updates the weight distribution W_t via a new scalable framework. During a boosting round, the easiest example x_i is given least weight if it is correctly classified across all views in previous iteration. Likewise, highest weight is assigned to the most onerous example. Intermediate weights of x_i are scaled according to cumulative misclassification occurances over the representative views. Difficulty of x_i is measured by the metric $\gamma_t(i)$, given by:

$$\gamma_t(i) = \frac{2j}{V} - 1; j \in [0, 1, 2, ...V] \tag{5}$$

where an example x_i has been misclassified on j views. Let

$$\beta_t = 0.5 * log\left(\frac{1 - \chi_t}{\chi_t}\right) \tag{6}$$

represents the learning weight of entire group. A low misclassification cost χ_t ensures high β_t. Then the weight distribution $W_t(i)$ is updated as:

$$W_{t+1}(i) = \frac{W_t(i) * exp(\beta_t * \gamma_t(i))}{N_t} \tag{7}$$

where N_t is a normalization constant to preserve $W_{t+1}(i)$ as a distribution. Such a scalable weight distribution ensures that an arduous example is collaboratively learnt by all views.

3.3 Conglomerating Ensemble Decisions

The paper presents a novel framework for combining decisions of local view hypotheses. Let $S_{t,v}$ be a set such that,

$$S_{t,v} = \{x_i| \ h_{t,v}(x_i) = y_i\} \tag{8}$$

Classification accuracy of $h_{t,v}(x)$ is given by $\eta_{t,v} = \ | \ S_{t,v}|/m$. Performace reward of $h_{t,v}(x)$ is formulated as $R_{t,v}$:

$$R_{t,v} = \sum_{i:h_{t,v}(x_i)=y_i} W_t(i) * |h_{t,v}(x_i)|$$

$$- \sum_{j:h_{t,v}(x_j)\neq y_j} (1 - W_t(j)) * |h_{t,v}(x_j)| \tag{9}$$

The overall performace metric of $h_{t,v}(x)$ is determined as:

$$P_{t,v} = \eta_{t,v} * (1 + R_{t,v}) \tag{10}$$

Such a reward based metric emphasizes those hypotheses which correctly classify difficult examples with high confidence than those which correctly classify easy examples with high confidence. High penalty is incurred on misclassifying an easy example with high confidence. Depending on the final classification space of $h_{t,v}(x)$, MA-AdaBoost has two variants: i. MA-AdaBoost.V1 and ii. MA-AdaBoost.V2.

3.4   MA-AdaBoost.V1

In this version the final output domain (D.V1) of $h_{t,v}(x)$ is defined as D.V1={1,2,3...K}. Final classifier is given by

$$F_{fin}(x) = \left\lfloor \frac{\sum_{t=1}^{T} \sum_{v=1}^{V} P_{t,v} * h_{t,v}(x)}{K * \sum_{t=1}^{T} P_{t,v}} \right\rfloor \tag{11}$$

where $\lfloor a \rfloor$ represents nearest integer to (a).

3.5   MA-AdaBoost.V2

In this version $h_{t,v}(x)$ yields confidence vector about each class instead of crisp labels. Thus $h_{t,v}(x) \in \mathbf{R}^{KX1}$ and output domain (D.V2) $\in$ [0,1]. Final classifier is given by

$$F_{fin}(x) = \underset{k \in L}{\operatorname{argmax}} \left[\frac{\sum_{t=1}^{T} \sum_{v=1}^{V} P_{t,v} * |h_{t,v}^{k}(x)|}{\sum_{t=1}^{T} P_{t,v}} \right] \tag{12}$$

where $|h_{t,v}^{k}(x)|$ is prediction confidence of class k. The sequential steps of MA-AdaBoost are showed in Algorithm 1.

Algorithm 1. MA-AdaBoost for Multiclass Classification

Input:

- Learning Space: X={(x_1,y_1), (x_2,y_2),..(x_m, y_m)}
- Label Space: L={1,2,.. K}
- View Space: VS={v_1, v_2,..v_V }
- Local View Hypothesis: $h_{t,v}(x)$
- Weight Distribution: W_1
- Total Boosting Rounds: T

For t=1 to T

1. Train local hypotheses on all views
2. Calculate misclassification cost of $h_{t,v}(x)$ from Equation (3)

3. Calculate χ_t from Equation (4)
4. Calculate β_t from Equation (6)
5. Calculate difficulty of x_i from Equation (5)
6. Update weight distribution $W_t(i)$ from Equation (7)
7. Evaluate performance of $h_{t,v}(x)$ from Equation (10)

END FOR

Output:
Use Equation (11) or (12) for final classifier $F_{fin}(x)$

---

4   Simulation Results

This section presents the classification performances of MA-AdaBoost and compares with Co-AdaBoost, Mumbo, and various boosting methods which use late fusion combination.

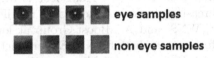

Fig. 1. Samples cut from FERET database for training ensemble classifiers.

4.1   Two Class Classification

For two class classification eye and non eye samples of 32×32 pixels are manually cut from FERET database [21,22]. Total 5923 eye samples and 6123 non eye samples are collected. Few examples are shown in Fig. 1. Each sample is transformed to gray scale space and 2D Haar transformation space. 2D Haar transformation of an image yields three matrices for emphasizing horizontal,vetical and diagonal edges and fourth matrix as an average image [23]. Without loss of generality we perform singular value decompositions of gray scale space and vertical edge space. 32 eigen values from gray scale space and 16 eigen values from vertical edge space act as two views of the system. We train a 2-layer back propagation ANN with one hidden layer on each view. We perform 10 rounds of boosting with 50 iterations of training ANN in each round.The training set, validation set and test set are divided in 60:20:20 proportions and we follow 5-fold validation for determing the optimum regularization parameter(λ) of ANN.

We report the training set performances in Table 1. At onset of boosting, WNS [24] creates a sub sample space by identifying the most informative training examples. WNS speeds up AdaBoost but tends to compromise on accuracy. AdaBoost.Group [25] proposes to train independent hypotheses on each view. The hypotheses are optimized by maximizing F_1 scores on respective views.

Table 1. Comparison of training set accuracy rates of different ensemble classifiers for eye classification on FERET database.

T	Iterations	WNS	AdaBoost.M2	AdaBoost.Group	Mumbo	Co-AdaBoost	V1[a]	V2[b]
2	05	66.0	67.8	69.3	67.6	62.4	60.0	64.0
	25	73.0	74.6	75.0	75.9	73.0	75.0	78.4
	50	75.0	76.2	77.2	78.0	75.8	79.8	82.4
5	05	68.2	70.2	71.2	69.2	65.6	63.4	67.8
	25	79.8	81.4	82.0	80.7	78.8	80.8	85.0
	50	83.2	85.6	86.2	88.0	87.5	87.8	92.0
10	05	74.8	77.9	80.0	79.0	75.2	75.0	76.4
	25	85.3	87.8	88.6	93.8	90.6	96.2	98.0
	50	86.0	88.0	91.0	94.0	93.2	97.0	99.0

[a]Proposed: **MA-AdaBoost.V1**
[b]Proposed: **MA-AdaBoost.V2**

Finally the local hypotheses are combined by majority voting. From Table 1 we see that MA-AdaBoost outperforms the traditional fused based boosting algorithms by considerable margins. At low iterations, due to dearth of training, the total misclassification cost χ_t of MA-AdaBoost is high and thus hinders the learning rate by increasing β_t. So MA-AdaBoost manifests inferior learning compared to AdaBoost, WNS, and AdaBoost.Group at low iterations. But β_t increases rapidly with further training of ANN. Experiments show that after 15 rounds of training, MA-AdaBoost starts yielding superior performance compared to boosting. During final combination, MA-AdaBoost.V1 allows combination of crisp labels from each local hypothesis but MA-AdaBoost.V2 allows combination over entire label space and is therefore more expressive and superior. On avarage, after 50 training iterations, MA-AdaBoost.V1 outperforms WNS, AdaBoost.M2 and AdaBoost.Group by 8.63 %, 7.1 %, and 6.93 % respectively and the corresponding margins for MA-AdaBoost.V2 are 10.95 %, 8.2 %, and 7.4 % respectively. Co-AdaBoost and Mumbo perform comparable to MA-AdaBoost.V1 and is outperformed by MA-AdaBoost.V2 by an average margin of 4.95 % and 4.63 % respectively. Mumbo tends to perform superior at low iterations. At low iterations, mislabelling cost is robustly dealt by Mumbo by maintaining 2 cost matrices and allowing only the best discriminative view to classify an example. Upper bound on training set error for MA-AdaBoost ϵ_{MA}: [26]

$$\epsilon_{MA} \leq 2^T \prod_{t=1}^{T} \sqrt{\chi_t (1 - \chi_t)} \tag{13}$$

while for AdaBoost.M2, WNS, and AdaBoost.Group, the error bound ϵ_A:

$$\epsilon_A \leq 2^T \prod_{t=1}^{T} \sqrt{\theta_t (1 - \theta_t)} \tag{14}$$

where $\theta_t = \left[\sum_{v=v_1}^{v_V} \sum_{t=1}^{T} \sum_{j:h_{t,v}(x_j) \neq y_j} W_{t,v}(x_j) \right]$ is misclassification cost on round (t) and $W_{t,v}(x)$ is the weight distribution on view (v) during boosting

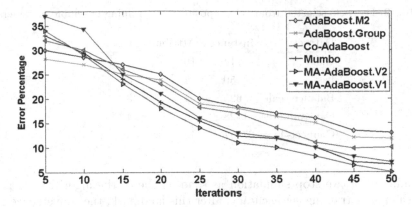

Fig. 2. Comparison of average generalization error rates of various ensemble classifiers trained for classification of eyes on FERET database. The classifiers are trained over 10 boosting rounds with 50 iterations of training per round.

round (t). Now, $\chi_t < \theta_t$, and thus $\epsilon_{MA} < \epsilon_A$. So the convergence rate of MA-AdaBoost is faster compared to traditional boosting.

In Fig. 2 we report the generalization error rates of the ensemble classifiers. In each boosting round, we increment ANN training by 5 iterations and study the effect on test set performances. Due to space scarcity we report the average over 10 boosting rounds. Horizontal axis represents number of times ANN is trained per boosting round while vertical axis delineates generalization error rates. We see that MA-AdaBoost offers better test set performance comapared to fusion based boosting. On average MA-AdaBoost has 4.6 % and 3.8 % less error rate than AdaBoost.M2 and AdaBoost.Group respectively while the same margins for MA-AdaBoost.V2 are 6.1 % and 4.2 % respectively. For visual clarity we did not plot the curve for WNS. Specifically, MA-AdaBoost.V1 and MA-AdaBoost.V2 outperforms WNS by 11.5 % and 13.2 % respectively. Mumbo and Co-AdaBoost yield comparable results.

4.2 Multiclass Classification

In this section we test our model on several datasets from the benchmark UCI database [27]. Co-AdaBoost and AdaBoost.Group cannot be compared with as those models are apt only for binary classes. Weighted majority voting(WMV) [28] is an enhanced boosting algorithm. WMV is based on *boosting by resampling* AdaBoost which selects a subspace of original sample distribution and formulates a hypothesis. A correction factor is introduced while updating weight distribution for enhancing accuracy of AdaBoost.

We select 5 datasets from UCI repository as shown in Table 2. The datasets span over domains such as biology, commerce, game playing, and forensics. We randomly divide a dataset into 2 views and train 2-layer backpropagation ANN with one hidden layer on each view. For investigating the rate of convergence

Table 2. Datasets selected from UCI repository for training ensemble classifiers

Dataset	Instances	Attributes	Classes
Glass	214	10	7
Iris	150	4	3
Balance scale	625	4	3
Car evaluate	1728	6	4
Connect-4	67557	42	3

of training error, we stop simulation as soon as one of the algorithms achieve more than 90 % training set accuracy; after this landmark, the convergence rate is sluggish for all algorithms. We report the training set performances in Table 3.

In each round of boosting we increment the training iterations in steps of 30 and investigate the classification spaces of competing algorithms. In Table 3, T denotes the boosting round at which we first achieve greater than 90 % accuracy from any one of the ensemble classifiers while N denotes the number of times ANNs are trained per boosting round. We note that convergence rates of multiview based collaborative algorithms are significantly higher than that of non-cooperative boosting algorithms.

Let after (t) rounds of boosting the final classifier be $H_{final}(X, t, v) = f(h_{t,v}(X))$, where X and Y represent training data set and label set respectively and $h_{t,v}(X)$ is the hypothesis on view (v). We define Γ as:

$$\Gamma = \operatorname*{argmin}_{t} \{P_r(H_{final}(X, t, v) \neq Y) < 10\%\} \tag{15}$$

i.e. Γ represents the minimum boosting required to acquire 90 % training set accuracy. If algorithms 1 and 2 have different Γ_1 and Γ_2 respectively, then we define *"edge-of-convergence"* e_{Γ_1, Γ_2} as:

$$e_{\Gamma_1, \Gamma_2} = \frac{\Gamma_1 - \Gamma_2}{\Gamma_2}; \quad \Gamma_1 > \Gamma_2 \tag{16}$$

$e_{\Gamma_1, \Gamma_2} \geq 0$ signifies faster convergence rate for algorithm 2. We report e_{Γ_1, Γ_2} in Fig. 3 with MA-AdaBoost.V2 as algorithm 2 and the competitors as algorithm 1. Mumbo performs comparable to MA-AdaBoost and is thus not compared in Fig. 3. We see that the boosting algorithms perform worst on Iris dataset. Due to scarcity of sufficient attributes on each view, the algorithms cannot train the independent hypotheses. The lack of proper training combined with dearth of collaboration leads to drastic drop of learing rate. Independent boosting algorithms fair best on Connect-4 dataset due to presence of plethora of data and attributes.

4.3   Kappa-Error Diversity Analysis

An ideal ensemble classifier should possess highly veracious members and should simultenously disagree within the group in most instances [29]. Such a requirement

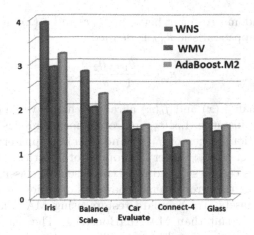

Fig. 3. Comparison of e_{Γ_1, Γ_2} (y axis) of MA-AdaBoost.V2 with variants of boosting on various UCI datasets (x axis).

Table 3. Study of training error convergence rates on UCI datasets. **T:** total boosting rounds elapsed before any one of the ensemble classifiers achieves 90% accuracy rate on a particular dataset. **N:** ANN training iterations per boosting round. The first classifier to achieve 90% accuracy on a particular dataset is marked in bold.

Dataset	(T,N)	WNS	AdaBoost.M2	WMV	Mumbo	V1[a]	V2[b]
Iris	(4,60)	55.0%	61.2%	63.4%	89.3%	88.0%	**93.2%**
Balance scale	(3,30)	65.4%	70.8%	72.9%	91.0%	87.4%	**92.6%**
Car evaluate	(5,60)	73.4%	81.8%	83.0%	89.3%	90.4%	**92.7%**
Glass	(4,30)	73.2%	78.3%	81.4%	**90.7%**	87.0%	88.7%
Connect-4	(7,90)	84.8%	88.2%	88.0%	90.5%	89.8%	**94.3%**

[a]**Proposed: MA-AdaBoost.V1**
[b]**Proposed: MA-AdaBoost.V2**

imposes a trade-off between miscellany and accuracy in a classifier space. Kappa-error diagram [30] is a visualization measure to study error-diversity trend of ensemble clasifiers. For two classifiers $f_a(x)$ and $f_b(x)$, a contingency table **A** is defined such that $\mathbf{A}(k, l) = 1$ whenever $f_a(x_i)$=k and $f_b(x_i)$=l; x_i is a training example and (k,l) are class labels. A high trace value of **A** manifests agreement between $f_a(x)$ and $f_b(x)$ on most instances. Define

$$\theta_1 = \frac{\sum_{l=1}^{K} \mathbf{A}(l, l)}{m}; K = number\ of\ classes \tag{17}$$

as probability of agreement between $f_a(x)$ and $f_b(x)$. Define

$$\theta_2 = \sum_{k=1}^{K} \left(\sum_{l=1}^{K} \frac{\mathbf{A}(k, l)}{m} \sum_{l=1}^{K} \frac{\mathbf{A}(l, k)}{m} \right) \tag{18}$$

as probabilty of random agreement between $f_a(x)$ and $f_b(x)$; m is the cardinality of sample space. Kappa statistic $\kappa_{a,b}$ is defined as

$$\kappa_{a,b} = \frac{\theta_1 - \theta_2}{1 - \theta_2} \tag{19}$$

$\kappa_{a,b} = 0$ signifies that $f_a(x)$ and $f_b(x)$ agree by chance while $\kappa_{a,b} = 1$ signifies agreement on every instance. Let $\epsilon_{a,b}$ represent mean misclassification cost on combined classification spaces of $f_a(x)$ and $f_b(x)$. Kappa-error diagram is a scatter plot of $\epsilon_{a,b}$ versus $\kappa_{a,b}$. After (n) rounds of boosting, $^nC_2$ combinations of pairwise classifiers can be selected from the ensemble classifier space.

In Fig. 4 we report the error-diversity patterns of various ensemble classifiers over the 5 UCI datasets. We compare results using MA-AdaBoost.V2 which gives slightly better result than MA-AdaBoost.V1. The scatter clouds of the classifiers are highly overlapping; hence we plot only the centroids of the cluster clouds. The horizontal and vertical axis represent $\kappa_{a,b}$ and $\epsilon_{a,b}$ respectively; both axes are scaled between [0,1] for visualization. An ideal ensemble classifier has low values for both $\epsilon_{a,b}$ and $\kappa_{a,b}$ and thus its centroid of scatter cloud should occupy the third quadrant of error-diversity diagram.We deduce the following inferences from Fig. 4.

- Ensemble spaces trained by collaborative learning possess more accurate member hypotheses compared to ensemble spaces trained by non communicating boosting algorithms. Conglomeration of more accurate member aids in better generalization ability and supports the results in Table 4 which reports test set performaces of ensemble classifiers.
- Scatter clouds of Mumbo and MA-AdaBoost.V2 tend to concentrate in the third quadrant of $\epsilon_{a,b} - \kappa_{a,b}$ space and thus tend towards realization of ideal ensemble learning.
- Inter hypothesis agreement is slightly more in Mumbo than in MA-AdaBoost.V2. In Mumbo, an arduous example x_i is removed from sample space of weak hypotheses and only the best hypotheses classify it; agreement thus increases among the best members. But as pointed out earlier, this increases computational and memory costs of Mumbo.
- Error clouds of WMV are usually concentrated below error clouds of AdaBoost.M2. WMV adaptively reduces probabilties of correctly classified examples so that classifiers can concentrate on hard examples. Such a modified weight distribution tends to enhance boosting classification accuracy.
- Members within WNS classifier space are least accurate. WNS forms a subspace from distribution space of AdaBoost by identifying the most discriminative examples. This reduced distribution subsapce reduces classification efficieny of WNS but aids in reduced execution time.

In Table 4 we report the generalization error rates of the ensemble classifiers after 10 rounds of boosting. The best results are marked in bold.

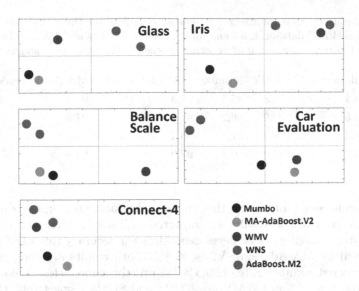

Fig. 4. Study of Kappaa-Error diagrams on 5 UCI datasets. Horizontal axis represents agreement metric $\kappa_{a,b}$. Vertical axis represents mean misclassification cost $\epsilon_{a,b}$. Both axes are scaled to span between [0,1]. The dots denote the centroids of error-diversity scatter clouds of various ensemble classifiers.

Table 4. Generalization error rates of various ensemble classifiers on UCI datasets.

Datasets / Algorithm	AdaBoost.M2	WNS	WMV	Mumbo	MA-AdaBoost.V2
Iris	33·5	35·1	20·3	7·3	**3·2**
Glass	19·8	21·3	15·8	**5·3**	5·9
Balance Scale	18·5	20·3	11·2	9·1	**4·1**
Connect-4	35·4	27·0	19·2	15·6	**14·3**
Car Evaluate	23·2	24·9	21·7	15·3	**9·2**

4.4   An Interesting Application in Computer Vision

"ONE HUNDRED SPECIES LEAVES" [31] is a challenging database in computer vision. The dataset contains 100 classes of leaves of different species. Sixteen different variants of each species are photographed as an RGB image against white background. Each of these samples is then characterized by three distinct 16D feature spaces: shape signature, texture histogram, and margin-feature histogram. Thus the sample space consists of 1600 samples; each sample is represented by a 64D feature vector.

The multiview setting of this dataset is apt to be applied on our model. We train 2-layer ANN with one hidden layer on each of these views for five rounds of boosting and hundred iterations of training ANN per round. We follow a sixteen fold evaluation to compare our results with [32], which reports the best

Table 5. Accuracy rates of various ensemble classifiers on the *"ONE HUNDRED SPECIES LEAVES"* dataset. Each ensemble classifier consists of ANN members which are trained 100 times per round of boosting on each of the three view spaces.

T	AdaBoost.M2	WMV	Mumbo	MA-AdaBoost.V1	MA-AdaBoost.V2
2	73.4	77.8	85.3	92.3	95.4
3	75.6	79.0	86.2	94.5	97.8
4	78.2	79.9	87.3	96.4	98.2
5	80.2	81.0	90.1	97.0	98.8

classification accuracy of 99.3 %, though their classification method is based on probabilistic K-NN. The results are reported in Table 5. After five rounds of boosting, MA-AdaBoost.V1 achieves generalization accuracy rate of 97 % while that achieved by MA-AdaBoost.V2 is 98.8 %. Both results are comparable to the best reported accuracy rate of 99.3 % [32]. At the same instant the accuracy rates of AdaBoost.M2 and WMV are 80.2 % and 81.3 % respectively. On average over five boosting rounds, MA-AdaBoost.V1 outperforms AdaBoost.M2 and WMV by an average margin of 18.2 % and 15.5 % respectively. The corresponding margins achieved by MA-AdaBoost.V2 are 20.4 % and 18.1 % respectively.

Note that performance of Mumbo deteriotes on this dataset compared to MA-AdaBoost. The three feature spaces are comparable to each other in clasification accuracy. But Mumbo requires a major view which will be assisted by several minor views. Absence of such a view arrangement minifies group learning in Mumbo, thereby reducing classification efficacy. MA-AdaBoost.V1 outperforms Mumbo by 7.8 % while MA-AdaBoost.V2 outperforms Mumbo by 10.3 %.

Experimental success on *"ONE HUNDRED SPECIES LEAVES"* dataset bolsters our claim that MA-AdaBoost is superior compared to other boosting based classification methods and is ready to be embraced in domains such as computer vision where an object of interst is frequently represented in multitude of view spaces.

5   Conclusion and Direction for Further Work

The paper presents a new algorithm, MA-AdaBoost in the context of multiview based multiclass classification for supervised learning. The core invigoration of MA-AdaBoost is to foster assistive learning across views. Importance of an example is ascertained based on its difficulties of classification on all the representative views. A single weight distribution is then updated based on importance of sample space across all view spaces. Such an update rule encourages that an example be learnt collaboratively by all views.

The paper then proposes a novel method for conglomerating decisions of hypotheses from multiple views. During combination, MA-AdaBoost assigns more importance to a hypothesis which correctly classifies a difficult example with high confidence than a hypothesis which correctly classifies an easy example with high confidence. Similarly, higher loss is suffered by a hypothesis if it misclassifies a naive example with high credence than misclassifying an arduous example with high conviction.

Experimental results confirm the boosting property of MA-AdaBoost; the training error decreases with increase of boosting rounds. The underlying assumption about the accuracy of an individual hypothesis trained on a view is much more relaxed in MA-AdaBoost compared to Mumbo and Co-AdaBoost. The rate of convergence of training set error is shown to be superior for MA-AdaBoost compared to Mumbo and Co-AdaBoost. Extensive simulations over samples from FERET, UCI and "ONE HUNDRED SPECIES LEAVES" databases manifest the superior generalization capability of MA-AdaBoost. The paper also studies Kappa-Error diagrams for analyzing performances of ensemble classifiers on test sets. The diagrams reveal that ensemble space on MA-AdaBoost consists of more accurate members compared to ensemble spaces of other algorithms such as WMV,WNS, Mumbo, and Co-AdaBoost.

In future we wish to perform a thorough mathematical analysis to comprehend the changes MA-AdaBoost renders to traditional boosting. Another interesting area of investigation is to compare the performances of MA-AdaBoost using other learning platforms such as SVM, C4.5, Bayesian Networks, etc.

Acknowledgement. The work is financially supported by Space Technology Cell, ISRO, Ahmedabad under the *"SVD"* project. The work is dedicated to our respected Lt. Prof. Somnath Sengupta, Dept. of E&ECE, IIT Kharagpur.

References

1. Freund, Y., Schapire, R., Abe, N.: A short introduction to boosting. J. Jpn. Soc. Artif. Intell. **14**, 1612 (1999)
2. Freund, Y., Schapire, R.E.: Experiments with a new boosting algorithm. ICML **96**, 148–156 (1996)
3. Zhang, H., Yang, Z., Gönen, M., Koskela, M., Laaksonen, J., Honkela, T., Oja, E.: Affective abstract image classification and retrieval using multiple kernel learning. In: Lee, M., Hirose, A., Hou, Z.-G., Kil, R.M. (eds.) ICONIP 2013, Part III. LNCS, vol. 8228, pp. 166–175. Springer, Heidelberg (2013)
4. Masulli, F., Mitra, S.: Natural computing methods in bioinformatics: a survey. Inf. Fusion **10**, 211–216 (2009)
5. Duangsoithong, R., Windeatt, T.: Relevant and redundant feature analysis with ensemble classification. In: Seventh International Conference on Advances in Pattern Recognition. ICAPR 2009, pp. 247–250. IEEE (2009)
6. Culp, M., Michailidis, G., Johnson, K.: On multi-view learning with additive models. Ann. Appl. Stat. **3**, 292–318 (2009)
7. Seung, H.S., Opper, M., Sompolinsky, H.: Query by committee. In: Proceedings of the Fifth Annual Workshop on Computational Learning Theory, pp. 287–294. ACM (1992)
8. Blum, A., Mitchell, T.: Combining labeled and unlabeled data with co-training. In: Proceedings of the Eleventh Annual Conference on Computational Learning Theory, pp. 92–100. ACM (1998)

9. Zhu, X.: Semi-supervised learning. In: Sammut, C., Webb, G.I. (eds.) Encyclopedia of Machine Learning, pp. 892–897. Springer, Heidelberg (2010)
10. Li, G., Chang, K., Hoi, S.C.: Multiview semi-supervised learning with consensus. IEEE Trans. Knowl. Data Eng. **24**, 2040–2051 (2012)
11. Cui, X., Huang, J., Chien, J.T.: Multi-view and multi-objective semi-supervised learning for hmm-based automatic speech recognition. IEEE Trans. Audio Speech Lang. Process. **20**, 1923–1935 (2012)
12. Wang, W., Zhou, Z.H.: On multi-view active learning and the combination with semi-supervised learning. In: Proceedings of the 25th International Conference on Machine Learning, pp. 1152–1159. ACM (2008)
13. Zhou, Z.H., Li, M.: Semi-supervised learning by disagreement. Knowl. Inf. Syst. **24**, 415–439 (2010)
14. Liu, W., Tao, D.: Multiview hessian regularization for image annotation. IEEE Trans. Image Process. **22**, 2676–2687 (2013)
15. Hady, M., Schwenker, F.: Co-training by committee: a new semi-supervised learning framework. In: IEEE International Conference on Data Mining Workshops. ICDMW 2008, pp. 563–572. IEEE (2008)
16. Snoek, C.G., Worring, M., Smeulders, A.W.: Early versus late fusion in semantic video analysis. In: Proceedings of the 13th Annual ACM International Conference on Multimedia, pp. 399–402. ACM (2005)
17. Liu, J., Li, J., Sun, X., Xie, Y., Lei, J., Hu, Q.: An embedded co-adaboost based construction of software document relation coupled resource spaces for cyber-physical society. Future Gener. Comput. Syst. **32**, 198–210 (2014)
18. Liu, J., Li, J., Xie, Y., Lei, J., Hu, Q.: An embedded co-adaboost and its application in classification of software document relation. In: 2012 Eighth International Conference on Semantics, Knowledge and Grids (SKG), pp. 173–180. IEEE (2012)
19. Koço, S., Capponi, C.: A boosting approach to multiview classification with cooperation. In: Gunopulos, D., Hofmann, T., Malerba, D., Vazirgiannis, M. (eds.) Machine Learning and Knowledge Discovery in Databases. Lecture Notes in Computer Science, vol. 6912, pp. 209–228. Springer, Heidelberg (2011)
20. Koço, S., Capponi, C., Béchet, F.: Applying multiview learning algorithms to human-human conversation classification. In: INTERSPEECH (2012)
21. Philips, P., Wechsler, H., Huang, J., Rauss, P.: The feret database and evaluation procedure for face recognition algorithms. Image Vis. Comput. **16**, 295–306 (1998)
22. Philips, P., Moon, H., Rizvi, S., Rauss, P.: The feret evaluation methodology for face recognition algorithms. IEEE Trans. Pattern Anal. Mach. Intell. **22**, 1090–1104 (2000)
23. Papageorgiou, C.P., Oren, M., Poggio, T.: A general framework for object detection. In: Sixth International Conference on Computer Vision, pp. 555–562. IEEE (1998)
24. Seyedhosseini, M., Paiva, A.R., Tasdizen, T.: Fast adaboost training using weighted novelty selection. In: The 2011 International Joint Conference on Neural Networks (IJCNN), pp. 1245–1250. IEEE (2011)
25. Ni, W., Huang, Y., Li, D., Wang, Y.: Boosting over groups and its application to acronym-expansion extraction. In: Tang, C., Ling, C.X., Zhou, X., Cercone, N.J., Li, X. (eds.) ADMA 2008. LNCS (LNAI), vol. 5139, pp. 27–38. Springer, Heidelberg (2008)
26. Freund, Y., Schapire, R.E.: A decision-theoretic generalization of on-line learning and an application to boosting. J. Comput. Syst. Sci. **55**, 119–139 (1997)
27. Bache, K., Lichman, M.: Uci machine learning repository (2013). http://archive.ics.uci.edu/ml

28. Zhang, C.X., Zhang, J.S., Zhang, G.Y.: An efficient modified boosting method for solving classification problems. J. Comput. Appl. Math. **214**, 381–392 (2008)
29. Rodriguez, J.J., Kuncheva, L.I., Alonso, C.J.: Rotation forest: a new classifier ensemble method. IEEE Trans. Pattern Anal. Mach. Intell. **28**, 1619–1630 (2006)
30. Margineantu, D.D., Dietterich, T.G.: Pruning adaptive boosting. ICML **97**, 211–218 (1997). Citeseer
31. Mallah, C., Cope, J., Orwell, J.: Plant leaf classification using probabilistic integration of shape, texture and margin features. In: Computer Graphics and Imaging/798: Signal Processing, Pattern Recognition and Applications (CGIM2013), pp. 2013–798. Acta Press (2013)
32. Mallah, C., Cope, J.: Probabilistic classification from a k-nearest-neighbour classifier. Comput. Res. **1**, 1–9 (2013)

Age Estimation by Multi-scale Convolutional Network

Dong Yi[✉], Zhen Lei, and Stan Z. Li

Center for Biometrics and Security Research and National Laboratory of Pattern
Recognition, Institute of Automation, Chinese Academy of Sciences, Beijing, China
dong.yi@nlpr.ia.ac.cn

Abstract. In the last five years, biologically inspired features (BIF) always held the state-of-the-art results for human age estimation from face images. Recently, researchers mainly put their focuses on the regression step after feature extraction, such as support vector regression (SVR), partial least squares (PLS), canonical correlation analysis (CCA) and so on. In this paper, we apply convolutional neural network (CNN) to the age estimation problem, which leads to a fully learned end-to-end system can estimate age from image pixels directly. Compared with BIF, the proposed method has deeper structure and the parameters are learned instead of hand-crafted. The multi-scale analysis strategy is also introduced from traditional methods to the CNN, which improves the performance significantly. Furthermore, we train an efficient network in a multi-task way which can do age estimation, gender classification and ethnicity classification well simultaneously. The experiments on MORPH Album 2 illustrate the superiorities of the proposed multi-scale CNN over other state-of-the-art methods.

1 Introduction

Human age estimation from face images is a young but hot research topic. The earliest work about age estimation was published in 1994 by Kwon and da Vitoria Lobo [1], in which the age was just classified into several ranges. After 2000, pushed by new models, features and classifiers in facial analysis, the field of age estimation started to flourish and the mean absolute error (MAE) on FG-NET database [2] was reduced from 9 to 5 years gradually. With moderate accuracy, age estimation can appeal the basic requirements of many applications, such as demographics analysis, commercial user management, and video security surveillance. Recently, Guo and Mu [3] first obtained a MAE below 4 years on the MORPH database [4]. This paper reduces the MAE further, which will supply a more stable age estimator for practical applications.

Like other facial analysis technics, age estimation is easily affected by many intrinsic and extrinsic factors. The most important factors include identity, gender and ethnicity. The face images of difference persons have different statistical properties, *i.e.,* For two persons of same age, maybe one has a young face, but another has an old face. The relationship between image pixels and age may be

© Springer International Publishing Switzerland 2015
D. Cremers et al. (Eds.): ACCV 2014, Part III, LNCS 9005, pp. 144–158, 2015.
DOI: 10.1007/978-3-319-16811-1_10

different when the face images come from different gender or ethnicity. Therefore, the age of face image is tightly coupled with its identity, gender and ethnicity. Other factors are similar to those in face recognition, such as pose, illumination and expression (PIE). Due to the above reasons, age estimation is a hard problem and the relation between face image to age is highly nonlinear. It's hard to find a robust and accurate function to map the image pixels to its corresponding age.

Most existing methods estimate the age of face image by two steps: local feature extraction and regression (or classification). The task of local feature extraction is to get a representation robust to irrelevant factors list above, such as identity, gender, ethnicity, PIE and so on. And the dimension of the local features are usually reduced by feature selection or down-sampling. Based on the low dimensional features, regression methods are used to predict the age of face image, such as SVR [5], PLS [6] and CCA [7]. In this framework, the most representative work is BIF + CCA (or rCCA, KCCA) [3], which includes three steps: Gabor filters [8], Max + Std pooling and CCA. With careful tuning, this method achieved very high performance, but we still have room to improve the performance further.

In this paper, we propose a novel age estimation method based on convolutional neural network (CNN). Compared with BIF + CCA, CNN has learnable parameters and there is no gap between the feature extraction step and the regression step. In CNN, all steps are optimized together to minimize the estimation error. Note that Yang et al. [9] has used CNN for age estimation under surveillance scenarios, but the focus of their work is face tracking. For the age estimation module in the system, they just use the original CNN without much modification, therefore the accuracy of [9] is lower than BIF [10].

To dig out the power of CNN, we incorporate the tricks in traditional facial analysis methods into it. (1) Several facial landmarks are used to generate many local aligned patches from a face image and feed them into CNN, which can make our method more robust to image translation and pose variations. (2) Face image is cropped into many multi-scale patches and a regression function is learned on these patches jointly. Due to the complementary information between different parts and scales, multi-scale analysis can improve the performance of CNN significantly. (3) Facial symmetry is used to augment the database, which improves the generalization of CNN. Finally, we train a multi-task CNN to illustrate the flexibility of the proposed network. The multi-task network can estimate the age, gender and ethnicity of face image simultaneously in high precision and speed.

Because the complexity of CNN is higher than traditional methods, large data are needed to train a good network. In existing age databases, MORPH Album 2 has the largest scale, containing more than 55,000 face images. To alleviate the over-fitting problem of CNN, we choose MORPH Album 2 as the database for experiments. On this database, we achieve a new state-of-the-art result: MAE = 3.63 years, which is better than 3.98 years of BIF + KCCA [3]. Meanwhile, the speed of CNN is much faster than KCCA because of its big kernel matrix.

2   Related Works

Human age estimation from face image has been studied for 20 years. Limited by the technology of facial analysis, early methods mainly used geometric features to judge the age range of face image, such as baby, young adult and senior adult. Popular geometric features included chin drop, nose drop and so on [1,11]. Geometry features can discriminate baby and adult easily but cannot distinguish adult and old man. Therefore, geometric and texture features were combined in some works. As the improvement of classification accuracy, researchers started to estimate the exact age instead of the coarse age range. Because AAM [12] was a natural tool to model the shape and texture of face image, many novel methods were proposed based on it, such as AAM + Quadratic Estimator [2], Aging Pattern Subspace (AGES) [13] and so on. By combing AGES and LDA [13], the MAE on FG-NET achieved 6.22 years. However, AAM is an pixel based method, which causes the AAM based methods unstable to environmental variations. After 2007, local features gradually became the mainstream in this field, such Gabor [14], LBP [15], Spatially Flexible Patch (SFP) [16], and BIF [10].

Based on these features, much attention were paid on the second step: age estimation by classification or regression. From the extracted features, we need predict the age range or the exact age from them. For classification, SVM and SVR are the most popular methods. Using BIF + SVM, [10] achieved MAEs of 3.47 and 3.91 years for male and female on YGA database [17]. In the same paper, the authors reported the MAE of 4.77 years on FG-NET by using BIF + SVR. In [18], Cao et al. formulated the age estimation as a ranking problem and proposed a novel method based on Rank-SVM [19]. On a subset of MORPH Album 2, they achieved a good result, MAE = 5.12 years. Recently, majority methods estimated age by regression, such as linear regression [17], SVR [10], PLS [20], and CCA [3]. Due to the ability of handling multiple tasks, PLS and CCA hold the best performance in the literature [3].

Among existing methods, BIF + CCA [3] was almost the best method for practical applications in terms of accuracy and speed. Generally speaking, we can see BIF + CCA as a 3-layered network composed by convolutional, pooling and full connected layers. Deep neural network has also been used for age estimation [9] and gender classification [21], but its potentials were not worked out completely. As described in the previous section, the biggest contribution of this paper is combing some strategies of traditional methods into CNN to improve the state-of-the-art.

This work is mainly inspired by CNN and the three tricks in traditional methods: multi-scale analysis, local aligned face patch, and facial symmetry. Compared with the proposed network, a similar multi-scale CNN was proposed for scene labeling [22] not long ago, but the multi-scale analysis in [22] was mainly used in testing stage while ours is used both in training and testing stages. Local aligned patch has succussed in many methods [23] for unconstrained face recognition problem. And facial symmetry is also a widely used trick to deal with pose problem [24] or reduce the dimension of face image and augment the database [25].

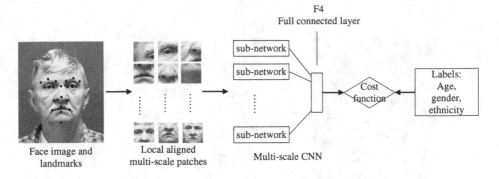

Fig. 1. The structure of the proposed network. The input face image is cropped into many local aligned patches. All patches are fed to the multi-scale convolutional network. The response of each patch are combined at the full connected layer to estimate the age, gender and ethnicity.

3   Multi-scale Convolutional Network

The structure of the proposed network is shown in Fig. 1, which includes many sub-networks for each patch. The details of the network are described in the following contents.

3.1   Local Aligned Face Patches

Facial landmarks are important for good face recognition algorithms, especially for unconstrained face recognition problem. Based on the precise facial landmarks, one can correct the pose of face image or build pose robust face descriptors. The most simple and effective method to use landmarks is local alignment. By cropping face patch around each landmark, we can get some patches aligned in the local coordinate system. For different face images, these patches have the same semantics, which are better than holistic face to learn high level tasks.

Due to the success of landmarks in face recognition, we crop face image into many local aligned patches as the input of our network. Given a face image, we first localize 21 facial landmarks by ASM [26]. The positions of the detected landmarks are shown in Fig. 2. According to facial symmetry, we group the landmarks into 13 pairs. The index of the landmark pairs are: (1, 2), (3, 4), (5, 6), (7, 8), (9, 10), (11, 12), (13, 14), (15, 16), (17, 17), (18, 18), (19, 19), (20, 20), (21, 21). For those points (17–20) on the middle line of face image, they form pairs to themselves.

In accordance with other papers, all color images are first converted into gray, because the color information is unstable and useless for age estimation. Before cropping image patches, the distance of reference landmarks 17 and 19 (*i.e.*, scale) of all face images are normalized to 60, 42, 30, 22 pixels in 4 scales. All landmarks are transformed along with the normalization of images. On the normalized images, several 48×48 patches are cropped in 4 scales (differing by

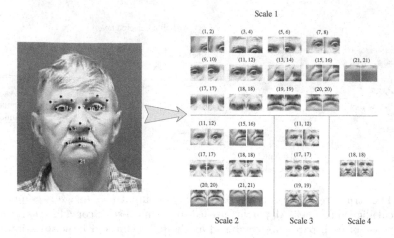

Fig. 2. 23×2 multi-scale patches cropped from a face image based on its corresponding landmarks. The resolution of all patches are 48×48. The patches from the right half of face are mirrored to augment the database.

half-octave) by taking the landmarks as center. The number of landmark pairs used in 4 scales are 13, 6, 3 and 1 from small to large scale, thus giving 23 multi-scale patch pairs. For the landmarks in the right half of face, the patches are mirrored to be consistent with the left half. In this way, we can get $23 \times 2 = 46$ local aligned, multi-scale image patches for a face image, which are shown in Fig. 2. The patches capture the appearance of the face image in multi-scale and are robust to rigid and non-rigid deformations.

3.2   Convolutional Network for Age Estimation

Figure 1 shows the architecture of the proposed network, the details of each layer is described in Fig. 3. For the 23 groups of image patches, we create 23 sub-networks to process them respectively and fuse their responses in the final full connected layer to estimate the age. This structure has two benefits: (1) 23 sub-networks can learn the particular features for each patch; (2) The final layer connects all sub-networks together, which can make them mutually complementary. Note that the parameters of the 23 sub-networks and the final layer in Figs. 1 and 3 are optimized in a whole process.

The sub-network for each patch is composed by a convolutional layer, a max pooling layer and a local layer (Locally-connected layer with unshared weights). The number of channels of the convolutional, pooling and local layers are both 16. Before convolution the input are padded by zero values, therefore the output have the same size with input. The filter size of C1 layer is 7×7 and the filter size of L3 layer is 3×3. ReLU neuron [27] is used as activation function for C1 and L3. The stride of S2 is 3 that means it down-samples the feature maps from 48×48 to 16×16 and S2 includes a cross-channel normalization unit. The output of the sub-network (L3) has $16 \times 16 \times 16 = 4096$ dimensions. Therefore

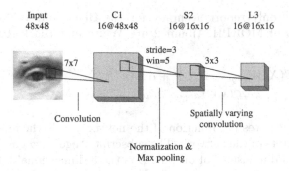

Fig. 3. The structure of sub-network for each patch. The input of sub-network are face patches and the output are sent to the F4 layer in Fig. 1.

the input of F4 has $4096 \times 23 = 94208$ dimensions. F4 uses square difference as cost function, so it can be seen as a linear regression layer. In practice, we should pay attention to the magnitude of F4's output and the target (age). Generally, we need introduce a scale factor to make them in the same order of magnitude. The network are optimized by Stochastic Gradient Descent (SGD).

Besides the learnable parameters, the proposed network has an extra local layer when compares with BIF + CCA [3]. As we know, convolution is appropriate to capture the statistics over the whole image, but the statistical properties of face image are not stationary with respect to the location in image. Thus we add a local layer to model the spatially varying statistics in the high level of network. The following experiments will illustrate the improvement produced by this layer.

3.3 Multi-task Learning

Age, gender and ethnicity are three close related traits of human. When we estimate them from face images, the three traits interact each other. Guo and Mu [28] first estimated the gender and ethnicity of a face image and then sent it to a gender-ethnicity group based age estimator, which obtained good results. References [20] and [3] used PLS and CCA to estimate the three traits simultaneously and obtained better results than previous methods. Jointly estimating age, gender and ethnicity has two advantages: (1) By sharing the model between the three tasks can improve the speed of learning and inference; (2) Multi-label can supply more information of the database to regularize the network during training.

Based on the proposed network, we extend it by a multi-task loss function to estimate age, gender and ethnicity of face image jointly. The output of F4 layer in Fig. 1 is modified from 1 to 3 dimensions, in which each dimension is corresponded to age, gender and ethnicity respectively. Our multi-task loss function is composed by three terms: a square loss for age, binomial deviance loss [29] (also known as cross-entropy) for gender and ethnicity. For ethnicity classification, we only report accuracy for the Black and White because the majority images of MORPH Album 2 are White and Black (96%). The loss function is

$$J = (C(X,W)_{age} - L_{age})^2 + \alpha \ln(e^{-2C(X,W)_{gender}L_{gender}} + 1)$$
$$+ \beta \ln(e^{-2C(X,W)_{ethnicity}L_{ethnicity}} + 1), \tag{1}$$

where $C(X,W)$ denotes the function of the network. X is the input face image. W is the parameters of the network. The subscripts "age", "gender" and "ethnicity" denote the 3 dimensions of output. L is the 3 dimensional label of training set. $L_{gender} \in (-1,1)$, -1 denotes Male and 1 denotes Female. $L_{ethnicity} \in (-1,1)$, -1 denotes Black and 1 denotes White. α and β are hyper-parameters to tune the importance of each term.

Because Eq. (1) is derivable, the objective can be easily optimized by SGD too. If need deal with multiple ethnicity classification on other databases, we can use softmax regression and negative log-likelihood as loss function.

4   Experiments

Large data is needed to train a good neural network, therefore we conduct the experiments on MORPH Album 2, which is the only large aging database we know. First, the information and setup of MORPH is described. Then, four networks with different architecture are compared to illustrate the superiority of the proposed network. And the benefits of multi-scale analysis and local alignment are verified by the results. Finally, the proposed network is compared with state-of-the-art methods and an efficient multi-task network is presented.

4.1   Database and Setup

MORPH Album 2 contains about 55,000 face images of more than 13,000 subjects. The capture time spans from 2003 to 2007. Age ranges from 16 to 77 years. Although it is a good and large database, the distributions of gender and ethnicity are uneven. The Male-Female ratio is about 5.5:1 and the White-Black ratio is about 4:1. Except for White and Black, the proportion of other ethnicity is very low (4%).

To use the database effectively, we follow the previous way [28] to preprocessing the database and split it into three non-overlapped subsets S_1, S_2 and S_3 randomly. First, all images in MORPH are processed by a face detector [30]. Because MORPH contains some non-face images (e.g., tattoo), they are removed from the database after this step. The number of face images in the processed database is 55244. Then the facial landmarks of face images are localized by ASM [26] and local aligned patches are cropped based on the landmarks described in Sect. 3.1. We construct the $S1$, $S2$ and $S3$ subsets by two rules: (1) Making Male-Female ratio ≈ 3; (2) Making White-Black ratio $= 1$. The information of the subsets are shown in Table 1. In all experiments, the

Table 1. The information of the pre-processed MORPH Album 2 and S1, S2, S3 subsets.

	Black			White			Other
Male	S1: 4012	S2: 4012	S3: 28835	S1: 4012	S2: 4012	S3: 0	S3: 1845
Female	S1: 1305	S2: 1305	S3: 3166	S1: 1305	S2: 1305	S3: 0	S3: 130

training and testing are repeated in two times: (1) training on $S1$, testing on $S2 + S3$ and (2) training on $S2$, testing on $S1 + S3$. The performance of the two experiments and their average are reported. For age and gender estimation, all images in Table 1 are used. For ethnicity classification, the images in "Other" column are neglected.[1]

4.2 Age Estimation

In the age estimation experiments, we will illustrate the advantages of the proposed network in three aspects: architecture, multi-scale analysis, and local alignment.

As described in Sect. 3.1, $23 \times 2 = 46$ multi-scale patches are generated for every face image. We call those not mirrored patches as left-patches (marked by blue box in Fig. 4), and the mirrored patches as right-patches (marked by red box). In the training stage, the left-patches and right-patches can be seen as a way to double the training set. In the test stage, we can get two predicts based on the left-patches and right-patches respectively and fuse the two predicts by average. The test process is shown in Fig. 4.

Architecture. The architecture of neural network determines the capacity of the model. How to choose a good architecture is a problem specific task and is also affected by the scale of training data. In this section, we compare 4 networks with various architectures from shallow to deep. The architectures for comparison are as follows.

1. C-P-F: convolution + max pooling + full connection;
2. C-P-L-F (proposed): convolution + max pooling + local layer (Locally-connected layer with unshared weights) + full connection;
3. C-P-C-F: convolution + max pooling + convolution + full connection;
4. C-P-C-P-L-F: convolution + max pooling + convolution + max pooling + local layer + full connection.

"C-P-L-F" is the proposed architecture which has been described in Sect. 3.2. In all networks, the number of filters are both 16. The number of training epoch is set to 30. Before training, all images subtract the mean value over the training set from each pixel.

The performance of age estimation of above 4 networks are shown in Table 2. From the table we can see many interesting results. The proposed architecture

---

[1] The detailed evaluation protocols and facial landmarks can be downloaded from http://www.cbsr.ia.ac.cn/users/dyi/agr.html.

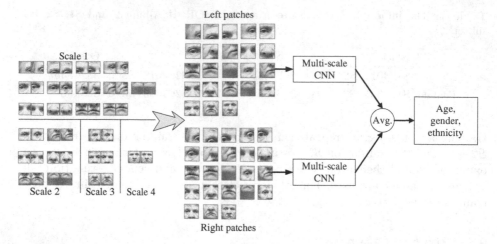

Fig. 4. The test process of the proposed network. For a face image, $23 \times 2 = 46$ multi-scale patches are divided into two groups "left patches"(blue box) and "right patches"(red box) and their predicts are fused by average (Color figure online).

Table 2. Comparison of 4 networks with different architectures.

Architecture	Training set	Test set	Age MAE	Average MAE
C-P-F	S1	S2 + S3	3.75	3.71
	S2	S1 + S3	3.66	
C-P-L-F (proposed)	S1	S2 + S3	3.63	**3.63**
	S2	S1 + S3	3.63	
C-P-C-F	S1	S2 + S3	3.94	3.93
	S2	S1 + S3	3.91	
C-P-C-P-L-F	S1	S2 + S3	3.85	3.78
	S2	S1 + S3	3.71	

"C-P-L-F" has lower error than other compared architectures. Using a local layer before the full connected layer can always improve the performance, *i.e.,* "C-P-L-F" is better than "C-P-F" and "C-P-C-P-L-F" is better than "C-P-C-F", which illustrate the importance of the local layer. Deeper architectures ("C-P-C-F" and "C-P-C-P-L-F") have worse performance than the shallow ones ("C-P-F" and "C-P-L-F"). The reason may be that the potentials of deeper architecture are not developed by the current scale of training data. In the following experiments, we will set the architecture as "C-P-L-F".

Multi-scale Analysis. As shown in Fig. 2, the patches are generated in 4 scales. And the number of patches in each scale are: 13, 6, 3, 1. To illustrate the advantage of multi-scale analysis in our network, we evaluate the performance of

Table 3. The performance of networks in single scale and multi-scale.

Scale	#Patches	Training set	Test set	Age MAE	Average MAE
Scale 1	13	S1	S2 + S3	3.84	3.87
		S2	S1 + S3	3.89	
Scale 2	6	S1	S2 + S3	4.39	4.41
		S2	S1 + S3	4.43	
Scale 3	3	S1	S2 + S3	4.44	4.36
		S2	S1 + S3	4.27	
Scale 4	1	S1	S2 + S3	5.53	5.45
		S2	S1 + S3	5.37	
Multi-scale (proposed)	23	S1	S2 + S3	3.63	**3.63**
		S2	S1 + S3	3.63	

Table 4. The performance of two networks trained on aligned and non-aligned patches.

	Training set	Test set	Age MAE	Average MAE
Non-aligned	S1	S2 + S3	3.87	3.79
	S2	S1 + S3	3.70	
Aligned (proposed)	S1	S2 + S3	3.63	**3.63**
	S2	S1 + S3	3.63	

each scale respectively. Except for the number of sub-networks, the architecture for each scale is as same as the multi-scale version. The results of each scale and multi-scale are shown in Table 3. Small scale generally has better performance than large scale. There are three possible reasons for this phenomenon: first, patches in small scale contain more texture information which are close related to human age; second, small scale patches are better aligned than large scale patches; third, the number of patches in small scale is more than large scale.

Although different scales have different performance, they are very complementary to each other. When fusing the 4 scales together, the MAE is reduced significantly from 3.87 to 3.63.

Local Aligned Patches. Besides of the multi-scale analysis, local alignment is our another contribution. Here, we conduct an experiment to verify the power of local alignment. For fairness, we crop patches for all face images again but based on a mean shape, which is generated by averaging the landmarks of all face images in MORPH Album 2. Because the mean shape cannot be accurate for every face image, the cropped patches are not aligned well. Then we use these not well aligned patches to train a network for comparison. We call these two networks as aligned network and non-aligned network. The two networks have the same structure and their inputs are both $23 \times 48 \times 48$ dimensions. Some aligned and non-aligned patches of a face image are shown in Fig. 5.

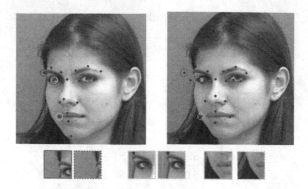

Fig. 5. Left: A face image and its corresponding landmarks. Right: The face image and the positions of the mean shape. Bottom: Some aligned and non-aligned patches of the face image. For abbreviation, just three patch pairs are shown (Color figure online).

Table 4 shows the performance of the aligned and non-aligned networks. Apparently, the MAE of the aligned network is lower than the non-aligned one. Due to the non-aligned patches have more variations in translation, the non-aligned network should pay more attention to learn the translation invariant feature, which reduces the performance of age estimation. On the contrary, the input patches of the aligned network are already aligned well, therefore the network can focus on age estimation better. Moreover, the non-aligned network need 35 epoches to converge, which is slightly more than 30 epoches of the aligned network.

The improvements of each module in the proposed method has been verified in the above paragraphs, including architecture, multi-scale analysis and local alignment. The overall performance of the proposed method is compared with state-of-the-art methods in Table 5. The comparison is done on MORPH Album 2 too, the largest public database for age estimation. From the last column of Table 5, we can see the existing lowest MAE = 3.98 is obtained by BIF + KCCA [3]. The proposed multi-scale CNN reduces the MAE to 3.63 significantly, and the relative reduction is 8.8 %. From the results, we can find another interesting thing for BIF, that is the kernel methods are consistently better than their linear version, such as KCCA > (r)CCA, KPLS > PLS and KSVM > LSVM. The observation indicates that the "convolution + pooling + kernel correlation" architecture is better than "convolution+pooling+linear transformation" in age estimation. In our intuition, the architecture of the proposed network, "C-P-L-F" (see Sect. 4.2), is very similar to "BIF + kernel method". By comparing Tables 5 and 3, we can see that even using a single scale our MAE = 3.87 is still lower than BIF + KCCA.

4.3 Joint Estimation of Age, Gender and Ethnicity

Finally, we train a multi-task network to estimate age, gender and ethnicity simultaneously from face image using the method described in Sect. 3.3. The training process is similar to the previous experiment, architecture = "C-P-L-F",

Table 5. The results of estimating age, gender and ethnicity on MORPH Album 2 and comparison of the proposed method to state-of-the-art methods.

Method	Tr. set	Test set	Gender Accu.	Ethnicity Accu.	Age MAE	Avg. MAE
CNN (Single-Task)	S1	S2 + S3	–	–	3.63	**3.63**
	S2	S1 + S3	–	–	3.63	
CNN (Multi-Task)	S1	S2 + S3	98.0%	99.1%	3.72	**3.63**
	S2	S1 + S3	97.8%	98.1%	3.54	
Baseline CNN [9][a]	S1	S2 + S3	–	–	4.64	4.60
	S2	S1 + S3	–	–	4.55	
BIF + CCA [3]	S1	S2 + S3	95.2%	97.8%	5.39	5.37
	S2	S1 + S3	95.2%	97.8%	5.35	
BIF + rCCA [3]	S1	S2 + S3	97.6%	98.7%	4.43	4.42
	S2	S1 + S3	97.6%	98.6%	4.40	
BIF + KCCA [3]	S1	S2 + S3	98.5%	98.9%	4.00	3.98
	S2	S1 + S3	98.4%	99.0%	3.95	
BIF + PLS [20]	S1	S2 + S3	97.4%	98.7%	4.58	4.56
	S2	S1 + S3	97.3%	98.6%	4.54	
BIF + KPLS [20]	S1	S2 + S3	98.4%	99.0%	4.07	4.04
	S2	S1 + S3	98.3%	99.0%	4.01	
BIF + 3Step [28]	S1	S2 + S3	98.1%	98.9%	4.44	4.45
	S2	S1 + S3	97.9%	98.8%	4.46	
BIF + LSVM [3]	S1	S2 + S3	–	–	5.06	5.09
	S2	S1 + S3	–	–	5.12	
BIF + KSVM [3]	S1	S2 + S3	–	–	4.89	4.91
	S2	S1 + S3	–	–	4.92	
CPNN [31]	10-fold CV		–	–	–	4.87

[a] This 5-layered baseline CNN is implemented by us according to the description in [9]. The dimension of face images to train and test the network is 64 × 64.

epoch = 30, and optimized by SGD, except for the label of training samples including extra gender and ethnicity information. The size of α and β in Eq. (1) just has a little influence to the performance of the multi-task network, so we set them as 1 in the experiment. The performance of the multi-task network is list in the second row of Table 5. When jointly optimizing with gender and ethnicity classification, the average MAE of age estimation is as same as the single-task network, which are both 3.63 years. And meanwhile, the accuracies of gender and ethnicity classification are comparable to state-of-the-art. Being consistent with other works, the accuracy of ethnicity classification is higher than gender. This may be a clue to design novel multi-task networks in the future.

Compared with the proposed method, the most competitive methods are BIF + KCCA and BIF + KPLS, but their test speed are slow. On a Intel Core 2 CPU@2.1 GHz, excluding the time of feature extraction, the test time of KCCA and KPLS are 72515.6 and 72516.4 s [3]. On a Tesla K20 GPU, the test time of our network on the whole test set is 87 s (44610 samples, 2 ms/sample), which is faster than kernel methods significantly. On a Intel Core i3-2370M@2.4 GHz (single thread), the test time of our CPU version is 8900 s (200 ms/sample), which is 100× slower than the GPU version, but still faster than KCCA and KPLS significantly. Note that our test time is measured from inputting the aligned patches to outputting the results.

5   Conclusions

We proposed a novel age estimation method based on CNN in this paper. Compared with the state-of-the-art BIF based methods, our method achieved significant lower error on MORPH Album 2 database due to its deeper structure and learnable parameters. To apply CNN effectively in age estimation, we carefully designed the architecture of the network and combined two important tricks into the network. Extensive experiments illustrated the improvements brought by our design principles, including "C-P-L-F" architecture, multi-scale analysis and local aligned patches. Furthermore, we constructed a novel loss function for age, gender and ethnicity joint estimation and trained a multi-task network. Experiments showed that our multi-task network achieved the same MAE with the single-task network and achieved high accuracies in gender and ethnicity classification at the same time. Future work will focus on how to design more reasonable multi-task architectures for age, gender and ethnicity joint estimation.

Acknowledgment. This work was supported by the Chinese National Natural Science Foundation Projects #61105023, #61103156, #61105037, #61203267, #61375037, #61473291, National Science and Technology Support Program Project #2013BAK02 B01, Chinese Academy of Sciences Project No. KGZD-EW-102-2, and AuthenMetric R&D Funds. The GPU was donated by NVIDIA.

References

1. Kwon, Y.H., da Vitoria Lobo, N.: Age classification from facial images. In: 1994 IEEE Computer Society Conference on Computer Vision and Pattern Recognition. Proceedings CVPR 1994, pp. 762–767 (1994)
2. Lanitis, A., Draganova, C., Christodoulou, C.: Comparing different classifiers for automatic age estimation. IEEE Trans. Syst. Man Cybern. B: Cybern. **34**, 621–628 (2004)
3. Guo, G., Mu, G.: Joint estimation of age, gender and ethnicity: CCA vs. PLS. In: FG, pp. 1–6 (2013)
4. Rawls, A.W., Ricanek Jr., K.: MORPH: development and optimization of a longitudinal age progression database. In: Fierrez, J., Ortega-Garcia, J., Esposito, A., Drygajlo, A., Faundez-Zanuy, M. (eds.) BioID MultiComm2009. LNCS, vol. 5707, pp. 17–24. Springer, Heidelberg (2009)

5. Basak, D., Pal, S., Patranabis, D.C.: Support vector regression. Neural Inf. Process. Lett. Rev. **11**, 203–224 (2007)
6. Geladi, P., Kowalski, B.R.: Partial least-squares regression: a tutorial. Anal. Chim. Acta **185**, 1–17 (1986)
7. Hardoon, D.R., Szedmak, S., Shawe-Taylor, J.: Canonical correlation analysis: an overview with application to learning methods. Neural Comput. **16**, 2639–2664 (2004)
8. Daugman, J.G.: Complete discrete 2D Gabor transforms by neural networks for image analysis and compression. IEEE Trans. ASSP **36**, 1169–1179 (1988)
9. Yang, M., Zhu, S., Lv, F., Yu, K.: Correspondence driven adaptation for human profile recognition. In: CVPR, pp. 505–512 (2011)
10. Guo, G., Mu, G., Fu, Y., Huang, T.S.: Human age estimation using bio-inspired features. In: CVPR. pp. 112–119 (2009)
11. Kwon, Y.H., da Vitoria Lobo, N.: Age classification from facial images. Comput. Vis. Image Underst. **74**, 1–21 (1999)
12. Cootes, T.F., Edwards, G.J., Taylor, C.J.: Active appearance models. In: Burkhardt, H., Neumann, B. (eds.) ECCV 1998. LNCS, vol. 1407, pp. 484–498. Springer, Heidelberg (1998)
13. Geng, X., Zhou, Z.H., Smith-Miles, K.: Automatic age estimation based on facial aging patterns. IEEE Trans. Pattern Anal. Mach. Intell. **29**, 2234–2240 (2007)
14. Gao, F., Ai, H.: Face age classification on consumer images with Gabor feature and fuzzy LDA method. In: Tistarelli, M., Nixon, M.S. (eds.) ICB 2009. LNCS, vol. 5558, pp. 132–141. Springer, Heidelberg (2009)
15. Gunay, A., Nabiyev, V.V.: Automatic age classification with LBP. In: 2008 23rd IEEE International Symposium on Computer and Information Sciences. ISCIS 2008, pp. 1–4 (2008)
16. Yan, S., Liu, M., Huang, T.S.: Extracting age information from local spatially flexible patches. In: 2008 IEEE International Conference on Acoustics, Speech and Signal Processing. ICASSP 2008, pp. 737–740 (2008)
17. Fu, Y., Huang, T.S.: Human age estimation with regression on discriminative aging manifold. IEEE Trans. Multimed. **10**, 578–584 (2008)
18. Cao, D., Lei, Z., Zhang, Z., Feng, J., Li, S.Z.: Human age estimation using ranking SVM. In: Zheng, W.-S., Sun, Z., Wang, Y., Chen, X., Yuen, P.C., Lai, J. (eds.) CCBR 2012. LNCS, vol. 7701, pp. 324–331. Springer, Heidelberg (2012)
19. Herbrich, R., Graepel, T., Obermayer, K.: Large margin rank boundaries for ordinal regression. In: Smola, A.J., et al. (eds.) Advances in Large Margin Classifiers. MIT Press, Cambridge (2000)
20. Guo, G., Mu, G.: Simultaneous dimensionality reduction and human age estimation via Kernel partial least squares regression. In: CVPR. pp. 657–664 (2011)
21. Duffner, S.: Face image analysis with convolutional neural networks. Ph.D. thesis (2008)
22. Farabet, C., Couprie, C., Najman, L., LeCun, Y.: Learning hierarchical features for scene labeling. IEEE Trans. Pattern Anal. Mach. Intell. **35**, 1915–1929 (2013)
23. Chen, D., Cao, X., Wen, F., Sun, J.: Blessing of dimensionality: high-dimensional feature and its efficient compression for face verification. In: CVPR, pp. 3025–3032 (2013)
24. ul Hussain, S., Wheeler, Napolon, T., Jurie, F.: Face recognition using local quantized patterns. In: Proceedings on British Machine Vision Conference, vol. 1, pp. 52–61 (2012)
25. Li, S.Z., Yi, D., Lei, Z., Liao, S.: The CASIA NIR-VIS 2.0 face database. In: CVPR Workshops, pp. 348–353 (2013)

26. Cootes, T.F., Taylor, C.J., Cooper, D.H., Graham, J.: Active shape models: their training and application. CVGIP: Image Underst. **61**, 38–59 (1995)
27. Krizhevsky, A., Sutskever, I., Hinton, G.E.: ImageNet classification with deep convolutional neural networks. In: NIPS, pp. 1106–1114 (2012)
28. Guo, G., Mu, G.: Human age estimation: What is the influence across race and gender? In: 2010 IEEE Computer Society Conference on Computer Vision and Pattern Recognition Workshops (CVPRW), pp. 71–78 (2010)
29. Friedman, J., Tibshirani, R., Hastie, T.: The Elements of Statistical Learning: Data Mining, Inference, and Prediction. Springer Series in Statistics. Springer, New York (2009)
30. Viola, P., Jones, M.: Rapid object detection using a boosted cascade of simple features. In: Proceedings of IEEE Computer Society Conference on Computer Vision and Pattern Recognition, Kauai, Hawaii (2001)
31. Geng, X., Yin, C., Zhou, Z.H.: Facial age estimation by learning from label distributions. IEEE Trans. Pattern Anal. Mach. Intell. **35**, 2401–2412 (2013)

Photorealistic Face De-Identification by Aggregating Donors' Face Components

Saleh Mosaddegh$^{(\boxtimes)}$, Loic Simon, and Frédéric Jurie

CNRS UMR 6072, University of Caen, ENSICAEN, Caen, France
{Saleh.Mosaddegh,Loic.Simon,Frederic.Jurie}@unicaen.fr

Abstract. With the adoption of pervasive surveillance systems and the development of efficient automatic face matchers, the question of preserving privacy becomes paramount. In this context, automated face de-identification is revived. Typical solutions based on eyes masking or pixelization, while commonly used in news broadcasts, produce very unnatural images. More sophisticated solutions were sparingly introduced in the literature, but they fail to account for fundamental constraints such as the visual likeliness of de-identified images. In contrast, we identify essential principles and build upon efficient techniques to derive an automated face de-identification solution meeting our predefined criteria. More specifically, our approach relies on a set of face donors from which it can borrow various face components (eyes, chin, *etc.*). Faces are then de-identified by substituting their own face components with the donors' ones, in such a way that an automatic face matcher is fooled while the appearance of the generated faces are as close as possible to original faces. Experiments on several datasets validate the approach and show its ability both in terms of privacy preservation and visual quality.

1 Introduction

A large number of cameras oversee public and semi-public spaces today. It raises concerns on the unintentional and unwarranted invasion of the privacy of individuals caught in the videos. To address these concerns, automated methods to de-identify individuals in these videos are necessary [1]. De-identification does not aim at removing all the information involving the individuals. Its ideal goals are to obscure the identity of the subject without obscuring the action or the rest of the scene.

Finding the right trade-off between privacy and awareness has a long history in the computer vision literature. As noted by Hudson and Smith [16], systems which attempt to support awareness in distributed media immediately face several important challenges. First among these is the widely recognized issue of privacy. They believe there is a fundamental trade-off between providing awareness information and preserving privacy. In general, the more information transmitted about one's actions, the more potential for awareness exists among those receiving the information. At the same time, however, the more information transmitted, the more potential for violation of one's privacy exists.

D. Cremers et al. (Eds.): ACCV 2014, Part III, LNCS 9005, pp. 159–174, 2015.
DOI: 10.1007/978-3-319-16811-1_11

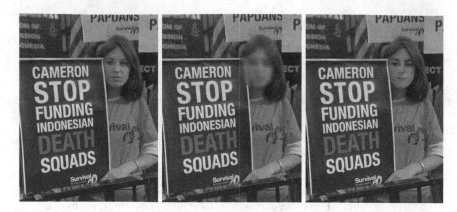

Fig. 1. Comparing blurring with our approach (from left to right): original image, image de-identified with naive blur, image automatically de-identified with our approach. While looking natural, the photo does not reveal explicitly the identity of the person.

Ideally, face, silhouette, gait and other characteristics need to be obscured. Our approach focuses however on face de-identification on a per-frame basis. Our main concern is to ensure privacy while preserving the likelihood of the produced de-identified image. One typical illustration of this process is illustrated in Fig. 1. The image looks natural but the face shown on the photo can not be identified because it has been replaced by an artificial computer-generated face. Obviously, the new face should not reveal the identity of someone else, which would be the case if using face swapping algorithms (*e.g.* using [19]). The new face must be a fully artificial face, looking natural and similar to the face to be de-identified.

We formulate this goal in a principled way by expressing our response as the solution of an optimization problem. Our approach relies on the use of a bank of face donors from which the algorithm is allowed to pick components (such as eyes, nose, *etc.*). The optimal face, for a given face matcher algorithm, is the image which fools the face matcher (*i.e.* the distance between the original face and the de-identified one is greater than a threshold) while the difference between the two images is visually as small as possible (in this paper the visual difference is computed as the PSNR). In addition, another constraint guarantees that the forged face is not recognized by the face matcher for any of the donors used to de-identify the image. The comparison of Fig. 1, obtained using our approach, with existing de-identification approaches shown Fig. 2 motivates this work. Besides, in order to make the solving tractable, we reduce the search space to faces that are likely to be relevant to our purposes using different heuristics.

Let us list several key aspects of our approach. First, the de-identification can be applied to faces outside the donor database (*e.g.* Fig. 1). Besides, the proposed approach does not requires having the best face matcher available at the moment. Indeed, the face matcher is meant to give the direction along which faces should be modified to make their recognition harder. Obviously, better face matchers can lead to de-identified images with smaller visual differences

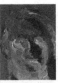

(a) De-indentification images from [10]: original image, pixelization with a block size of 16, Gaussian blur with a standard deviation $\sigma = 8$, scrambling by random sign inversion, scrambling by random permutation.

(b) Original/de-identified image, live-shadow algorithm of [29].

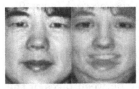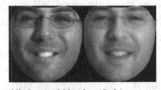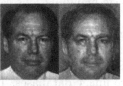

(c) Original/deidentified image, k-same algorithm of [23].

(d) Original/de-identified image, multifactor $(\epsilon; k)$-map algorithm algorithm of [12].

(e) Original/de-identified image, Driessen and Durmuth's algorithm [9].

Fig. 2. Visual comparison of recently published de-identification approaches.

(in terms of PSNR). Another strong aspect of the method is the lack of required pre-processing. In other words, the queried image does not need to be normalized beforehand.

The rest of the paper is organized as follows: after presenting the related work (Sect. 2) the details of our formulation are presented in Sect. 3, followed by an experimental validation (Sect. 4) in which the proposed approach is validated using images from three different datasets.

2   Related Work

Enforcing privacy by de-identifying faces in images has a long history in the computer vision literature. As noted by [5], one common technique, often seen on news broadcasts, is to *pixelize* people's faces, replacing them by large pixels (squares). More advanced and general techniques have also been developed *e.g.* Hudson and Smith [16] who described a shadow-view filter giving the visual impression of ghostly shadow moving in a static scene, or Crowley *et al.* [8] who used eigen-filters to analyze a scene and reconstruct its images in a *socially-correct* way.

While identity masking techniques have been widely used in the media, there has been little empirical investigation of their effectiveness in protecting the identity of innocent passers-by children or crime witnesses from people familiar with them. Zhao and Stasko [29] examined four filters by asking volunteers to identify which of five actors were featured. Before the experiment started, volunteers were shown portraits of the actors. In [5], Boyle *et al.* analyzed how a blur and a pixelize image filter might impact both awareness and privacy in images. They examined how well observers of several filtered video scenes extract particular awareness cues. Their results suggest that the blur filter, and to a lesser extent the pixelize filter, have a level suitable for providing awareness information while safeguarding privacy. More recently, Lander et al. [18] evaluated the effectiveness of pixelization and blurring on masking the identity of familiar faces. They concluded that privacy may not be fully preserved depending on whose identity is being concealed. Another important issue is to ensure anonymity while preserving the rest of the information [1]. Finally, it is worth noting that simple image manipulations can be retro engineered, allowing to reconstruct faces [6].

Besides these simple blurring and pixelization techniques, more advanced techniques have been introduced, most of them based on the well-known eigenfaces representation [9,23], or some variants [12]. Newton et al. [23] proposed k-Same, a privacy enhancing algorithm based on the concept of k-anonymity to face image databases. The algorithm determines similarity between faces of the database, clusters similar faces, and creates a new face by aggregating the faces of a cluster. Gross et al. [12] proposed a factorization approach to separate identity and non-identity related factors, allowing to only replace the factors expressing the identity by the cluster's aggregation, while keeping the non-identity factors untouched to better preserve facial expressions. Dufaux and Ebrahimi [10] present an effective scrambling techniques to foil face recognition. Very recently, Driessen and Dürmuth [9] focussed on the preservation of the human recognition as a top requirement, by finding the modification of the image which has the lowest distortion (in the image space) while changing the signature to a desired value. This is done by projecting the face on the manifold spanned by some eigenfaces. Then, modifying the signature amounts to changing this projection. And since this is a linear process, mapping back this modification into the image space is simply achieved by modulating the eigenfaces components. The image part orthogonal to the space spanned by the eigenfaces is kept untouched.

The approaches mentioned in the previous paragraphs present two drawbacks. First, they do not produce photorealistic face images; they all look unnatural and attract the attention (see Fig. 2). Second, the k-Same principle is addressing a question which is very different from ours: the goal is to sanitize a database before publishing it, in such a way that searching for the most similar face to a query image will output k identities. Our approach is different as we assume the social network has already published a collection of pictures, and it is up to the user to process any novel picture before posting it.

Face swapping can be seen as an interesting solution for addressing the aforementioned limitations. In [3], given an input image, Bitouk et al. detect all the faces occurring in the image, align them, select candidate face images from a face library, adjust the pose, lighting, and color of the candidate face images to match the appearance of those in the input image, and seamlessly blend in the results. A user study validates the high quality of the replacement results. Zhu et al. [30] extended the approach by proposing a better alignment approach. Lin et al. [19] addressed the case of face replacement with large-pose differences. However, face swapping raises other issues related to privacy, as the face template used for the replacement can easily be recognized.

Face synthesis provides yet another way to produce de-identified images. Taking inspiration from exemplar-based texture synthesis [11], Mohammed *et al.* [22] generated realistic images of faces using a model trained from real examples, describing textures with local non-parametric models. This approach paves the way to very realistic faces with interesting inpainting applications. The approach is however limited to frontal views and the use of such a technique for face de-identification has not been investigated so far. A somehow similar approach was introduced in [28] in the context of face hallucination.

In addition, several loosely related techniques may prove useful in improving the status of face de-identification. For instance, approaches based on landmark detection [31] such as active appearance models [7,20] provide effective ways to align faces with different poses, hence alleviating the frontal view restriction. Parsing a face into meaningful components has been addressed in different ways, *e.g.* in [26]. Based on parsing, exemplar-based synthesis can be adapted into replacing parts of a face with corresponding components taken from a database. Eventually, leveraging seamless blending [25] allows to avoid artefacts.

In conclusion, despite the existence of a large body of related techniques, face de-identification remains insufficiently explored. We argue that at least two fundamental principles should be endorsed, namely (i) face de-identification should be guided by face matching, as face matching algorithms are getting closer and closer to human performance [27] and (ii) faces should look natural and artefact-free. To the best of our knowledge, the question of ensuring both criteria has not been satisfactorily addressed in the literature. Therefore we build upon powerful techniques such as automatic landmark detection, exemplar-based synthesis and seamless blending to provide an adapted solution to face de-identification.

3   A New Method for Synthesizing Artificial Faces Using Face Component Donations

3.1   Problem Statement

Let I be loosely defined as the set of images containing one single face per image. We also assume that we have at our disposal a face matcher, *i.e.* a function $F(x_s, x_m)$ from $I \times I$ to $\mathbb{R}$, associating two images x_s and x_m with a scalar value such that $F(x_s, x_m) > \mu$ if and only if the two faces are believed to represent different persons. We also assume that a set of N face images of different people acting as *face donors* is available from which we can harvest face components (eyes, noses, *etc.*). This set is denoted by $\mathcal{FD}$.

Starting with an image x_o to be de-identified, our objective is to produce a modified image x_m by minimizing the following problem:

$$x_m^* = \underset{x_m \in I}{\operatorname{argmin}} \quad \|x_m - x_o\|$$
$$\text{subject to} \quad F(x_m, x_o) > \mu \tag{1}$$
$$\forall x_i \in \mathcal{FD}, F(x_m, x_i) > \mu$$

In other words, we want to produce a novel face that meets several criteria. First it must not be confused by the face matcher with any of the donors nor with the original face. Second, it must remain as similar to the original face as allowed by the previous constraints.

In some applications (*e.g.* social networks), another exemplar x'_o of the same person as x_o may be available and published already. In that case, we introduce a slight modification where we verify that the face matcher does not recognize x'_o instead of x_o which is not meant to be published. The new variant is as follows:

$$x_m^* = \underset{x_m \in I}{\operatorname{argmin}} \quad \|x_m - x_o\|$$
$$\text{subject to} \quad F(x_m, x'_o) > \mu \tag{2}$$
$$\forall x_i \in \mathcal{FD}, F(x_m, x_i) > \mu$$

To distinguish between the two formulations we will refer to them as self-identification for the former $(x'_o = x_o)$ and pairwise de-identification for the later. For the sake of generality, our approach will be described for a generic x'_o.

3.2 Overview of the Approach

We address the previous problem by using a face component cloning algorithm. We assume that faces are made of a set of C spatially delimited face components that can be cloned individually. Let $c = (c_1, \cdots, c_i, \cdots, c_c) \in [\![0, N]\!]^C$ an index vector expressing the origin within the donor bank of the different components of the artificially generated face. More precisely, $c_i = 0$ means the face component i is unchanged, $c_i = k$ with $0 < k \leq N$ means that the i-th component of the face has to be cloned from the k-th image of the face donor bank.

Let's denote by $FG(x_o, c, \mathcal{FD})$ a face generator algorithm that can generate an image from a source image x_o by cloning the face components indexed in c from the donor bank. The previous problem is then made simpler by restricting the search space from I to the range of faces created by FG when starting from the original face. It yields the following approximation:

$$x_m^* = \underset{x_m \in FG(x_o)}{\operatorname{argmin}} \quad \|x_o - x_m\|$$
$$\text{subject to} \quad F(x_m, x'_o) > \mu \tag{3}$$
$$\forall x_i \in \mathcal{FD}(x_m, x_i) > \mu$$

where with a slight abuse of notation $FG(x_o) = \{FG(x_o, c, \mathcal{FD})/c \in [\![0, N]\!]^C\}$.

3.3 Optimization Strategy

The optimization problem in Eq. 3 cannot easily be solved by using standard optimization toolboxes let alone brute force. It has the form of a constrained problem, where the energy functional is admittedly convex, but where the constraints can display any intricate behaviour. As a matter of fact, these constraints

input: $x_o, x'_o, \mathcal{FD}$
output: x^*_m

function OPTIMIZE($x_o, x'_o, \mathcal{FD}$)
    $x^*_m \leftarrow x_o$
    $\forall 1 \leq i \leq C,\ K_i \leftarrow [\![1, N]\!]$ *keep track of candidate donors for each component*
    while $\exists i$ s.t. $K_i \neq \emptyset$ and not CHECKCONSTRAINT($x^*_m, x'_o, \mathcal{FD}$) **do**   *Main Loop*
        for $i := 1$ to C **do**   *Loop on components*
            $k_i \leftarrow \underset{k \in K_i}{\operatorname{argmin}} \| x_o - FG(x^*_m, e_{i,k}, \mathcal{FD}) \|$ *First heuristic*
            $y_i \leftarrow FG(x^*_m, e_{i,k_i}, \mathcal{FD})$
        end for
        $i^* \leftarrow \underset{1 \leq i \leq C}{\operatorname{argmax}} F(x_0, y_i)$ *Second heuristic*
        $K_{i^*} \leftarrow K_{i^*} \setminus \{k_{i^*}\}$
    end while
    return x^*_m
end function

Algorithm 1: Optimization routine.

involve $F(x_m, x'_o)$ and despite this latter being often interpreted as a distance function, it is actually a black-box on which we do not exert any control.

Instead of falling back on brute force, that would be overly inefficient, we propose a greedy alternative presented in Algorithm 1. We iteratively replace one new component at a time, using one particular donor. We denote by $e_{i,k} = (0, \cdots, 0, k, 0, \cdots, 0)$ the index vector corresponding to the substitution of component i from donor k. Two greedy heuristics are implemented for the selection of the component and the donor. More precisely, the donor choice is leveraged in order to keep the energy functional small, and the component choice is meant to maximize our chances to de-identify the original face. The iterations continue until the de-identification constraints are met or if there is no donor left for any of the components. In the latter case, the optimization has failed.

3.4 Face Generator

The overall working of the face generator is depicted in Fig. 3. For a given target image, we use up to 4 donors in order to replace the content of different regions of interest (ROI) associated with the components. There is a single connected ROI for three components, namely the mouth+chin component, the nose+cheeks one and the eyebrows. For the eyes on the other hand two connected ROIs are extracted. To perform the replacement of a given ROI we first cleanly align the donor image with the target inside the ROI and then we apply Poisson blending [25].

Landmark detection. We start our process by automatically detecting landmarks. They will be used in the alignment procedure and in generation of the ROIs. In our current implementation, the landmarks are detected following the approach

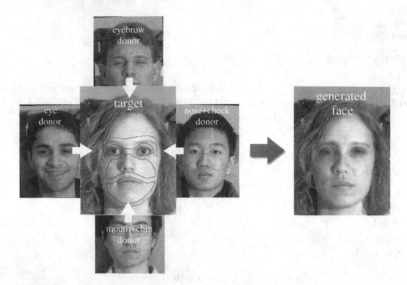

Fig. 3. The face generator implemented in this article. All the components are being replaced using a different donor. Each donor image is registered so that the region of interest (ROI) of the concerned component (red contour) is cleanly aligned with the same ROI in the target image. Artefacts are mitigated thanks to Poisson blending (Color figure online).

of [31]. In total, the set of landmarks is composed of 68 points. As shown in Fig. 4(a) each one of the 4 components is attached a fixed subset of the landmarks. This association is represented through a color code in the figure.

Face alignment. In order to improve accuracy, the alignment phase is performed per ROI. It is guided by the subset of relevant landmarks. More precisely, we estimate an optimal similarity transformation to register the target landmarks contained inside the ROI with their corresponding landmarks in the donor. The optimal transformation is obtained through classical Procrustes analysis. The obtained registration process is similar to the approach of [4].

Composing faces. So far we did not explain how the ROIs are actually built. The leading purpose here is to create a set of non overlapping ROIs covering most of the features of the face while leaving narrow bands of the original face uncovered. Such bands are useful to ensure the overall consistency among the blended donor components. The process to generate the ROIs is described in Fig. 4. This process is entirely automated and is composed of 4 steps. Step (a) corresponds to the landmark detection. In (b), we generate additional landmarks bound to define the contours of a first version of the ROIs depicted in (c). In this first version, the ROIs are tightly joined at some locations. We therefore shrink them by applying a morphological erosion with a 6 pixel disk. This is not applied to the eyes ROI, because it is actually well separated from the surrounding ROIs.

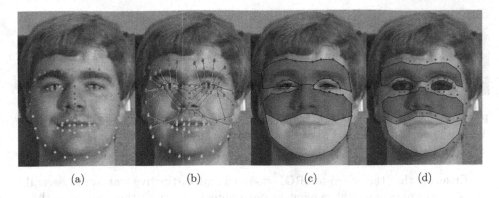

| (a) | (b) | (c) | (d) |

Fig. 4. Mask creation is conducted in 4 steps: (a) Landmarks detection and association with the face components (color coded) - (b) Landmark completion by barycentric averages - (c) mask initialization based on a predefined subset of landmarks - (d) Final mask creation by erosion or dilation. Two color codes are used in this picture (see the text for details) (Color figure online).

On the contrary, we apply a dilation in that case. The final ROIs are depicted in (d) using the same color code as in (a) and (c): green for the forehead, gray for the eyes, purple for the nose and cheeks, and yellow for mouth and chin.

The process to generate the additional landmarks (step (b)) is slightly technical. They are produced by using barycentric averages between two existing landmarks (original ones or already generated new landmarks). The weights used in the barycentric operations and the pairs of landmarks have been hand-tuned once for all in order to maximize the chance to capture meaningful textures in each ROI. The chosen segments and the produced landmarks are depicted in Fig. 4(b). The new landmarks are filled in red. And the color of the link between the support pairs of landmarks represents the value of the weights. Each weight is chosen among a list of 5 possible values $\frac{1}{5}$ (green), $\frac{1}{4}$ (orange), $\frac{1}{2}$ (light-blue), $\frac{2}{3}$ (yellow) and $-\frac{2}{3}$ (dark blue). In the last case, the generated landmark is actually extrapolated rather than interpolated.

Additional remarks. At this point, it may appear odd that the eyes are handled in a different way compared to the other components. This is true in several respects. First, the component is broken in two separate ROIs. This choice is justified by the goal of generating a natural looking face. Such a purpose requires that both eyes are accurately located and scaled. Performing the alignment separately on each eye greatly simplifies that task. Furthermore, the initial ROI of each eye is fixed in a conservative way (that is tightly around the original landmarks) and then scaled up while the exact opposite strategy is applied to the other components. The rationale here is that the original eyes landmarks are much more reliably located around the actual boundary of the eye than the generated ones. It is therefore easier to capture the whole shape of the eye by dilating the region delimited by the original landmarks.

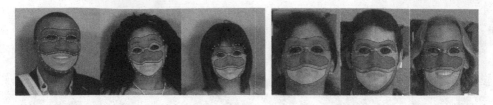

Fig. 5. A few examples of face component's ROIs generated on faces from MUCT database (left-hand side) and MULTIPIE database (right-hand side).

Ensuring that the generated ROIs do not break distinctive features in several parts is an important achievement in our context. It brings the guarantee that in most situations, the collage will not produce structural artefacts. To illustrate the visual performance of the ROIs extraction process, we show in Fig. 5 several examples selected from two different databases.

4   Experimental Results

The objective of the experimental validation is twofold: one one hand, we want to show that the optimization algorithm is working as expected *i.e.* that at each iteration the distance from the original face is monotonically increased (from the perspective of the face matcher) while the modifications of the image are as small as possible (from the perspective of the PSNR). On the other hand, we want to show that resulting images are visually plausible and artifact free.

4.1   Experimental Settings

The experimental validation is mostly done on a subset of the MultiePie dataset [13] containing 2184 frontal images of 346 people (men and women), with 11 images for each individual, under different facial expressions and illuminations. The choice of this database is led by the higher image quality compared to more common datasets such as LFW [15] which is an inevitable requirement for donor database. The images are annotated based on whether the person is wearing sun glasses (*i.e.* the eyes are visible or not). We also present some experiments on images drawn from the MUCT [21] (3755 images of 276 different subjects) and PUT [17] (9971 images of 100 subjects) datasets (using similar settings to MultiePie). During the component replacement we use MultiPie's annotations to reject eye and eyebrows components covered by sunglasses hence only using mouths and noses. In addition, we do not consider the donors with glasses while replacing eyes. Finally, we reject any donor images belonging to the target image. The set of donors contains around 100 faces in the presented experiments.

The face matcher used throughout our approach is inspired by [24] and computes face signatures as histograms of LBP descriptors [2]. Once the descriptors of two images are computed, the distance of the two faces is evaluated as the cosine distance. In other words, if we denote by ϕ and ϕ' the descriptors of

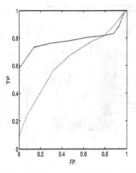

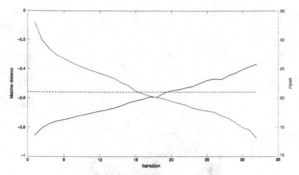

(a) ROC profile for the face matcher before (red) and after (green) applying our approach.

(b) Evolutions of the PSNR (green) and the face matcher distance (blue) with the iterations. The dashed line indicates the value of the de-identification threshold μ.

Fig. 6. Face matcher's de-identification performance (Color figure online).

the images x and x', then $F(x, x') := \frac{\langle \phi | \phi' \rangle}{\|\phi\| \|\phi'\|}$. As mentioned in the introduction, while more recent methods (*e.g.* [27]) give better performances, this simple verification pipeline has the great advantage of being much faster to compute (which is an important advantage when working with a large donor data-set), while being good enough for giving the direction in which an image should be modified to alter the identity as much as possible without altering the image too much. The threshold μ (see Sect. 3) is set using a validation set.

4.2 Quantitative Results and Algorithm's Convergence

To demonstrate the de-identification power of our approach we first present ROC profiles in Fig. 6(a). In order to produce these curves, 262 positive pairs (2 images of the same person) and the same number of negative pairs (two images of different persons) were randomly selected from the MULTIPIE dataset. In each positive pair, one of the two images is de-identified with our approach while negative pairs are untouched. The red curve shows the true positive detection rate against the false positive one, as obtained by the face matcher, before de-identification. The alternate curve (in green) shows the same statistics when the face matcher is applied after de-identification of the database. As expected, de-identification effectively renders the face matcher inefficient since the ROC profile becomes closer to the top-right diagonal curve. Such a profile is typical of a system that provides purely random outputs.

Our optimization is guided by the aim of applying as mild visual degradations to the original image as is allowed by the de-identification itself. Although PSNR is a debatable choice for measuring the amount of visual perturbation, it is the one that we have favored in our formulation. Therefore Fig. 6(b) presents the evolution of the PSNR and of the face matcher distance against the number of iterations of the optimization process. The curves are actually obtained by

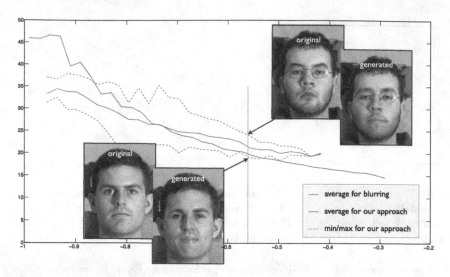

Fig. 7. PSNR against face matcher distance. The solid curves correspond to average performance on the MULTIPIE database, and the dashed ones to the best and worst cases (maximum and minimum PSNR). The blue curve corresponds to de-identification by blurring, and the red one to our approach. The threshold μ is indicated via the green line. For this value of the face Matcher, we show the original and de-identified faces corresponding to the worst and best PSNR (Color figure online).

averaging 132 different runs. As expected, the face matcher distance increases with the iterations while the PSNR decreases. Interestingly, in average, de-identification requires around 20 iterations. This means that for each component there are several donors which look very similar to the subject under consideration.

In Fig. 7, we refine our analysis by comparing the needed amount of texture deformation to reach a certain face matcher distance with our method and with naive blurring. The relevant part of the curves is the rightmost one, since it corresponds to the highest level of de-identification. In particular, one should focus on the curves behavior near and beyond the de-identification threshold μ. From that perspective our method is uniformly superior to blurring. To emphasize the fact that our approach performs evenly in all experiments, we have also added worst and best case curves in dash. In both cases, the original and de-identified face corresponding to the de-identification threshold are also presented.

4.3 Visual Inspection of Output Images

Although the good behavior of a de-identification method with respect of PSNR is a desirable property, it is actually much more important to assess if the produced images are visually realistic. Making quantitative assessment about such realism is not an easy task. Instead, we provide in Fig. 8 a selection of examples (the first 2 rows are from MULTIPIE, the next 3 ones from MUCT and the

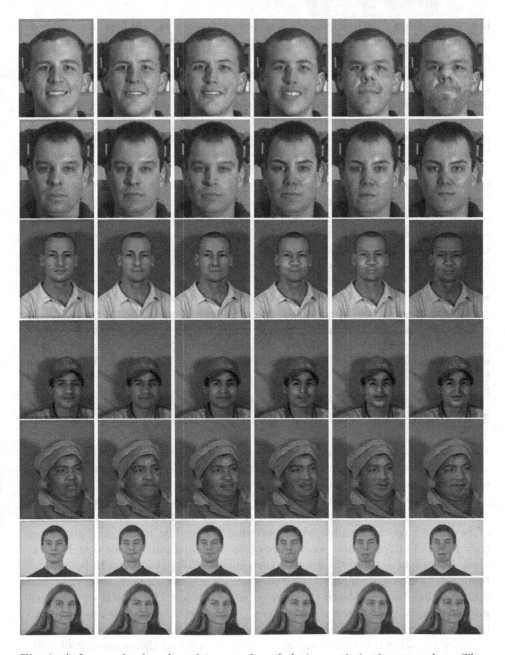

Fig. 8. A few randomly selected images forged during optimization procedure. The faces are presented in the same order as they were produced during the iterations. The original image is marked with a blue frame. Similarly the forged face that passes the de-identification test is marked with a yellow frame. The right-most faces give a glimpse of the degree of de-identification possibly achieved by letting the algorithm run further (or equivalently by imposing a more challenging de-identification threshold μ) (Color figure online).

last 2 ones from PUT). For each example, a sequence of 6 images is presented. Among such a sequence, the original image is marked with a blue frame and the first to reach the prescribed de-identification level is marked with a yellow frame. The remaining four images were picked randomly and were placed accordingly to their iteration. Amazingly, even long after de-identification is reached the generated faces continue to look very convincing.

Some examples demonstrate a striking versatility of the face generator. For instance in the third row, the subject was gradually transformed into an individual of seemingly different ethnic origin without noticeable artefacts. As a side note, the presented sequences suggest the creation of criminal identikits as an unexpected application of our method. In such a scenario, a witness would start from an exemplar face looking globally similar to the target criminal (similar face silhouette and global features). Then, the profiled face would be refined by iteratively replacing the components of the current image with those of a selection of donors. The set of donors would be determined under the guidance of the witness and based on appropriate criteria.

As a more conventional application of our work, we consider now the typical situation where a user of a social network is about to share a photo and wants to prevent the faces from being tagged. Figure 1 presented on the first page serves as a good example. The same principle could be also applied to web-services such as Google Streetview. Indeed, for legal reasons, such services are bound to occult the identity of the passers-by. So far, this is done based on aggressive blurring so that the images do not remain realistic.

5   Conclusions

Relying on a bank of face components from which face elements can be borrowed, and exploiting the power of Poisson editing techniques, this paper presents a simple yet very efficient and fully automatic pipeline for the de-identification of face images. The proposed algorithm produces optimally de-identified faces with respect to a given face matcher. The so-obtained faces have the property of being as close as possible to the original ones while having the guarantee they fool the face matcher. As a proof of concept a standard face matcher was used, but recent state-of-the art matchers such as [27], considered to be close to human performance, would allow to produce even more convincing images. The approach has been validated on three different datasets for which we obtained impressive results. Without requiring any prior normalization, our approach can handle arbitrary faces provided that it is within 15 degrees from the frontal pose. In order to tackle this limitation, an extension based on the extraction of a 3D template similar to [14] is currently studied.

Acknowledgments. This work was partly supported by the ANR-SECULAR project.

References

1. Agrawal, P., Narayanan, P.J.: Person de-identification in videos. IEEE Trans. Circuits Syst. Video Technol. **21**(3), 299–310 (2011)
2. Ahonen, T., Hadid, A., Pietikainen, M.: Face description with local binary patterns: Application to face recognition. IEEE Trans. Pattern Anal. Mach. Intell. **28**(12), 2037–2041 (2006)
3. Bitouk, D., Kumar, N., Dhillon, S., Belhumeur, P., Nayar, S.K.: Face swapping: automatically replacing faces in photographs. ACM Trans. Graphics (TOG) **27**, 39 (2008)
4. Bonnen, K., Klare, B.F., Jain, A.K.: Component-based representation in automated face recognition. IEEE Trans. Inf. Forensics Secur. **8**(1), 239–253 (2013)
5. Boyle, M., Edwards, C., Greenberg, S.: The effects of filtered video on awareness and privacy. In: ACM Conference on Computer Supported Cooperative Work, New York, USA, pp. 1–10 (December 2000)
6. Cavedon, L., Foschini, L., Vigna, G.: Getting the face behind the squares: Reconstructing pixelized video streams. In: Proceedings of the 5th USENIX Conference on Offensive Technologies, WOOT 2011, p.5. USENIX Association, Berkeley (2011)
7. Cootes, T.F., Edwards, G.J., Taylor, C.J., et al.: Active appearance models. IEEE Trans. Pattern Anal. Mach. Intell. **23**(6), 681–685 (2001)
8. Crowley, J.L., Coutaz, J., Bérard, F.: Perceptual user interfaces: things that see. Commun. ACM **43**(3), 54–60 (2000)
9. Driessen, B., Dürmuth, M.: Achieving anonymity against major face recognition algorithms. In: De Decker, B., Dittmann, J., Kraetzer, C., Vielhauer, C. (eds.) CMS 2013. LNCS, vol. 8099, pp. 18–33. Springer, Heidelberg (2013)
10. Dufaux, F., Ebrahimi, T.: A framework for the validation of privacy protection solutions in video surveillance. In: IEEE International Conference on Multimedia and Expo (ICME), pp. 66–71 (2010)
11. Efros, A.A., Freeman, W.T.: Image quilting for texture synthesis and transfer. In: Proceedings of the 28th Annual Conference on Computer Graphics and Interactive Techniques, pp. 341–346 (2001)
12. Gross, R., Sweeney, L., De la Torre, F., Baker, S.: Semi-supervised learning of multi-factor models for face de-identification. In: IEEE Conference on Computer Vision and Pattern Recognition, pp. 1–8 (2008)
13. Gross, R., Matthews, I., Cohn, J., Kanade, T., Baker, S.: Multi-pie. Image Vis. Comput. **28**(5), 807–813 (2010)
14. Hassner, T.: Viewing real-world faces in 3d. In: IEEE International Conference on Computer Vision, pp. 3607–3614 (2013)
15. Huang, G.B., Ramesh, M., Berg, T., Learned-Miller, E.: Labeled faces in the wild: A database for studying face recognition in unconstrained environments. Tech. Rep. 07–49, University of Massachusetts, Amherst (October 2007)
16. Hudson, S.E., Smith, I.: Techniques for addressing fundamental privacy and disruption tradeoffs in awareness support systems. In: ACM Conference on Computer Supported Cooperative Work, New York, USA, pp. 248–257 (1996)
17. Kasinski, A., Florek, A., Schmidt, A.: The put face database. Image Proc. Commun. **13**(3–4), 59–64 (2008)
18. Lander, K., Bruce, V., Hill, H.: Evaluating the effectiveness of pixelation and blurring on masking the identity of familiar faces. Appl. Cogn. Psychol. **15**(1), 101–116 (2001)

19. Lin, Y., Lin, Q., Tang, F., Wang, S.: Face replacement with large-pose differences. In: ACM International Conference on Multimedia, pp. 1249–1250. ACM, New York (October 2012)
20. Matthews, I., Xiao, J., Baker, S.: 2d vs. 3d deformable face models: Representational power, construction, and real-time fitting. Int. J. Comput. Vision **75**(1), 93–113 (2007)
21. Milborrow, S., Morkel, J., Nicolls, F.: The muct landmarked face database. Pattern Recognition Association of South Africa (2010)
22. Mohammed, U., Prince, S.J., Kautz, J.: Visio-lization: generating novel facial images. ACM Trans. Graphics (TOG) **28**, 57 (2009)
23. Newton, E.M., Sweeney, L., Malin, B.: Preserving privacy by de-identifying face images. IEEE Trans. Knowl. Data Eng. **17**(2), 232–243 (2005)
24. Nguyen, H.V., Bai, L.: Cosine similarity metric learning for face verification. In: Kimmel, R., Klette, R., Sugimoto, A. (eds.) ACCV 2010, Part II. LNCS, vol. 6493, pp. 709–720. Springer, Berlin Heidelberg (2011)
25. Pérez, P., Gangnet, M., Blake, A.: Poisson image editing. ACM Trans. Graphics (TOG) **22**, 313–318 (2003)
26. Smith, B.M., Zhang, L., Brandt, J., Lin, Z., Yang, J.: Exemplar-based face parsing. In: IEEE Conference on Computer Vision and Pattern Recognition, pp. 3484–3491 (2013)
27. Taigman, Y., Yang, M., Ranzato, M., Wolf, L.: Deepface: Closing the gap to human-level performance in face verification. In: IEEE Conference on Computer Vision and Pattern Recognition (2014)
28. Yang, C.Y., Liu, S., Yang, M.H.: Structured face hallucination. In: IEEE Conference on Computer Vision and Pattern Recognition, pp. 1099–1106 (2013)
29. Zhao, Q.A., Stasko, J.T.: Evaluating image filtering based techniques in media space applications. In: ACM Conference on Computer Supported Cooperative Work, New York, USA, pp. 11–18(November 1998)
30. Zhu, J., Van Gool, L., Hoi, S.C.: Unsupervised face alignment by robust nonrigid mapping. In: IEEE 12th International Conference on Computer Vision, pp. 1265–1272. IEEE (2009)
31. Zhu, X., Ramanan, D.: Face detection, pose estimation, and landmark localization in the wild. In: IEEE Conference on Computer Vision and Pattern Recognition, pp. 2879–2886 (2012)

Which Image Pairs Will Cosegment Well? Predicting Partners for Cosegmentation

Suyog Dutt Jain[✉] and Kristen Grauman

University of Texas at Austin, Austin, USA
suyog@cs.utexas.edu

Abstract. Cosegmentation methods segment multiple related images *jointly*, exploiting their shared appearance to generate more robust foreground models. While existing approaches assume that an oracle will specify which pairs of images are amenable to cosegmentation, in many scenarios such external information may be difficult to obtain. This is problematic, since coupling the "wrong" images for segmentation—even images of the same object class—can actually deteriorate performance relative to single-image segmentation. Rather than manually specify partner images for cosegmentation, we propose to automatically *predict* which images will cosegment well together. We develop a learning-to-rank approach that identifies good partners, based on paired descriptors capturing the images' amenability to joint segmentation. We compare our approach to alternative methods for partnering images, including basic image similarity, and show the advantages on two challenging datasets.

1 Introduction

In the cosegmentation problem, we are given two or more images containing related content, and must segment them each into regions. Because the inputs are known to share some visual relationship—for example, they contain the same foreground object, or instances of the same object class—the algorithm has valuable cues about which pixels might go together. At a high level, the idea is to detect any common appearance/shapes, exploit that association to determine likely foreground regions, then use a "shared" foreground model to jointly guide the region estimates in all input images [1–8]. In contrast, such cues are not available in the traditional single-image segmentation task, where the system must rely solely on bottom-up features to perform the grouping.

Methods for cosegmentation have a variety of potential applications. They are valuable when working with "weakly supervised" data for object recognition, since they make it possible to automatically isolate the foreground object in training images in spite of cluttered backgrounds. This is quite practical given the availability of tagged Web photos, which are often curated to form recognition

Electronic supplementary material The online version of this chapter (doi:10.1007/978-3-319-16811-1_12) contains supplementary material, which is available to authorized users.

© Springer International Publishing Switzerland 2015
D. Cremers et al. (Eds.): ACCV 2014, Part III, LNCS 9005, pp. 175–190, 2015.
DOI: 10.1007/978-3-319-16811-1_12

| Query | Source | Cosegmentation | Query | Source | Cosegmentation |

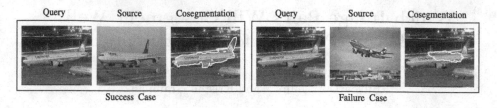

Success Case   Failure Case

Fig. 1. Motivation for our approach. When an image pair share strong foreground similarity, their cosegmentation is successful (left). However, when incompatible images are used—even from the same object category—cosegmentation fails and can even deteriorate the single-image results (right).

datasets but lack foreground annotations. Furthermore, cosegmentation methods can be applied to discover the re-occurring patterns in an image database and summarize its key visual themes, or focus on the foreground for content-based image retrieval tasks. Cosegmentation of batches of related photos (or video frames) can help initialize an interactive method for rotoscoping, allowing designers to composite the foreground object onto novel backgrounds.

Researchers have made substantial progress on the cosegmentation problem in recent years. While initially the problem was defined to entail two input images showing very same object against distinct backgrounds [1], recent work broadens the problem definition to include batches of input images known only to contain instances of the same object class [2–10]. This is also referred to as *weakly supervised* or *joint foreground segmentation*: each input image is known to contain an instance from the same object category, but its localization within the background is unknown.[1] Some work further relaxes the two-region (foreground/background) assumption to tackle k-region segmentation [6,7,11]. Furthermore, eager to capitalize on large collections of weakly labeled images, methods are being developed to account for both noisily labeled instances [8,11] and scalable optimization [6,7,12].

Nonetheless, intra-class appearance variation remains a major obstacle to accurate cosegmentation. In the ideal "clean" scenario, the input batch of images would contain very similar-looking objects, making each image mutually valuable to the rest for building a shared foreground model. However, in many realistic scenarios, the input batch is not so clean. The foreground object may actually look quite different in some images, whether due to image tagging errors, viewpoint variations, or simply diversity in that category's visual appearance. As a result, *not all images are mutually valuable for cosegmentation*. In fact, for this very reason, recent studies report the discouraging outcome that, on some datasets, standard single-image segmentation actually exceeds its cosegmentation counterpart—despite the latter's presumed advantage of having access to a batch of weakly labeled data [4,8]. See Fig. 1.

---

[1] We use the terms *cosegmentation*, *joint segmentation*, and *weakly supervised segmentation* interchangeably.

This motivates us to reconsider the standard assumption that all images are created equal for cosegmentation. Instead, we propose to *predict* which pairs of images are likely to successfully cosegment together. Given an input image and a pool of candidate images sharing the same weak label (e.g., a batch of "car" images), the goal is to find the candidate that, when coupled with the input image, will most boost its foreground accuracy if they are jointly segmented. To this end, we introduce a learning approach that uses a paired description of two images to predict their degree of cosegmentation success. The paired description captures not only to what extent the images seem to agree in appearance, but also the uncertainty resulting from their shared foreground model. We formulate the task in a learning-to-rank objective, where successful pairs are constrained to rank higher than those that cosegment poorly together.

Our approach offers a novel way to automatically "partner" images for cosegmentation. Existing methods assume that the "what to cosegment?" question is already answered by some external oracle [1–10], or else use image similarity alone to gauge compatibility [8,11]. In contrast, we show how to explicitly *learn* how well image pairs are likely to cosegment together. We demonstrate our approach on two challenging datasets, and show there is great potential to focus joint segmentation only on images where it is most valuable.

2   Related Work

Methods to jointly segment images vary foremost in what they assume about the input images. At one end of the spectrum are methods that assume strong agreement in the inputs' foregrounds, i.e., that the two images contain the same exact object against differing backgrounds [1]. This setting continues to be developed, e.g., for greater efficiency [12] and multi-image collections with interactive user input [13]. In the middle of the spectrum is the *weakly supervised* scenario, where the input images are assumed to contain instances of the same object category [2–10], and the goal is to extract the foreground per image (or possibly multiple foreground objects [6,7]). At the other end of the spectrum are unsupervised methods, which permit the input images to come from multiple categories. These methods attempt to simultaneously discover the object region boundaries and the category groupings [11,14,15]. We apply our method in the middle scenario, where we have a pool of candidate partners that are likely to contain the same object, but they may vary significantly in appearance.

Prior methods assume that all the input images are amenable to cosegment together. In the strict same-object cosegmentation setting, this is assured by manually selecting the input pair (or set). For example, a designer may supply a set of images to be rotoscoped [1], or an analyst may gather aligned brain images from which to segment pathologies [12], or a consumer may group a burst of photos at an event (e.g., a soccer game) into a mini-album [13]. In the weakly supervised setting, the related images often originate from Internet search for an object's name. In this case, the majority of methods assume that all images are mutually amenable to a joint segmentation [2–7,9,10]. In contrast, we propose to automatically determine which among the plausible candidates would serve as the most effective partners for cosegmentation.

To our knowledge, the only prior work that specifically avoids jointly segmenting all input images does so on the basis of a manually defined (i.e., non-learned) image similarity metric [8,11]. In [11], regions are clustered using a context-based descriptor, and a fixed number of the top clusters are used for joint graph-cut segment refinement. In [8], the joint segmentation is restricted to an image and a fixed number of its K nearest neighbors using global descriptor (GIST) similarity. In that work, the motivation for paring down the neighbors happens to be computational cost—not accuracy—since it uses inter-image dense correspondences, which are prohibitive to perform on all pairs of examples for large datasets. In both existing methods, the assumption is that image similarity alone is sufficient to predict cosegmentation success. In contrast, our approach learns the behavior of the cosegmentation algorithm, and thus can predict its success for a novel input pair.

There is limited prior work on predicting the quality of a segmentation, and all of it targets the single-image segmentation problem [16–20]. Given the output of a bottom-up segmentation, various methods attempt to classify or rank the regions by their "object-like" quality, having learned the properties of true object segmentations [17–19]. The method of [16] aims to predict the segmentation accuracy of an algorithm on a novel image based on its global descriptor, while the interactive approach of [20] estimates how much user input is required to sufficiently segment a novel input. Unlike any of the above, our method predicts the extent to which a *joint* segmentation will succeed based on the paired relationship of two candidate images.

3   Approach

As input, our approach takes a **"query"** image I^q and a pool of candidate partner images $\mathcal{P} = \{I^1, \ldots, I^N\}$. Among those N candidates, our method selects the best partner image for I^q, that is, the image that when paired with I^q for cosegmentation is expected to produce the most accurate result. Then, as output, our method returns the result of cosegmenting I^q with its selected partner, namely, a foreground mask for I^q. In the following, we refer to a candidate partner image as a **"source"** image, denoted $I^s \in \mathcal{P}$.

In our implementation, we study the weakly supervised setting, where images in $\mathcal{P}$ contain the same object category as I^q. This forces our method to perform fine-grained analysis to select among all the possibly relevant partners. Even with weak supervision, not all images are satisfactory cosegmentation partners, since they contain objects exhibiting complex appearance and viewpoint variations, as discussed above.

In the following, we first define a basic single-image segmentation algorithm (Sect. 3.1). We then expand that basic engine to handle cosegmentation of a pair of images (Sect. 3.2). Finally, we introduce our ranking approach to predict the compatibility of two images for cosegmentation (Sect. 3.3).

3.1   Single-Image Segmentation Engine

We first describe an approach to perform *single-image* segmentation. In addition to serving as a baseline for the cosegmentation methods, we will also use the output of the single-image segmentation when we predict cosegmentation compatibility (cf. Sect. 3.3). The method below produces good foreground initializations, though alternative single-image methods could also be plugged into our framework.

Given an image I^i, the goal is to estimate a label matrix L^i of the same dimensions, where $L^i(p) = y_p^i$ denotes the binary label for the pixel p, and $y_p^i \in \{0, 1\}$. The label 0 denotes background (bg) and 1 denotes foreground (fg). We use a standard Markov Random Field (MRF) approach, where each pixel p is a node connected to its spatial neighbors.

We define the MRF's unary potentials using saliency and a foreground color model, as follows. Since this is a single-image segmentation, there is no external knowledge about where the foreground is. Thus, we rely on a generic saliency metric to estimate the plausible foreground region, then boostrap an approximate foreground color model from those pixels. Specifically, for image I^i we first compute its pixel-wise saliency map S^i using a state-of-the-art algorithm [21]. We threshold that real-valued map by its average, yielding an initial estimate for the foreground mask. Then, we use the pixels inside (outside) that mask to learn a Gaussian mixture model (GMM) for the foreground (background) in RGB space. Let G_{fg}^i and G_{bg}^i denote those two mixture models.

The single-image MRF energy function uses these color models and the saliency map:

$$E_{sing}(L^i) = \sum_p A_p^i(y_p^i) + \sum_p X_p^i(y_p^i) + \sum_{p,p' \in \mathcal{N}} T_{p,p'}^i(y_p^i, y_{p'}^i), \qquad (1)$$

where A_p^i and X_p^i are unary terms, $T_{p,p'}^i$ is a pairwise term, and $\mathcal{N}$ consists of all 4-connected neighborhoods. We define the *appearance likelihood* term as:

$$A_p^i(y_p^i) = -\log P(F^i(p)|G_{y_p^i}^i), \qquad (2)$$

where $F^i(p)$ denotes the RGB color for pixel p in image I^i. This term reflects the cost of assigning a pixel as fg (bg) according to the GMM models. We define the *saliency prior* unary term as:

$$X_p^i(y_p^i = 1) = -\log P(S^i(p)), \qquad (3)$$

where $S^i(p)$ denotes the saliency value for pixel p. This term reflects the cost of assigning a pixel as fg, where more salient pixels are assumed more likely to be foreground. For the background label, we have the corresponding term, $X_p^i(y_p^i = 0) = -\log(1 - P(S^i(p)))$. Finally, the pairwise term,

$$T_{p,p'}^i(y_p^i, y_{p'}^i) = \delta(y_p^i \neq y_{p'}^i) \exp(-\beta \|F^i(p) - F^i(p')\|), \qquad (4)$$

is a standard smoothness prior that penalizes assigning different labels to neighboring pixels that are similar in color, where β is a scaling parameter.

We employ graph cuts to efficiently minimize Eq. 1 and apply five rounds of iterative refinement (as in GrabCut [22]), alternating between learning the likelihood functions and obtaining the label estimates. The result is a label matrix $L_{sing}^{i^*} = \arg\min_{L^i} E_{sing}(L^i)$.

3.2 Paired-Image Cosegmentation Engine

Next we define the cosegmentation engine we use in our implementation, which expands on the single-image approach above. During training, our method targets a given cosegmentation algorithm, as we will see in the next section. Any existing cosegmentation algorithm could be plugged in; the role of our method is to improve its results by focusing on the most compatible image partners.

Given a query and source image pair, I^q and $I^s \in \mathcal{P}$, we define an energy function over their joint labeling. This model is initialized using GMM appearance models learned from $L_{sing}^{q^*}$ and $L_{sing}^{s^*}$, the single-image results for the two inputs obtained by optimizing Eq. (1). Specifically, we pool the foreground (background) pixels from both label masks to learn the joint GMM G_{fg}^{qs} (G_{bg}^{qs}) in RGB space. Here and below, the superscript qs denotes a joint term that is a function of both the query and source images.

Let L^{qs} be shorthand for the two label matrices output by the cosegmentation, $L^{qs} = (L^q, L^s)$. Our joint energy function takes the following form:

$$E_{coseg}(L^{qs}) = E_{sing}(L^q) + E_{sing}(L^s) + \Theta_{app}^{qs}(L^{qs}) + \Theta_{match}^{qs}(L^{qs}), \quad (5)$$

where the first two terms refer to the single-image energy for either output, as defined in Eq. (1), and Θ_{app}^{qs} and Θ_{match}^{qs} capture the energy of a joint label assignment based on appearance and matching terms, respectively (and will be defined next). Note that even though the energy function contains terms for individual label matrices, they are optimized *jointly* to minimize Eq. (5).

The *joint appearance likelihood* term is defined as

$$\Theta_{app}^{qs}(L^{qs}) = \sum_{p \in I^q} A_p^{qs}(y_p^q) + \sum_{r \in I^s} A_r^{qs}(y_r^s), \quad (6)$$

and it captures the extent to which the two output masks deviate from the expected foreground/background appearance discovered with saliency. As before, each A_p^{qs} term is defined as the negative log likelihood over the GMM probabilities; however, here it uses the joint GMM appearance models G_{fg}^{qs} and G_{bg}^{qs} obtained by pooling pixels from the two images' initial foreground estimates.

The *matching likelihood* term $\Theta_{match}^{qs}(L^{qs})$ leverages a dense pixel-level correspondence to establish pairwise links between the two input images. Let $\mathcal{F}_{qs}(p)$ denote the 2D flow vector from pixel p in image I^q to its match in image I^s. We introduce an edge in the cosegmentation MRF connecting each pixel $p \in I^q$ to its matching pixel $r \in I^s$, where $r = p + \mathcal{F}_{qs}(p)$. Using these correspondences, the matching likelihood is a contrast-sensitive smoothness potential over linked (matched) pixels in the two images:

$$\Theta_{match}^{qs}(L^{qs}) = \sum_{p \in I^q, r \in I^s} \delta(y_p^q \neq y_r^s) \exp(-\beta\|D^q(p) - D^s(r)\|), \quad (7)$$

where $D^i(p)$ is a local image descriptor computed at pixel p (we use dense SIFT), and β is a scaling constant. This energy term encourages similar-looking *matched* pixels between the query and source to take the same fg/bg label.

The matching in Eq. (7) helps cosegmentation robustness. We compute $\mathcal{F}_{qs}$ using the Deformable Spatial Pyramid (DSP) matching algorithm [23], an efficient method that regularizes match consistency across a pyramid of spatial regions and permits cross-scale matches. By linking $p \in I^q$ to $r \in I^s$—rather than naively linking $p \in I^q$ to $p \in I^s$—we gain robustness to the translation and scale of the foreground object in the two input images. This is valuable when the inputs do share a similar-looking object, but its global placement or size varies. Notably, this flexibility is lacking in a strictly image-based global comparison approach (like GIST and the scale-sensitive SIFT Flow as used in [8]). It thus enables mutual discovery of the object between the two images.

To optimize Eq. (5), we again employ graph cuts with iterative updates. This yields the cosegmented output image pair, $(L^{q^*}_{coseg}, L^{s^*}_{coseg}) = \arg \min_{L^{qs}} E_{coseg}(L^{qs})$.

3.3   Learning Cosegmentation Compatibility to Predict Partners

Having defined the underlying single-image and paired-image segmentation algorithms, we can now present our approach to predict which partner image is best suited for cosegmentation with a novel query image. There are two main components: (1) extracting features that are suggestive of cosegmentation success, and (2) training a ranking function to prioritize successful partners.

We are given a training set $\mathcal{T} = \{(T^1, L^1), \ldots, (I^M, L^M)\}$ of M images labeled with their ground truth foreground masks, where T^i denotes an image and L^i denotes its mask. This set is not only disjoint from the candidate partner set $\mathcal{P}$ defined above, it also does *not* contain images of the same object category as what appears in $\mathcal{P}$ or the eventual novel queries. This is important, since it means our approach is required to learn generic cues indicative of cosegmentation compatibility, as opposed to object-specific cues. While object-specific cues are presumably easier to exploit, it may be impractical to train a model for every new object class of interest. Instead, all learning is done on data and classes disjoint from the weakly supervised image set $\mathcal{P}$.

Training a ranker for cosegmentation compatibility. First, we apply the cosegmentation algorithm (Sect. 3.2) to every pair of images in $\mathcal{T}$. Each image in the training set acts as a "query" in turn, while the remaining images act as its candidate source images. Let (T^i_q, T^j_s) denote one such query-source pair comprised of training images T^i and T^j. For each pairing, we record the cosegmentation quality that results for T^i_q, that is, the intersection-over-union overlap score between the ground truth L^i and the cosegmentation estimate $L^{i^*}_{coseg}$ that results from optimizing Eq. (5) with T^i as the query and T^j as the source. After computing these scores for all training pairs $(i, j) \in \{1, \ldots, M\}$, we have a set of training tuples $\langle T^i, T^j, o_{ij} \rangle$, where o_{ij} denotes the overlap score for pair i, j. The scores will vary across pairs depending on their compatibility.

Next, we generate a ranked list of source images for each training example. We use these M-length ranked lists to train a ranking function. As input, the learned ranking function f takes features computed on an image pair $\phi(I^q, I^s)$ (to be defined below), and it returns as output a score predicting their cosegmentation compatibility. For simplicity we train a linear ranking function:

$$f(\phi(I^q, I^s)) = \boldsymbol{w}^T \phi(I^q, I^s), \tag{8}$$

where $\boldsymbol{w}$ is a vector of the same dimensionality as the feature space. To learn $\boldsymbol{w}$ from the training tuples, we want to constrain it to return higher scores for more compatible pairs. Let $\mathcal{O}$ be the set of *pairs* of all training tuples $\{(i, j), (i, k)\}$ for which $o_{ij} > o_{ik}$, for all $i = 1, \ldots, M$. Using the SVM Rank formulation of [24], we seek the projection of the data that preserves these training set orders, with a regularizer that favors a large margin between nearest-projected pairs:

$$\text{minimize} \quad \frac{1}{2}||\boldsymbol{w}||_2^2 + C \sum \xi_{ijk}^2 \tag{9}$$
$$\text{s.t.} \quad \boldsymbol{w}^T \phi(T^i, T^j) \geq \boldsymbol{w}^T \phi(T^i, T^k) + 1 - \xi_{ijk}$$
$$\forall (i, j, k) \in \mathcal{O},$$

where the constant C balances the regularizer and constraints. In other words, the model should score a training pair with greater overlap higher than one with lower overlap.[2]

Defining features indicative of compatibility. Next we define the features $\phi(I^q, I^s)$. Their purpose is to expose the images' compatibility for cosegmentation. We define features of two types: (1) *source image features* meant to capture the quality of the source in general, and (2) *inter-image features* meant to capture the likelihood of success in coupling a particular source and query. The former makes use of the single-image segmentation mask $L_{sing}^{s^*}$ from Sect. 3.1; the latter makes use of the cosegmentation estimates $L_{coseg}^{q^*}$ and $L_{coseg}^{s^*}$ from Sect. 3.2.

Source image features. Ideally, we would like to cosegment with a source image that is easy to segment on its own, since then it has better ability to guide the foreground (when the query is compatible). Thus, our three source features aim to expose the predicted quality of the source's single-image segmentation:

- *Foreground-background separability:* We use $L_{sing}^{s^*}$ to compute separate color histograms for the (estimated) fg and bg regions, then record the χ^2 distance between the two histograms as a feature. More distinctive foregrounds will yield higher χ^2 distances.

---

[2] Alternatively, one could use regression. However, ranking has the advantage of giving us more control over which training tuples are enforced, and it places emphasis only on the relative scores (not absolute values), which is what we care about for deciding which partner is best.

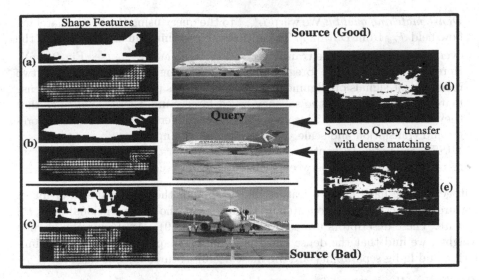

Fig. 2. Feature illustration. **Center:** an example query and two candidate source images. **(a-c):** Cropped single-image segmentation masks (top) and corresponding HOGs (bottom). These features are good indicators of foreground shape similarity, as we see by comparing the query (b) to its good and bad source partners (a) and (c), respectively. **(d-e):** Results of mask transfer with dense matching from the source image to the query image. The success of this transfer clearly depends on the compatibility between the query and source (i.e., it succeeds in (d) but fails in (e)).

- *Graph cuts uncertainty:* We use dynamic graph cuts [25] to measure each pixel's graph cut uncertainty. We bin these uncertainties from the foreground pixels of $L^{s^*}_{sing}$ into 5 bins and record this distribution as the feature. It captures how uncertain the single image segmentation is.
- *Number of connected components:* We record the number of connected components in $L^{s^*}_{sing}$ as a measure of how coherent the source's single-image segmentation is.

Inter-image features. To detect good partner candidates, the quality of the source image alone is insufficient; we also want to look explicitly at the compatibility of the particular input pair. Thus, our three inter-image features aim to reveal the predicted success of the pair's cosegmentation:

- *Foreground similarity:* We compute the foreground similarity between the source and query using their estimated foregrounds from single-image segmentation. Specifically, we record two χ^2 distances: one between their color histograms, and one between their SIFT bag-of-words histograms. By excluding background from this feature, we leave open the possibility to discover compatible partners with varying backgrounds.
- *Shape similarity:* We resize the cropped foreground region from $L^{s^*}_{sing}$ to the size of the cropped foreground region from $L^{q^*}_{sing}$. To gauge shape similarity, we record both the overlap between those masks as well as the L_2 distance on the HOG features computed on the original images at those masked positions (see Fig. 2(a-c)).

- *Dense matching quality:* We warp $L^{s^*}_{sing}$ to the query using the dense matching flow field $\mathcal{F}_{qs}$ from DSP [23]. To capture the matching quality, we record the overlap score between the transferred source mask and $L^{q^*}_{sing}$ (see Fig. 2(d-e)). Here the saliency-driven foreground masks and dense matching serve as two independent signals of alignment. If the two images permit an accurate dense match that agrees with the saliency-based foreground, there is evidence that they are closely related. This compatibility cue offers some tolerance to foreground translation and scale variation in the two inputs.
- *GIST similarity:* To capture global layout similarity of the image pair, we record the L_2 distance between their GIST [26] descriptors.

Altogether, we have 7 and 6 feature dimensions for the source and inter-image features, respectively. We concatenate them to form the 13-dimensional $\phi(I^q, I^s)$ feature. These descriptors are used in training (Eq. (9)). Analyzing the learned weights, we find that the dense matching quality, shape similarity, GIST similarity, and fg-bg separability are the most useful features for our task.

Predicting the partner for a novel image. At test time, we are given a novel image I^q and the partner candidate set $\mathcal{P}$. We compute its descriptor $\phi(I^q, I^s)$ for every $I^s \in \mathcal{P}$, apply the learned ranking function, and select as its partner the one that maximizes the predicted cosegmentation compatibility:

$$I^{p^*} = \arg \max_{I^s \in \mathcal{P}} f(\phi(I^q, I^s)). \tag{10}$$

Finally, we return the foreground segmentation for I^q that results from cosegmenting the pair (I^q, I^{p^*}) using the algorithm in Sect. 3.2.

4   Results

Datasets: We evaluate our approach on two challenging publicly available datasets. The first is **MIT Object Discovery** (MIT), a dataset recently introduced for evaluating object foreground discovery through cosegmentation [8].[3] It consists of Internet images of objects from three classes: Airplane, Car, and Horse. The images within a class contain significant appearance and viewpoint variation. We use the 100-image per class subset designated by the authors to enable comparisons with multiple other existing methods. The second dataset is the **Caltech-28**, a subset of 28 of the Caltech-101[4] classes designated by [3] for study in weakly supervised joint segmentation. The 30 images per class originate from Internet search and cover an array of different objects.

Methods compared: We compare to results reported by a number of state-of-the-art cosegmentation techniques, namely [5–8] on MIT and [3,9,22,27] on Caltech-28. In addition, we implement several baseline techniques:

---

[3] http://people.csail.mit.edu/mrub/ObjectDiscovery/.

[4] http://www.vision.caltech.edu/ImageDatasets/Caltech101/.

Table 1. Overlap accuracy on the MIT Object Discovery dataset.

	Single-Seg	Rand-Coseg	GIST-Coseg	Ours	Ours-Best k	Upper bound
Airplane	39.14	42.22	42.34	**45.81**	46.26	57.39
Car	46.76	52.47	50.95	**53.63**	54.31	61.81
Horse	49.82	51.69	**52.73**	50.18	52.86	63.52

- **Single-Seg:** the saliency-based single-image approach defined in Sect. 3.1. This baseline reveals to what extent a query benefits at all from cosegmentation.
- **Rand-Coseg:** the cosegmentation approach defined in Sect. 3.2 applied with a random image *from the same object category* as the partner source image, averaged over 20 trials. This baseline helps illustrate the need to actively choose a cosegmentation partner among a weakly labeled dataset.
- **GIST-Coseg:** the same cosegmentation approach is applied using the source image that looks most similar to the query, in terms of GIST descriptors. This baseline highlights how image similarity alone—used in existing work [8, 11]—can be insufficient to determine good partners for cosegmentation.
- **Ours-Best k:** we apply our method, but instead of choosing the single maximally ranked image for cosegmentation, we refer to ground truth to pick the best partner from among the $k = 5$ source images our method ranks most highly.
- **Upper bound:** the upper bound for cosegmentation accuracy. We use ground truth to select the partner leading to the maximum overlap score for each query. This reveals the best accuracy any method could possibly attain for the cosegmentation partner selection problem.

As discussed above, we consider the weakly supervised setting. All baselines reference the exact same candidate set $\mathcal{P}$ as our method. Our method's training set $\mathcal{T}$ is always disjoint from $\mathcal{P}$, and furthermore $\mathcal{P}$ and $\mathcal{T}$ never overlap in object class. For example, when applying our method to Cars in the MIT data, we train it using only images of Airplanes and Horses.

To quantify segmentation accuracy, we use the standard intersection-over-union **overlap** accuracy score (Jaccard index), unless otherwise noted.

Implementation details: The color model GMMs consist of 5 mixture components. The scale parameters β are set automatically as the inverse of the mean of all individual distances. We use 50 visual words for the SIFT bag-of-words used in the inter-image foreground similarity, and 11 bins per color channel in all color histograms. The approximate run time per pair is between 10–12 s, which is dominated by the SIFT extraction step.

4.1 Results on MIT Object Discovery Dataset

Table 1 shows our results against the baselines on all 3 classes in the MIT dataset. We observe several things from this result. First, the large gap between

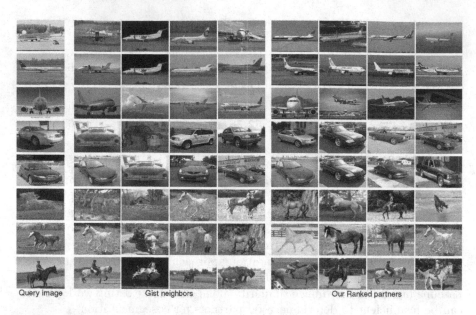

Query image   Gist neighbors   Our Ranked partners

Fig. 3. Examples of the four top-ranked neighbors for a novel query, using either the GIST nearest neighbors (center block) or our learned ranking function (right block). Best viewed in color. While both methods can identify similar-looking source images among their top-ranked set, our method identifies partners that are more closely aligned in viewpoint or appearance and thus amenable to cosegmentation (Color figure online).

Table 2. Comparison to state-of-the-art cosegmentation methods on the MIT Object Discovery dataset, in terms of average overlap.

	Joulin et al. [5]	Joulin et al. [6]	Kim et al. [7]	Ours	Rubinstein et al. [8]
Airplane	15.26	11.72	7.9	45.81	**55.81**
Car	37.15	35.15	0.04	53.63	**64.42**
Horse	30.16	29.53	6.43	50.18	**51.65**

Single-Seg and the Upper bound underscores the fact that cosegmentation can indeed exceed the accuracy of single-image segmentation on challenging images— *if* suitable partners are used. Despite the images' diversity within a single class, the shared appearance in the optimally chosen partner is beneficial. Second, we see that our approach outperforms the baselines in nearly every case. This supports our key claim: it is valuable to actively choose an appropriate coseg-mentation partner by learning the cues for success/failure. In two of three classes we outperform the GIST-Coseg baseline, showing that off-the-shelf image simi-larity is inferior to our learning approach for this problem. The Horse class is an exception, where we underperform the GIST-Coseg baseline. This is likely due to weak saliency priors in some of the more cluttered Horse images. Third, the fact that the Rand-Coseg approach does as well as it does (in fact, nearly as good as the GIST-Coseg method for Airplanes) indicates that many images of the

Table 3. Accuracy on the Caltech-28 dataset, in terms of average overlap. We show the 10 best and 4 worst performing classes (see Supp. for all classes).

		Single-Seg	Rand-Coseg	GIST-Coseg	Ours	Ours-Best k	Upper bound
Best	brain	73.31	72.43	72.54	**75.73**	76.09	76.22
	ferry	54.99	55.87	55.23	**57.64**	57.71	58.02
	dalmatian	39.58	39.13	38.15	**40.23**	40.94	41.59
	ewer	63.87	62.58	63.87	**65.86**	66.18	66.53
	joshua tree	53.04	54.05	54.45	**56.21**	57.12	57.52
	cougar face	58.19	57.39	56.51	**58.25**	58.53	59.05
	sunflower	70.48	70.10	69.77	**71.29**	72.07	73.48
	motorbike	**57.38**	55.86	55.79	57.21	58.12	58.59
	euphonium	57.72	57.25	58.32	**59.45**	60.27	60.28
	kangaroo	59.79	59.26	59.13	**60.24**	60.57	61.81
Worst	lotus	76.71	75.98	**78.38**	77.59	79.51	80.16
	grand piano	67.21	67.28	**67.93**	66.58	67.01	68.33
	crab	61.86	62.25	**62.11**	61.23	62.3	62.46
	watch	55.00	56.4	**57.72**	56.11	56.16	58.30

same class offer *some* degree of help with cosegmentation. Hence, our method's gain is due to its fine-grained analysis of the candidate source images. Finally, the bump in accuracy we achieve if considering the k top-ranked source images (Ours-Best k) indicates that future refinements of our method should consider ways to exploit the ranked partners beyond the top-ranked example.

Figure 3 shows examples of the top-ranked partner images produced by the GIST-Coseg baseline and our approach, for a variety of query images in the MIT dataset. We see how our method's learning strategy pays off: it focuses on source images that have more fine-grained compatability with the query image. The GIST neighbors are globally similar, but can be too distinct in viewpoint or appearance to assist in cosegmenting the query. In contrast, the partner source images retrieved by our ranking algorithm are better equipped to share a foreground model due to their viewpoint, appearance, and/or individual saliency.

Table 2 compares our result to several state-of-the-art cosegmentation methods.[5] Our method outperforms all the existing methods by a large margin, except the method of [8]. Our disadvantage in that case may be due to the fact that [8] operates over a joint graph of all images in the class at once, whereas we consider pairs of images for cosegmentation. This suggests future work to extend our algorithm, e.g., by using our compatibility predictions as weights within a multi-image cosegmentation graph.

4.2 Results on Caltech-28 Dataset

Table 3 shows the results for the Caltech-28 dataset, in the same format as Table 1 above. Due to space constraints, we show just a sample of the 28 classes.

---

[5] These are the overlap accuracies reported in [8], where the authors applied the public source code to generate results for [5–7].

Specifically, we display the top 10 cases where we most outperform GIST-Coseg and the bottom 4 cases where we most underperform GIST-Coseg. See the Supp. file for all classes.

The analysis is fairly similar to our MIT dataset results. We again see good support for actively selecting a cosegmentation partner: our method outperforms the Rand-Coseg and GIST-Coseg baselines in most cases. Overall, we outperform GIST-Coseg in 23 of the 28 classes, and Single-Seg in 20 of the 28 classes. Our method is also quite close to the Upper bound on this dataset, only 1.5 points away on average.

However, for the Caltech data, the gap between Single-Seg and the Upper bound—while still noticeably wider than the gap between our method and the Upper bound—is also narrowed considerably compared to the MIT data. This indicates that the Caltech images have greater regularity within a class and/or more salient foregrounds (both of which we find true upon visual inspection). In fact, Single-Seg can even outperform the cosegmentation methods in some cases (e.g., see motorbike). This finding agrees with previous reports in [4,8]; while one hopes to see gains from the "more supervised" cosegmentation task, single-image segmentation can be competitive either when the intra-class variation is too high or the foreground is particularly salient.

Table 4. Comparison to state-of-the-art cosegmentation algorithms on the Caltech-28 dataset.

Method	Average precision
Spatial Topic Model-Coseg [9]	67
Single-Seg	82.71
GrabCut-Coseg (see [3])	81.5
ClassCut-Coseg [3]	83.6
BPLR-Coseg [27]	85.6
Ours	**85.81**

Finally, we compare our method to state-of-the-art cosegmentation methods using their published numbers on the Caltech-28. Table 4 shows the results, in terms of average precision (the metric reported in the prior work). Our method is more accurate than all the previous results. Notably, all the prior cosegmentation results ([3,9,27] and the multi-image GrabCut [22] extension defined in [3]) indiscriminately use all the input images for joint segmentation, whereas our method selects the single most effective partner per query. This result is more evidence for the advantage of doing so.

5   Conclusions

Cosegmentation injects valuable implicit top-down information for segmentation, based on commonalities between related input images. Rather than assume that useful partners for cosegmentation will be known in advance, we propose to predict which pairs will work well together. Our results on two challenging datasets are encouraging evidence that it is worthwhile to actively focus cosegmentation on relevant pairs.

While so far we have focused on the weakly supervised setting—in which it is arguably harder to see impact, due to the potential relevance of *any* candidate partner—the approach is also applicable to the fully unsupervised setting, as we will explore in future work. We also plan to extend the algorithm from pairs to the multi-image joint segmentation scenario.

Acknowledgements. This research is supported in part by ONR award N00014-12-1-0068.

References

1. Rother, C., Minka, T., Blake, A., Kolmogorov, V.: Cosegmentation of image pairs by histogram matching - incorporating a global constraint into MRFs. In: CVPR (2006)
2. Winn, J., Jojic, N.: LOCUS: learning object classes with unsupervised segmentation. In: ICCV (2005)
3. Alexe, B., Deselaers, T., Ferrari, V.: ClassCut for unsupervised class segmentation. In: Daniilidis, K., Maragos, P., Paragios, N. (eds.) ECCV 2010, Part V. LNCS, vol. 6315, pp. 380–393. Springer, Heidelberg (2010)
4. Vicente, S., Rother, C., Kolmogorov, V.: Object cosegmentation. In: CVPR (2011)
5. Joulin, A., Bach, F., Ponce, J.: Discriminative clustering for image co-segmentation. In: CVPR (2010)
6. Joulin, A., Bach, F., Ponce, J.: Multi-class cosegmentation. In: CVPR (2012)
7. Kim, G., Xing, E., Fei Fei, L., Kanade, T.: Distributed cosegmentation via submodular optimization on anisotropic diffusion. In: ICCV (2011)
8. Rubinstein, M., Joulin, A., Kopf, J., Liu, C.: Unsupervised joint object discovery and segmentation in internet images. In: CVPR (2013)
9. Cao, L., Fei-Fei, L.: Spatially coherent latent topic model for concurrent segmentation and Classification of objects and scenes. In: ICCV (2007)
10. Todorovic, S., Ahuja, N.: Unsupervised category modeling, recognition, and segmentation in images. PAMI **30**, 2158–2174 (2008)
11. Lee, Y.J., Grauman, K.: Collect-cut: segmentation with top-down cues discovered in multi-object images. In: CVPR (2010)
12. Hochbaum, D., Singh, V.: An efficient algorithm for co-segmentation. In: ICCV (2009)
13. Batra, D., Kowdle, A., Parikh, D., Luo, J., Chen, T.: iCoseg: interactive cosegmentation with intelligent scribble guidance. In: CVPR (2010)
14. Russell, B., Efros, A., Sivic, J., Freeman, W., Zisserman, A.: Using multiple segmentations to discover objects and their extent in image collections. In: CVPR (2006)
15. Faktor, A., Irani, M.: "Clustering by composition" – unsupervised discovery of image categories. In: Fitzgibbon, A., Lazebnik, S., Perona, P., Sato, Y., Schmid, C. (eds.) ECCV 2012, Part VII. LNCS, vol. 7578, pp. 474–487. Springer, Heidelberg (2012)

16. Liu, D., Xiong, Y., Pulli, K., Shapiro, L.: Estimating image segmentation difficulty. In: Machine Learning and Data Mining in Pattern Recognition (2011)
17. Carreira, J., Sminchisescu, C.: CPMC: automatic object segmentation using constrained parametric min-cuts. PAMI **34**, 1312–1328 (2012)
18. Endres, I., Hoiem, D.: Category independent object proposals. In: Daniilidis, K., Maragos, P., Paragios, N. (eds.) ECCV 2010, Part V. LNCS, vol. 6315, pp. 575–588. Springer, Heidelberg (2010)
19. Ren, X., Malik, J.: Learning a classication model for segmentation. In: ICCV (2003)
20. Jain, S., Grauman, K.: Predicting sufficient annotation strength for interactive foreground segmentation. In: ICCV (2013)
21. Jiang, B., Zhang, L., Lu, H., Yang, C., Yang, M.H.: Saliency detection via absorbing markov chain. In: ICCV (2013)
22. Rother, C., Kolmogorov, V., Blake, A.: Grabcut -interactive foreground extraction using iterated graph cuts. In: SIGGRAPH (2004)
23. Kim, J., Liu, C., Sha, F., Grauman, K.: Deformable spatial pyramid matching for fast dense correspondences. In: CVPR (2013)
24. Joachims, T.: Optimizing search engines with clickthrough data. In: KDD (2002)
25. Kohli, P., Torr, P.H.S.: Measuring uncertainty in graph cut solutions. CVIU **112**, 30–38 (2008)
26. Torralba, A.: Contextual priming for object detection. Int. J. Comput. Vis. **53**, 169–191 (2003)
27. Kim, J., Grauman, K.: Boundary preserving dense local regions. In: CVPR (2011)

Image Restoration via Multi-prior Collaboration

Feng Jiang[1,2]([⊠]), Shengping Zhang[1], Debin Zhao[1], and S.Y. Kung[2]

[1] School of Computer Science, Harbin Institute of Technology, Harbin, China
fjiang@hit.edu.cn
[2] School of Electrical Engineering, Princeton University, Princeton, USA

Abstract. This paper proposes a novel multi-prior collaboration framework for image restoration. Different from traditional non-reference image restoration methods, a big reference image set is adopted to provide the references and predictions of different popular prior models and accordingly further guide the subsequent multi-prior collaboration. In particular, the collaboration of multi-prior models is mathematically formulated as a ridge regression problem. Due to expensive computation complexity of handling big reference data, scatter-matrix-based kernel ridge regression is proposed, which achieves high accuracy while low complexity. Additionally, an iterative pursuit is further proposed to obtain refined and robust restoration results. Five popular prior methods are applied to evaluate the effectiveness of the proposed multi-prior collaboration framework. Compared with the state-of-the-art image restoration approaches, the proposed framework improves the restoration performance significantly.

1 Introduction

Mathematically, image restoration aims to reconstruct the original high quality image u from its observed degradation y, which is a typical ill-posed linear inverse problem and can be generally formulated as

$$y = Hu + n, \tag{1}$$

where $u \in \mathbb{R}^d$ and $y \in \mathbb{R}^d$ are lexicographically stacked representations of the original image and the degraded image, respectively, $H \in \mathbb{R}^{d \times d}$ is a matrix representing a non-invertible linear degradation operator and $\in \mathbb{R}^d$ is usually additive Gaussian white noise. When H is an identity matrix, the problem becomes image denoising [1]; when H is a blur operator, the problem becomes image deblurring [2]; when H is a mask, that is, H is a diagonal matrix whose diagonal entries are either 1 or 0, the problem becomes image inpainting [3]; when H is a set of random projections, the problem becomes compressive sensing [4,5]. To cope with the ill-posed nature of image restoration, one type of scheme in the literature employs image prior knowledge for regularizing the solution to the following minimization problem

$$\arg\min_u \frac{1}{2} \|Hu - y\|_2^2 + \lambda\Psi(u), \tag{2}$$

© Springer International Publishing Switzerland 2015
D. Cremers et al. (Eds.): ACCV 2014, Part III, LNCS 9005, pp. 191–204, 2015.
DOI: 10.1007/978-3-319-16811-1_13

where $\frac{1}{2}\|Hv - y\|_2^2$ is the ℓ_2-norm based data-fidelity term, $\Psi(u)$ denotes image prior (also called the regularization term) and λ is the regularization parameter. In fact, the above regularization-based minimization can be strictly derived from Bayesian inference with prior knowledge in image generation models [6]. Many optimization approaches for regularization-based image inverse problems have been developed [7–9].

It has been widely recognized that image prior knowledge plays a critical role for image restoration approaches. Therefore, designing effective regularization terms to reflect intrinsic image prior models is at the core of image restoration. Classical regularization terms utilize local structural patterns and are built on the assumption that images are locally smooth except at edges. Several representative work in the literature includes half quadrature formulation [10], Mumford-Shah (MS) model [11] and total variation (TV) models [12]. These regularization terms demonstrate high effectiveness in preserving edges and recovering smooth regions. However, they usually smear out image details and cannot deal well with fine structures since they only exploit local statistics, neglecting nonlocal statistics of nature images.

In recent years, the most significant nonlocal statistics in image processing is perhaps the nonlocal self-similarity exhibited by natural images. The nonlocal self-similarity depicts the repetitiveness of higher level patterns (e.g., textures and structures) globally positioned in images. A representative work is the popular nonlocal means (NLM) [13], which takes advantage of this image property to conduct a type of weighted filtering for denoising tasks. This simple weighted approach is quite effective in generating sharper image edges and preserving more image details. Later, inspired by the success of nonlocal means (NLM) denoising filter, a series of nonlocal regularization terms have been proposed [14], which can be roughly divided into two categories according to their formulations. The first one is directly derived from NLM [15], since nonlocal filtering can essentially be understood as a quadratic regularization based on a nonlocal graph, as detailed for instance in the geometric diffusion framework in [16]. The other one goes one step further to solve general inverse problems by incorporating nonlocal graph into traditional regularization terms, such as nonlocal total variation (NL/TV) [17] and nonlocal Mumford-Shah (NL/MS) [18]. Due to the utilization of self-similarity prior by adaptive nonlocal graph, nonlocal regularization terms produce superior performance over the local ones, with the ability of preserving sharper image edges and more image details [19]. Nonetheless, there are still plenty of image details and structures that cannot be recovered accurately. The reason is that the above nonlocal regularization terms depend on the weighted graph, while it is inevitable that the weighted manner gives rise to disturbance and inaccuracy [20].

Vision information in natural images is extremely complex. Although many statistical priors have been explored from distinctive viewpoints, each prior model has its shortcomings especially for a specific applications. Intuitively, it is natural to consider to combine the existing prior models and let them collaborate to result in a better solution. However, from point of view of theory, is difficult to propose a general collaboration framework that combines multiple prior models. Some previous work incorporates two or more prior models into a regularization-based framework for image restoration [21–23]. In [21], the local total variation model and nonlocal adaptive 3-D sparse representation model are combined to solve image restoration from partial random samples in spatial domain. In CS-MRI (Compressive Sensing Magnetic Resonance Imaging) models, the linear combination of total variation and wavelet sparse regularization is popular [22,23].

The existing methods of combining multiple prior models mainly add the prior knowledge as a regularization term in the objective function to be optimized. Although some improvements have been reported, the complex objective function with pre-defined weights of different priors and the high computation complexity in the optimization process restrict the regularization methods from being a general framework. The regularization terms depend on the weighted graph, however it is inevitable that the weighted manner gives rise to disturbance and inaccuracy. In this paper, a novel and general multi-prior collaboration framework is proposed as shown in Fig. 1. Instead of merging multi-prior in a traditional predefined regularization term, we evaluated the potential of the prior models on current degraded images as well as their coupling dynamically. The collaboration of multiple priors is mathematically formulated as a ridge regression problem. Due to the computation complexity of dealing with big reference data, scatter-matrix-based kernel ridge regression (KRR) is proposed. Compared with the traditional KRR, scatter-matrix-based KRR achieves relative low computation cost and ensures accuracy and robustness at the same time.

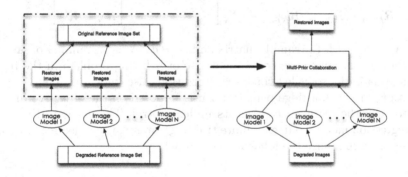

Fig. 1. The proposed multi-prior collaboration framework.

2 Kernel Ridge Regression Based Multi-Prior Collaboration Model

Given the prior model set $\mathbb{P} = \{\mathcal{P}_1, \ldots, \mathcal{P}_M\}$ and a degraded image I', we can obtain the restored images $\{I'_{r\oplus 1}, \ldots, I'_{r\oplus M}\}$ with M prior models respectively. let I denote the non-degraded image corresponding to the degraded image I'.

It is reasonable to assume the residual $\boldsymbol{I} - \boldsymbol{I}'$ has a linear relationship with the innovation brought by each prior model $\{\boldsymbol{I}'_{r\oplus 1} - \boldsymbol{I}', \dots, \boldsymbol{I}'_{r\oplus M} - \boldsymbol{I}'\}$, which can be expressed as

$$\boldsymbol{I} - \boldsymbol{I}' = [\boldsymbol{I}'_{r\oplus 1} - \boldsymbol{I}', \boldsymbol{I}'_{r\oplus 2} - \boldsymbol{I}', \dots, \boldsymbol{I}'_{r\oplus M} - \boldsymbol{I}']\boldsymbol{\omega} = \boldsymbol{\Gamma}\boldsymbol{\omega} \tag{3}$$

where $\boldsymbol{\Gamma} = [\boldsymbol{I}'_{r\oplus 1} - \boldsymbol{I}', \dots, \boldsymbol{I}'_{r\oplus M} - \boldsymbol{I}'] \in \mathbb{R}^{d \times M}$ and $\boldsymbol{\omega} \in \mathbb{R}^M$ is the weight vector for the restoration which can be obtained by a regression process. The final restoration image $\hat{\boldsymbol{I}}$ can be obtained as

$$\hat{\boldsymbol{I}} = \boldsymbol{I}' + \boldsymbol{\Gamma}\boldsymbol{\omega} . \tag{4}$$

In the multi-prior collaboration, the training data, i.e., the reference images, are used to predict the restoration performance with respect to the current degraded image. Ideally, a reference images set with the similar content and category can evaluate the restoration capability of the different priors when applied to the current degraded image.

Define $\mathcal{R} = \{\boldsymbol{R}_1, \dots, \boldsymbol{R}_N\}$ is the set of reference nature images with the similar content and category with the current degraded image $\boldsymbol{I}'$, and their corresponding degraded images consist of the set of reference degraded images $\mathcal{R}' = \{\boldsymbol{R}'_1, \dots, \boldsymbol{R}'_N\}$. For each degraded image $\boldsymbol{R}'_n \in \mathbb{R}^d$, a restored result $\boldsymbol{R}'_{n\oplus m}$ can be obtained with prior $\mathcal{P}_m$. Obviously, according to Eq. 3, the reference images should satisfy

$$\begin{bmatrix} \boldsymbol{R}'_{1\oplus 1} - \boldsymbol{R}'_1 & \cdots & \boldsymbol{R}'_{1\oplus M} - \boldsymbol{R}'_1 \\ \vdots & \ddots & \vdots \\ \boldsymbol{R}'_{N\oplus 1} - \boldsymbol{R}'_N & \cdots & \boldsymbol{R}'_{N\oplus M} - \boldsymbol{R}'_N \end{bmatrix} \boldsymbol{\omega} = \boldsymbol{X}^\top \boldsymbol{\omega} = \begin{bmatrix} \boldsymbol{R}_1 - \boldsymbol{R}'_1 \\ \vdots \\ \boldsymbol{R}_N - \boldsymbol{R}'_N \end{bmatrix} = \boldsymbol{y} , \tag{5}$$

where $\boldsymbol{X} \in \mathbb{R}^{M \times \hat{N}}$ is the sample matrix and $\hat{N} = d \times N$ is the number of samples.

A classic solution to overcome the above over-fitting problem in the regression analysis is the so-called ridge regularization, also known as Tikhonov regularization, in which a ridge penalty term is imposed on the objective function so as to keep the regressor coefficients under control. This leads to the classic ridge regression method. Given a finite training dataset, the objective of a linear regressor is to minimize the following cost function

$$E_{RR}(\boldsymbol{\omega}) = \sum_{i=1}^{\hat{N}} \epsilon_i^2 + \rho\|\boldsymbol{\omega}\|^2 , \tag{6}$$

where $\epsilon_i = \boldsymbol{\omega}^\top \boldsymbol{x}_i - y_i$ and $\boldsymbol{x}_i$ is the i-th column of matrix $\boldsymbol{X}$ and y_i is the i-th element of vector $\boldsymbol{y}$ and ρ is the ridge parameter. The principle of ridge regression lies in the incorporation of a penalty term into the loss function to control the regressor coefficients. Being adjustable by the ridge parameter ρ, the penalty term can effectively mitigate the over-fitting problem and thus enhance the robustness of the learned classifier.

2.1   Kernel Based Approach: Learning Models in Empirical Space

With a kernel function $\phi : \mathbb{R}^M \rightarrow \mathbb{R}^J$ mapping a sample $\boldsymbol{x}_i$ from the M-dimensional space to the J-dimensional space, the objective is to find the decision vector $\boldsymbol{u} \in \mathbb{R}^J$ and the threshold b such that

$$\min_{\boldsymbol{u},b} E_{KRR}(\boldsymbol{u},b) = \min_{\boldsymbol{u},b}\{\sum_{i=1}^{\hat{N}} \epsilon_i^2 + \rho\|\boldsymbol{u}\|_2^2\} , \tag{7}$$

where

$$\epsilon_i = \boldsymbol{u}^\top\phi(\boldsymbol{x}_i) + b - y_i , \forall i = 1,\ldots,N . \tag{8}$$

In matrix notation,

$$E_{KRR}(\boldsymbol{u},b) = \|\boldsymbol{\Phi}^\top\boldsymbol{u} + b\boldsymbol{e} - \boldsymbol{y}\|_2^2 + \rho\|\boldsymbol{u}\|_2^2 . \tag{9}$$

where $\boldsymbol{\Phi} = [\phi(\boldsymbol{x}_1),\ldots,\phi(\boldsymbol{x}_{\hat{N}})] \in \mathbb{R}^{J\times\hat{N}}$. The zero-gradient point of $E_{KRR}(\boldsymbol{u},b)$ with respect to $\boldsymbol{u}$ can be obtained as

$$\frac{\partial E_{KRR}(\boldsymbol{u},b)}{\partial \boldsymbol{u}} = 2\boldsymbol{\Phi}(\boldsymbol{\Phi}^\top\boldsymbol{u} + b\boldsymbol{e} - \boldsymbol{y}) + 2\rho\boldsymbol{u} = 0 . \tag{10}$$

By Eq. 10, we have

$$\boldsymbol{u} = -\rho^{-1}\boldsymbol{\Phi}(\boldsymbol{\Phi}^T\boldsymbol{u} + b\boldsymbol{e} - \boldsymbol{y}) . \tag{11}$$

Thus, there exists an $\hat{N}$-dimensional vector $\boldsymbol{a}$ such that $\boldsymbol{u} = \boldsymbol{\Phi}\boldsymbol{a}$. This establishes the validity of LSP, *i.e.* $\boldsymbol{u} \in \text{span}[\boldsymbol{\Phi}]$. The knowledge of the LSP is instrumental for the actual solution for $\boldsymbol{u}$. More exactly, on plugging the LSP, $\boldsymbol{u} = \boldsymbol{\Phi}\boldsymbol{a}$ into Eq. 9, we obtain

$$E'_{KRR}(\boldsymbol{a},b) = \|\boldsymbol{\Phi}^\top\boldsymbol{\Phi}\boldsymbol{a} + b\boldsymbol{e} - \boldsymbol{y}\|_2^2 + \rho\boldsymbol{a}^\top\boldsymbol{\Phi}^\top\boldsymbol{\Phi}\boldsymbol{a} \tag{12}$$

$$= \|\boldsymbol{K}\boldsymbol{a} + b\boldsymbol{e} - \boldsymbol{y}\|_2^2 + \rho\boldsymbol{a}^\top\boldsymbol{K}\boldsymbol{a} . \tag{13}$$

where $\boldsymbol{K} = \boldsymbol{\Phi}^\top\boldsymbol{\Phi} \in \mathbb{R}^{\hat{N}\times\hat{N}}$. The zero-gradient point of $E'_{KRR}(\boldsymbol{a},b)$ with respect to $\boldsymbol{a}$ leads to

$$\begin{bmatrix} \boldsymbol{K}+\rho\boldsymbol{I} & \boldsymbol{e} \\ \boldsymbol{e}^\top & 0 \end{bmatrix} \begin{bmatrix} \boldsymbol{a} \\ b \end{bmatrix} = \begin{bmatrix} \boldsymbol{y} \\ \boldsymbol{0} \end{bmatrix} , \tag{14}$$

2.2   Scatter-Matrix Based Approach: Multi-Prior Models Collaboration in the Intrinsic Space

By Eq. 10, we have the following optimal decision vector

$$\boldsymbol{u} = (\boldsymbol{\Phi}\boldsymbol{\Phi}^\top + \rho\boldsymbol{I})^{-1}\boldsymbol{\Phi}(\boldsymbol{y} - b\boldsymbol{e}) \tag{15}$$

$$= (\boldsymbol{S} + \rho\boldsymbol{I})^{-1}\boldsymbol{\Phi}(\boldsymbol{y} - b\boldsymbol{e}) . \tag{16}$$

where $S = \Phi\Phi^\top \in \mathbb{R}^{J \times J}$. The first-order gradient of $E'_{KRR}(u, b)$ with respective to b leads to

$$\frac{\partial E'_{KRR}(u, b)}{\partial b} = e^\top \Phi^\top u + be^\top e - e^\top y \tag{17}$$

$$= e^\top \Phi^\top u + \hat{N} \times b - e^\top y \tag{18}$$

Let the first-order gradient be zero, the solution for KRR may be derived from the matrix system

$$\begin{bmatrix} S + \rho I & \Phi e \\ e^\top \Phi^\top & \hat{N} \end{bmatrix} \begin{bmatrix} u \\ b \end{bmatrix} = \begin{bmatrix} \Phi y \\ e^\top y \end{bmatrix}, \tag{19}$$

We have so far independently derived the optimal KRR solutions both for the intrinsic space and for the empirical-space formulation. Logically, both approaches should lead to the same solutions. However, as an alternative verification, we shall now provide an algebraic method to directly connect the two solutions. For the kernel-matrix-based solution (Eq. 20), note that $K = \Phi^\top \Phi$, we obtain

$$\begin{bmatrix} e^\top & -\rho \end{bmatrix} \begin{bmatrix} K + \rho I & e \\ e^\top & 0 \end{bmatrix} \begin{bmatrix} a \\ b \end{bmatrix} = \begin{bmatrix} e^\top & -\rho \end{bmatrix} \begin{bmatrix} y \\ 0 \end{bmatrix} \tag{20}$$

$$\begin{bmatrix} e^\top K + e^\top \rho I - \rho e^\top & e^\top e \end{bmatrix} \begin{bmatrix} a \\ b \end{bmatrix} = e^\top y \tag{21}$$

$$\begin{bmatrix} e^\top K & e^\top e \end{bmatrix} \begin{bmatrix} a \\ b \end{bmatrix} = e^\top y \tag{22}$$

$$e^\top K a + e^\top e b = e^\top y \tag{23}$$

$$e^\top \Phi^\top \Phi a + \hat{N} b = e^\top y \tag{24}$$

$$e^\top \Phi^\top u + \hat{N} b = e^\top y \tag{25}$$

By Woodbury's matrix identity [24], we have

$$(K + \rho I)^{-1} = \rho^{-1} I - \rho^{-1} \Phi^T (\rho I + S)^{-1} \Phi \tag{26}$$

and it follows that

$$\Phi(K + \rho I)^{-1} = \rho^{-1} \Phi - \rho^{-1} S(\rho I + S)^{-1} \Phi = (\rho I + S)^{-1} \Phi . \tag{27}$$

We can obtain

$$u = \Phi a = \Phi(K + \rho I)^{-1}(y - be) = (\rho I + S)^{-1} \Phi(y - be) . \tag{28}$$

On pre-multiplying the above by $(\rho I + S)$, we arrive at

$$(\rho I + S)u = \Phi y - \Phi e b \tag{29}$$

By combining Eqs. 25 and 29, which is equivalent to the formulation given in Eq. 19 derived for the original space.

3 Iterative Pursuit Degraded Image Restoration

In order to obtain more refined restoration results, an iterative pursuit is provide to guide the restoration process. This process is based on the following assumptions: the reference big data simulate the restoration process and their performance will give a reliable prediction of the current restoration, which will provide the restoration for each single prior models. Firstly, in each iterative step each image in reference image set is restored with prior models respectively and the results and the corresponding residual with the ground truth is then used to get the multi prior model corporation rule; then, each image in the reference degraded set is further updated with the same rule. A simple illustration is shown as Fig. 2. In each step of the iterative process, for each reference image R'_n, M restored images $\{R'_{n\oplus 1}, \ldots, R'_{n\oplus M}\}$ are obtained, then projected to $\{\widetilde{R}'_{n\oplus 1}, \ldots, \widetilde{R}'_{n\oplus J}\}$ where $\widetilde{R}'_{n\oplus j}(m, n) = \phi_j(R'_{n\oplus 1}(m, n), \ldots, R'_{n\oplus M}(m, n))$. The ground truth R_n is also projected into $\{\widetilde{R}_{n\oplus 1}, \ldots, \widetilde{R}_{n\oplus J}\}$ where $\widetilde{R}_{n\oplus j}(m, n) = \phi_j(R_{n\oplus 1}(m, n), \ldots, R_{n\oplus M}(m, n))$.

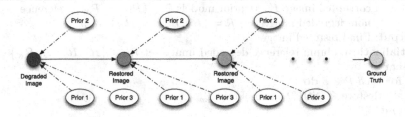

Fig. 2. An illustration of the proposed multi-prior collaboration framework.

In the situation of linear regression, for each prior model $\mathcal{P}_m$, it has N restoration results when applied to the set $\mathcal{R}'$. The divergent of PSNR of these N restored images reflects the prediction certainty of $\mathcal{P}_m$. Supposed for degraded images $\mathcal{R}'$, $\mathcal{P}_m$ gets the prediction certainty, i.e., the variation of Peak Signal to Noise Ratio (PSNR) as σ_m^2, then in the linear collaboration, the total certainty can be expressed as $\sum_{m=1}^{M} \omega_m^2 \sigma_m^2$ Since a prior model performs restoration differently for different images, we hope the restored results of each prior model has least divergent.

Similarly, in the nonlinear situation, the prediction certainty can be introduced into Eq. 7 and resulting the following objective function

$$E'_{KRR}(\boldsymbol{u}, b) = \sum_{i=1}^{\hat{N}} \epsilon_i^2 + \rho\|\boldsymbol{u}\|_2^2 + \lambda \sum_{j=1}^{J} u_j^2 \sigma_j^2 , \tag{30}$$

where $\sigma_j^2 = var(PSNR(\widetilde{R}'_{1\oplus j}, \widetilde{R}_{1\oplus j}), \ldots, PSNR(\widetilde{R}'_{N\oplus j}, \widetilde{R}_{N\oplus j}))$.

In matrix notation,

$$E'_{KRR}(\boldsymbol{u}, b) = \|\boldsymbol{\Phi}^\top \boldsymbol{u} - \boldsymbol{y}\|_2^2 + \rho\|\boldsymbol{u}\|_2^2 + \boldsymbol{u}^\top \boldsymbol{U}\boldsymbol{u} . \qquad (31)$$

where $\boldsymbol{U} = diag(\sigma_1^2, \sigma_2^2, \ldots, \sigma_M^2)$ is a diagonal matrix.

The zero-gradient point of $E'_{KRR}(\boldsymbol{u}, b)$ with respect to $\boldsymbol{u}$ can be obtained as

$$\frac{\partial E_{KRR}(\boldsymbol{u}, b)}{\partial \boldsymbol{u}} = 2\boldsymbol{\Phi}(\boldsymbol{\Phi}^\top \boldsymbol{u} - \boldsymbol{y}) + 2(\rho\boldsymbol{I} + \boldsymbol{U}) = 0 . \qquad (32)$$

The solution is

$$\boldsymbol{u} = (\boldsymbol{\Phi}\boldsymbol{\Phi}^\top + \rho\boldsymbol{I} + \boldsymbol{U})^{-1}\boldsymbol{\Phi}(\boldsymbol{y} - b\boldsymbol{e}) = (\boldsymbol{S} + \rho\boldsymbol{I} + \boldsymbol{U})^{-1}\boldsymbol{\Phi}(\boldsymbol{y} - b\boldsymbol{e}) . \qquad (33)$$

The detailed procedure of the proposed image restoration is summarized in Algorithm 1.

Algorithm 1. The proposed multi-prior collaboration and degraded image restoration

---

Input   : corrupted image $\boldsymbol{I}'$, M prior models $\mathbb{P} = \{\mathcal{P}_1, \ldots, \mathcal{P}_M\}$, reference
             non-degraded images set $\mathcal{R} = \{\boldsymbol{R}_1, \boldsymbol{R}_2, \ldots, \boldsymbol{R}_N\}$, λ, ρ
Output: Final restored image
Initialization: obtain reference degraded image set $\mathcal{R}_d = \{\boldsymbol{R}'_1, \boldsymbol{R}'_2, \ldots, \boldsymbol{R}'_N\}$
repeat
    for *each* $\mathcal{P} \in \mathbb{P}$ **do**
     | Restore $\boldsymbol{I}'$ with $\mathcal{P}_m$ and obtain $\boldsymbol{I}'_m$
    end
    Obtain $\phi_{I'} = \phi(I'_1 - I', I'_2 - I', \cdots, I'_M - I') \in \mathbb{R}^{d \times J}$
    for *each* $\boldsymbol{R}'_n \in \mathcal{R}_d$ **do**
     | **for** *each* $\mathcal{P} \in \mathbb{P}$ **do**
     | | Restore $\boldsymbol{R}'_n$ with $\mathcal{P}_m$ and obtain $\boldsymbol{R}'_{n\oplus m}$
     | **end**
     | Obtain $\phi_{R'_n} = \phi(\boldsymbol{R}'_{n\oplus 1} - \boldsymbol{R}'_n, \boldsymbol{R}'_{n\oplus 2} - \boldsymbol{R}'_n, \cdots, \boldsymbol{R}'_{n\oplus M} - \boldsymbol{R}'_n) \in \mathbb{R}^{d \times J}$
     | project $\{\boldsymbol{R}'_{n\oplus 1}, \ldots, \boldsymbol{R}'_{n\oplus M}\}$ to $\{\widetilde{\boldsymbol{R}}'_{n\oplus 1}, \ldots, \widetilde{\boldsymbol{R}}'_{n\oplus J}\}$ with
     | $\widetilde{\boldsymbol{R}}'_{n\oplus j}(m, n) = \phi_j(\boldsymbol{R}'_{n\oplus 1}(m, n), \ldots, \boldsymbol{R}'_{n\oplus M}(m, n))$
     | Translate $\boldsymbol{R}_n$ to $\{\widetilde{\boldsymbol{R}}_{n\oplus 1}, \ldots, \widetilde{\boldsymbol{R}}_{n\oplus J}\}$ with
     | $\widetilde{\boldsymbol{R}}_{n\oplus j}(m, n) = \phi_j(\boldsymbol{R}_{n\oplus 1}(m, n), \ldots, \boldsymbol{R}_{n\oplus M}(m, n))$
    end
    Obtain $\boldsymbol{U}$ and $\boldsymbol{\Phi} = (\phi_{R'_1}^\top, \phi_{R'_2}^\top, \ldots, \phi_{R'_N}^\top)^\top$
    Compute $\boldsymbol{u}$ using Eq. 33
    Update $\boldsymbol{I}' = \boldsymbol{u}^\top \phi_{I'} + \boldsymbol{I}'$
    for *each* $\boldsymbol{R}'_n \in \mathcal{R}_d$ **do**
     | Update $\boldsymbol{R}'_n = \boldsymbol{u}^\top \phi_{R'_n} + \boldsymbol{R}'_n$
    end
until *Stopping criterion is satisfied*

---

4   Experiments

To evaluate the performance of the proposed framework, we take 5 classical priors: TV, BM3D [25], FOE [26], KSVD [27], BLSGSM [28]. The total variation (TV) model [29] has been quite successful used in many aspects of the image processing. TV model favors the piecewise smoothness, and it represents a local prior. In this approach, TV model serve as a regularizer in an unconstrained convex minimization problem, and the parameter before TV model controls the tradeoff between the regularity and fidelity terms. And the Block-matching 3D (BM3D) [25] algorithm is based on the phenomenon that a patch (block) tends to recur in a natural image. Denoising process is mainly that grouping similar 2D image blocks into 3D data arrays then through the procedure of collaborative filtering. Obviously, this method is based on a nonlocal prior. The Fields of Experts(FOE) [26] that extends traditional Markov Random Field (MRF) models by learning potential functions over extended pixel neighborhoods is a classic method, The approach develop a framework for learning generic, expressive image priors that capture the statistics of natural scenes. And the approach of KSVD [27] taken is based on sparse representation over the trained overcomplete dictionary. In the sparse representation modeling the choice of dictionary is an important issue, and there has been much effort in learning dictionaries from a set of example image patches [27]. In the algorithm of BLS-GSM [28], the authors describe the method for removing noise from digital images, based on a statistical model of the coefficients of an overcomplete multi-scale oriented basis.

In experimental settings, the type and intensity of noise is known, that is, the noise model is determined. So almost all the proposed algorithms rely on some explicit or implicit assumptions about the true(noise free) image. The experimental results of TV, BM3D, KSVD, BLSGSM and FOE are all generated by the original authors' codes, with the corresponding parameters manually optimized.

4.1   Linear Collaboration of Multi-Prior Models

Because of the fact that the content of the image affect restoration effect, eight training (and test) images are come from a similar certain class of textured images. These eight images are shown in Fig. 3.

Table 1 lists PSNR results of TV model and BM3D model collaboration. All the images are degraded by additive Gaussian noise $\sigma = 12$. The coefficients of each image is obtained by leave-one-out cross validation. That means,in order to obtain the coefficient of an image we train the other 7 images (Fig. 4).

In the Table 1, the second and third rows represent the restoration results from TV and BM3D models respectively. The fourth and fifth rows represent the coefficients of each image. The sixth row reports the performance of the collaboration of the TV and BM3D with the proposed method. Generally, BM3D method can get a better result than TV model in this image training set, so we list the gain between BM3D result and combination result in seventh row. From Table 1, we could find that the coefficients of TV part are in the range of (0.1280,

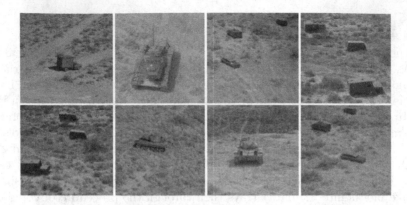

Fig. 3. Images used for evaluation and reference set (grey, 512 × 512).

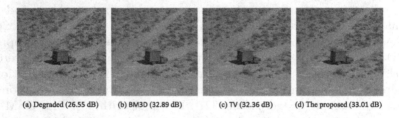

(a) Degraded (26.55 dB)   (b) BM3D (32.89 dB)   (c) TV (32.36 dB)   (d) The proposed (33.01 dB)

Fig. 4. comparison of Gaussian noise removal.

Table 1. TV and BM3D priors collaboration performance (PSNR).

Priors	img1	img2	img3	img4	img5	img6	img7	img8
TV	32.36	32.14	32.73	30.39	30.42	30.78	31.00	32.56
BM3D	32.89	32.37	33.26	30.79	30.84	31.03	31.52	33.06
Coef_of TV	0.1299	0.1280	0.1325	0.1362	0.1369	0.1352	0.1383	0.1331
Coef_of BM3D	0.7735	0.7802	0.7701	0.7768	0.7755	0.7780	0.7720	0.7698
The proposed	33.01	32.60	33.35	30.99	31.03	31.25	31.70	33.15
Gain	0.12	0.23	0.09	0.20	0.19	0.22	0.18	0.09

0.1383) and the coefficients of BM3D part are in the range of (0.7698, 0.7802). The coefficients are relatively stable.

4.2 Nonlinear Collaboration of Multi-Prior Models

One of the distinct difference of our method is the introduction of reference data in the image restoration process. The proposed multi-prior collaboration framework is expected a better performance on a bigger reference data set. To verify the learning efficiency of nonlinear collaboration of multi-prior models with big data, we use the INRIA Holiday dataset [29], which has 1491 images in total. One advantage of this data set is that there are multiple images in the same scene captured at different viewpoints and focal lengths, which ensure the contained images have the similar content and category. 8 images are selected as test images and the rest are used as reference images. These same scene and category images are used to simulate the similar images obtained form a big training data for the degraded images. All the test images are degraded by additive Gaussian noise $\sigma = 12$. We used iterative pursuit restoration and TRBF3 kernel in this experiment and the results are shown as Table 2. Nine configurations are used to evaluate our proposed multi-prior model collaboration.

Table 2. TV and BM3D priors collaboration performance (PSNR).

Priors		img1	img2	img3	img4	img5	img6	img7	img8	Gain
1	T&F	32.65	32.35	32.97	30.77	30.79	30.97	31.40	32.80	0.29
2	T&K	32.12	32.48	33.08	30.93	30.95	31.16	31.54	32.92	0.31
3	T&BL	32.86	32.45	33.11	30.81	30.83	31.07	31.52	32.95	0.14
4	BM&F	32.98	32.58	33.33	30.98	31.02	31.23	31.69	33.14	0.15
5	BM&K	33.39	32.98	33.73	31.38	31.42	31.64	32.10	33.54	0.55
6	BM&BL	33.15	32.72	33.46	31.11	31.14	31.36	31.83	33.27	0.28
7	F&K	32.86	32.52	33.13	31.05	31.06	31.22	31.66	32.98	0.39
8	F&BL	32.98	32.56	33.24	30.97	30.99	31.19	31.67	33.08	0.27
9	K&BL	32.89	32.46	33.12	30.90	30.92	31.12	31.58	32.96	0.18

T: TV prior; **K**: K-SVD prior; **BL**: BLS-GSM prior;
BM: BM3D prior. **Training data**: INRIA Holiday dataset

Obviously in all the configuration, the collaborated prior models considerably outperforms the unique prior restoration in all the cases, with the highest PSNR, achieving the average PSNR improvements over the performance of unique prior adopted is 0.55 dB. With the adopted of big reference data set, the proposed scatter-matrix-based KRR have a significant improvement in the collaboration of multi-prior. An average of 0.28 DB improvement is obtain in the image restoration.

In the configuration of BLS_GSM prior and K-SVD prior, FoE prior and K-SVD prior, the proposed method get the most significant improvement 0.55 and 0.39 DB. It can be seen that BLS_GSM and K-SVD, FOE and KSVD models have less coupled, while in the configuration of TV and BLS_GSM, only 0.14 DB is got, it implied that there were prior coupled in these two prior models.

If a TRBF3 kernel is adopted, the scatter-matrix-based KRR has an overwhelming speed advantage over direct KRR. While the conventional KRRs complexity is N^3, the complexity of the scatter-matrix-based KRR is $\max\{J^3, NJ^2\}$. This represents a major saving in computational time. This shows that when N is huge, the learning complexity becomes very costly both for direct KRR. In contrast, the scatter-matrix based KRR has a complexity with a growth rate proportional to N. It allows a super-saving when N becomes enormously large. It effectively overcomes the curse of empirical degree.

The large-scale database of images plays important role in the quality of reconstructed images. For an input image, if we cannot find highly correlated images in the cloud, the scheme cannot output a satisfying quality reconstruction. Although in our experiment, we used a predefined reference data set, significant improvement is achieved compared with the unique prior. A refined data set with more similar content is expected to further improve the restoration performance.

5   Conclusions

In this paper we present a novel framework for image restoration by combining multiple prior models. An iterative procedure is adopted in which the reference data are used for evaluation and prediction in each step. Different prior models are assessed based on their performance on reference data dynamically and scatter-matrix-based KRR is adopted to collaborate the multi-prior models with liner computational complexity with the size of reference data set, which applies to the bid data situation. Our proposed method not only provides an effective way to collaborate multiple prior models, but also demonstrates the coupling relationship of the exiting prior models. It provides a metric for the further prior model design. Besides, the scatter-matrix-based KRR shows significant capability of solving large-scale image restoration while with relative low computation complexity.

Acknowledgement. This work was supported in part by the Major State Basic Research Development Program of China (973 Program 2015CB351804) and the National Natural Science Foundation of China under Grant No. 61272386, 61100096 and 61300111.

References

1. Bioucas-Dias, J., Figueiredo, M.: A new twIST: Two-step iterative shrinkage/thresholding algorithms for image restoration. IEEE Trans. Image Process. **16**, 2992–3004 (2007)
2. Dong, W., Zhang, L., Shi, G., Wu, X.: Image deblurring and super-resolution by adaptive sparse domain selection and adaptive regularization. IEEE Trans. Image Process. **20**, 1838–1857 (2011)
3. Mairal, J., Bach, F., Ponce, J., Sapiro, G.: Online learning for matrix factorization and sparse coding. J. Mach. Learn. Res. **11**, 19–60 (2010)
4. Donoho, D.L.: Compressed sensing. IEEE Trans. Inf. Theory **52**, 1289–1306 (2006)
5. Candès, E., Romberg, J., Tao, T.: Robust uncertainty principles: Exact signal reconstruction from highly incomplete frequency information. IEEE Trans. Inf. Theory **52**, 489–509 (2006)
6. Olshausen, B., Field, D.: Emergence of simple-cell receptive field properties by learning a sparse code for natural images. Nature **381**, 607–609 (1996)

7. Eckstein, J., Bertsekas, D.: On the douglas rachford splitting method and the proximal point algorithm for maximal monotone operators. Math. Program. **55**, 293–318 (1992)
8. Yin, W., Osher, S., Goldfarb, D., Darbo, J.: Bregman iterative algorithms for L1-minimization with applications to compressed sensing. SIAM J. Imag. Sci. **1**, 142–168 (2008)
9. Setzer, S.: Operator splittings, bregman methods and frame shrinkage in image processing. Int. J. Comput. Vis. **92**, 265–280 (2011)
10. Geman, D., Reynolds, G.: Constrained restoration and the recovery of discontinuitie. IEEE Trans. Pattern Anal. Mach. Intell. **14**, 367–383 (1992)
11. Mumford, D., Shah, J.: Optimal approximation by piecewise smooth functions and associated variational problems. Commun. Pure Appl. Math. **42**, 577–685 (1989)
12. Chan, R., Dong, Y., Hintermuller, M.: An efficient two-phase L1-TV method for restoring blurred images with impulse noise. IEEE Trans. Image Process. **19**, 1731–1739 (2010)
13. Efros, A.A., Leung, T.K.: Texture synthesis by non-parametric sampling. In: ICCV, vol. 2, pp. 1022–1038 (1999)
14. Buades, A., Coll, B., Morel, J.M.: Image enhancement by non-local reverse heat equation. CMLA Technical Report 22 (2006)
15. Zhang, J., Liu, S., Xiong, R., Ma, S., Zhao, D.: Improved total variation based image compressive sensing recovery by nonlocal regularizatio. In: IEEE International Symposium on Circuits and Systems, pp. 2836–2839 (2013)
16. Coifman, R.R., Lafon, S., Lee, A.B., Maggioni, M., Nadler, B., Warner, F., Zucker, S.W.: Geometric diffusions as a tool for harmonic analysis and structure definition of data: Diffusion maps. In: Proceedings of the National Academy of Sciences, vol. 102, pp. 7426–7431 (2005)
17. Gilboa, G., Osher, S.: Nonlocal operators with applications to image processing. CMLA Technical Report 23 (2007)
18. Jung, M., Bresson, X., Chan, T.F., Vese, L.A.: Nonlocal mumford-shah regularizers for color image restoration. IEEE Trans. Image Process. **20**, 1583–1598 (2011)
19. Kindermann, S., Osher, S., Jones, P.: Deblurring and denoising of images by nonlocal functionals. Multiscale Model. Simul. **4**, 1091–1115 (2005)
20. Zhang, X., Burger, M., Bresson, X., Osher, S.: Bregmanized nonlocal regularization for deconvolution and sparse reconstruction. SIAM J. Imag. Sci. **3**, 253–276 (2010)
21. Zhang, J., Xiong, R., Ma, S., Zhao, D.: High-quality image restoration from partial random samples in spatial domain. In: VCIP, pp. 1–4 (2011)
22. Ma, S., Yin, W., Zhang, Y., Chakraborty, A.: An efficient algorithm for compressed mr imaging using total variation and wavelets. In: CVPR, pp. 1–8 (2008)
23. Chen, C., Huang, J.: Compressive sensing mri with wavelet tree sparsity. In: NIPS, pp. 1124–1132 (2012)
24. Woodbury, M.A.: Inverting Modified Matrices. Princeton University, Princeton (1950)
25. Dabov, K., Foi, A., Katkovnik, V., Egiazarian, K.: Image denoising by sparse 3-d transform-domain collaborative filtering. IEEE Trans. Image Process. **16**, 2080–2095 (2007)
26. Roth, S., Black, M.J.: Fields of experts: A framework for learning image priors. In: IEEE Computer Society Conference on Computer Vision and Pattern Recognition, CVPR 2005, vol. 2, pp. 860–867. IEEE (2005)
27. Aharon, M., Elad, M., Bruckstein, A.: K-svd: An algorithm for designing overcomplete dictionaries for sparse representation. IEEE Trans. Sig. Process. **54**, 4311–4322 (2006)

28. Portilla, J., Strela, V., Wainwright, M.J., Simoncelli, E.P.: Image denoising using scale mixtures of gaussians in the wavelet domain. IEEE Trans. Image Process. **12**, 1338–1351 (2003)
29. Jegou, H., Douze, M., Schmid, C.: Inria holidays dataset (2008)

Modeling the Temporality of Saliency

Ye Luo[1], Loong-Fah Cheong[1]([✉]), and John-John Cabibihan[2]

[1] Department of Electrical and Computer Engineering,
National University of Singapore, Singapore, Singapore
eleclf@nus.edu.sg
[2] Mechanical and Industrial Engineering Department,
Qatar University, Doha, Qatar

Abstract. Dynamic cues have until recently been usually considered as a simple extension of the static saliency, usually in the form of optic flow between two frames. The evolution of stimuli over a period longer than two frames has been largely ignored in saliency research. We argue that considering temporal evolution of trajectory even for a relatively short period can significantly extend the kind of meaningful regions that can be extracted from videos, without resorting to higher-level processes. Our work is a systematic and principled investigation of the temporal aspect of saliency under a dynamic setting. Departing from the majority of works where the dynamic cue is considered as an extension of the static saliency, our work places central importance on temporality. We formulate both intra- and inter-trajectory saliency to measure relationships within and between trajectories respectively. Our inter-trajectory saliency formulation also represents the first attempt among computational saliency works to look beyond the immediate neighborhood in space and time, utilizing the perceptual organization rule of common fate (temporal synchrony) to make a group of trajectories stand out from the rest. At the technical level, our use of the superpixel trajectory representation captures the detailed dynamics of superpixels as they progress in time. This allows us to better measure changes such as sudden movement or onset compared to other representations. Experimental results show that our method achieves state-of-the-art performance both quantitatively and qualitatively.

1 Introduction

Salient objects capture attention by coming to the foreground in perception. The process is apparently a bottom-up effect that begins at early level in perception. Traditionally, something can only be salient if it is considered unpredictable within some local or global context. When the scene contains strong semantic objects such as faces, texts, or other socially salient contents [1,2], improved models have been proposed to better predict human fixations by integrating higher-level features such as face, horizon [3–6], etc. The most common approach is to add object-specific detectors but this has an unsatisfactory piecemeal quality given that there are thousands of object categories. Lately deep learning framework has been used to discover non-object-specific features [7].

© Springer International Publishing Switzerland 2015
D. Cremers et al. (Eds.): ACCV 2014, Part III, LNCS 9005, pp. 205–220, 2015.
DOI: 10.1007/978-3-319-16811-1_14

When we consider saliency in the context of every day dynamic activity (aka dynamic saliency or video saliency), the issues seem more complex but less well-explored. At the most basic level, reacting quickly to unexpected changes (something with strong temporal contrast) is clearly important. Beyond this most basic level of temporal stimuli, all animals are probably highly sensitive to the difference between animate and inanimate motions (agents vs non-agents), given the importance of this distinction to their survival. At an even higher level, they would also be sensitive to the intent of these moving agents or meaning of these actions, be it in the timeless drama played out between predators and preys, or in a social interaction setting for a social animal like us. Our eyes and brains have evolved in a dynamic visual world, so why should not vision be designed by evolution to exploit this rich source of information that reveals itself through time?

Despite their importance, motion cues have until recently been usually considered as an extension of the static saliency (usually in the form of optic flow between two frames). The evolution of stimuli over a period longer than two frames has been largely ignored in saliency research. Even if some newer datasets contain video clips, they mainly comprise of short video clips strung together by abrupt transitions (jump cuts), in order to avoid high-level influence. This precludes analyzing those attributes of motion cues mentioned in the preceding paragraph. We argue that considering temporal evolution of trajectory even for

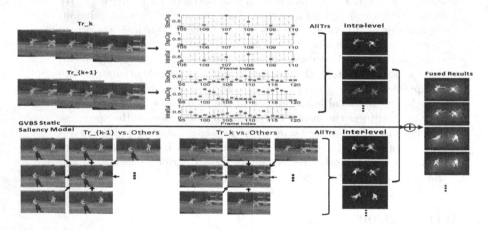

Fig. 1. Illustrations of the proposed video saliency estimation method. The upper part depicts saliency estimation at the intra-trajectory level (from left to right): the depiction of the thrust movement of the corresponding superpixels k and $k+1$ (in red), the intra-trajectory saliency profile of the two superpixels, with the peak indicating a thrust movement, and the intra-trajectory saliency maps of three of the frames, with brighter values indicating higher saliency. The lower part depicts saliency estimation at the inter-trajectory level (from left to right): the superpixel k-1 and k (in red) found to have strong correlations with 7 other superpixels depicted in different colors, and the inter-trajectory saliency maps of three of the frames. The middle line represents the static image saliency model, and the rightmost figure shows some overall video saliency results after fusion from all three levels. Best viewed in color (Color figure online).

a relatively short period can significantly extend the kind of meaningful regions that can be extracted from videos, without resorting to higher-level processes.

This is akin to the development of object-level attributes in image saliency works: one looks beyond the immediate spatial neighborhood of a pixel to compute mid-level visual cues such as convexity, surroundings, symmetry, etc. [8,9]. In the temporal domain, there exist similar perceptual organization cues such as common fate or temporal synchrony. Indeed, there is abundant psychophysical evidence that the brain can exploit these temporal structures so that certain features stand out as a group (for review, see [10]). In this paper, we propose a principled hierarchical framework that jointly utilizes low-level temporal and spatial cues to define a more comprehensive range of salient objects in videos.

At the most basic level of this hierarchy, we have the Harel and Koch's graph-based visual saliency model (GVBS) [1] with its static spatial features. In addition to this static level, we have two further levels to incorporate dynamic cues: the intra-trajectory and finally the inter-trajectory levels. We then propose a simple scheme to naturally integrate these various levels together. Figure 1 illustrates the ideas of our framework and some results are shown in the rightmost of the figure. In the following, we will briefly explicate the information extracted from the intra-trajectory and the inter-trajectory levels, and discuss the motivations behind some of our designs.

1.1   Intra-trajectory Level

There is much information residing in a single trajectory that is related to the distinction between agents and non-agents, and between entities capable of intentionality or not. Of cues that make the object's movements appear goal-directed include sudden direction and speed change, rational interactions with spatial contexts and other objects, apparent violations of Newtonian mechanics [11]. For this work, we wish to eschew the use of high-level semantics and non-visual cue such as gravity direction. Thus, we only adopt the "sudden direction and speed change" cue to model these intentionality attributes. In addition, we also model human's sensitivity to onset and offset (when a particular spatial region appears or disappears over time). Specifically, we look out for any sudden change in the size and the displacement of a superpixel. Referring to the upper part of Fig. 1, where the temporal evolution of the intra-trajectory saliency of the fencer's right hand has been depicted as a plot, it is clear that the right hand catches our attention when it makes the sudden cut and thrust movement.

1.2   Inter-trajectory Level

There are motions that might not be considered particularly meaningful individually, but when they exhibit temporal synchrony with other motions, they become salient. These well-synchronized movements might be between various body parts of the same person or even from different persons. At the coarsest level, they alert us to the presence of purposive behaviors and encode causality. At a more fine-grained level, it could signify something socially relevant and govern our interaction with others, or it could even be maneuvers perceived as threatening (either in real physical combats or in sports). To detect temporal correlation, we use mutual information between each pair of trajectories. Using fencing as an example again (Fig. 1, lower part), we can see that the pair of fencers are more salient than the judge (especially during the cut and thrust movement); our scheme captures the fact that we feel in the coordinated movements of the hands and the legs a sense of purpose (threatening in this case), and in the coordinated offense and defense movements a sense of cause and effect.

In sum, the main contribution of our work is a systematic and principled investigation of the temporal aspect of saliency under a dynamic setting. Departing from the majority of works where dynamic cue is considered as an extension of the static saliency, our work places central importance on temporality, as it is mainly through time that intentionality (clearly salient to us as social beings) is expressed. Being able to detect regions that carry meaningful actions has implications for the design of action recognition algorithms; one can use the dynamic saliency proposed here to drive the pooling step [12] as it has a more intrinsic relationship with the semantics of the actions. At the technical level, our use of the superpixel trajectory representation captures the detailed dynamics of superpixels as they progress in time. This allows us to better measure changes such as sudden movement compared to other representations such as video cube [13] or site entropy [14]. Our inter-trajectory saliency formulation also represents the first attempt among computational saliency works to look beyond the immediate neighborhood in space and time, utilizing the perceptual organization rule of common fate to make a group of trajectories stand out from the rest.

2   Related Work

Despite a spate of recent works on dynamic visual saliency (e.g. [14–19]), they do not depart from the various traditional notions used in image saliency works. These works are either based on extending center-surround saliency [13,18–21], and those with an information-theoretic slant [17,22]. The center-surround scheme with optic flow as one of the feature channels was first proposed by Itti in [20]. This basic idea has since been implemented in various different ways for video: the statistical likelihood of a voxel to its near surroundings [13], the error of reconstructing a patch from its spatial and temporal surrounding patches [21], and the contrast between the center and the surround regions [18,19]. Then there are those measures which are rooted in an information-theoretic interpretation of perception, such as the mutual information which is maximized to discriminate the salient and the non-salient classes [17], and saliency regarded as a kind of maximum information sampling [22,23].

While the first two levels proposed in our framework are similarly based on the notion of distinctiveness, our trajectory representation substantially deviates from the above approaches in terms of implementation and allows us to capture much more of the temporal structure. Various dynamic saliency works [18,19] utilize the motion between a pair of frames (e.g. optical flow) as one of the low-level features and compute the local distinctiveness of the flow in a spatial neighborhood. The flow's variation in time is ignored. Works such as [14,24] look at the feature evolution in time at a site (pixel or patch) or globally [23]. Unlike our trajectory representation, these measurements are rooted either at a site or global, and hence they do not track the motion characteristics of a specific point or region over a longer interval of time.

The most important difference with the aforementioned computational saliency works lies in the third level of saliency cue proposed in our framework. As far as we are aware, it is the first attempt to formulate saliency based on temporal synchrony, which is not rooted in the traditional concept of conspicuity or distinctiveness. Furthermore, by favoring those synchronous trajectories that exhibit goal-directedness, our work also represents the first attempt to encode movements that are likely to be socially salient in our interaction with other animate agents.

Our work is also related to the "objectness" works [25,26], especially those that also include saliency. Specifically, objectness can be viewed as a mid-level concept that should include classical perceptual grouping cues such as convexity, symmetry, etc. (besides the enclosedness cue used in [26]). Similarly, our work can be considered as a kind of perceptual grouping but based on temporal cues. Due to the different grouping cues used, our temporal grouping may yield different "objects" from those of spatial grouping. For instance, a group of objects interacting together will be regarded as temporally salient due to their synchrony. This could include a person and the object he or she holds, say, a handphone, even though the latter might not be salient in the spatial sense. Conversely, in a sport video with multiple people, the objectness approach might return all people as objects, even though not all are salient, whereas our approach will only return those with strong dynamic interaction. We argue that it is such dynamic saliency rather than objectness per se that is more appropriate in a dynamic video setting.

In a similar vein, video segmentation works [27–29] might appear related but their objective is quite different. They focus on dividing the video into motion layers, and in the simple case (e.g. planar scenes or rigid motions), such motion layers yield foreground objects and the background. However, even if this simple scenario holds, the distinction between objects and saliency as objective mentioned in the preceding paragraph still holds. Another important difference lies in that our work attempts to capture general temporal synchrony, not just the specific form of synchrony arising from rigid motions. Thus two persons shaking hands would be regarded as an ensemble exhibiting dynamic saliency due to the correlation in their movements. We also favor those movements that exhibit goal-directedness because they are socially salient; these aspects are what distinguish us from pure video segmentation works.

In the psychophysics community, alternative models of gaze allocation in complex dynamic scenes are emerging (for a review, see [30]). This is because conspicuity-based models are found to lack explanatory power in the context of dynamic vision under natural viewing. So far, such deviation of viewing behavior from the conspicuity-based theoretical models are primarily explained as coming from higher level factors, such as the influence of tasks [2,30]. While there might have been a few works that explore low-level dynamic cues such as flicker and motion contrast [30], on the whole, there has been a lack of systematic investigation of how various facets of low-level dynamic cues can be used to better account for how we distribute attention in a dynamic environment.

3   The Proposed Method

In this section, the details of the proposed framework for video saliency are introduced, with emphasis given to the dynamic part. For the static part, it suffices to note that given a video clip V with T frames, for the $t^{th}(t \in [1,T])$ frame, we obtain its image saliency map S_I^t by the well-known GVBS algorithm [1]. Since GVBS is pixel based, we take the average saliency value within a superpixel as the saliency value of the superpixel in S_I.

To better describe the long term motion cues, we first employ [31] to obtain the so-called temporal superpixels. We denote the ith superpixel trajectory as a sequence of superpixel locations:

$$Tr_i = \{(x_i^k, y_i^k, t_i^k), k = t_i^s \cdots t_i^e\}, \quad i = 1 \cdots n, \tag{1}$$

where (x_i^k, y_i^k, t_i^k) is the spatiotemporal position of the centroid of the ith superpixel R_i^k at frame k, t_i^s and t_i^e are the start and the end time indices of Tr_i, with $[t_i^s, t_i^e]$ being an interval inside $[1, T]$, and n is the number of detected trajectories in V. Based on this temporal superpixel representation, we can now proceed to estimate the intra-trajectory and the inter-trajectory components of the dynamic saliency.

3.1   Intra-trajectory Level

At this level, we want to first capture any significant change in the size of the superpixel, including outright appearance and disappearance, as a measurement of the onset/offset phenomenon. We also want to capture any sudden direction or speed change in the superpixel displacement. For the former, we describe the size change of a superpixel i between two consecutive frames k and $k - 1$ as $\Delta R_{sz}^k = abs\left(|R_i^k| - |R_i^{k-1}|\right)$, where $|R_i^k|$ is the cardinality of the superpixel R_i^k, and $abs()$ returns the absolute value. For the latter, we describe the displacement change as $\Delta R_{disp}^k = d\left(R_i^k, R_i^{k-1}\right)$, where $d()$ returns the Euclidean distance between the centroids of R_i^k and R_i^{k-1}. The intra-trajectory saliency for the ith trajectory at frame k (or equivalently, R_i^k) can then be estimated as follows, with both the ΔR_{sz}^k and ΔR_{disp}^k weighted equally with a suitable normalization:

$$S_{intra}(R_i^k) = \begin{cases} \frac{1}{2}\left(\frac{\Delta R_{sz}^k}{\Delta R_{sz}^{Max}} + \frac{\Delta R_{disp}^k}{\Delta R_{disp}^{Max}}\right) & t_i^s < k < t_i^e \\ 1 & k = t_i^s \text{ or } k = t_i^e. \end{cases} \tag{2}$$

Here ΔR_{sz}^{Max} and ΔR_{disp}^{Max} are the maximum size and displacement change over all the trajectories in the current video clip V. The second condition represents the instant when the ith superpixel appears or disappears (onset and offset respectively), during which we give maximum intra-saliency. Note that we do not want to consider the appearance and disappearance of superpixels at the image boundary as salient in that it is simply an artificial onset/offset caused by the image boundary. Furthermore, sudden change in speed or direction is also difficult to ascertain at the image boundary. Thus, in addition to the above, we also remove all those trajectories currently lying close to the image boundaries from consideration. Saliency estimation results at the intra-trajectory level for a football video are shown in Fig. 2. As can been seen from Fig. 2, the superpixels with significant changes stand out from others and are estimated with large values in the intra-trejecory level saliency maps.

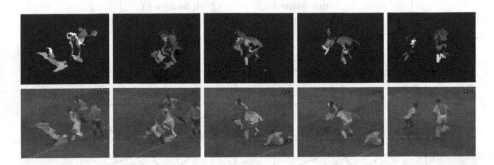

Fig. 2. Intra-trajectory saliency estimation for a football video. The intral-trajectory saliency maps and their corresponding heat maps are shown in the first and second rows, respectively. In the heat map, warm colors indicate large saliency values. Best viewed in color (Color figure online).

3.2   Inter-trajectory Level

Two trajectories $Tr_i = \{(x_i^k, y_i^k, t_i^k), k = t_i^s \cdots t_i^e\}$ and $Tr_j = \{(x_j^k, y_j^k, t_j^k), k = t_j^s \cdots t_j^e\}$ are potentially interesting to us if they are temporally synchronized. We use mutual information (MI) to measure the synchronization between these two trajectories over the time interval during which they overlap. We denote this overlapping time interval between Tr_i and Tr_j by $[t^s, t^e] = [t_i^s, t_i^e] \cap [t_j^s, t_j^e]$, assuming $[t^s, t^e] \neq \emptyset$. For simplicity, we use the Gaussian distribution to model the probability of motion vectors from a trajectory. That is $(v_x^i, v_y^i) \sim N(\mu_i, \Sigma_i)$, where $\mu_i = [\mu_x^i \quad \mu_y^i]^T$ and $\Sigma_i = C_{ii} = diag(\sigma_x^i, \sigma_y^i)$. Similarly, for Tr_j, we have another Gaussian $N(\mu_j, \Sigma_j)$, where $\mu_j = [\mu_x^j \quad \mu_y^j]^T$ and $\Sigma_j = C_{jj} = diag(\sigma_x^j, \sigma_y^j)$. The mutual information between Tr_i and Tr_j can then be estimated as [32]:

$$MI(Tr_i, Tr_j) = \begin{cases} \frac{1}{2} \log \frac{|C_{ii}| \cdot |C_{jj}|}{|C|} & Tr_j \notin \mathcal{N}(Tr_i) \text{ and } |\{t^s, \cdots, t^e\}| \geq 3 \\ 0 & \text{Otherwise} \end{cases}, \quad (3)$$

where $|.|$ is the determinant of a matrix, $C = \begin{bmatrix} C_{ii} & C_{ij} \\ C_{ji} & C_{jj} \end{bmatrix}$, and $C_{ij} = C_{ji}^T$ is the between-sets covariance matrix computed as $C_{ij} = \begin{bmatrix} cov(v_x^i, v_x^j) & cov(v_x^i, v_y^j) \\ cov(v_y^i, v_x^j) & cov(v_y^i, v_y^j) \end{bmatrix}$.

$\mathcal{N}(Tr_i)$ in the first condition is the spatial-temporal neighborhood of Tr_i used to enforce a mutual inhibition zone: the reason being that we should be allocating more attention only if the temporally synchronous trajectories are not originating from superpixels immediately adjacent to one another (immediately adjacent superpixels exhibiting synchrony would be less surprising). More specifically, $\mathcal{N}(Tr_i)$ is defined as all the trajectories which are spatially connected to Tr_i at some point in time. An example can be seen in Fig. 3, in which the spatial-temporal neighbors of Tr_5 originating from frames k and $k+1$ are illustrated, i.e.

$$\mathcal{N}(Tr_5) = \left\{ \cdots, \underbrace{Tr_1, Tr_2, Tr_3, Tr_6, Tr_7, Tr_8}_{\text{from frame } k}, \underbrace{Tr_9, Tr_{10}}_{\text{from frame } k+1}, \cdots \right\}. \text{ The condition}$$

$|\{t^s, \cdots, t^e\}| \geq 3$ aims to measure MI only for those trajectories which have temporal intersection of at least three frames.

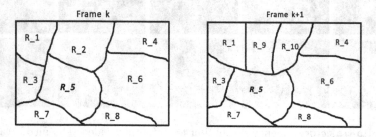

Fig. 3. The spatial-temporal neighbors of Tr_5 at frame k and frame $k+1$.

From the MI computed between all pairwise trajectories, a mutual informa-tion matrix $G \in R^{n \times n}$ with $G(i,j) = MI(Tr_i, Tr_j)$ can be obtained between all trajectories. The inter-trajectory saliency of Tr_i should then be the maximum MI values in row i of G. However, we also want to put into context the value of this MI. For instance, the temporal synchrony exhibited between two ballet dancers involved in complex *pas de deux* sequence should have higher value than that between two parallel linear trajectories. Thus we use the entropy of motion vectors from Tr_i itself to weigh the inter-trajectory level saliency as:

$$S_{inter}(Tr_i) = max_j (G(i,j)) \times H_i, \tag{4}$$

where $H_i = \sum_{k=t_i^s}^{t_i^e}(-p_k \log(p_k))$ is the entropy of motion vectors of Tr_i, and p_k, the probability of the motion vector at frame k, can be obtained from $N(\mu_i, \Sigma_i)$. This saliency value is defined at the level of trajectory; thus all superpixels on the trajectory Tr_i are assigned the same value. Figure 4 shows the inter-trajectory saliency results for a skiing video clip. As can be seen, the strong movement cor-relations among different parts of the skier make him stand out from the back-ground.

3.3   Fusion and Others

Thus far, we have obtained saliency values from all three levels, with the value of the static and intra-trajectory saliency already normalized to between $[0, 1]$

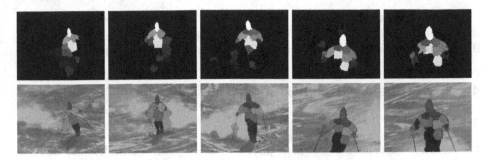

Fig. 4. Inter-trajectory saliency estimation for a skiing video. The inter-trajectory saliency maps and their corresponding heat maps are shown in the first and last rows, respectively. In the heat map, warm colors indicate large saliency values. Best viewed in color (Color figure online).

on a per image and per-video basis respectively. To recap, the maximum value used for normalization in the intra-trajectory level is sought over all values in a particular video. We now also normalize the inter-trajectory level saliency to $[0, 1]$ on a per video basis for the final fusion step. While there might be reasons to perform normalization over the entire video corpus, we stick to the aforementioned simple scheme, in keeping with the normalization practice for static saliency computation (whereby the normalization for each feature channel is usually done on a per-image basis, not over the entire image dataset).

Without any particular reason to favor the saliency values of one level over the other, we perform a simple weighted combination of the normalized saliency values of all three levels, with the weights equal to $\frac{1}{3}$:

$$SM(R_i^k) = \frac{1}{3} \left(S_I(R_i^k) + S_{intra}(R_i^k) + S_{inter}(R_i^k) \right). \tag{5}$$

where $SM(R_i^k)$ is the fused saliency map value indexed by the ith superpixel at the kth frame.

Several other points should be noted. Firstly, the background motion induced by camera movement could significantly affect both the intra- and the inter-trajectory saliency computation. Thus, we first estimate the background model with a simple homography model, using RANSAC to mark out the outliers (i.e. the objects of interest). The background motion is then removed before the intra- and the inter-trajectory saliency are computed.

Secondly, our work is meant to capture the salient aspects of trajectories over a relatively short period of time. Clearly, there must be some upper limit to the length of the video clips T, in accordance with human's short-term memory. In practice, we did not split our videos into shorter clips, as the datasets used in our experiments usually consist of video clips between 5 to 12 s, which we consider to be short enough. An exception is some of the long surveillance video clips. But even in the latter, objects do not appear in the videos for long duration (unless they are not moving, in which case their saliency would be attenuated by their high entropy).

Lastly, for simplicity, we did not consider the inhibition-of-return (IOR) mechanism in our model. In fact, under a dynamic setting, it is not even clear if there is a transient inhibition at attended locations for humans [30].

4   Experimental Results and Analysis

4.1   Datasets

We conduct experiments on three public datasets and one additional dataset compiled by us: respectively, UCF-Sports dataset [33], ASCMN [15], Ten-video dataset [34] and Interaction dataset. As the name implies, our own Interaction dataset contains video clips depicting human-human interaction, which has been not the primary focus of those currently available public datasets but is of interest to us.

1. UCF-Sports dataset consists of 150 video sequences of 10 different sports action classes. The averaged length of videos is between 5 to 12 s. Four subjects (2 males and 2 females) were asked to freely view videos and the eye tracker data recorded include the fixation points and the saccade movements.
2. ASCMN dataset contains 5 classes of videos: videos with abnormal motions, surveillance videos, videos with crowd motions, videos with moving camera and videos with sudden motions. Several participants were asked to freely view all the videos and the gaze points were recorded and then blurred by a low-pass Gaussian filter, the output of which serves as the ground truth. Due to the difficulties to extract trajectories from videos with crowd motions, videos except for ones with crowd motions are used on this dataset.
3. Ten-Video-Clips dataset contains 10 short video clips of 5 to 10 s each. Every video clip has the camera focused on one major object in the scene. The ground truths are taken to be the manually defined object masks.
4. Interaction dataset (to be released later) consists of 8 video clips with 2 fencing videos, 2 boxing videos, 1 ice dancing videos, 1 American football videos and 2 soccer videos. We manually define the ground truths in terms of object masks. While there might be multiple persons interacting in these clips, we choose a maximum of 3 objects for masking, governed by the accepted view that human short-term memory has a capacity of 3–4 items. This choice also helps to reduce the arbitrariness of the ground truth creation process, in that it is usually the pair of persons directly involved in the interaction (e.g. the forward and the immediate defender in a football video), and often a target object (e.g. the ball) that are selected.

4.2   Evaluation Metrics

Various measures can be used to evaluate a particular saliency model against some ground truth data. Each measure has its own strengths and drawbacks depending on the form of the ground truths [35,36].

For the UCF-Sport dataset and the ASCMN dataset where the ground truths are given in terms of the eye fixations, the Normalized Scanpath Saliency (NSS) [37], the Linear Correlation Coefficients (CC) [38] and the Area under the Receiver Operating Characteristics Curve (AUC-ROC) [39] are employed for evaluation. Readers are referred to the references for details of these measures, but basically NSS is the average of the response values obtained by using the fixation points to index into the estimated saliency map, and CC measures the linear correlation between the estimated saliency map and the Gaussian-smoothed fixation map. For both measures, larger values indicate better prediction of the saliency model. We adopt the implementations in [36] for all these three measurements.

For the Ten-Video-Clips dataset and our Interaction dataset, where human-labeled masks of the attended regions are provided, the ROC curve is more appropriate for comparison. The ROC curve is generated by plotting the true positive rate against the false positive rate for different values of threshold.

4.3   Results Comparison

We compare the performance of our proposed method with three state-of-the-art methods (Seo et al. [13], Rahtu et al. [18] and Guo et al. [40]) in the four video datasets mentioned above. We did not compare with [19] since the algorithm works only on videos without camera motions. Further experiments are also performed to analyse the different components of our proposed method. In our method, the number of temporal superpixels for the initial frame of each video is set as 100 — as a result, more than 500 trajectories can be extracted for a video. The threshold for the RANSAC algorithm is empirically set, its values ranging from 0.01 to 0.001 (pixel unit in the normalized coordinate), depending on the motion magnitudes of the video. We deem a trajectory as belonging to the background if the optical flows along the trajectory are grouped into the background for more than half of its duration. For other methods chosen for comparison, we use the codes released by the authors as well as their default parameter settings.

We first show the results of UCF-Sports dataset and ASCMN dataset in Fig. 5. As can be seen, our proposed method outperforms the other methods on all three metrics employed: NSS, CC and AUC-ROC. The estimated video saliency maps for one of the clips from UCF-Sports dataset are also provided in the top half of Fig. 9, from which it can be seen that our results are qualitatively closest to the human fixations among all methods. Both riders have been successfully detected by our method as salient objects due to their high correlation in movement, whereas all other methods primarily focus on the more conspicuous (static-feature-wise) rider on the left.

Next, we show in Fig. 6 the results of Ten-Video-Clips dataset and Interaction dataset, plotted in terms of the ROC curve (or the hit-miss curve) for different threshold values and matched against the manually specified ground truth information. Direct comparisons with the AUC values of all methods on the two databsets can been in Table 1. The estimated saliency maps for one of the clips in the Interaction dataset are also shown in the bottom half of Fig. 9. As can be

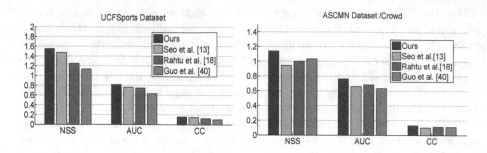

Fig. 5. Results on UCF-Sports dataset and ASCMN dataset respectively.

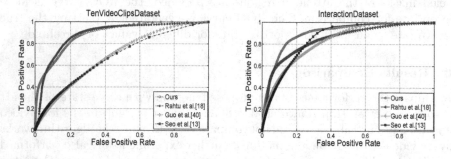

Fig. 6. Results on the Ten-Video-Clips dataset and the Interaction dataset respectively.

Table 1. AUC values comparisons on Ten-Video-Clips dataset and Interaction dataset.

AUC	Our Method	Rahtu et al. [18]	Guo et al. [40]	Seo et al. [13]
Ten-Video-Clips	0.8903	0.8861	0.6870	0.6768
Interaction	0.9007	0.8472	0.8284	0.8485

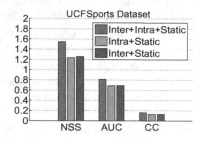

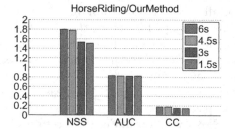

Fig. 7. Results of our method on UCF-Sports dataset at the individual levels, and those obtained from fusion of selected and all the components.

Fig. 8. Results for the proposed method on 12 *horse-riding* videos from UCF-Sports dataset at the individual time lengths.

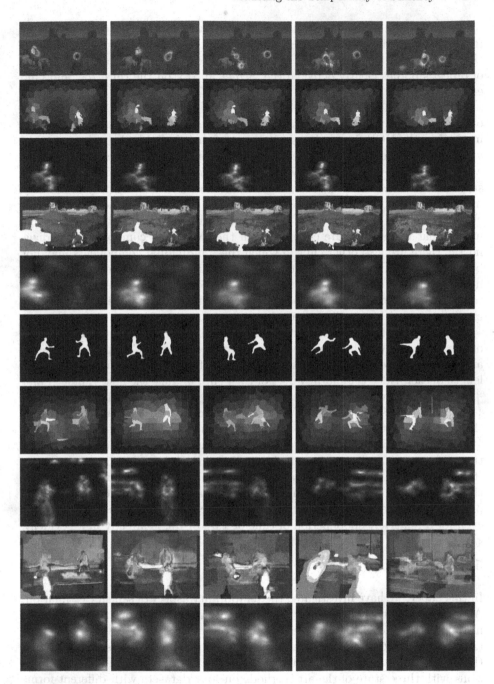

Fig. 9. A qualitative comparison of our method with four other video saliency estimation methods, using clips from the UCF sports dataset (top half) and the Interaction dataset (bottom half) respectively. For each half, from top to bottom: the original frames, ground truth (Gaussian-smooth eye fixations overlaid on the original frames for the top half and object masks for the bottom half), our results, results from Seo et al. [13], Rahtu et al. [18] and Guo et al. [40] respectively. In the heat map, warm colors indicate large saliency values.

seen, the strong movement correlations among two fencers make them stand out from the judge and others in background while the other methods either detect the judge (i.e. Rahtu et al. [18] on the fourth row) or do not have the shapes of object's bodies clearly detected (i.e. Seo et al. [13] on the third row and Guo et al. [40] on the fifth row).

The remaining experiments aim to shed light on the different components of our proposed method. First we show in Fig. 7 the performance of the proposed method on the UCF-Sports dataset in terms of their individual components, and various ways of combining these components. From the figure, it can be seen that when the intra- and the inter-level saliency are individually combined with the static saliency (i.e. intra + static, inter + static), they seem to only marginally improve the performance of the resulting algorithm. However, when all three levels are combined together, there is a substantial increase in performance. This means that while there are clips in which the individual components are diagnostic, there are also other clips in which these individual components may not be useful or even counter-productive (thus resulting in only a marginal improvement). However, the intra- and the inter-level seem to complement each other well so that when all three components are fused together, there is a significant improvement with regarding to all three metrics.

Last but not least, we analyse the effect of clip length on the performance of our method. We use the twelve *horse-riding* videos from UCF-Sports dataset as an example. For each video, the frame rate is 10 frames per second and the total length of each video is uniformly 6 s. For each clip, we take the first $\frac{1}{4}$, first $\frac{1}{2}$, first $\frac{3}{4}$ of the clip, as well as the full clip, resulting in four videos with the lengths of $\{1.5\,\text{s}, 3\,\text{s}, 4.5\,\text{s}, 6\,\text{s}\}$ respectively. We then run our algorithm on these videos and the average results over the 12 videos for each time duration are shown in Fig. 8.

From Fig. 8, it can be noted that longer time durations generally improves the performance, at least up to maximum time length tested in this experiment. It is beyond the scope of this paper to determine if human can keep track of these temporal correlations for an indefinite amount of time, but it suffices for the purpose of this paper to note that the beneficial effect of temporal consideration, even for a relatively short period of time of 1.5 s or 3 s, is already quite evident.

5   Conclusion

In this paper, we have investigated the temporality aspect of saliency estimation. A principled method based on three levels of saliency has been proposed: the intra-trajectory level, the inter-trajectory level and the static level. Experimental results validate the concepts put forth in the paper, as well as characterizing the effects of time, and the contributions made by individual levels. Comparisons with three state-of-the-art methods on four datasets with different forms of ground truth demonstrate the superiority of the proposed method.

Acknowledgement. This work was partially supported by the Singapore PSF grant 1321202075 and the NUS AcRF grant R-263-000-A21-112.

References

1. Harel, J., Koch, C., Perona, P.: Graph-based visual saliency. In: NIPS, pp. 545–552 (2007)
2. Einhauser, W., Spain, M., Perona, P.: Objects predict fixations better than early saliency. J. Vis. **8**, 1–26 (2008)
3. Judd, T., Ehinger, K., Durand, F., Torralba, A.: Learning to predict where humans look. In: ICCV, pp. 2106–2113 (2009)
4. Cerf, M., Harel, J., Einhaeuser, W., Koch, C.: Predicting human gaze using low-level saliency combined with face detection. In: NIPS, pp. 241–248 (2008)
5. Zhao, Q., Koch, C.: Learning a saliency map using fixated locations in natural scenes. J. Vis. **11**, 1–15 (2011)
6. Cerf, M., Koch, C.: Faces and text attract gaze independent of the task: experimental data and computer model. J. Vis. **9**, 1–15 (2009)
7. Shen, C., Mingli, S., Zhao, Q.: Learning high-level concepts by training a deep network on eye fixations. In: Deep Learning and Unsupervised Feature Learning Workshop, in Conjunction with NIPS (2012)
8. Fowlkes, C.C., Martin, D.R., Malik, J.: Local figure-ground cues are valid for natural images. J. Vis. **7**, 1–9 (2007)
9. Xu, J., Jiang, M., Wang, S., Kankanhalli, M.S., Zhao, Q.: Predicting human gaze beyond pixels. J. Vis. **14**, 1–20 (2014)
10. Blake, R., Lee, S.H.: The role of temporal structure in human vision. Behav. Cogn. Neurosci. Rev. **4**, 21–42 (2005)
11. Gao, T., Scholl, B.: Chasing vs. stalking: Interrupting the perception of animacy. J. Exp. Psychol. **37**, 669–684 (2011)
12. Ballas, N., Yang, Y., Lan, Z.Z., Delezoide, B., Preteux, F., Hauptmann, A.: Space-time robust representation for action recognition. In: ICCV, pp. 2704–2711 (2013)
13. Seo, H.J.J., Milanfar, P.: Static and space-time visual saliency detection by self-resemblance. J. Vis. **9**, 1–27 (2009)
14. Wang, W., Wang, Y., Huang, Q., Gao, W.: Measuring visual saliency by site entropy rate. In: CVPR, pp. 2368–2375 (2010)
15. Riche, N., Mancas, M., Culibrk, D., Crnojevic, V., Gosselin, B., Dutoit, T.: Dynamic saliency models and human attention: a comparative study on videos. In: Lee, K.M., Matsushita, Y., Rehg, J.M., Hu, Z. (eds.) ACCV 2012, Part III. LNCS, vol. 7726, pp. 586–598. Springer, Heidelberg (2013)
16. Borji, A., Itti, L.: State-of-the-art in visual attention modeling. T-PAMI **35**, 185–207 (2013)
17. Mahadevan, V., Vasconcelos, N.: Spatiotemporal saliency in dynamic scenes. T-PAMI **32**, 171–177 (2010)
18. Rahtu, E., Kannala, J., Salo, M., Heikkilä, J.: Segmenting salient objects from images and videos. In: Daniilidis, K., Maragos, P., Paragios, N. (eds.) ECCV 2010, Part V. LNCS, vol. 6315, pp. 366–379. Springer, Heidelberg (2010)
19. Zhou, F., Kang, S.B., Cohen, M.F.: Time-mapping using space-time saliency. In: CVPR (2014)
20. Itti, L., Koch, C., Niebur, E.: A model of saliency-based visual attention for rapid scene analysis. T-PAMI **20**, 1254–1259 (1998)
21. Li, Y., Zhou, Y., Xu, L., Yang, X., Yang, J.: Incremental sparse saliency detection. In: ICIP, pp. 3093–3096 (2009)
22. Zhang, L., Tong, M.H., Cottrell, G.W.: SUNDAy: saliency using natural statistics for dynamic analysis of scenes. In: The Thirty-First Annual Cognitive Science Society Conference, pp. 1–6 (2009)

23. Hou, X., Zhang, L.: Dynamic visual attention: searching for coding length increments. In: NIPS, pp. 681–688 (2008)
24. Itti, L., Baldi, P.: A principled approach to detecting surprising events in video. In: CVPR, pp. 631–637 (2005)
25. Alexe, B., Deselaers, T., Ferrari, V.: Measuring the objectness of image windows. T-PAMI **34**, 2189–2202 (2012)
26. Bergh, M.V.D., Roig, G., Boix, X., Manen, S., Gool, L.V.: Online video seeds for temporal window objectness. In: ICCV, pp. 377–384 (2013)
27. Brox, T., Malik, J.: Object segmentation by long term analysis of point trajectories. In: Daniilidis, K., Maragos, P., Paragios, N. (eds.) ECCV 2010, Part V. LNCS, vol. 6315, pp. 282–295. Springer, Heidelberg (2010)
28. Ochs, P., Brox, T.: Object segmentation in video: a hierarchical variational approach for turning point trajectories into dense regions. In: ICCV, pp. 1583–1590 (2011)
29. Zhang, D., Javed, O., Shah, M.: Video object segmentation through spatially accurate and temporally dense extraction of primary object regions. In: CVPR, pp. 628–635 (2013)
30. Tatler, B.W., Hayhoe, M.M., Land, M.F., Ballard, D.H.: Eye guidance in natural vision: Reinterpreting salience. J. Vis. **11**, 1–23 (2011)
31. Chang, J., Wei, D., III, J.W.F.: A video representation using temporal superpixels. In: CVPR, pp. 2051–2058 (2013)
32. Borga, M.: Learning Multidimensional Signal Processing. Ph.D. thesis, Linköping University, Sweden, SE-581 83 Linköping, Sweden (1998)
33. Shapovalova, N., Raptis, M., Sigal, L., Mori, G.: Action is in the eye of the beholder: eye-gaze driven model for spatio-temporal action localization. In: NIPS, pp. 2409–2417 (2013)
34. Fukuchi, K., Miyazato, K., Kimura, A., Takagi, S., Yamato, J.: Saliency-based video segmentation with graph cuts and sequentially updated priors. In: Proceeding of International Conference on Multimedia and Expo (ICME), pp. 638–641 (2009)
35. Riche, N., Duvinage, M., Mancas, M., Gosselin, B., Dutoit, T.: Saliency and human fixations: state-of-the-art and study of comparison metrics. In: ICCV (2013)
36. Borji, A., Sihite, D.N., Itti, L.: Quantitative analysis of human-model agreement in visual saliency modeling: a comparative study. TIP **1**, 55–69 (2012)
37. Peters, R.J., Iyer, A., Itti, L., Koch, C.: Components of bottom-up gaze allocation in natural images. Vision. Res. **45**, 2397–2416 (2005)
38. Jost, T., Ouerhani, N., von Wartburg, R., Muri, R., Hugli, H.: Assessing the contribution of color in visual attention. CVIU **100**, 107–123 (2005)
39. Green, D.M., Swets, J.A.: Signal Detection Theory and Psychophysics. Wiley, New York (1966)
40. Guo, C., Zhang, L.: A novel multiresolution spatiotemporal saliency detection model and its applications in image and video compression. TIP **57**, 1856–1866 (2010)

Salient Object Detection Using Window Mask Transferring with Multi-layer Background Contrast

Quan Zhou[1]([⊠]), Shu Cai[1], Shaojun Zhu[2], and Baoyu Zheng[1]

[1] College of Telecommunication and Information Engineering,
Nanjing University of Posts and Telecommunications,
Nanjing, People's Republic of China
quan.zhou@njupt.edu.cn
[2] Department of Computer and Information Science,
University of Pennsylvania, Philadelphia, PA, USA

Abstract. In this paper, we present a novel framework to incorporate bottom-up features and top-down guidance to identify salient objects based on two ideas. The first one automatically encodes object location prior to predict visual saliency without the requirement of center-biased assumption, while the second one estimates image saliency using contrast with respect to background regions. The proposed framework consists of the following three basic steps: In the top-down process, we create a specific location saliency map (SLSM), which can be identified by a set of overlapping windows likely to cover salient objects. The binary segmentation masks of training windows are treated as high-level knowledge to be transferred to the test image windows, which may share visual similarity with training windows. In the bottom-up process, a multi-layer segmentation framework is employed, which is able to provide vast robust background candidate regions specified by SLSM. Then the background contrast saliency map (BCSM) is computed based on low-level image stimuli features. SLSM and BCSM are finally integrated to a pixel-accurate saliency map. Extensive experiments show that our approach achieves the state-of-the-art results over MSRA 1000 and SED datasets.

1 Introduction

The human visual system (HVS) has an outstanding ability to quickly detect the most interesting regions in a given scene. In last few decades, the highly effective attention mechanisms of HVS have been extensively studied by researchers in the fields of physiology, psychology, neural systems, image processing, and computer vision [1–8], The computational modeling of HVS enables various vision applications, e.g., object detection/recognition [9,10], image matching [2,11], image segmentation [12], and video tracking [13].

Visual saliency can be viewed from different perspectives. Top-down (supervised) and bottom-up (unsupervised) are two typical categories. The first category often describes the saliency by the visual knowledge constructed from the

© Springer International Publishing Switzerland 2015
D. Cremers et al. (Eds.): ACCV 2014, Part III, LNCS 9005, pp. 221–235, 2015.
DOI: 10.1007/978-3-319-16811-1_15

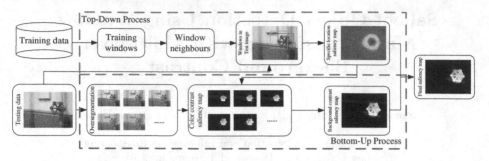

Fig. 1. Our approach consists of two components: (1) Top-down process. Given the training data consists of images with annotated binary segmentation masks, we first employ the technique of [9] to detect windows likely to contain salient objects on all training images and testing images. Then the binary segmentation masks of training windows are transferred to each detective windows in testing image with the most similar appearance (window neighbours). The transferred segmentation masks are used to derive the specific location saliency map (SLSM); (2) Bottom-up process. Using the over-segmentation technique of [25], an input testing image is first partitioned to multi-layer segmentation in a coarse to fine manner. Given the SLSM as prior map, a set of robust background regions are abstracted, and then the color-based contrast saliency maps are created for each layer of segmentation. These saliency maps are combined to form our background contrast saliency map (BCSM). SLSM and BCSM are finally integrated to a pixel-accurate saliency map. (Best viewed in color) (Colour figure online)

training process, and then uses such knowledge for saliency detection on the test images [14,15]. Based on the biological evidence that the human visual attention is often attracted to the image center [16], the center-biased assumption is often employed as the location prior for estimating visual saliency in top-down models [15,17].

While the salient regions are mostly located in the image center, the inverse might not necessarily be true [18,19]. Not all image center regions tend to be more salient. The salient object might be located far away from image center, even on the image boundary. Furthermore, a center-biased assumption always supposes that there is only one salient object within each image, yet it often fails when nature image contains two or more salient objects [19]. Thus, to detect salient regions without center-biased constrains, some semantic knowledge (e.g., face and pedestrian) are integrated in a top-down process, which is mostly based on object detectors [14,17,20]. The integration, however, acts rather more general on object category level than at the saliency-map level.

On the other hand, the bottom-up models are mainly motivated from the *contrast* formulation. For example, Itti *et al.* [1,21] proposed a set of pre-attentive features including local center-surround intensity, color and direction contrasts. These contrasts were then integrated to compute image saliency through the winner-take-all competition. Cheng *et al.* [22] and Achanta *et al.* [23] utilize the global contrast with respect to the entire scene to estimate visual saliency. Recently, Borji and Itti [24] combine local and global patch rarities as contrast to measure saliency for eye-fixation task. We argue that the contrast based on background regions also plays an important role in such processes.

In this paper, we propose a novel method to integrate bottom-up, lower-level features and top-down, higher-level priors for salient object detection. Our approach is fully automatic and requires no center-biased assumption. The key idea of our top-down process is inspired by [26], where the binary segmentation masks are treated as prior information to be transferred from the supervised training image set to the testing image set. Then, the transferred segmentation masks are used to derive specific location prior of salient object in the test image.

Figure 1 illustrates the overview of our method. The basic intuition is that the windows with similar visual appearance often share similar binary segmentation masks. Since these transferred windows exhibit less visual variability than the whole scenes and are often centered on the salient regions, they are much suitable for location transfer with better support regions. As a result, we utilize the method of [9] to extract candidate windows that are likely to contain salient objects, and then transfer training window segmentation masks that share visual similarity to windows in the test image. Afterwards, the bottom-up saliency map is computed based on low-level image stimuli features. In nature images, although the salient regions and backgrounds may also tend to be perceptually heterogeneous, the appearance cues (e.g., color and texture) of the salient object region are still quite different from the backgrounds. Therefore, different from the previous methods that mainly utilize the local central-surround contrast [1,15,24] and global contrast [22,23,27] to encode saliency, our framework estimates visual saliency using the appearance-based contrast with respect to the background candidate regions. In order to automatically abstract robust background regions, we employ the multi-layer segmentation framework, which is able to provide large amount of background candidates within different sizes and scales.

The contributions of our approach are three-fold:

(1) In the top-down process, it proposes a specific location prior for salient object detection. Through window mask transferring, our method is able to provide more accurate location prior to detect salient regions, which results in more accurate and reliable saliency maps than the models using center-biased assumptions, such as [16] and [17];

(2) In the bottom-up process, unlike the previous approaches that utilize the local and global contrast to predict visual saliency, we attempt to estimate visual saliency using the contrast with respect to the background regions;

(3) Compared with most competitive models [1,14,17,18,22,23,27–31], our method achieves the state-of-the-art results over MSRA 1000 and SED datasets.

2   Related Work

In this section, we focus on reviewing the existing work for salient object detection, which can be roughly classified into two categories: bottom-up and top-down models.

The bottom-up approaches select the unique or rare subsets in an image as the salient regions [1,28,32,33]. As a pioneer work, Itti *et al.* [1] introduced a biologically inspired saliency model based on the center-surround operation. Graph-based models [29,34] are suggested to predict saliency following the principle of Markov random walk theory. Some researchers attempt to detect irregularities as visual saliency in the frequency domain [23,27,35]. Bruce and Tsotsos [36] established a bottom-up model following the principle of maximizing information sampled from a scene. Sparsity models [17,37] are also employed to encode saliency, where the salient regions are identified as sparse noises when recovering the low-rank matrix.

Despite the success of these models, they are difficult to generalize to real-word scenes. Instead, some researchers attempt to incorporate the top-down priors for salient object detection [10,15,20]. Li *et al.* [38] and Ma *et al.* [39] formulate the top-down factors as high level semantic cues (e.g., faces and pedestrian). Alternatively, Navalpakkam and Itti [40] modeled the top-down gain optimization as maximizing the signal-to-noise ratio (SNR). Liu *et al.* [15] proposed to adopt a conditional random field (CRF) model for predicting visual saliency. Bayesian modeling is also used for combining sensory evidence with prior constrains. In these models, the prior knowledge (such as scene context [14] or gist descriptors [41]) and sensory evidence (such as target features [42]), are probabilistically combined according to Bayesian rule. Different from these methods, our method employs the specific location prior as top-down knowledge by transferring window segmentation masks.

3   Our Approach

In this section, we elaborate on the details of our method. We first introduce how to obtain the specific location saliency map (SLSM) by transferring window masks. Given the multi-layer segmentations and SLSM on hand, we select a series of background regions that are used to compute background contrast saliency map (BCSM). Finally, two maps are incorporated to generate pixel-wised saliency.

3.1   Specific Location Saliency Map (SLSM)

Finding Similar Windows. In order to utilize the prior knowledge of annotated binary segmentation mask in the training set, we first detect windows likely to contain an object using the "objectness" technique of [9]. It tends to return more windows covering an object with a well-defined boundary, rather than amorphous background elements. In our experiments, sampling only $\mathcal{N}$ windows per image (e.g., $\mathcal{N} = 100$) seems enough to cover most salient objects. Putting all the training windows together, we obtain the training window set $\{W_t\}$. This leads to retrieving much better neighborhood windows with similar appearance, whose segmentation masks are more suitable to transfer for test image. Given a

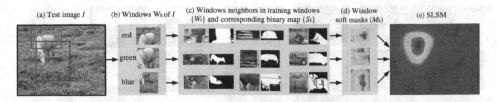

Fig. 2. An example of the full pipeline for producing SLSM. Given a test image I in (a), three top windows (denoted as red, green and blue rectangles) are highlighted out of $\mathcal{N}$ windows, as shown in (b). The window neighbors are displayed in (c). It is shown that green window is tightly centered on an object and gets very good neighbors, while for red and blue windows, the neighbors are good matches for transferring segmentation mask, even though these windows do not cover the "horse" perfectly. This results in an accurate transfer mask for each window of I, as illustrated in (d). On the rightmost column of (e), we integrate the soft mask M_k from all windows into a soft mask for the whole scene, which is used to derive the SLSM. Note blue color denotes low saliency, while red color represents high saliency (Best viewed in color)(Colour figure online)

new test image I as illustrated in Fig. 2(a), the $\mathcal{N}$ number of "objectness" windows are also extracted using [9] as well as for the training images. Figure 2(b) shows top three "objectness" windows in the test image I, and it is observed that many detective windows are centered on the salient object "horse". For one specific test window $W_k, k = \{1, 2, \cdots, \mathcal{N}\}$, we compute GIST feature [43] inside W_k to describe its appearance, and compare GIST descriptors with the ℓ^2-norm distance to all training windows $\{W_t\}$ to find window neighbors. Thus, the set $\{S_k^j\}, j = \{1, 2, \cdots, \mathcal{M}\}$ containing the segmentation masks of the top $\mathcal{M}$ training windows most similar to W_k is used for transferring. Figure 2(c) illustrates that the nearest neighbor windows accurately depict similar animals in similar poses, resulting in well-matched binary segmentation masks.

Segmentation Transfer. Let $S_T(x, y)$ be the SLSM, which defines the probability of pixel at location (x, y) to be salient. We construct $S_T(x, y)$ for each pixel from the segmentation masks transferred from all windows containing it.

(1) Soft masks for windows. For the kth test window W_k, we have a set of binary segmentation masks $\{S_k^j\}$ of neighbor windows from the training set. Here we compute a soft segmentation mask M_k for each W_k as the pixel-wise mean of the masks in $\{S_k^j\}$. To this end, all masks in $\{S_k^j\}$ are resized to the resolution of W_k. Let $\{S_k^{j'}\}$ be the resized masks, then the soft mask M_k for window W_k is defined as:

$$M_k = \frac{1}{\mathcal{M}} \sum_{j'=1}^{\mathcal{M}} S_k^{j'} \tag{1}$$

In this aligned space, a pixel value in M_k corresponds to the probability for it to be a salient object in $\{S_k^{j'}\}$. Figure 2(d) shows the corresponding M_k for the detected windows. Note the resolution of each soft window mask M_k is the same as the one of detected window in Fig. 2(b).

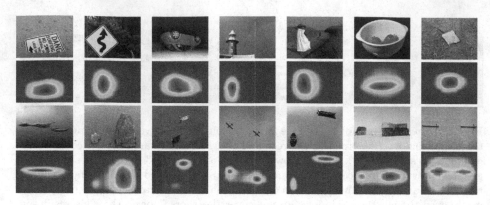

Fig. 3. Illustration of SLSM. The first and third rows are the example images form MSRA 1000 and SED dataset, respectively. The second and fourth rows are the corresponding SLSM, where blue color denotes low saliency, while red color represents high saliency. (Best viewed in color) (Colour figure online)

(2) Soft mask for the test image. After obtaining soft masks M_k, we integrate M_k for all windows into a single soft segmentation mask $M(x,y)$ for the test image I. For each window W_k, we place its soft mask M_k at the image location (x,y) defined by W_k. The soft mask $M(x,y)$ of the test image is the pixel-wise mean of all $\mathcal{N}$ placed masks $M_k(x,y)$:

$$M(x,y) = \frac{1}{\mathcal{N}} \sum_{k=1}^{\mathcal{N}} M_k(x,y) \tag{2}$$

A pixel value in $M(x,y)$ is the probability for it to be salient, according to all transferred segmentations (as illustrated in Fig. 2(d)). Therefore, we define the SLSM $S_T(x,y)$ as

$$S_T(x,y) = M(x,y) \tag{3}$$

Due to the integration of all soft segmentation masks $M_k(x,y)$ from the individual windows, our approach achieves even more robust results. The key step of our approach is that we extract many windows (e.g., 100 per image) overlapping salient object. One effect is that a certain window might not have good neighbors in the training set, leading to transferring an inaccurate or even completely incorrect mask $M_k(x,y)$. However, other overlapping windows will probably have good neighbors, diminishing the effect of the inaccurate $M_k(x,y)$ in the integration step. Another effect may happen when the transferred windows may not cover a salient object, (e.g., detecting a patch on the backgrounds, as the blue window shown in Fig. 1). This does not pose a problem to our approach, as the training images are decomposed in the same type of windows [9]. Therefore, a background window will probably also has similar appearance neighbors on backgrounds in the training images, resulting in correctly transferring a background binary segmentation mask. As a result, our approach is fully symmetric over salient and background windows. Figure 3 exhibits some SLSMs of nature images over MSRA 1000 and SED datasets.

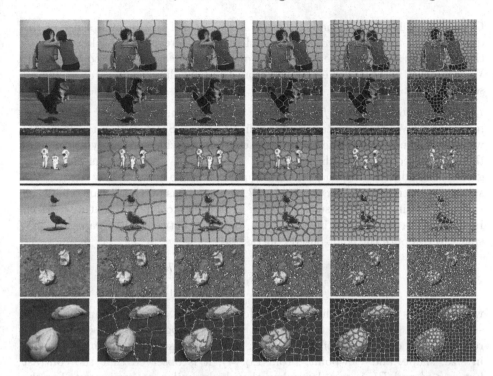

Fig. 4. Image representation by multi-layer segmentation. The upper panel shows the examples from MSRA dataset, while the bottom panel illustrates the examples from SED dataset. From left to right are the original images and their over-segmentation results in a coarse to fine manner. Different segments are separated by white boundaries.

3.2 Background Contrast Saliency Map (BCSM)

No matter where the salient object locates, it often exhibits quite different appearance cues (e.g., color and texture) within the entire scene. We thus build our background contrast saliency map (BCSM) guided by the global color-based contrast measurement [22]. Instead of computing saliency based on an entire image, here we calculate the contrast based on background candidates.

Multi-layer Segmentation. In order to make full use of background candidate regions, we employ the multi-layer segmentation framework.

Traditionally, an image is typically represented by a two-dimensional array of RGB pixels. With no prior knowledge of how to group these pixels, we can compute only local cues, such as pixel colors, intensities or responses to convolution with bank of filters [44,45]. Alternatively, we use the SLIC algorithm [25] to implement over-segmentation, since it performs more efficiently. In practice, we partition test image I into J layers of segmentations. There are two parameters to be tuned for this segmentation algorithm, namely (rgnSize, regularizer), which denote the number of segments used for over-segmentation and the trade-off appearance for spatial regularity, respectively. As shown in Fig. 4, the advantages of using this technique are that it can often group the homogeneous regions with similar appearance and preserve the true boundary of objects.

Computing BCSM. Denote $S_B(x, y)$ as the BCSM to convey a sense of the dissimilarity of a pixel based on its local feature with respect to backgrounds, so that $S_B(x, y)$ also gives the probability of pixel at location (x, y) to be salient. We construct $S_B(x, y)$ for each pixel from the multi-layer segmentation via all segments containing it.

(1) Color contrast saliency for each layer segmentation. Let r_i^j be i^{th} specific segment in j^{th} layer of segmentation. According to the SLSM, we select the segments with low saliency value to be background candidates, which are ready to compute the color-based contrast saliency. Let $\mathcal{B}^j = \{B_1^j, B_2^j, \cdots, B_M^j\}$ be selected background candidate regions in j^{th} layer segmentation. To measure how distinct the salient region is with respect to $B_m^j \in \mathcal{B}^j$, we can measure the distance between r_i^j and B_m^j using various visual cues such as intensity, color, and texture/texton. In this paper, we use the inverse cosine distance between histograms of HSV space to compute the color-based contrast:

$$C_{i,m}^j(\mathcal{H}(r_i^j), \mathcal{H}(B_m^j)) = 1 - \frac{\mathcal{H}(r_i^j)^T \mathcal{H}(B_m^j)}{||\mathcal{H}(r_i^j)|| \cdot ||\mathcal{H}(B_m^j)||} \qquad (4)$$

where $\mathcal{H}(\cdot)$ is the binned histogram calculated from all color channels of one segment, and $|| \cdot ||$ denotes the ℓ^2 norm. We use histograms because they are a robust global description of appearance. They are insensitive to small changes in size, shape, and viewpoint. From Eq. (4), it is observed that the contrast between r_i^j and B_m^j is very low when they look similar, otherwise not. For the given segment r_i^j, its color contrast saliency $S_B(r_i^j)$ is computed as the mean of L smallest contrasts in $\{C_{i,m}^j(\cdot, \cdot)\}, m = 1, 2, \cdots, M$

$$S_B(r_i^j) = \frac{1}{L} \sum_{m=1}^L C_{i,m}^j(\cdot, \cdot) \qquad (5)$$

As will be seen, when r_i^j is truly a salient region, the L smallest contrasts always get large value with respect to the background regions, resulting in high saliency for $S_B(r_i^j)$. The saliency map $S_B(r_i^j)$ is normalized to a fixed range $[0, 255]$, and $S_B(r_i^j)$ is assigned to each image pixel belonging to r_i^j with the saliency value as $S_B^j(x, y)$.

(2) BCSM for testing image. We now incorporate the $S_B^j(x, y)$ for all segmentation layers into a single saliency map for the test image I. Then the BCSM $S_B(x, y)$ is defined as:

$$S_B(x, y) = \frac{1}{J} \sum_{j=1}^J S_B^j(x, y) \qquad (6)$$

$S_B(x, y)$ is also normalized to a fixed range $[0, 255]$.

3.3   Combined Saliency

We integrate SLSM and BCSM to produce our final saliency map $S(x, y)$ with a linearly combination model

$$S(x, y) = \eta \cdot S_T(x, y) + (1 - \eta) \cdot S_B(x, y) \tag{7}$$

where η is the harmonic parameter to balance the top-down SLSM and bottom-up BCSM. Then $S(x, y)$ is normalized to a fixed range $[0, 255]$.

4 Experimental Results

To validate our proposed method, we carried out several experiments on two benchmark datasets using the Precision-Recall curve and F-measure described below. The main reason behind employing several datasets is that current datasets have different image and feature statistics, stimulus varieties, and center-biases. Hence, it is necessary to employ several datasets as models leverage different features that their distribution varies across datasets.

Datasets. We test our proposed model on two datasets: (1) Microsoft Research Asian (MSRA) 1000 dataset [23] is the most widely used and as baseline benchmark for evaluating salient object detection models. It contains 1000 images with resolution of approximate 400×300 or 300×400 pixels, which only have one salient object per image and provides accurate object-contour-based ground truth. (2) The SED [19] dataset is a smaller dataset only containing 100 images with resolution ranged from 300×196 to 225×300 pixels. The reason to employ this dataset lies in that it is not center-biased and there are two salient objects in each image. Therefore, this dataset is more challenging for the task of salient object detection.

Baselines. To show the advantages of our method, we selected 12 state-of-the-art models as baselines for comparison, which are spectral residual saliency (SR [27]), spatiotemporal cues (LC [31]), visual attention measure (IT [1]), graph-based saliency (GB [29]), frequency-tuned saliency (FT [23]), salient region detection (AC [30]), context-aware saliency (CA [14]), global-contrast saliency (HC and RC [22]), saliency filter (SF [28]), low rank matrix recovery (LR [17]), and geodesic saliency (SP [18]). In practice, we implemented all the 12 state-of-the-art models using a Dual Core 2.6 GHz machine with 4GB memory over two datasets to generate saliency maps.

Evaluation Metrics. In order to quantitatively evaluate the effectiveness of our method, we conducted experiments based on the following widely used criteria. The precision-recall curve (PRC) is used to evaluate the similarity between the predicted saliency maps and the ground truth. Precision corresponds to the percentage of salient pixels correctly assigned, while recall corresponds to the fraction of detected salient pixels in relation to the ground truth number of salient pixels. Another criterion to evaluate the overall performance is the F-measure [22,23], which is used to weight harmonic mean measurement of precision and recall. The F-measure is defined as

$$F_\beta = \frac{(1 + \beta^2) \times Precision \times Recall}{\beta^2 \times Precision + Recall} \tag{8}$$

where $\beta^2 = 0.3$ following [22,23].

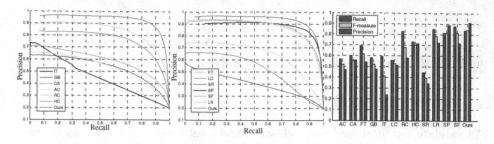

Fig. 5. Quantitative comparison for all algorithms with naive thresholding of saliency maps using 1000 publicly available benchmark images. Left and middle: PRC of our method compared with CA [14], AC [30], IT [1], LC [31], SR [27], GB [29], SF [28], LR [17], FT [23], SP [18], HC and RC [22]. Right: Average precision, recall and F-measure with adaptive-thresholding segmentation. Our method shows high precision, recall, and F_β values on the MSRA 1000 dataset. (Best viewed in color) (Colour figure online)

Implemented Details. In order to make our approach work well, it is important to establish a large and diverse training set, which is able to provide sufficient appearance statistics to distinguish salient regions and background. In our implementation, we employ the full PASCAL VOC 2006 [46] as our training dataset, since it includes more than 5000 images with accurate annotated object-contour-based ground truth.

The parameter settings are: $\mathcal{N} = 100$ for sampling windows per image, $\mathcal{M} = 100$ for window neighbors for one sampling window, $J = 5$ for segmentation layers in a coarse to fine manner, $L = 5$ for computing color contrast saliency involved in Eq. (5), (rgnSize, regularizer) are initialized as $\{25, 10\}$, and rgnSize is updated as $\{25, 50, 100, 200, 400\}$ with fixed regularizer, $\eta = 0.6$ to balance SLSM and BCSM for producing final saliency map.

We follow two widely used methodologies [17,23] to implement our experiments. In the first implementation, we adopt the scheme that segments image according to the saliency values with a fixed threshold. Given a threshold $T \in [0, 255]$, the regions whose saliency values are higher than threshold are marked as a salient object. The segmented image is then compared with the ground truth to obtain the precision and recall. We draw the PRC using a series of precision-recall pairs by varying T from 0 to 255.

In the second implementation, the test image is segmented by an adaptive threshold method [17]. Given the over-segmented image, an average saliency is calculated for each segment. Then an overall mean saliency value over the entire image is obtained as well. If the saliency in this segment is larger than twice of the overall mean saliency value, the segment is marked as foreground. Precision and recall values are sequentially calculated, and F-measure is finally computed for evaluation.

Overall Results. The average PRC and F-measure on MSRA 1000 dataset are illustrated in Fig. 5. It clearly shows that our method outperforms other approaches. It is interesting to note that the minimum recall value of our methods

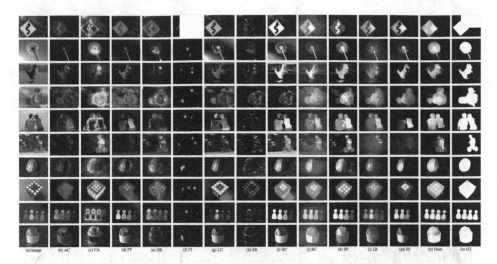

Fig. 6. Visual comparison of previous approaches with our method. See the legend of Fig. 5 for the references to all methods.

starts from 0.08, and the corresponding precision is higher than those of the other methods, probably because the saliency maps computed by our methods contain more pixels with the saliency value 255. The improvement of recall over other methods is more significant, which means our method are likely to detect more salient regions, while keeping a high accuracy.

We also evaluate our method on SED dataset and compare it with other 12 models. Figure 7(a) reports the comparison results in terms of F-measure. Our method achieves the state-of-the-art results and higher F-measure value (ours = 0.763) than other competitive models (SF = 0.739, LR = 0.68, RC = 0.62, and HC = 0.60), which clearly shows the validity of our approach in the case of more than one salient object within each image.

Visual comparison with different methods on MSRA 1000 dataset are shown in Fig. 6, and some qualitative results on SED dataset are displayed in Fig. 8. Compared with other models, our method is very effective in eliminating the cluttered backgrounds, and uniformly highlighted salient regions with well-defined object shapes, no matter whether salient objects locate in image center, or far away from image center, even on the image boundary.

Analysis of Implemental Efficiency. In order to evaluate the implemental efficiency of our method, we compare the average running time with some competitive models, and report the results in Table 1. Our method is slower than HC and FT, and faster than SR, IT, GB, SP, SF, RC, LR. The majority of this time is spent performing multi-layer segmentation, producing detected window, and computing window neighbours (about 80 %), and only 20 % account for the actual saliency computation.

Table 1. Average running time of different methods on MSRA 1000 dataset.

Method	SR [27]	IT [1]	GB [29]	FT [23]	SP [18]
Time(s)	0.064	0.611	1.614	0.016	1.213
Code	Matlab	Matlab	Matlab	C++	Matlab
Method	HC [22]	RC [22]	SF [28]	LR [17]	ours
Time(s)	0.019	0.253	0.153	1.748	0.759
Code	C++	C++	C++	Matlab	Matlab

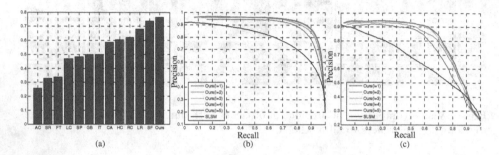

Fig. 7. Left: From left to right: (a) F-measure of the different saliency models to ground truth on SED dataset. (b) and (c) The comparison of PRC by gradually increasing the layers of segmentation on MSRA 1000 and SED dataset, respectively. In (b) and (c), the performance of individual SLSM is also included. (Best viewed in color) (Colour figure online)

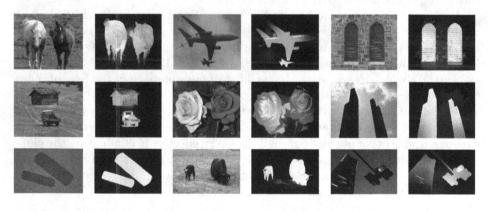

Fig. 8. Some visual examples on SED dataset. The first, third and fifth columns are original images, and the second, fourth and sixth columns are the corresponding saliency maps. (Best viewed in color) (Colour figure online)

Analysis of Parameter Setting and Individual Saliency Map. One factor affecting the performance is the layers of over-segmentation. Figure 7(b) and (c) exhibit the plot of PRC with different number of segmentation layers on the

MSRA 1000 and SED datasets, respectively. It is observed that better performance can be achieved along with the increasement of segmentation layers, and no further improvement after 5 layer segmentations. This demonstrates that our method performs robustly over a wide range of segmentation layers.

In order to evaluate the contributions of each individual saliency map, the PRC of SLSM is also included for comparison in Fig. 7(b) and (c). The performance of SLSM is already better than most of the competitive models, whose results are shown in Fig. 5. Using BCSM noticeably improves the performance for both two datasets, which indicates the importance of measuring visual saliency using contrast with respect to background regions.

5   Conclusion and Future Work

In this paper, we propose a novel framework for salient object detection based on two key ideas: (1) using specific location information as top-down prior by transferring segmentation masks from windows in the training images that are visually similar to windows in the test image; (2) using the contrast based on the background candidates in bottom-up process makes our method more robust than methods estimating contrast on the entire image. Compared with existing competitive models, the extensive experiments show that our approach achieves the state-of-the-art results over MSRA 1000 and SED datasets. In the future, we would like to combine two saliency maps, SLSM and BCSM, with adaptive weights using learning technique, as well as [47] does.

Acknowledgement. The authors would like to thank all the anonymous reviewers valuable comments. We would like to thank Prof. Liang Zhou for his valuable comments to improve the readability of the whole paper. This work was supported by NSFC 61201165, 61271240, 61401228, 61403350, PAPD and NY213067.

References

1. Itti, L., Koch, C., Niebur, E.: A model of saliency-based visual attention for rapid scene analysis. TPAMI **20**, 1254–1259 (1998)
2. Zhao, R., Ouyang, W., Wang, X.: Person re-identification by salience matching. In: ICCV, pp. 73–80 (2013)
3. Jiang, H., Wang, J., Yuan, Z., Wu, Y., Zheng, N., Li, S.: Salient object detection: a discriminative regional feature integration approach. In: CVPR, pp. 2083–2090 (2013)
4. Yan, Q., Xu, L., Shi, J., Jia, J.: Hierarchical saliency detection. In: CVPR, pp. 1155–1162 (2013)
5. Borji, A., Tavakoli, H.R., Sihite, D.N., Itti, L.: Analysis of scores, datasets, and models in visual saliency prediction. In: CVPR, pp. 921–928 (2013)
6. Li, X., Lu, H., Zhang, L., Ruan, X., Yang, M.H.: Saliency detection via dense and sparse reconstruction. In: ICCV (2013)
7. Yang, C., Zhang, L., Lu, H., Ruan, X., Yang, M.H.: Saliency detection via graph-based manifold ranking. In: CVPR, pp. 3166–3173 (2013)

8. Marchesotti, L., Cifarelli, C., Csurka, G.: A framework for visual saliency detection with applications to image thumbnailing. In: ICCV, pp. 2232–2239 (2009)
9. Alexe, B., Deselaers, T., Ferrari, V.: What is an object? In: CVPR, pp. 73–80 (2010)
10. Gao, D., Han, S., Vasconcelos, N.: Discriminant saliency, the detection of suspicious coincidences, and applications to visual recognition. TPAMI **31**, 989–1005 (2009)
11. Toshev, A., Shi, J., Daniilidis, K.: Image matching via saliency region correspondences. In: CVPR, pp. 1–8 (2007)
12. Jung, C., Kim, C.: A unified spectral-domain approach for saliency detection and its application to automatic object segmentation. TIP **21**, 1272–1283 (2012)
13. Mahadevan, V., Vasconcelos, N.: Saliency-based discriminant tracking. In: CVPR, pp.1007–1013 (2009)
14. Goferman, S., Zelnik-Manor, L., Tal, A.: Context-aware saliency detection. In: CVPR, pp. 2376–2383 (2010)
15. Liu, T., Yuan, Z., Sun, J., Wang, J., Zheng, N., Tang, X., Shum, H.: Learning to detect a salient object. TPAMI **33**, 353–367 (2011)
16. Tatler, B.: The central fixation bias in scene viewing: selecting an optimal viewing position independently of motor biases and image feature distributions. J. Vis. **7**, 1–17 (2007)
17. Shen, X., Wu, Y.: A unified approach to salient object detection via low rank matrix recovery. In: CVPR, pp. 853–860 (2012)
18. Wei, Y., Wen, F., Zhu, W., Sun, J.: Geodesic saliency using background priors. In: Fitzgibbon, A., Lazebnik, S., Perona, P., Sato, Y., Schmid, C. (eds.) ECCV 2012, Part III. LNCS, vol. 7574, pp. 29–42. Springer, Heidelberg (2012)
19. Borji, A., Sihite, D.N., Itti, L.: Salient object detection: a benchmark. In: Fitzgibbon, A., Lazebnik, S., Perona, P., Sato, Y., Schmid, C. (eds.) ECCV 2012, Part II. LNCS, vol. 7573, pp. 414–429. Springer, Heidelberg (2012)
20. Judd, T., Ehinger, K., Durand, F., Torralba, A.: Learning to predict where humans look. In: ICCV, pp. 2106–2113 (2009)
21. Itti, L., Koch, C.: A saliency-based search mechanism for overt and covert shifts of visual attention. Vis. Res. **40**, 1489–1506 (2000)
22. Cheng, M., Zhang, G., Mitra, N., Huang, X., Hu, S.: Global contrast based salient region detection. In: CVPR, pp. 409–416 (2011)
23. Achanta, R., Hemami, S., Estrada, F., Susstrunk, S.: Frequency-tuned salient region detection. In: CVPR, pp. 1597–1604 (2009)
24. Borji, A., Itti, L.: Exploiting local and global patch rarities for saliency detection. In: CVPR, pp. 478–485 (2012)
25. Achanta, R., Shaji, A., Smith, K., Lucchi, A., Fua, P., Süsstrunk, S.: Slic superpixels. EPEL. Technical report 149300 (2010)
26. Kuettel, D., Ferrari, V.: Figure-ground segmentation by transferring window masks. In: CVPR, pp. 558–565 (2012)
27. Hou, X., Zhang, L.: Saliency detection: a spectral residual approach. In: CVPR, pp. 1–8 (2007)
28. Perazzi, F., Krahenbuhl, P., Pritch, Y., Hornung, A.: Saliency filters: contrast based filtering for salient region detection. In: CVPR, pp. 733–740 (2012)
29. J., H., C., K., P., P.: Graph-based visual saliency, pp. 545–552. In: NIPS (2006)
30. Achanta, R., Estrada, F.J., Wils, P., Süsstrunk, S.: Salient region detection and segmentation. In: Gasteratos, A., Vincze, M., Tsotsos, J.K. (eds.) ICVS 2008. LNCS, vol. 5008, pp. 66–75. Springer, Heidelberg (2008)
31. Zhai, Y., Shah, M.: Visual attention detection in video sequences using spatiotemporal cues. In: ACMMM, pp. 815–824 (2006)

32. Parkhurst, D., Law, K., Niebur, E.: Modeling the role of salience in the allocation of overt visual attention. Vis. Res. **42**, 107–124 (2002)
33. Wang, W., Wang, Y., Huang, Q., Gao, W.: Measuring visual saliency by site entropy rate. In: CVPR, pp. 2368–2375 (2010)
34. Gopalakrishnan, V., Hu, Y., Rajan, D.: Random walks on graphs for salient object detection in images. TIP **19**, 3232–3242 (2010)
35. Guo, C., Ma, Q., Zhang, L.: Spatio-temporal saliency detection using phase spectrum of quaternion fourier transform. In: CVPR, pp. 1–8 (2008)
36. Bruce, N., Tsotsos, J.: Saliency based on information maximization. In: NIPS, pp. 155–162 (2006)
37. Lang, C., Liu, G., Yu, J., Yan, S.: Saliency detection by multi-task sparsity pursuit. TIP **21**, 1327–1338 (2012)
38. Li, J., Tian, Y., Huang, T., Gao, W.: Probabilistic multi-task learning for visual saliency estimation in video. IJCV **90**, 150–165 (2010)
39. Ma, Y.F., Hua, X.S., Lu, L., Zhang, H.J.: A generic framework of user attention model and its application in video summarization. TMM **7**, 907–919 (2005)
40. Navalpakkam, V., Itti, L.: Search goal tunes visual features optimally. Neuron **53**, 605–617 (2007)
41. Torralba, A., Oliva, A., Castelhano, M., Henderson, J.: Contextual guidance of eye movements and attention in real-world scenes: the role of global features in object search. Psychol. Rev. **113**, 766–786 (2006)
42. Zhang, L., Tong, M., Marks, T., Shan, H., Cottrell, G.: Sun: a bayesian framework for saliency using natural statistics. J. Vis. **8**, 1–20 (2008)
43. Oliva, A., Torralba, A.: Modeling the shape of the scene: a holistic representation of the spatial envelope. IJCV **42**, 145–175 (2001)
44. Comaniciu, D., Meer, P.: Mean shift: a robust approach toward feature space analysis. TPAMI **24**, 603–619 (2002)
45. Shi, J., Malik, J.: Normalized cuts and image segmentation. TPAMI **22**, 888–905 (2000)
46. Everingham, M., Zisserman, A., Williams, C.K.I., Van Gool, L.: The PASCAL visual object classes challenge (VOC2006) results 2006. (http://www.pascal-network.org/challenges/VOC/voc2006/results.pdf)
47. Itti, L., Koch, C.: Feature combination strategies for saliency-based visual attention systems. J. Electron. Imaging **10**, 161–169 (2001)

A Patch Aware Multiple Dictionary Framework for Demosaicing

Meiqing Zhang[✉] and Linmi Tao

Department of Computer Science and Technology, Tsinghua University,
Beijing, China
zhang-mq12@mails.tsinghua.edu.cn, ime.ting@hotmail.com

Abstract. Most digital cameras rely on demosaicing algorithms to restore true color images. Data captured by these cameras is reduced by two thirds because a Color Filter Array (CFA) allows only one particular channel go through at each pixel. This paper proposes a Patch Aware Multiple Dictionary (PAMD) framework for demosaicing. Instead of using a common dictionary, multiple dictionaries are trained for different classes of signals. These class-specific dictionaries comprise a super overcomplete dictionary. The most suitable dictionary would be adaptively selected based on the patch class, determined by the *Energy Exclusiveness Feature* (EEF) which measures the degree of energy domination in the representation code. In this way, candidate atoms are constrained in a set of atoms with low correlations; and meanwhile, the signal would have sparser representation over this adapted dictionary than over the common one, making the fixed sample rate relatively high and thus, accomplishing satisfying restoration according to the compressive sensing theory. Extensive experiments demonstrated that PAMD outperforms traditional Single Dictionary (SD) based approach as well as leading algorithms in diffusion-based family significantly, with respect to both PSNR and visual quality. Especially, the general artifact by Bayer CFA, Moiré Pattern, is dramatically reduced. Furthermore, on several images, it also significantly outperforms the state-of-the-art algorithms which are also sparse coding based but very complicated. PAMD is a general framework which can cooperate with existing demosaicing algorithms based on sparse coding.

1 Introduction

Demosaicing is a key technique in most digital cameras to recover true color images from data mosaiced by Color Filter Array (CFA) which allows only one channel go through at each pixel. Its great impact on numerous consumer cameras (especially on medium- and low-end devices such as mobiles) has drawn great attentions to demosaicing research in the past decade [1–6]. Numerous algorithms have been proposed for demosaicing. They can be roughly categorized as classical diffusion-based [7–9] or sparse coding based [1,10–12]. Diffusion-based approaches perform filling-in at pixel level by diffusing information from known

© Springer International Publishing Switzerland 2015
D. Cremers et al. (Eds.): ACCV 2014, Part III, LNCS 9005, pp. 236–251, 2015.
DOI: 10.1007/978-3-319-16811-1_16

regions to missing parts, typical examples include the widely used interpolation family algorithms such as OAP [4], refined ACPI [13] and kernel regression based interpolation [14].

Sparse coding based approaches treat the demosaicing problem from a different perspective. Prior knowledge is packed in dictionaries and under the assumption that signals of interests can be represented using a small number of atoms (i.e., sparsely representsable). Compressive sensing theory [15], on the other hand, provides solid theory foundations for accurate recovery of sparse signal from only a few observations [1,16]. Generally, the dictionary can be comprised with mathematically pre-defined bases (e.g., [1]) or learnt from training samples (e.g., [10,11]). One of the advantages of educated dictionary is that its knowledge is from domain-specific training samples thus can be particularly efficient [17]. This kind of approaches has achieved stat-of-the-art demosaicing results [1,10].

The success of sparse coding based approaches evidences that sparsity should be learned for specific signal. Guided by this philosophy, this paper proposes the Patch Aware Multiple Dictionary (PAMD) framework for demosaicing. In learning stage, patches are classified and a dictionary is trained for each class; then in demosaicing stage, the most suitable dictionary would be automatically selected according to the patch class. In this way, it makes the selected dictionary adaptive to the signal characteristic and improves the sparsity level of the representation code, as evidenced by our experiments. Consequently, better demosaicing performance is achieved.

PAMD allows multiple dictionaries, rather than one, to be trained from numerous samples, thus can pack more knowledge. These dictionaries comprise a super overcomplete dictionary; and meanwhile, candidate atoms for sparse coding are still constrained in a set where low correlation between atoms is ensured, which is a basic premise of most sparse coding algorithms. Our extensive experiments demonstrated that PAMD outperforms traditional Single Dictionary (SD) based approach as well as leading algorithms in diffusion-based family significantly, with respect to both PSNR and visual quality. Furthermore, on several images, it also significantly outperforms the state-of-the-art algorithms which are also sparse coding based but very complicated. Especially, the general artifact by Bayer CFA, Moiré Pattern, is dramatically reduced. PAMD is a general framework which can cooperate with current sparse coding based state-of-the-art algorithms.

2   Problem Formulation, Related Work and Contributions

2.1   Problem Formulation

Suppose that the initial color image X is mosaiced to be Y, as formulated in Eq. (1). M is a known matrix determined by the spatial layout of missing pixels (e.g., Bayer pattern).

$$Y = MX \tag{1}$$

Demosaicing aims to estimate $\hat{X}$ from Y. It is usually performed in vectorized patch space. Patch vector $\hat{x} \in R^{3n}$ is estimated based on the observation $y \in R^n$.

The core assumption used in estimating $x \in R^{3n}$ is that it has a sparse representation over a dictionary $D \in R^{3n \times L}$ ($L \geq 3n$), a sparse coding problem as formulated in Eq. (2) where $||s||_0$ is the ℓ^0 norm (i.e., the sparsity).

$$x \approx Ds \text{ subject to } ||s||_0 \ll L \tag{2}$$

Suppose that y can be written as $y = M_t x$, then combining Eq. (2) we have Eq. (3).

$$y = M_t x \approx M_t Ds, \quad subject \ to \ ||s||_0 \ll L \tag{3}$$

Sparse representation code $\hat{s}$ of y over the dictionary $M_t D$ can be first computed as shown in Eq. (4). Then $\hat{x}$ can be estimated as $D\hat{s}$.

$$\hat{s} = \arg\min ||s||_p \ subject \ to \ ||y - (M_t D)s||_2^2 < \xi \tag{4}$$

Equation (4) can be written in the regularized form as Eq. (5).

$$\hat{s} = \arg\min ||y - (M_t D)s||_2^2 + \lambda ||s||_p \tag{5}$$

Ideally, p in Eq. (4) should be taken as 0, the same as that in Eq. (3). However, directly minimizing the ℓ^0 norm is NP-hard. Alternatives include the Smoothed L0 algorithm (SL0) [18], which tries to directly minimize the ℓ^0 norm by using a continuous smooth function to approximate the discrete ℓ^0 norm; and greedy methods such as Orthogonal Matching Pursuit (OMP) [19]. Other classical alternative solutions are ℓ^1 norm based approaches such as L1 magic [20], feature-sign search [21] and LASSO [22].

Though efficient sparse coding algorithms are critical, the most fundamental ingredient is the basis set, i.e., the dictionary. For example, if the cosine distances between the signal and all of the bases are large, it would make most coefficients large and sparse representation is hardly possible.

Consequently, it is better to learn the dictionary D from samples than to use pre-defined mathematical bases [11,23], so that the signals of the specific class are sparse in the space spanned by these bases.

Generally, ℓ^0 regularization based applications (e.g., sparse classification) is more eager for a data-class-specific and educated dictionary than ℓ^1 and ℓ^2, because the number of its activated atoms is limited, the fitting error would be large if there are no bases which are cosine similar to the signal. Popular algorithms for obtaining an educated dictionary from training sample matrix include K-SVD [11], NMF [24] and Independent Component Analysis (ICA) [25,26].

Besides learning from samples, another method to improve the sparsity level is increasing the number of atoms, constructing an overcomplete dictionary ($L > 3n$). However, the fatal counterproductive effect is the increasing of correlations among atoms, which breaks the premise of most sparse coding algorithms.

PAMD tackles this problem by patch classification and training a dictionary for each class. Candidate atoms for sparse coding are still constrained in only one of the dictionaries thus low correlations are ensured. Meanwhile, in class-specific dictionary, it is more possible to fit the signal using only a small number of atoms, thus improving the sparsity level of the representation code.

2.2 Relation with Previous Work and Contributions

The leading demosaicing algorithms in diffusion based family include OAP [4], DL [12], LPA [27], CAD [3] and regularization based approach [28]. The *a priori* about natural images used in these approaches are usually based on pre-defined rules, rather than data driven. For example, the assumptions of channel smoothness [28] and local similarity [27]. A comprehensive survey can be found in [29].

Sparse coding and Compressive Sensing (CS) theory [15,30] provide a different perspective for demosaicing [1,10]. Sparse coding based approaches exploit the *a priori* that natural images are sparse after suitable transformation. Standard CS theory has shown that robust reconstruction of full signal s (or x) from y which contains only a few observations is possible, as long as the transformation and observation matrices satisfy certain conditions and the number of measurements m meets the criterion that

$$m > c||s||_0 log(L/||s||_0), \qquad (6)$$

where c is a small constant [16]. If the signal is not sparse enough in the transformed space, or the sample rate is too low, the sparse coding based demosaicing approaches would not yield satisfying results [1].

The sparsity assumption is found to be very efficient for demosaicing, and has achieved state-of-the-art results [1,10]. According to Eq. (6), because educated dictionary from samples can provide sparser representation than pre-defined mathematical bases, the fixed sample rate 1/3 would become relatively high, so satisfying restoration performance can be achieved.

The successes of current state-of-the-art algorithms [1,10] rely on various techniques. In [10], an online learning algorithm [31] is exploited to train a highly optimized dictionary from numerous samples (more than 2×10^7 patches); then another dictionary which packs the non-local similarity and group sparsity constraints is trained on-the-fly based on patches in the test image which are similar to the patch to be demosaiced. These two dictionaries are concatenated for restoring the patch. This approach provides a more overcomplete dictionary and meanwhile, imposes the non-local similarity constraints on the sparse coding, thus it would be very efficient for images which contain many similar patches. However, it will cause heavy computation overhead in testing stage.

In [1], adaptive patch sizes are used, rather than fixed. It is observed that small patch size is more suitable for singular area while large size for texture and smooth areas [1]. A high-pass filter is trained to filter each large patch, to detect whether it should be divided into small patches based on the energy of the filtered patch.

PAMD is much simpler than them and has low computation overhead in testing stage. No training is needed in testing. Based on the simple *Energy*

Exclusiveness Feature (EEF) and fast classification method, it trains a dictionary for each class using samples falling in the same class, and the mosaiced patch is restored using the dictionary corresponding to its class.

To reveal the relationship between our approach and previous work, we interpret [1,10] also from the perspective of PAMD. In [1,10], the concept of patch class only exists in testing stage. In [10], patches in the test image are clustered into many classes based on intensities, and a dictionary is trained using patches in each class. Multiple dictionary training while testing involves additional high computation load. Moreover, the amount of patches used in LSSC is very large, more than 2×10^7, significantly larger than the average number of about 4×10^4 for each dictionary in PAMD. In [1], adaptive patch size is initially introduced to reduce the artifacts. From the view of PAMD, in the test image, high-pass filtered patches having the energy above the threshold would be in one class while others below the threshold are in the other class.

To sum up, the main contributions of this paper can be outlined as below.

(a) The PAMD framework is proposed to furthermore refine the patch class in both training and testing stages, so that the representation coefficient vector would become sparser, making the fixed sample rate relatively higher and then yielding more satisfying restoration.
(b) The *Energy Exclusiveness Feature* (EEF) is proposed for patch classification. EEF is a scalar so simple that classification just involves bin location. PAMD has low computation overhead in testing.
(c) Extensive experiments showed that PAMD significantly improves the demosaicing performance over the single dictionary based approach on standard benchmark, with respect to both PSNR and visual quality. Especially, the general artifact by Bayer CFA, Moiré Pattern, is dramatically reduced. It also outperforms the leading algorithms in diffusion based algorithm family. Furthermore, though PAMD is very simple, its performance is comparable with the complicated state-of-the-art algorithms based on sparse coding, and even better than them on several images.

Moreover, PAMD can corporate with existing sparse coding based algorithms. Based on patch classification, they can be performed in each class. Sparser representation is a common advantage, PAMD is a general framework and can be potentially utilized in other fields of applications.

3 Patch Aware Multiple Dictionary Framework

3.1 Energy Exclusiveness Feature and Patch Classification

Energy Exclusiveness Feature (EEF) is a scalar f which measures the magnitude of a patch follows the power law phenomenon after the sparse transformation, i.e., a small number of sparse representation coefficients dominate most of the energy. Suppose that the coefficient vector of the patch over the dictionary is $s = (s_1, \cdots, s_L)^T$, and $(d_1, \cdots, d_L)$ is the index permutation so that $|s_{d_i}|^p \ (p > 0)$

is monotone non-increasing, and $\tau \in (0,1)$ is a threshold, then f is defined as Eq. (7).

$$f \triangleq k/L \ , k = \arg\min \frac{\sum_{i=1}^{k}|s|_{d_i}^{p}}{\sum_{i=1}^{L}|s|_{d_i}^{p}} \geq \tau \tag{7}$$

The parameter p exponentially magnifies (when $p > 1$) or shrinks ($p < 1$) the difference between coefficients. In our experiments, p is set as 2.0 and τ is taken as 0.7. It can be seen that $f \in [\frac{1}{L}, 1.0]$. Based on EEF, patch classification is very simple. By defining threshold intervals $[\zeta_0, \zeta_1), [\zeta_1, \zeta_2), \cdots, [\zeta_n, 1]$, the class of a patch is determined by the interval in which its EEF falls.

EEF measures the sparsity degree of a patch over the common dictionary. Higher sparsity (smaller f) is important for good reconstruction performance because it means lower minimum sample rate, then the fixed sample rate $1/3$ in the demosaicing application would become relatively higher. Our experiments found that a common dictionary is not optimal to provide sparse representation for various patches. Separately training a dictionary for each patch class using samples from the same class would improve the dictionary expression capability for patches in this class, yielding small f.

3.2   EEF Based Dictionary Learning and Demosaicing

In the learning stage, vectorized patch samples are concatenated, yielding a whole sample matrix which will be factorized to obtain the common dictionary D_{all}. All of the patch samples will be classified into one of r classes based on the EEF of the mosaiced patch over the $M_{rggb}D_{all}$. Here M_{rggb} means "RGGB" mosaic pattern for a patch. Samples in each class j will be used to train a corresponding dictionary D_j. Then $[D_1, \cdots, D_r]$ comprise a super overcomplete dictionary. In demosaicing stage, patch class J is determined by the EEF of the mosaiced patch y_t over $M_t D_{all}$. Then dictionary D_J is selected to restore y_t, which yields the final demosaiced patch $\hat{x}_t$. Patches are aggregated to a true color image by averaging overlapped pixels. Though atom correlations across $[D_1, \cdots, D_r]$ may be high, PAMD will *adapt* to the patch automatically by constraining candidate atoms within a low-correlated dictionary D_J.

The detailed demosaicing algorithm is interpreted as Algorithm 1. Because in training stage, all patches are mosaiced using M_{rggb}, however, at each step t in the demosaicing procedure, M_t for the corresponding patch may be not "RGGB" pattern[1]. Our solution is first restoring the whole image using D_{all}; secondly, the patch classification is based on the EEF of $M_{rggb}x$ over the dictionary $M_{rggb}D_{all}$, then we compute the code $\hat{s}$ of $M_t x$ over dictionary $M_t D_J$; finally, the patch is estimated as $\hat{x}_t = D_J \hat{s}_t^1$.

---

[1] In the setting of Bayer "RGGB" CFA, if the sliding-window moves forward by odd number pixel(s) at each step, then there would be 4 patterns for M_t as "RGGB", "GRBG", "GBRG", and "BGGR". However, if by even number pixels per step, there would be only one pattern as "RGGB", then in this case, we do not have to first restore the whole image using D_{all} in Algorithm 1.

Traditionally, averaging weights for a pixel in several sliding windows are the same as $w_t = 1$. However, we propose that the weights can be associated with the EEF f_t as Eq. (8).

$$w_t = (1/f_t)^\beta \tag{8}$$

It means that larger weights are given to restored pixels within windows in which patches can be more sparsely represented. The benefits of adaptive weighting policy would be presented and discussed in the experiment Sect. 4.3.

Algorithm 1. PAMD based Demosaicing

Input: D_{all}, D_j $(j = 1, \cdots, r)$, mosaiced image Y, mosaic matrix M (determined by Bayer CFA), EEF threshold intervals $[\zeta_{j-1}, \zeta_j)$
Output: Demosaiced image $\hat{X}$
1: Pre-restoration: Restore the whole image first using D_{all}
    ▷ `Patch classification is based on the EEF`
    of $M_{rggb}x$, `so this pre-restoration is necessary ONLY when the sliding`
    `window moves forward by odd number pixel(s) per step.`
2: **for** each patch y_t in Y **do**
3:     Compute corresponding EEF over $M_{rggb}D_{all}$ and classify this patch as class J
4:     Compute $\hat{s}_t$ of y_t over $M_t D_J$ by solving Eq. (4)
5:     Estimate the patch as $\hat{x}_t = D_J \hat{s}_t$
6: **end for**
7: Aggregate patches $\hat{x}_t$ to obtain $\hat{X}$
    ▷ `Overlapped pixels would be averaged with weights` w_t.

---

4   Experimental Results

4.1   Settings

Bayer CFA of "RGGB" pattern is used in our experiments, which determines M_{rggb}, M in Eq. (1) and M_t in Eq. (3). Specially, suppose that the patch is of size $2 \times 2 \times 3$ and vectorized to $x \in R^{12}$ in the order as $x = (R_1, R_2, R_3, R_4, G_1, G_2, G_3, G_4, B_1, B_2, B_3, B_4)^T$. Then the mask M_{rggb} is as Eq. (9) and $y = (R_1, G_2, G_3, B_4)^T$.

$$M_t = \begin{pmatrix} 1\,0\,0\,0\,0\,0\,0\,0\,0\,0\,0\,0 \\ 0\,0\,0\,0\,0\,1\,0\,0\,0\,0\,0\,0 \\ 0\,0\,0\,0\,0\,0\,1\,0\,0\,0\,0\,0 \\ 0\,0\,0\,0\,0\,0\,0\,0\,0\,0\,0\,1 \end{pmatrix} \tag{9}$$

In practice, Y and $M_t D$ are obtained by removing corresponding channels from X and rows from D respectively, instead of constructing the huge M.

Training patches of size $p \times q \times 3 = 10 \times 10 \times 3$ are randomly sampled from 122 natural images mainly from McGill Colour Image Database [32]. The average number of training patches for each class is about 4×10^4, a rather small number compared with that of more than 2×10^7 in complicated LSSC [10] whose dictionary training in testing stages causes additional computation overhead.

A common dictionary $D_{all} \in R^{300 \times 300}$ is factorized using FastICA algorithm [33], an efficient ICA implementation. Then the *energy exclusiveness feature* f is computed from the mosaiced patch over the dictionary $M_{rggb}D_{all} \in R^{100 \times 300}$. Patches are classified into 4 classes, corresponding f would fall into one of the four bins as $[0, 0.25)$, $[0.25, 0.45)$, $[0.45, 0.65)$ and $[0.65, +\infty)$. So, 4 dictionaries $D_j \in R^{300 \times 300} (j = 1, \cdots, 4)$ are learned, one for a class.

SL0 [18] is used as the sparse coding algorithm and the decrease factor σ is empirically chosen as 0.4 while the σ_{min} which determines the coding accuracy is set as 0.3. As for PAMD with adaptive averaging weight in Eq. (8), parameter β is set as 2.0. Similar with most existing works and for fair comparisons, a boarder of 15 pixels is excluded when calculating PSNR (dB). Test images are from Kodak PhotoCD benchmark [34] which includes 24 color images of 768×512 size. Source code (MatLab implementation) can be found at http://media.cs.tsinghua.edu.cn/~cvg/zhangmeiqing/PAMD.html.

4.2 Numerical Results and Visual Quality

The numerical comparisons on Kodak PhotoCD benchmark with respect to PSNR (dB) between our PAMD, Single Dictionary based approach (SD), CAD [3], DL [12] and LPA [27] are presented in Table 1. The images on which PAMD outperforms CD [1] and LSSC [10] can be found in Tables 2 and 3 respectively. In these tables, SD_1 stands for single dictionary with averaging weight $w_t = 1$ while SD_β means single dictionary with averaging weight $w_t = (1/f_t)^\beta, \beta = 2.0$. It is similar for $PAMD_1$ and $PAMD_\beta$.

Besides higher PSNR, results by PAMD also have better visual quality than those by SD and the state-of-the-art (e.g., LSSC), including significantly less Moiré Pattern (Figs. 2, 3 and 5) and sharper edges (Figs. 4 and 6).

4.3 Discussions

It can be seen that PAMD significantly outperforms single dictionary based approach with 0.46 dB PSNR improvement on average when $w_t = 1$, as shown in Table 1. Moreover, PAMD also outperforms the leading algorithms including CDM [35], RI [36], CAD [3], OAP [4], DL [12] and LPA [27] in non-sparse-coding family, on average with 2.94, 1.98, 1.41, 1.27, 0.52 and 0.08 dB PSNR improvement respectively when $\beta = 2.0$. On several images, PAMD also outperforms the complicated CD [1] and LSSC [10] with respect to both PSNR (Tables 2 and 3) and visual quality (Fig. 2). Especially, the general artifact by Bayer CFA, Moiré Pattern, is dramatically eliminated.

The success can be partly explained as that patch aware dictionary for each patch class can improve the sparsity level of the representation coefficient vector, i.e., yielding smaller EEF. This is evidenced in Fig. 1, which demonstrates that sparser coefficients are accomplished in PAMD framework. As aforementioned, sparser coefficient means that the minimum sample rate required by the compressive theory for good restoration would be lower, then the fixed sample rate 1/3 would become relatively higher. Another interesting finding is that the

M. Zhang and L. Tao

Table 1. Demosaicing results with respect to PSNR (dB). Test images are from the True Color Kodak Images dataset [34]. It can be seen that PAMD framework significantly improves the demosaicing performance over Single Dictionary (SD) based approach, leading algorithms including CDM [35], RI [36], CAD [3], OAP [4], DL [12] and LPA [27]. In this table, the subscript 1 in SD_1 and $PAMD_1$ means averaging weight $w_t = 1$ while β in SD_β and $PAMD_\beta$ means adaptive averaging weight $w_t = (1/f_t)^\beta$. Visual quality comparisons are presented in Figs. 2, 3, 4, 5, and 6. A 15-pixels boarder is excluded for all results.

Img	CDM [35]	RI [36]	CAD [3]	OAP [4]	DL [12]	LPA [27]	SD_1	SD_β	$PAMD_1$	$PAMD_\beta$	$PAMD_1 - SD_1$
01	34.38	35.50	34.91	37.94	38.46	39.45	40.74	40.49	**41.71**	41.69	0.97
02	39.76	39.56	41.14	39.50	40.89	41.36	40.51	40.21	41.39	**41.52**	0.88
03	41.79	41.14	43.36	41.47	42.66	**43.47**	41.52	41.18	42.36	42.17	0.84
04	39.59	40.12	**42.11**	40.00	40.49	40.84	40.70	40.54	40.99	41.18	0.29
05	35.69	36.66	35.57	37.47	38.07	37.51	37.44	37.30	37.91	**37.93**	0.47
06	35.70	38.39	37.72	38.74	40.19	40.92	40.67	40.56	**41.31**	41.29	0.64
07	41.45	41.92	42.11	41.81	42.35	**43.06**	42.01	41.79	42.59	42.62	0.58
08	32.49	34.18	35.12	35.43	35.58	37.13	37.11	36.96	37.43	**37.58**	0.32
09	40.45	41.26	41.14	41.85	43.05	**43.50**	42.13	41.95	42.89	42.93	0.76
10	40.82	41.69	41.14	42.13	42.54	**42.77**	42.29	42.19	42.59	42.58	0.30
11	36.84	38.11	38.59	39.32	40.01	40.51	40.19	40.13	**40.68**	40.64	0.49
12	40.94	42.21	42.11	42.66	43.45	44.01	43.76	43.54	44.34	**44.35**	0.58
13	0.62	31.96	32.95	34.45	34.75	36.08	36.54	36.50	**36.78**	36.75	0.24
14	36.13	36.36	**37.72**	35.70	36.91	36.86	35.45	35.20	36.20	36.51	0.75
15	38.45	38.84	40.35	39.28	39.82	40.09	39.75	39.64	40.27	**40.38**	0.52
16	38.95	42.18	42.11	42.07	43.75	44.02	44.12	43.92	**44.71**	44.66	0.59
17	38.88	40.10	39.68	41.39	41.68	**41.75**	41.37	41.39	41.42	41.35	0.05
18	34.82	35.64	36.67	37.53	37.64	37.59	37.64	37.64	**37.72**	37.69	0.08
19	37.43	39.13	39.10	40.00	41.01	**41.55**	41.18	41.06	41.26	41.47	0.08
20	39.32	39.99	40.35	40.70	41.24	41.48	40.90	40.71	41.38	**41.53**	0.48
21	35.83	37.23	37.72	38.82	39.10	39.61	40.15	40.01	40.65	**40.66**	0.50
22	37.02	37.42	**38.59**	37.67	38.37	38.44	37.77	37.73	38.01	38.06	0.24
23	42.17	41.95	43.36	41.88	43.22	**43.92**	42.31	42.01	42.73	42.75	0.42
24	33.24	34.17	35.34	34.88	**35.55**	35.44	34.87	34.89	34.93	34.83	0.06
Avg	37.61	38.57	39.12	39.28	40.03	40.47	40.05	39.90	40.51	**40.55**	0.46

Table 2. PSNR (dB) comparison with complicated CD [1].

Image	CD [1]	$PAMD_1$	$PAMD_\beta$
01	41.51	**41.71**	41.69
02	41.27	41.39	**41.52**
04	40.86	40.99	**41.18**
07	42.58	42.59	**42.62**
13	36.43	**36.78**	36.75
15	39.77	40.27	**40.38**

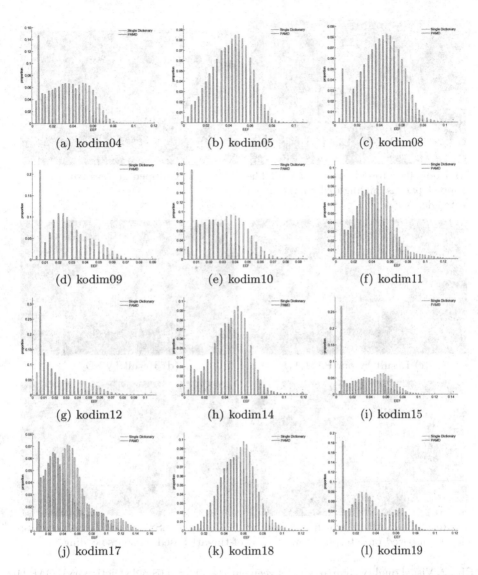

(a) kodim04 (b) kodim05 (c) kodim08

(d) kodim09 (e) kodim10 (f) kodim11

(g) kodim12 (h) kodim14 (i) kodim15

(j) kodim17 (k) kodim18 (l) kodim19

Fig. 1. Histograms of EEFs for patches in several test images. For each image, 96393 patches are used for building the histogram. The horizonal axis is the EEF f. The smaller f, the sparser the representation coefficient vector is. The vertical axis is the proportion (normalized, between 0 and 1) of patches whose EEFs fall in certain bin. The blue one is for Single Dictionary (SD) while the red one is for PAMD framework. Note that the red and blue histograms have the same total area (1.0). It can be seen that significantly sparser coefficients are accomplished in PAMD framework. Visually, the red area prevails in the left area (small f) while the blue area prevails in the right area (large f). It partly explains the success of PAMD (Colour figure online).

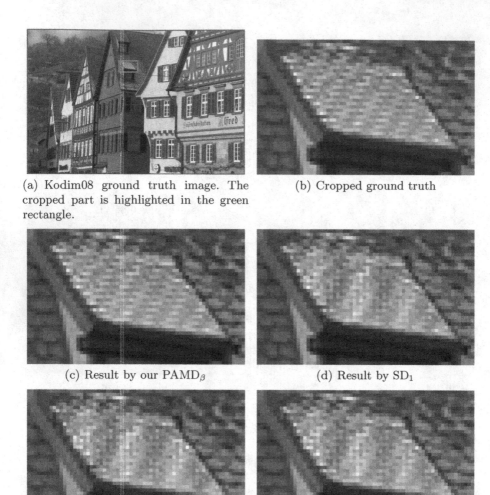

(a) Kodim08 ground truth image. The cropped part is highlighted in the green rectangle.

(b) Cropped ground truth

(c) Result by our PAMD$_\beta$

(d) Result by SD$_1$

(e) Result by OAP [4] which is a leading algorithm based on interpolation.

(f) Result by LSSC [10] which is the state-of-the-art based on sparse coding.

Fig. 2. Visual quality comparison between our PAMD, SD (Single Dictionary), OAP [4] and LSSC [10]. OAP is one of the leading algorithms in interpolation family. LSSC is the state-of-the-art and sparse coding based, which involves an online dictionary learning algorithm, more than 10^6 training patches, clustering, on-the-fly training from testing image patches, and group sparsity constrain techniques. LSSC is complicated and requires heavy computation overhead in demosaicing stage. PAMD is very simple and the average number of training samples for each class is only about 4×10^4, with low computation overhead in testing stage. It can be seen that by our PAMD framework, **the general artifact by Bayer CFA, Moiré Pattern, is dramatically eliminated.**

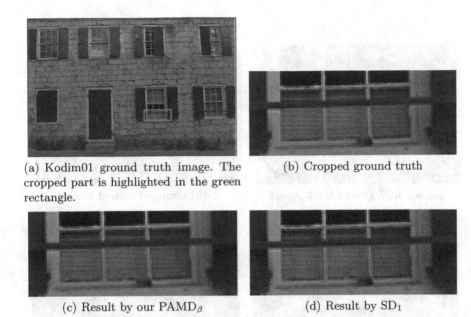

(a) Kodim01 ground truth image. The cropped part is highlighted in the green rectangle.

(b) Cropped ground truth

(c) Result by our PAMD$_\beta$

(d) Result by SD$_1$

Fig. 3. Visual quality comparison. PAMD greatly reduces **Moiré Pattern artifact**.

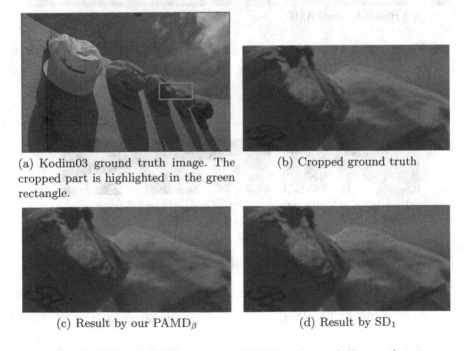

(a) Kodim03 ground truth image. The cropped part is highlighted in the green rectangle.

(b) Cropped ground truth

(c) Result by our PAMD$_\beta$

(d) Result by SD$_1$

Fig. 4. Visual quality comparison. PAMD achieves **sharper edges**.

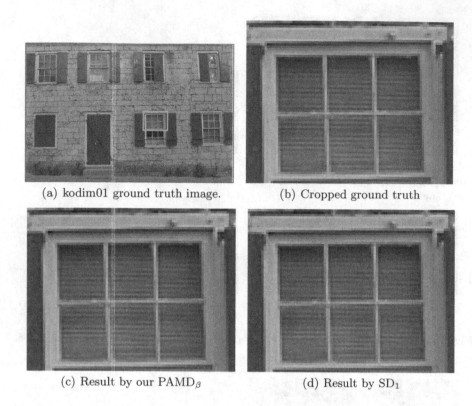

(a) kodim01 ground truth image.   (b) Cropped ground truth

(c) Result by our PAMD$_\beta$ (d) Result by SD$_1$

Fig. 5. Visual quality comparison. PAMD greatly reduces **Moiré Pattern artifact**.

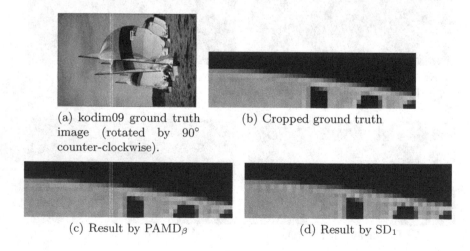

(a) kodim09 ground truth image (rotated by 90° counter-clockwise).   (b) Cropped ground truth

(c) Result by PAMD$_\beta$ (d) Result by SD$_1$

Fig. 6. Visual quality comparison. PAMD achieves **sharper edges**.

Table 3. PSNR (dB) comparison with complicated LSSC [10]. The number of training samples in PAMD for each class is about 4×10^4 while it is more than 2×10^7 for LSSC. Visual quality comparisons can be found in Fig. 2.

Image	LSSC [10]	$PAMD_1$	$PAMD_\beta$
01	41.36	**41.71**	41.69
08	37.57	37.43	**37.58**
13	36.35	**36.78**	36.75
21	40.65	40.65	**40.66**

adaptive weight $w_t = (1/f_t)^\beta$ accomplishes better result than that by $w_t = 1.0$ in PAMD framework while on the contrary in single dictionary framework.

Generally, sparse coding based approaches take longer time than interpolation based methods. Some interpolation based algorithms also take quite a long time such as approximately 1950 s per image (768×512) for CDM [35]. Currently, PAMD is implemented serially using MatLab without optimization nor parallel processing. When window steps are 10 pixels (even number, so no need for pre-restoration), PAMD only costs 8 s. When the step is 1 pixel, it achieves best restoration with about 700 s per image while SD with 500 s. Great speed-up can be accomplished by parallel processing.

5   Conclusion

A Patch Aware Multiple Dictionary (PAMD) framework for demosaicing is proposed to improve the sparsity level over dictionaries so that the fixed sample rate would become relatively high, yielding satisfying restoration. Based on the *Energy Exclusiveness Feature* (EEF), PAMD framework classifies patches in both training and testing stages. A dictionary would be trained for each class; and candidate atoms for sparse coding would be constrained within a class-specific dictionary so that low atom correlations are ensured. Multiple dictionaries pack more prior knowledge from a large number of training samples than single dictionary. As evidenced by our extensive experiments, class-specific dictionaries in PAMD framework significantly improve the sparsity level of patches and accomplish much better results than single dictionary based approach, with respect to both PSNR and visual quality. Especially, the general artifact by Bayer CFA, Moiré Pattern, is dramatically eliminated. PAMD also significantly outperforms many leading algorithms and outshines the complicated state-of-the-arts on several images. PAMD is very simple and can corporate with the existing state-of-the-arts. Particularly, based on patch classification, existing sparse coding based algorithms can be performed in each class. Moreover, sparser representation is an advantage for many sparse coding based applications to which PAMD is potentially able to be applied.

Acknowledgement. This work was supported in part by the National Natural Science Foundation of China under Grants 61272232 and MOST under Grants 2012AA011602.

References

1. Moghadam, A., Aghagolzadeh, M., Kumar, M., Radha, H.: Compressive framework for demosaicing of natural images. IEEE Trans. Image Process. **22**, 2356–2371 (2013)
2. Shao, L., Rehman, A.U.: Image demosaicing using content and colour-correlation analysis. Signal Process. **103**, 84–91 (2013)
3. Rehman, U.: A., Shao, L.: Classification-based de-mosaicing for digital cameras. Neurocomputing **83**, 222–228 (2012)
4. Lu, Y., Karzand, M., Vetterli, M.: Demosaicking by alternating projections: theory and fast one-step implementation. IEEE Trans. Image Process. **19**, 2085–2098 (2010)
5. Gunturk, B., Glotzbach, J., Altunbasak, Y., Schafer, R., Mersereau, R.: Demosaicking: color filter array interpolation. IEEE Signal Process. Mag. **22**, 44–54 (2005)
6. Gunturk, B., Altunbasak, Y., Mersereau, R.: Color plane interpolation using alternating projections. IEEE Trans. Image Process. **11**, 997–1013 (2002)
7. Menon, D., Calvagno, G.: Regularization approaches to demosaicking. IEEE Trans. Image Process. **18**, 2209–2220 (2009)
8. Ferradans, S., Bertalmío, M., Caselles, V.: Geometry-based demosaicking. IEEE Trans. Image Process. **18**, 665–670 (2009)
9. Malvar, H.S., He, L.w., Cutler, R.: High-quality linear interpolation for demosaicing of bayer-patterned color images. In: 2004. Proceedings IEEE International Conference on Acoustics, Speech, and Signal Processing (ICASSP 2004), vol. 3. IEEE (2004)
10. Mairal, J., Bach, F., Ponce, J., Sapiro, G., Zisserman, A.: Non-local sparse models for image restoration. In: IEEE 12th International Conference on Computer Vision, pp. 2272–2279 (2009)
11. Mairal, J., Elad, M., Sapiro, G.: Sparse representation for color image restoration. IEEE Trans. Image Process. **17**, 53–69 (2008)
12. Zhang, D., Wu, X.: Color demosaicking via directional linear minimum mean square-error estimation. IEEE Trans. Image Process. **14**, 2167–2178 (2005)
13. Chung, K.H., Chan, Y.H.: Color demosaicing using variance of color differences. IEEE Trans. Image Process. **15**, 2944–2955 (2006)
14. Tanaka, M., Okutomi, M.: Color Kernel regression for robust direct upsampling from raw data of general color filter array. In: Kimmel, R., Klette, R., Sugimoto, A. (eds.) ACCV 2010, Part III. LNCS, vol. 6494, pp. 290–301. Springer, Heidelberg (2011)
15. Candes, E., Romberg, J., Tao, T.: Robust uncertainty principles: exact signal reconstruction from highly incomplete frequency information. IEEE Trans. Inf. Theory **52**, 489–509 (2006)
16. Candes, E., Wakin, M.: An introduction to compressive sampling. IEEE Signal Process. Mag. **25**, 21–30 (2008)
17. Zhang, M., Tao, L.: Volume reconstruction for MRI. In: 2014 22nd International Conference on Pattern Recognition (ICPR), ICPR 2014, pp. 3351–3356. IEEE (2014)
18. Mohimani, H., Babaie-Zadeh, M., Jutten, C.: A fast approach for overcomplete sparse decomposition based on smoothed ℓ^0 norm. IEEE Trans. Signal Process. **57**, 289–301 (2009)

19. Tropp, J., Gilbert, A.: Signal recovery from random measurements via orthogonal matching pursuit. IEEE Trans. Inf. Theory **53**, 4655–4666 (2007)
20. Candes, E., Romberg, J.: l1-magic: Recovery of sparse signals via convex programming (2005). www.acm.caltech.edu/l1magic/downloads/l1magic.pdf
21. Lee, H., Battle, A., Raina, R., Ng, A.Y.: Efficient sparse coding algorithms. In: Schölkopf, B., Platt, J., Hoffman, T. (eds.) Advances in Neural Information Processing Systems, vol. 19, pp. 801–808. MIT Press, Cambridge (2007)
22. Tibshirani, R.: Regression shrinkage and selection via the lasso. J. Roy. Stat. Soc. Ser. B (Methodolog.) **58**, 267–288 (1996)
23. Aharon, M., Elad, M., Bruckstein, A.: k-svd: an algorithm for designing overcomplete dictionaries for sparse representation. IEEE Trans. Signal Process. **54**, 4311–4322 (2006)
24. Dhillon, I.S., Sra, S.: Generalized nonnegative matrix approximations with bregman divergences. In: Neural Information Processing Systems, pp. 283–290 (2005)
25. Bach, F.R., Jordan, M.I.: Kernel independent component analysis. J. Mach. Learn. Res. **3**, 1–48 (2003)
26. Filipovic, M., Kopriva, I., Cichocki, A.: Inpainting color images in learned dictionary. In: 2012 Proceedings of the 20th European Signal Processing Conference (EUSIPCO), pp. 66–70. IEEE (2012)
27. Paliy, D., Katkovnik, V., Bilcu, R., Alenius, S., Egiazarian, K.: Spatially adaptive color filter array interpolation for noiseless and noisy data. Int. J. Imaging Syst. Technol. **17**, 105–122 (2007)
28. Menon, D., Calvagno, G.: Regularization approaches to demosaicking. IEEE Trans. Image Process. **18**, 2209–2220 (2009)
29. Li, X., Gunturk, B., Zhang, L.: Image demosaicing: a systematic survey. In: Electronic Imaging 2008, International Society for Optics and Photonics, pp. 68221J–68221J (2008)
30. Donoho, D.L.: Compressed sensing. IEEE Trans. Inf. Theory **52**, 1289–1306 (2006)
31. Mairal, J., Bach, F., Ponce, J., Sapiro, G.: Online dictionary learning for sparse coding. In: ICML, p. 87 (2009)
32. Olmos, A., et al.: A biologically inspired algorithm for the recovery of shading and reflectance images. Perception **33**, 1463–1473 (2003)
33. Hyvärinen, A., Oja, E.: A fast fixed-point algorithm for independent component analysis. Neural Comput. **9**, 1483–1492 (1997)
34. Kodak: Kodak lossless true color image suite (2004). http://r0k.us/graphics/kodak
35. Zhang, L., Wu, X., Buades, A., Li, X.: Color demosaicking by local directional interpolation and nonlocal adaptive thresholding. J. Electron. Imaging **20**, 023016 (2011)
36. Kiku, D., Monno, Y., Tanaka, M., Okutomi, M.: Residual interpolation for color image demosaicking. In: IEEE International Conference on Image Processing, ICIP 2013, pp. 2304–2308, Melbourne, Australia, 15–18 September 2013

Large Margin Multi-metric Learning for Face and Kinship Verification in the Wild

Junlin Hu[1][✉], Jiwen Lu[2], Junsong Yuan[1], and Yap-Peng Tan[1]

[1] School of EEE, Nanyang Technological University, Singapore, Singapore
`JHU007@e.ntu.edu.sg`
[2] Advanced Digital Sciences Center, Singapore, Singapore

Abstract. Metric learning has been widely used in face and kinship verification and a number of such algorithms have been proposed over the past decade. However, most existing metric learning methods only learn one Mahalanobis distance metric from a single feature representation for each face image and cannot deal with multiple feature representations directly. In many face verification applications, we have access to extract multiple features for each face image to extract more complementary information, and it is desirable to learn distance metrics from these multiple features so that more discriminative information can be exploited than those learned from individual features. To achieve this, we propose a new large margin multi-metric learning (LM^{3}L) method for face and kinship verification in the wild. Our method jointly learns multiple distance metrics under which the correlations of different feature representations of each sample are maximized, and the distance of each positive is less than a low threshold and that of each negative pair is greater than a high threshold, simultaneously. Experimental results show that our method can achieve competitive results compared with the state-of-the-art methods.

1 Introduction

Metric learning techniques have been widely used in many visual analysis applications such as face recognition [5,9,21], image classification [28], human activity recognition [27], and kinship verification [17]. Over the past decade, a large number of metric learning algorithms have been proposed and some of them have been successfully applied to face and kinship verification [5,9,17,21]. In face image analysis, we usually have access to multiple feature representations for each face image and it is desirable to learn distance metrics from these multiple feature representations such that more discriminative information can be exploited than those learned from individual features. A possible solution is to concatenate different features together as a new feature vector and then apply existing metric learning algorithms directly on the concatenated vector. However, this concatenation is not physically meaningful because each feature has its own statistical characteristic, and such a concatenation ignores the diversity of multiple features and cannot effectively explore their complementary information.

© Springer International Publishing Switzerland 2015
D. Cremers et al. (Eds.): ACCV 2014, Part III, LNCS 9005, pp. 252–267, 2015.
DOI: 10.1007/978-3-319-16811-1_17

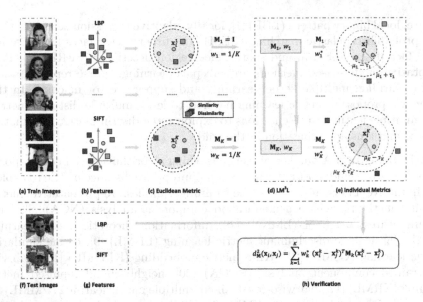

Fig. 1. Illustration of our large margin multi-metric learning method for face verification, which jointly learns multiple distance metrics, one for each feature descriptor, and collaboratively optimizes the objective function over different features. (a) A training face image set; (b) The extracted K different feature sets; (c) The distribution of these multiple feature representations in the Euclidean metric space; (d) Our LM^3L learning procedure; (e) The learned multiple distance metrics; (f) The test face image pair; (g) The extracted multiple feature descriptors of the test face pairs; (h) The overall distance by fusing the multiple distance metrics learned by our method.

In this paper, we propose a new large margin multi-metric learning (LM^3L) method for face and kinship verification in the wild. Instead of learning a distance metric with concatenated feature vectors, we jointly learn multiple distance metrics from multiple feature representations, where one metric is learned for each feature and the correlations of different feature representations of each sample are maximized, and the distance of each positive face pair is less than a smaller threshold and that of each negative pair is higher than a larger threshold, respectively. Experimental results on three widely used face datasets show that our method can obtain competitive results compared with the state-of-the-art methods. Figure 1 illustrates the working flow of our method.

2 Related Work

Face and Kinship Verification in the Wild: In recent years, many approaches have been proposed for face and kinship verification in the wild, and they can be mainly classified into two categories: feature-based [7,10,37,38] and model-based [17,18,33,34]. Feature-based methods represent each face image by using a hand-crafted or learned descriptor. State-of-the-art descriptors include Gabor feature, local binary pattern (LBP) [1], locally adaptive regression kernel (LARK) [23], probabilistic elastic matching (PEM) [15], fisher vector faces [25], discriminant face descriptor [14], and spatial face region descriptor (SFRD) [5]. Representative model-based methods are subspace learning, sparse representation, metric learning, multiple kernel learning, and support vector machine. In this paper, we propose a metric learning method to learn multiple distance metrics with multiple feature representations to exploit more discriminative information for face and kinship verification in the wild.

Metric Learning: A number of metric learning algorithms have been proposed in the literature, and most of them seek an appropriate distance metric to exploit discriminative information from the training samples. Representative metric learning methods include neighborhood component analysis (NCA) [8], large margin nearest neighbor (LMNN) [29], information theoretic metric learning (ITML) [6], logistic discriminant metric learning (LDML) [9], cosine similarity metric learning (CSML) [21], KISS metric embedding (KISSME) [13], pairwise constrained component analysis (PCCA) [20], neighborhood repulsed metric learning (NRML) [17], pairwise-constrained multiple metric learning (PMML) [5], and similarity metric learning (SML) [3]. While these methods have achieved encouraging performance in face and kinship verification, most of them learn a distance metric from single feature representation and cannot deal with multiple features directly. Different from these methods, we propose a multi-metric learning method by collaboratively learning multiple distance metrics, one for each feature, to better exploit more complementary information from multiple feature representations for face and kinship verification in the wild.

3   Proposed Method

Before detailing our method, we first list the notations used in this paper. Bold capital letters, e.g., $\mathbf{X}_1$, $\mathbf{X}_2$, represent matrices, and bold lower case letters, e.g., $\mathbf{x}_1$, $\mathbf{x}_2$, represent column vectors. Given a multi-feature data set with N training samples, i.e., $\mathbf{X} = \{\mathbf{X}_k \in \mathbb{R}^{d_k \times N}\}_{k=1}^K$, where $\mathbf{X}_k = [\mathbf{x}_1^k, \mathbf{x}_2^k, \cdots, \mathbf{x}_N^k]$ is the feature matrix extracted from the kth feature descriptor; $\mathbf{x}_i^k$ is the feature vector of the sample $\mathbf{x}_i$ in the kth feature space, $k = 1, 2, \cdots, K$; K is the total number of features; and d_k is feature dimension of $\mathbf{x}_i^k$.

3.1   Problem Formulation

Let $\mathbf{X}_k = [\mathbf{x}_1^k, \mathbf{x}_2^k, \cdots, \mathbf{x}_N^k]$ be a feature set from the kth feature representation, the squared Mahalanobis distance between a pair of samples $\mathbf{x}_i^k$ and $\mathbf{x}_j^k$ can be computed as:

$$d_{\mathbf{M}_k}^2(\mathbf{x}_i^k, \mathbf{x}_j^k) = (\mathbf{x}_i^k - \mathbf{x}_j^k)^T \mathbf{M}_k (\mathbf{x}_i^k - \mathbf{x}_j^k), \tag{1}$$

where $\mathbf{M}_k \in \mathbb{R}^{d_k \times d_k}$ is a positive definite matrix.

We seek a distance metric $\mathbf{M}_k$ such that the squared distance $d^2_{\mathbf{M}_k}(\mathbf{x}^k_i, \mathbf{x}^k_j)$ for a face pair $\mathbf{x}^k_i$ and $\mathbf{x}^k_j$ in the kth feature space should be smaller than a given threshold $\mu_k - \tau_k$ ($\mu_k > \tau_k > 0$) if two samples are from the same subject, and larger than a threshold $\mu_k + \tau_k$ if these two samples are from different subjects, which can be formulated as the following constraints:

$$y_{ij}\big(\mu_k - d^2_{\mathbf{M}_k}(\mathbf{x}^k_i, \mathbf{x}^k_j)\big) > \tau_k, \tag{2}$$

where $y_{ij} = 1$ if $\mathbf{x}^k_i$ and $\mathbf{x}^k_j$ are from the same person, otherwise $y_{ij} = -1$.

To learn $\mathbf{M}_k$, we define the constraints in Eq. (2) by a hinge loss function, and formulate the following objective function to learn the kth distance metric:

$$\min_{\mathbf{M}_k} I_k = \sum_{i,j} h\big(\tau_k - y_{ij}\big(\mu_k - d^2_{\mathbf{M}_k}(\mathbf{x}^k_i, \mathbf{x}^k_j)\big)\big), \tag{3}$$

where $h(x) = \max(x, 0)$ represents the hinge loss function.

Then, our large margin multi-metric learning (LM^{3}L) method aims to learn K distance metrics $\{\mathbf{M}_k \in \mathbb{R}^{d_k \times d_k}\}^K_{k=1}$ for a multi-feature dataset, such that

1. The discriminative information from each single feature can be exploited as much as possible;
2. The differences of different feature representations of each sample in the learned distance metrics are minimized, because different features of each sample share the same semantic label.

Since the difference computation of the sample $\mathbf{x}_i$ from the kth and ℓth ($1 \leq k, \ell \leq K$, $k \neq \ell$) feature representations relies on the distance metrics $\mathbf{M}_k$ and $\mathbf{M}_\ell$, which could be different in dimensions, it is infeasible to compute them directly. To address this, we use an alternative constrain to reflect the relationships of different feature representations. Since the difference of $\mathbf{x}^k_i$ and $\mathbf{x}^\ell_i$, and that of $\mathbf{x}^k_j$ and $\mathbf{x}^\ell_j$ are expected to be minimized as much as possible, the distance between $\mathbf{x}^k_i$ and $\mathbf{x}^k_j$, and that of $\mathbf{x}^\ell_i$ and $\mathbf{x}^\ell_j$ are also expected to be as small as possible. Hence, we formulate the following objective function to constrain the interactions of different distance metrics in our LM^{3}L method:

$$\min_{\mathbf{M}_1, \cdots, \mathbf{M}_K} J = \sum_{k=1}^K w_k\, I_k + \lambda \sum_{k,\ell=1, k<\ell}^K \sum_{i,j} \big(d_{\mathbf{M}_k}(\mathbf{x}^k_i, \mathbf{x}^k_j) - d_{\mathbf{M}_\ell}(\mathbf{x}^\ell_i, \mathbf{x}^\ell_j)\big)^2,$$

$$\text{s.t.} \quad \sum_{k=1}^K w_k = 1, \; w_k \geq 0, \; \lambda > 0, \tag{4}$$

where w_k is a nonnegative weighting parameter to reflect the importance of the kth feature in the whole objective function, and λ weights the pairwise difference of the distance between two samples $\mathbf{x}_i$ and $\mathbf{x}_j$ in the learned distance metrics $\mathbf{M}_k$ and $\mathbf{M}_\ell$. The physical meaning of Eq. (4) is that we aim to learn K distance metrics $\{\mathbf{M}_k\}^K_{k=1}$ under which the difference of feature representations of each pair of face samples is enforced to be as small as possible, which is consistent to the canonical correlation analysis-based multiple feature fusion approach [24].

Having obtained multiple distance metrics $\{\mathbf{M}_k\}_{k=1}^{K}$, the distance between two multi-feature data $\mathbf{x}_i$ and $\mathbf{x}_j$ can be computed as

$$d_{\mathbf{M}}^2(\mathbf{x}_i, \mathbf{x}_j) = \sum_{k=1}^{K} w_k (\mathbf{x}_i^k - \mathbf{x}_j^k)^T \mathbf{M}_k (\mathbf{x}_i^k - \mathbf{x}_j^k). \tag{5}$$

The trivial solution of Eq. (4) is $w_k = 1$, which corresponds to the minimum I_k over different feature representations, and $w_k = 0$ otherwise. This solution means that only one single feature that yields the best verification accuracy is selected, which does not satisfy our objective on exploring the complementary property of multi-feature data.

To address this shortcoming, we modify w_k to be w_k^p ($p > 1$), then the new objective function is rewritten as:

$$\min_{\mathbf{M}_1, \cdots, \mathbf{M}_K} J = \sum_{k=1}^{K} w_k^p I_k + \lambda \sum_{k,\ell=1, k<\ell} \sum_{i,j} \left(d_{\mathbf{M}_k}(\mathbf{x}_i^k, \mathbf{x}_j^k) - d_{\mathbf{M}_\ell}(\mathbf{x}_i^\ell, \mathbf{x}_j^\ell) \right)^2,$$

$$\text{s.t.} \quad \sum_{k=1}^{K} w_k = 1, \ w_k \ge 0, \ \lambda > 0. \tag{6}$$

3.2 Alternating Optimization

To our best knowledge, it is non-trivial to seek a global optimal solution to Eq. (6) because there are K metrics to be learned simultaneously. In this work, we employ an iterative method by using the alternating optimization method to obtain a local optimal solution. The alternating optimization learns $\mathbf{M}_k$ and w_k in an iterative manner. In our experiments, we randomly select the order of different features to start the optimization procedure and our tests show that the influence of this order is not critical to the final verification performance.

Fix $\mathbf{w} = [w_1, w_2, \cdots, w_K]$, **update** $\mathbf{M}_k$. With the fixed $\mathbf{w}$, we can cyclically optimize Eq. (6) over different features. We sequentially optimize $\mathbf{M}_k$ with the fixed $\mathbf{M}_1, \cdots, \mathbf{M}_{k-1}, \mathbf{M}_{k+1}, \cdots, \mathbf{M}_K$. Hence, Eq. (6) can be rewritten as:

$$\min_{\mathbf{M}_k} J = w_k^p I_k + \lambda \sum_{\ell=1, \ell \ne k} \sum_{i,j} \left(d_{\mathbf{M}_k}(\mathbf{x}_i^k, \mathbf{x}_j^k) - d_{\mathbf{M}_\ell}(\mathbf{x}_i^\ell, \mathbf{x}_j^\ell) \right)^2 + A_k, \tag{7}$$

where A_k is a constant term.

To learn metric $\mathbf{M}_k$, we employ a gradient-based scheme. After some algebraic simplification, we can obtain the gradient as:

$$\frac{\partial J}{\partial \mathbf{M}_k} = w_k^p \sum_{i,j} y_{ij} h'(z) \mathbf{C}_{ij}^k + \lambda \sum_{\ell=1, \ell \ne k}^{K} \sum_{i,j} \left(1 - \frac{d_{\mathbf{M}_\ell}(\mathbf{x}_i^\ell, \mathbf{x}_j^\ell)}{d_{\mathbf{M}_k}(\mathbf{x}_i^k, \mathbf{x}_j^k)} \right) \mathbf{C}_{ij}^k, \tag{8}$$

where $z = \tau_k - y_{ij} \left(\mu_k - d_{\mathbf{M}_k}^2(\mathbf{x}_i^k, \mathbf{x}_j^k) \right)$ and $\mathbf{C}_{ij}^k = (\mathbf{x}_i^k - \mathbf{x}_j^k)(\mathbf{x}_i^k - \mathbf{x}_j^k)^T$. The $\mathbf{C}_{ij}^k$ denotes the outer product of pairwise differences. $h'(x)$ is the derivative of $h(x)$, and we handle the non-differentiability of $h(x)$ at $x = 0$ by adopting a smooth hinge function as in [22,26]. In addition, we use some derivations given as:

$$\frac{\partial}{\partial \mathbf{M}_k} d_{\mathbf{M}_k}(\mathbf{x}_i^k, \mathbf{x}_j^k) = \frac{1}{2 \, d_{\mathbf{M}_k}(\mathbf{x}_i^k, \mathbf{x}_j^k)} \, \mathbf{C}_{ij}^k, \tag{9}$$

$$\frac{\partial}{\partial \mathbf{M}_k} \left(d_{\mathbf{M}_k}(\mathbf{x}_i^k, \mathbf{x}_j^k) - d_{\mathbf{M}_\ell}(\mathbf{x}_i^\ell, \mathbf{x}_j^\ell) \right)^2$$

$$= 2 \left(d_{\mathbf{M}_k}(\mathbf{x}_i^k, \mathbf{x}_j^k) - d_{\mathbf{M}_\ell}(\mathbf{x}_i^\ell, \mathbf{x}_j^\ell) \right) \frac{\partial}{\partial \mathbf{M}_k} d_{\mathbf{M}_k}(\mathbf{x}_i^k, \mathbf{x}_j^k)$$

$$= \left(1 - \frac{d_{\mathbf{M}_\ell}(\mathbf{x}_i^\ell, \mathbf{x}_j^\ell)}{d_{\mathbf{M}_k}(\mathbf{x}_i^k, \mathbf{x}_j^k)} \right) \mathbf{C}_{ij}^k. \tag{10}$$

Then, matrix $\mathbf{M}_k$ can be obtained by using a gradient descent algorithm:

$$\mathbf{M}_k = \mathbf{M}_k - \beta \, \frac{\partial J}{\partial \mathbf{M}_k}, \tag{11}$$

where β is the learning rate.

In practice, directly optimizing the Mahalanobis distance metric $\mathbf{M}_k$ may suffer slow convergence and overfitting problems if data is very high-dimensional and the number of training samples is insufficient. Therefore, we propose an alternative method to jointly perform dimensionality reduction and metric learning, which means a low-rank linear projection matrix $\mathbf{L}_k \in \mathbb{R}^{s_k \times d_k}$ $(s_k < d_k)$ is learned to project each sample $\mathbf{x}_i^k$ from the high-dimensional input space to a low-dimensional embedding space, where the distance metric $\mathbf{M}_k = \mathbf{L}_k^T \mathbf{L}_k$. Then, we differentiate the objective function J with respect to $\mathbf{L}_k$, and obtain the gradient as follows:

$$\frac{\partial J}{\partial \mathbf{L}_k} = 2\mathbf{L}_k \left[w_k^p \sum_{i,j} y_{ij} h'(z) \mathbf{C}_{ij}^k + \lambda \sum_{\ell=1, \ell \neq k}^{K} \sum_{i,j} \left(1 - \frac{d_{\mathbf{M}_\ell}(\mathbf{x}_i^\ell, \mathbf{x}_j^\ell)}{d_{\mathbf{M}_k}(\mathbf{x}_i^k, \mathbf{x}_j^k)} \right) \mathbf{C}_{ij}^k \right]. \tag{12}$$

Lastly, the matrix $\mathbf{L}_k$ can be obtained by using a gradient descent rule:

$$\mathbf{L}_k = \mathbf{L}_k - \beta \, \frac{\partial J}{\partial \mathbf{L}_k}. \tag{13}$$

Fix $\mathbf{M}_k$, $k = 1, 2, \cdots, K$, update w. Now, we update $\mathbf{w}$ with the fixed $\{\mathbf{M}_k\}_{k=1}^K$. We construct a Lagrange function as follows:

$$La(\mathbf{w}, \eta) = \sum_{k=1}^{K} w_k^p \, I_k + \lambda \sum_{k,\ell=1, k<\ell}^{K} \sum_{i,j} \left(d_{\mathbf{M}_k}(\mathbf{x}_i^k, \mathbf{x}_j^k) - d_{\mathbf{M}_\ell}(\mathbf{x}_i^\ell, \mathbf{x}_j^\ell) \right)^2$$

$$- \eta \left(\sum_{k=1}^{K} w_k - 1 \right). \tag{14}$$

Algorithm 1. LM^{3}L

Input: Training set $\{\mathbf{X}_k\}_{k=1}^K$ from K views; Learning rate β; Parameter p, λ,
    μ_k and τ_k; Total iterative number T; Convergence error ε.
Output: Multiple metrics: $\mathbf{M}_1, \mathbf{M}_2, \cdots, \mathbf{M}_K$; and weights: $w_1, w_2, \cdots, w_K$.
Step 1 (Initialization):
    Initialize $\mathbf{L}_k = \mathbf{E}^{s_k \times d_k}$,
    $w_k = 1/K$, $k = 1, \cdots, K$.
Step 2 (Alternating optimization):
    for $t = 1, 2, \cdots, T$, do
        for $k = 1, 2, \cdots, K$, do
            Compute $\mathbf{L}_k$ by Eqs. (12) and (13).
        end for
        Compute $\mathbf{w}$ according to Eq. (17).
        Computer $J^{(t)}$ via Eq. (6).
        If $t > 1$ and $|J^{(t)} - J^{(t-1)}| < \varepsilon$
            Go to **Step 3**.
        end if
    end for
Step 3 (Output distance metrics and weights):
    $\mathbf{M}_k = \mathbf{L}_k{}^T \mathbf{L}_k$, $k = 1, 2, \cdots, K$.
    Output $\mathbf{M}_1, \mathbf{M}_2, \cdots, \mathbf{M}_K$ and $\mathbf{w}$.

Let $\frac{\partial La(\mathbf{w}, \eta)}{\partial w_k} = 0$ and $\frac{\partial La(\mathbf{w}, \eta)}{\partial \eta} = 0$, we have

$$\frac{\partial La(\mathbf{w}, \eta)}{\partial w_k} = p \, w_k^{p-1} \, I_k - \eta = 0, \tag{15}$$

$$\frac{\partial La(\mathbf{w}, \eta)}{\partial \eta} = \sum_{k=1}^K w_k - 1 = 0. \tag{16}$$

According to Eqs. (15) and (16), w_k can be updated as follows:

$$w_k = \frac{\left(1/I_k\right)^{1/(p-1)}}{\sum\limits_{k=1}^K \left(1/I_k\right)^{1/(p-1)}}. \tag{17}$$

We repeat the above two steps until the algorithm meets a certain convergence condition. The proposed LM^{3}L algorithm is summarized in Algorithm 1, where $\mathbf{E} \in \mathbb{R}^{s_k \times d_k}$ is a matrix with 1's on the diagonal and zeros elsewhere.

4 Experiments

To evaluate the effectiveness of our LM^{3}L method, we conduct face and kinship verification in the wild experiments on three real-world face datasets including the Labeled Faces in the Wild (LFW) [12], the YouTube Faces (YTF) [30],

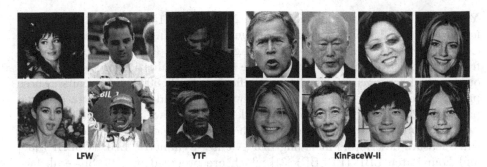

Fig. 2. Some sample positive pairs from the LFW, YTF and KinFaceW-II datasets.

and the KinFaceW-II [17]. Figure 2 shows some sample images from these three datasets. The parameters p, β, λ, μ_k and τ_k of our LM^3L method were empirically set as 2, 0.001, 0.1, 5 and 1 for all $k = 1, 2, \cdots, K$, respectively. The following details the experiments and results.

4.1 Datasets and Settings

LFW. The LFW dataset [12] contains more than 13000 face images of 5749 subjects collected from the web with large variations in expression, pose, age, illumination, resolution, and so on. There are two training paradigms for supervised learning on this dataset: *image-restricted* and *unrestricted*. In our experiments, we use the *image-restricted* setting where only the pairwise label information is required to train our method. We follow the standard evaluation protocol on the "View 2" dataset [12] which includes 3000 matched pairs and 3000 mismatched pairs and is divided into 10 folds with each fold consisting of 300 matched (positive) pairs and 300 mismatched (negative) pairs. We use the aligned LFW-a dataset[1] for our evaluation, and crop each image into 80 × 150 to remove the background information. For each face image, we extracted three different features: (1) Dense SIFT (DSIFT) [16]: We densely sample SIFT descriptors on each 16 × 16 patch without overlapping and obtain 45 SIFT descriptors. Then, we concatenate these SIFT descriptors to form one 5,760-dimensional feature vector; (2) LBP [1]: We divide each image into 8 × 15 non-overlapping blocks, where the size of each block is 10 × 10. Then, we extract a 59-dimensional uniform pattern LBP feature for each block and concatenate them to form a 7080-dimensional feature vector; (3) Sparse SIFT (SSIFT): We use the SSIFT feature provided by [9], which first localizes nine fixed landmarks in each image and extracts SIFT features over three scales at these landmarks, then concatenates these SIFT descriptors to form one 3456-dimensional feature vector. For these three features, we performed whitened PCA (WPCA) to project each feature into a 200 dimensional feature subspace, respectively.

---

[1] Available: http://www.openu.ac.il/home/hassner/data/lfwa/.

YTF. The YTF dataset [30] contains 3425 videos of 1595 different people collected from YouTube site. There are large variations in pose, illumination, and expression in each video, and the average length of each video clip is 181.3 frames. In our experiments, we follow the standard evaluation protocol and test our method for unconstrained face verification with 5000 video pairs. These pairs are equally divided into 10 folds with each fold has 250 intra-personal pairs and 250 inter-personal pairs. Similar to LFW, we also adopt the *image restricted* protocol to evaluate our method. For this dataset, we directly use three feature descriptors including LBP, Center-Symmetric LBP (CSLBP) [30] and Four-Patch LBP (FPLBP) [31] which are provided by [30]. Since all face images have been aligned by the detected facial key points, we average all the feature vectors within one video clip to form a mean feature vector. Lastly, we also use WPCA to map each feature into a 200-dimensional feature vector.

KinFaceW-II. The KinFaceW-II [17] is a kinship face dataset collected from the public figures or celebrities and their parents or children. There are four kinship relations in the KinFaceW-II datasets: Father-Son (F-S), Father-Daughter (F-D), Mother-Son (M-S) and Mother-Daughter (M-D), and each relation contains 250 pairs of kinship images. Following the experimental settings in [17], we construct 250 positive pairs (with kinship) and 250 negative pairs (without kinship) for each relation. For each face image, we also extract four types of features: LEarning-based descriptor (LE) [4], LBP, TPLBP and SIFT, and their dimensions are 200, 256, 256 and 200, respectively. We adopted the 5-fold cross validation strategy for each of the four subsets in this dataset and the finial results are reported by the mean verification accuracy.

4.2 Experimental Results on LFW

Comparison with Different Metric Learning Strategies: We first compare our method with three other different metric learning strategies: (1) Single Metric Learning (SML): we learn a single distance metric by using Eq. (3) with each feature representation; (2) Concatenated Metric Learning (CML): we first concatenate different features into a longer feature vector and then apply Eq. (3) to learn a distance metric; (3) Individual Metric Learning (IML): we learn the distance metric for each feature representation by using Eq. (3) and then use the equal weight to compute the similarity of two face images with Eq. (5). Table 1 records the verification rates with standard error of different metric learning strategies on the LFW dataset under the image restricted setting. We can see that our LM^3L consistently outperforms the other compared metric learning strategies in terms of the mean verification rate. Compared to SML, our LM^3L learns multiple distance metrics with multi-feature representations, such that more discriminative information can be exploited for verification. Compared with CML and IML, our LM^3L can jointly learn multiple distance metrics such that the distance metrics learned for different features can interact each other such that more complementary information can be extracted for verification.

Table 1. Comparisons of the mean verification rate (%) with different metric learning strategies on the LFW under image-restricted setting with label-free outside data.

Method	Feature	Accuracy (%)
SML	DSIFT	84.30 ± 2.17
SML	LBP	83.83 ± 1.31
SML	SSIFT	84.58 ± 1.14
CML	All	82.40 ± 1.62
IML	All	87.78 ± 1.83
LM^{3}L	All	**89.57 ± 1.53**

Table 2. Comparisons of the mean verification rate (%) with the state-of-the-art results on the LFW under image-restricted setting with label-free outside data, where NoF denotes the number of feature used in each method.

Method	NoF	Accuracy (%)
PCCA [20]	1	83.80 ± 0.40
PAF [35]	1	87.77 ± 0.51
CSML+SVM [21]	6	88.00 ± 0.37
SFRD+PMML [5]	8	89.35 ± 0.50
Sub-SML [3]	6	89.73 ± 0.38
DDML [11]	6	90.68 ± 1.41
VMRS [2]	10	91.10 ± 0.59
LM^{3}L	3	**89.57 ± 1.53**

Comparison with the State-of-the-Art Methods: We compare our LM^{3}L method with the state-of-the-art methods on the LFW dataset[2]. These compared methods can be categorized into metric learning based methods such as LDML [9], PCCA [20], CSML+SVM [21], DML-eig combined [36], SFRD+ PMML [5], Sub-SML [3], and discriminative deep metric learning (DDML) [11]; and descriptor based methods such as Multiple LE+comp [4], Pose Adaptive Filter (PAF) [35], and high dimensional vector multiplication (VMRS) [2]. Table 2 tabulates the mean verification rate with standard error and Fig. 3 shows the ROC curves of different methods on this dataset, respectively. We can see that our LM^{3}L achieves competitive results with these state-of-the-art methods except VMRS [2] and DDML [11], where they run on the 10 and 6 kinds of feature, respectively.

Comparison with the Latest Multiple Metric Learning Method: We compare our LM^{3}L method with the latest multiple metric learning method called PMML [5]. The standard implementation of PMML was provided by the original authors. Table 3 tabulates the mean verification rate with standard error

---

[2] Available: http://vis-www.cs.umass.edu/lfw/results.html.

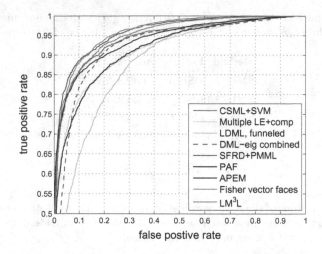

Fig. 3. Comparisons of ROC curves between our LM³L and the state-of-the-art methods on the LFW under image-restricted setting with label-free outside data.

Table 3. Comparison with the latest multiple metric learning method on the LFW under image-restricted setting with label-free outside data.

Method	Accuracy (%)
PMML [5]	85.23 ± 1.69
LM³L	**89.57 ± 1.53**

on this dataset. We can clearly see that our LM³L significantly outperforms PMML on the LFW dataset. This is because our LM³L can adaptively learn different weights to reflect the different importance of different features while PMML assigns equal weights to different features, such that our method can better exploit the complementary information.

4.3   Experimental Results on YTF

Comparison with Different Metric Learning Strategies: Similar to LFW, we also compare our method with different metric learning strategies such as SML, CML, and IML on the YTF dataset. Table 4 records the verification rates of different metric learning strategies on the YTF dataset under the image restricted setting. We can also see that our LM³L consistently outperforms the other metric learning strategies in terms of the mean verification rate.

Comparison with the State-of-the-Art Methods: We compare our method with the state-of-the-art methods on the YTF dataset. These compared methods include Matched Background Similarity (MBGS) [30], APEM [15], STFRD+ PMML [5], MBGS+SVM⊖ [32], VSOF+OSS (Adaboost) [19], and DDML [11]. Table 5 records the mean verification rate with the standard error, and Fig. 4

Table 4. Comparison of the mean verification rate with standard error (%) with different metric learning strategies on the YTF under the image restricted setting.

Method	Feature	Accuracy (%)
SML	CSLBP	73.66 ± 1.52
SML	FPLBP	75.02 ± 1.67
SML	LBP	78.46 ± 0.94
CML	All	75.36 ± 2.37
IML	All	80.12 ± 1.33
LM^{3}L	All	**81.28 ± 1.17**

Table 5. Comparisons of the mean verification rate with standard error (%) with the state-of-the-art results on the YTF under the image restricted setting.

Method	Accuracy (%)
MBGS (LBP) [30]	76.40 ± 1.80
APEM (LBP) [15]	77.44 ± 1.46
APEM (fusion) [15]	79.06 ± 1.51
STFRD+PMML [5]	79.48 ± 2.52
MBGS+SVM⊖ [32]	79.48 ± 2.52
VSOF+OSS (Adaboost) [19]	79.70 ± 1.80
DDML (combined) [11]	82.34 ± 1.47
LM^{3}L	**81.28 ± 1.17**

shows the ROC curves of our LM^{3}L and the state-of-the-art methods on the YTF dataset, respectively. We can observe that our LM^{3}L method achieves competitive result compared with these state-of-the-art methods on this dataset under the image restricted setting.

Comparison with the Latest Multiple Metric Learning Method: Table 6 shows the mean verification rate with standard error of our proposed method and PMML method on the YTF dataset. We can clearly see that our LM^{3}L outperforms PMML on this dataset.

4.4   Experimental Results on KinFaceW-II

Comparison with Different Metric Learning Strategies: We first compare our method with SML, CML, and IML on the KinFaceW-II dataset. Table 7 records the mean verification rates of different metric learning strategies on the KinFaceW-II dataset for four relations, respectively. We can also see that our LM^{3}L consistently outperforms the other compared metric learning strategies in terms of the mean verification rate.

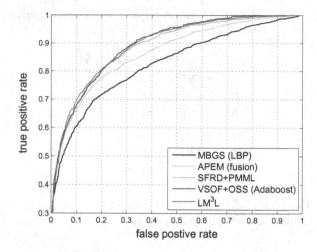

Fig. 4. Comparisons of ROC curves between our LM³L and the state-of-the-art methods on the YTF under the image restricted setting.

Table 6. Comparison with the existing multiple metric learning method on the YTF under the image restricted setting.

Method	Accuracy (%)
PMML [5]	76.60 ± 1.62
LM³L	**81.28 ± 1.17**

Table 7. Comparisons of the mean verification rate (%) with different metric learning strategies on the KinFaceW-II dataset.

Method	Feature	F-S	F-D	M-S	M-D	Mean
SML	LE	76.2	70.1	72.4	71.8	72.6
SML	LBP	66.9	65.5	63.1	68.3	66.0
SML	TPLBP	71.8	63.3	63.0	67.6	66.4
SML	SIFT	68.1	63.8	67.0	63.9	65.7
CML	All	76.3	67.5	74.3	75.4	73.4
IML	All	79.4	71.5	76.3	77.3	76.1
LM³L	All	**82.4**	**74.2**	**79.6**	**78.7**	**78.7**

Table 8. Comparisons of the mean verification rate (%) with the state-of-the-art methods on the KinFaceW-II dataset.

Method	Feature	F-S	F-D	M-S	M-D	Mean
PMML [5]	All	77.7	72.4	76.3	74.8	75.3
MNRML [17]	All	76.9	74.3	77.4	77.6	76.5
LM³L	All	**82.4**	**74.2**	**79.6**	**78.7**	**78.7**

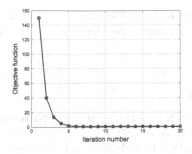

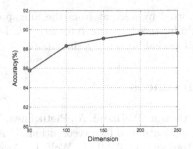

Fig. 5. The value of objective function of LM^{3}L versus different number of iterations on the LFW dataset.

Fig. 6. The mean verification rate of LM^{3}L versus different feature dimensions on the LFW dataset.

Comparison with the State-of-the-Art Methods: We compare our method with the state-of-the-art methods on the KinFaceW-II dataset. These compared methods include MNRML [17] and PMML [5]. Table 8 reports the mean verification rates of our method and these methods. We can observe that our LM^{3}L achieves about 2.0 % improvement over the current state-of-the-art result on this dataset for kinship verification.

4.5 Parameter Analysis

Since LM^{3}L is an iterative algorithm, we first evaluate its convergence with different number of iterations. Figure 5 shows the value of the objective function of LM^{3}L versus different number of iterations on the LFW dataset. We can see that the convergence speed of LM^{3}L is fast and it converges in 5–6 iterations.

Lastly, we evaluate the performance of LM^{3}L versus different feature dimensions. Figure 6 shows the mean verification rate versus different feature dimensions on the LFW dataset. We can see that the proposed LM^{3}L method can achieve stable performance when the feature dimension reaches 150.

5   Conclusion and Future Work

In this paper, we have proposed a large margin multi-metric learning (LM^{3}L) method for face and kinship verification. Our method has jointly learned multiple distance metrics under which more discriminative and complementary information can be exploited. Experimental results show that our method can achieve competitive results compared with the state-of-the-art methods. For future work, we are interested to apply our method to other computer vision applications such as visual tracking and action recognition to further show its effectiveness.

Acknowledgement. This work was carried out at the Rapid-Rich Object Search (ROSE) Lab at the Nanyang Technological University, Singapore. The ROSE Lab is supported by a grant from the Singapore National Research Foundation. This grant is administered by the Interactive & Digital Media Programme Office at the Media Development Authority, Singapore.

References

1. Ahonen, T., Hadid, A., Pietikainen, M.: Face description with local binary patterns: application to face recognition. TPAMI **28**, 2037–2041 (2006)
2. Barkan, O., Weill, J., Wolf, L., Aronowitz, H.: Fast high dimensional vector multiplication face recognition. In: ICCV, pp. 1960–1967 (2013)
3. Cao, Q., Ying, Y., Li, P.: Similarity metric learning for face recognition. In: ICCV, pp. 2408–2415 (2013)
4. Cao, Z., Yin, Q., Tang, X., Sun, J.: Face recognition with learning-based descriptor. In: CVPR, pp. 2707–2714 (2010)
5. Cui, Z., Li, W., Xu, D., Shan, S., Chen, X.: Fusing robust face region descriptors via multiple metric learning for face recognition in the wild. In: CVPR, pp. 3554–3561 (2013)
6. Davis, J.V., Kulis, B., Jain, P., Sra, S., Dhillon, I.S.: Information-theoretic metric learning. In: ICML, pp. 209–216 (2007)
7. Fang, R., Tang, K., Snavely, N., Chen, T.: Towards computational models of kinship verification. In: ICIP, pp. 1577–1580 (2010)
8. Goldberger, J., Roweis, S.T., Hinton, G.E., Salakhutdinov, R.: Neighbourhood components analysis. In: NIPS, pp. 513–520 (2004)
9. Guillaumin, M., Verbeek, J.J., Schmid, C.: Is that you? metric learning approaches for face identification. In: ICCV, pp. 498–505 (2009)
10. Guo, G., Wang, X.: Kinship measurement on salient facial features. TIM **61**, 2322–2325 (2012)
11. Hu, J., Lu, J., Tan, Y.P.: Discriminative deep metric learning for face verification in the wild. In: CVPR, pp. 1875–1882 (2014)
12. Huang, G.B., Ramesh, M., Berg, T., Learned-Miller, E.: Labeled faces in the wild: a database for studying face recognition in unconstrained environments. Technical report 07–49, University of Massachusetts, Amherst (2007)
13. Köstinger, M., Hirzer, M., Wohlhart, P., Roth, P.M., Bischof, H.: Large scale metric learning from equivalence constraints. In: CVPR, pp. 2288–2295 (2012)
14. Lei, Z., Pietikainen, M., Li, S.Z.: Learning discriminant face descriptor. TPAMI **36**, 289–302 (2014)
15. Li, H., Hua, G., Lin, Z., Brandt, J., Yang, J.: Probabilistic elastic matching for pose variant face verification. In: CVPR, pp. 3499–3506 (2013)
16. Lowe, D.G.: Distinctive image features from scale-invariant keypoints. IJCV **60**, 91–110 (2004)
17. Lu, J., Hu, J., Zhou, X., Shang, Y., Tan, Y.P., Wang, G.: Neighborhood repulsed metric learning for kinship verification. In: CVPR, pp. 2594–2601 (2012)
18. Lu, J., Zhou, X., Tan, Y.P., Shang, Y., Zhou, J.: Neighborhood repulsed metric learning for kinship verification. TPAMI **36**, 331–345 (2014)
19. Mendez-Vazquez, H., Martinez-Diaz, Y., Chai, Z.: Volume structured ordinal features with background similarity measure for video face recognition. In: ICB, pp. 1–6 (2013)
20. Mignon, A., Jurie, F.: Pcca: A new approach for distance learning from sparse pairwise constraints. In: CVPR, pp. 2666–2672 (2012)

21. Nguyen, H.V., Bai, L.: Cosine similarity metric learning for face verification. In: Kimmel, R., Klette, R., Sugimoto, A. (eds.) ACCV 2010, Part II. LNCS, vol. 6493, pp. 709–720. Springer, Heidelberg (2011)
22. Rennie, J.D.M., Srebro, N.: Fast maximum margin matrix factorization for collaborative prediction. In: ICML, pp. 713–719 (2005)
23. Seo, H.J., Milanfar, P.: Face verification using the lark representation. TIFS **6**, 1275–1286 (2011)
24. Sharma, A., Kumar, A., Daume III, H., Jacobs, D.: Generalized multiview analysis: a discriminative latent space. In: CVPR, pp. 1867–1875 (2012)
25. Simonyan, K., Parkhi, O.M., Vedaldi, A., Zisserman, A.: Fisher vector faces in the wild. In: BMVC, pp. 1–12 (2013)
26. Torresani, L., Lee, K.C.: Large margin component analysis. In: NIPS, pp. 1385–1392 (2006)
27. Tran, D., Sorokin, A.: Human activity recognition with metric learning. In: Forsyth, D., Torr, P., Zisserman, A. (eds.) ECCV 2008, Part I. LNCS, vol. 5302, pp. 548–561. Springer, Heidelberg (2008)
28. Wang, Z., Hu, Y., Chia, L.-T.: Image-to-class distance metric learning for image classification. In: Daniilidis, K., Maragos, P., Paragios, N. (eds.) ECCV 2010, Part I. LNCS, vol. 6311, pp. 706–719. Springer, Heidelberg (2010)
29. Weinberger, K.Q., Blitzer, J., Saul, L.K.: Distance metric learning for large margin nearest neighbor classification. In: NIPS (2005)
30. Wolf, L., Hassner, T., Maoz, I.: Face recognition in unconstrained videos with matched background similarity. In: CVPR, pp. 529–534 (2011)
31. Wolf, L., Hassner, T., Taigman, Y.: Descriptor based methods in the wild. In: ECCVW (2008)
32. Wolf, L., Levy, N.: The svm-minus similarity score for video face recognition. In: CVPR, pp. 3523–3530 (2013)
33. Xia, S., Shao, M., Fu, Y.: Kinship verification through transfer learning. In: IJCAI, pp. 2539–2544 (2011)
34. Xia, S., Shao, M., Luo, J., Fu, Y.: Understanding kin relationships in a photo. TMM **14**, 1046–1056 (2012)
35. Yi, D., Lei, Z., Li, S.Z.: Towards pose robust face recognition. In: CVPR, pp. 3539–3545 (2013)
36. Ying, Y., Li, P.: Distance metric learning with eigenvalue optimization. JMLR **13**, 1–26 (2012)
37. Zhou, X., Hu, J., Lu, J., Shang, Y., Guan, Y.: Kinship verification from facial images under uncontrolled conditions. In: ACM MM, pp. 953–956 (2011)
38. Zhou, X., Lu, J., Hu, J., Shang, Y.: Gabor-based gradient orientation pyramid for kinship verification under uncontrolled environments. In: ACM MM, pp. 725–728 (2012)

A Three-Color Coupled Level-Set Algorithm for Simultaneous Multiple Cell Segmentation and Tracking

Jierong Cheng[✉], Wei Xiong, Ying Gu, Shue-Ching Chia,
Yue Wang, and Joo-Hwee Lim

Institute for Infocomm Research, 1 Fusionopolis Way,
#21-01 Connexis (South Tower), Singapore 138632, Singapore
chengjr@i2r.a-star.edu.sg

Abstract. High content computational analysis of time-lapse microscopic cell images requires accurate and efficient segmentation and tracking. In this work, we introduce "3LS", an algorithm using only three level sets to segment and track arbitrary number of cells in time-lapse microscopic images. The cell number and positions are determined in the first frame by extracting concave points and fitting ellipses after initial segmentation. We construct a graph representing cells and the background with vertices and their adjacency relationships with edges. Each vertex of the graph is assigned with a color tag by applying a vertex coloring algorithm. In this way, the boundary of each cell can be embedded in one of three level set functions. The "3LS" algorithm is implemented in an existing coupled active contour framework (nLS) [1] to handle overlapped cells during segmentation. However, we improve nLS using a new volume conservation constraint (VCC) to prevent shrinkage or expansion on whole cell boundaries and produce more accurate segmentation and tracking of touching cells. When tested on four different time-lapse image sequences, the 3LS outperforms the original nLS and other relevant state-of-the-art counterparts in both segmentation and tracking however with a notable reduction in computational time.

1 Introduction

High throughput microscopy provides an unprecedented opportunity to visualize cellular events at high resolutions over time. Time-resolved microscopic imaging has become popular in studying basic cellular processes such as motility, migration, deformation, population dynamics, etc. However, increasing quantity of images of high throughput readouts coupled with complexity of the underlying information makes manual analysis of such images prohibitive.

Commercial microscopy software packages generally feature tools for object segmentation and tracking [2]. However, simple intensity based thresholding fails for cells observed in nonfluorescent imaging modes and for cells in contact. Likewise, standard correlation matching cannot keep track of cells that change their shapes. Such limitations are often partly compensated by graphical user interfaces

© Springer International Publishing Switzerland 2015
D. Cremers et al. (Eds.): ACCV 2014, Part III, LNCS 9005, pp. 268–283, 2015.
DOI: 10.1007/978-3-319-16811-1_18

that allow users to manually correct processing errors, but at the expense of speed and reproducibility – the main benefits of automation.

Existing cell tracking methods can be divided into two main classes. Algorithms in the first class perform cell detection and linking between cells from different frames separately. The linking process is usually based on certain criteria of the similarities in spatial positions and appearance of the cells. A typical method is "favorite matching" through a distance matrix computed from the Euclidean distance of the cell centroids and the sizes [3–5]. In [6], a dissimilarity measure was designed based on the spatial distribution, nuclei morphological appearance, migration, and intensity information. In [7], the similarities were calculated from object center coordinates, size, and total intensity. For tracking of mitotic cell nuclei, object correspondences were determined by searching for trajectories with maximum smoothness [8]. A framework combining mean shift and Kalman filters was designed for cell tracking [9]. The main difficulty of this type of methods is to split or merge the tracks in the event when the total number of objects is changed.

Algorithms in the second class integrate cell segmentation and tracking in a model evolution approach [2]. Mostly based on active contours or deformable models, they extend from segmentation to tracking by using the extracted contours of objects in the previous frame as initialization for the segmentation of the current frame. In [10], a parametric active contour based method was presented for the tracking of cell migrations in microscopy videos. Due to the inability of parametric contours to handle cell interactions, topological operators had to be introduced to handle cell divisions. In addition, the concept of repulsive contours were proposed to handle cell contact. It is notable that the initialization of the parametric active contours must be done manually on the first frame of the temporal sequence. Geometric active contour approaches based on level sets neither require any explicit parameterization nor suffer from any constraints on the topology. Such approaches have been used for segmenting and tracking cells in 2D images [11–14] and dynamic 3D images [1,15]. The main disadvantage of the model evolution approaches is the computational cost: to prevent cell fusion, each cell i has to be represented by its own level set function ϕ_i; a pair-wise coupling constraint is introduced to prevent neighbouring contours from overlapping each other (the details can be found in Sect. 2.1). Hence, if an image contains N cells, N level set functions $\phi_i, i = 1, 2, ..., N$ will be needed and the number of such coupling constraint terms will be N^2.

To reduce the number of level set functions representing multiple objects, vertex coloring has been proposed in a four-color level set algorithm [16] where a graph is constructed with vertices used for representing cells and edges used for their adjacency relationships. It is noted that, in all existing relevant approaches, the image background is not represented explicitly. In the present work, we choose to represent each background explicitly with a fixed vertex in the graph. With these concepts in mind, we introduce our 3LS algorithm which uses only three level set functions to tackle the problem of segmenting and tracking multiple cells simultaneously.

Besides cell overlapping in microscopic images, cells of similar intensity levels may touch and this causes errors in level set based cell tracking. To handle this, Dufour introduced a volume conservation constraint (VCC) term in his algorithms presented in [1]. However, the VCC term results in shrinkage or expansion on whole cell boundary. To avoid this undesirable effect, we introduce an improved VCC and combine it with a pair-wise coupling term. With these modifications, we propose a three-color coupled level set algorithm for the segmentation and tracking of arbitrary number of cells in time-lapse microscopic images with overlapping and touching cells. Notably, the proposed algorithm can reduce computational costs significantly while achieving better segmentation and tracking accuracy. This is validated by our numerical experiments.

2   Related Work

2.1   N-Coupled Level Sets

The tracking algorithms using coupled implicit active contours [11]/surfaces [1] are an extension to Chan and Vese's two-phase model in the level-set framework [17]. In order to track each cell separately, one level set function ϕ_i is assigned to each cell, $i = 1, 2, .., n$. In the 2D model, the total energy function for the n level sets (nLS) is given by

$$
E(\phi_1, ..., \phi_n, c_O, c_{I,1}, ..., c_{I,n}) = \iint_\Omega \sum_{i=1}^n \left[\alpha \delta(\phi_i)|\nabla \phi_i| + \lambda_I H(\phi_i)(I - c_{I,i})^2 \right.
$$

$$
\left. + \frac{\lambda_O}{n} \prod_j (1 - H(\phi_j)) \, (I - c_O)^2 + \gamma \sum_{i<j} H(\phi_i)H(\phi_j) \right] dxdy
$$

$$
+ \frac{1}{2} \sum_{i=1}^n \eta_i \left(\iint_\Omega H(\phi_i)dxdy - V_i^0 \right)^2 \quad (1)
$$

In this expression, $c_{I,i}$ and c_O are the mean intensity of voxels inside the ith level set ϕ_i and outside all the current level sets respectively. $\delta(\phi)$ and $H(\phi)$ are the Dirac and Heaviside functions, respectively. $I = I(x, y)$ is the image intensity at $(x, y) \in \Omega, \Omega \subset \mathbb{R}^2$. The term weighted by γ penalizes the pair-wise overlaps between distinct contours. The last term is the volume (or area in 2D) conservation constraint (VCC) introduced in [1] by Dufour which helps to improve the segmentation of touching cells. $V_i^0 = \iint_\Omega H(\phi_i^0)dxdy$ is the volume of cell i segmented from the first frame. When cells of similar intensity levels touch, the image dependent terms (the first three terms) are insufficient to determine the boundary between cells correctly. Without the VCC, the active contour evolution will depend primarily on the initialization and result in one contour engulfing the other contour.

From Eq. (1), for each ϕ_i, one can derive a time t indexed surface evaluation equation as follows:

$$\frac{\partial \phi_i}{\partial t} = \left[\alpha \nabla \cdot \frac{\nabla \phi_i}{|\nabla \phi_i|} - \lambda_I (I - c_{I,i})^2 + \lambda_O \prod_{j \neq i} (1 - H(\phi_j)) (I - c_O)^2 \right. $$
$$\left. -\gamma \sum_{j \neq i} H(\phi_j) - \eta_i \left(\iint_\Omega H(\phi_i) dx dy - V_i^0 \right) \right] \delta(\phi_i) \qquad (2)$$

where

$$c_{I,i}(t) = \langle H(\phi_i) \rangle; \quad c_O(t) = \left\langle \prod_j (1 - H(\phi_i)) \right\rangle \qquad (3)$$

A shortcoming of Dufour's VCC is that the resultant shrinking or expanding force applies not only on the portion of cell boundary where the cell touches or resides inside another cell, but also on the whole boundary of a cell. Therefore, undesirable shrinkage or expansion may be caused on the whole cell boundary. For isolated cells, the image dependent terms—the second and third terms on the right side of Eq. (1), are sufficient for correct segmentation. Cells and nuclei change their shapes dramatically during cell division. When tracking cell mitosis events applying Dufour's approach, one may obtain inaccurate results due to such effects of the VCC term.

2.2   Four-Coupled Level Sets

To reduce computational costs for segmenting of N objects, a four-color level set (4LS) algorithm based on graph vertex coloring was presented in [16]. The authors use the Delaunay graph to capture spatial relationship of cells, with each vertex of the graph representing a cell. By applying a vertex coloring processing on the graph, each vertex is tagged with a color which is different from those of its adjacent vertices in the graph. Therefore, cells can be divided into groups, according to the colors assigned to them. Since cells in the same group/color are not adjacent spatially, one can assign a single level set function to handle the processing of all cells with the same color tag. The famous "four-color theorem" states that any planar graphs can be colored with at most four colors and no two neighboring vertices are assigned with the same color [18]. Hence, one requires only four level set functions and six coupling constraint terms for the processing of N cells. This dramatically reduces the computational cost.

The four evolution equations are as follows ($i = 1, 2, 3, 4$):

$$\frac{\partial \phi_i}{\partial t} = \left[\alpha \nabla \cdot \frac{\nabla \phi_i}{|\nabla \phi_i|} - \lambda_I (I - c_{I,i})^2 + \lambda_O \prod_{j=1, j \neq i}^{4} (1 - H(\phi_j)) (I - c_O)^2 \right. $$
$$\left. -\gamma \sum_{j=i+1}^{4} H(\phi_j) \right] \delta(\phi_i) + \zeta \left[\Delta \phi_i - \nabla \cdot \frac{\nabla \phi_i}{|\nabla \phi_i|} \right] \qquad (4)$$

where the last term enforces the constraint of $|\nabla \phi_i| = 1$.

In addition to the pair-wise coupling constraint weighted by γ in Eq. (4), they also used an explicit coupling rule during the narrow-band evolution to penalize overlaps between level sets: a pixel on the front of a current level sets ($\delta(\phi_i) > s_{thresh}$) is updated only if its saliency is highest among all four level sets, i.e. $\delta(\phi_i) > \delta(\phi_j)$, for given i and for all $j \neq i$.

3   Methodology

This section describes in detail our segmentation/clump separating method and three-color coupled level set (3LS) algorithm for cell tracking.

The main steps of the proposed segmentation and tracking algorithm are summarized as follows:

(1) Segment the first frame of the sequence using Chan and Vese's two-phase level set algorithm [17].
(2) Determine the cell number and positions by extracting concave points and performing ellipse fitting after initial segmentation. Produce a label map where each cell is represented by a unique label.
(3) Use the label map to initialize three level set functions based on vertex coloring result.
(4) Update $c_{I,i}$ and c_O and evolve each level set function according to Eq. (11) until convergence.
(5) Determine whether there are new objects entering the current frame by applying two-phase level set algorithm.
(6) If there is a next frame, obtain a label map from the converged level set functions and go to step 3. Otherwise stop the algorithm.

We elaborate essential components of the algorithm as follows.

3.1   Concave Point Extraction and Ellipse Fitting

In level set based tracking methods, a good segmentation of the first frame is very important to perform correct tracking as it provides the information about the positions and the number of objects to be tracked [15]. At the beginning of our method, the first frame is binarized by Chan and Vese's approach [17] of active contours without edges in the level-set framework. Such initial segmentation tends to group close/touching cells together. Next, we use the derived *concave* points and ellipse fitting to separate clumped cells. Our concave point extraction and ellipse fitting method uses three parameters (d, $h_{\min}$, and f_{th}), comparing to Bai's popular method using seven parameters [19]. Let $\mathcal{B}$ be the binary image obtained. The output exterior boundaries of $\mathcal{B}$ are used to extract concave points. Let $p_c(x_c, y_c)$ be the point at order index $c, c = 1, 2, ..., N$ in a sequence of ordered points on a close boundary. $\theta(p_c)$, the degree of concavity of p_c is measured by the angle between the two vectors defined by three consecutive points (p_{c-1}, p_c, p_{c+1}):

$$\theta(p_c) = \begin{cases} a(p_{c-1}, p_c) - a(p_{c+1}, p_c), & \text{if } a(p_{c-1}, p_c) - a(p_{c+1}, p_c) > 0 \\ a(p_{c-1}, p_c) - a(p_{c+1}, p_c) + 2\pi, & \text{else} \end{cases} \quad (5)$$

where

$$a(p_{c-1}, p_c) = \arctan(y_{c-1} - y_c, x_{c-1} - x_c) \tag{6}$$
$$a(p_{c+1}, p_c) = \arctan(y_{c+1} - y_c, x_{c+1} - x_c) \tag{7}$$

The concave points are the local maxima of $\theta(p_c), c = 1, 2, ..., N$, with minimum peak separation distance of d and minimum peak height of $h_{\min}$.

$$p_{\text{concave}} = \{p_{c^*} | \theta(p_{c^*}) \geq \theta(p_c) \quad \forall \quad |c - c^*| \leq d \text{ and } \theta(p_{c^*}) \geq h_{\min}\} \tag{8}$$

where d is minimum peak separation distance and $h_{\min}$ are the minimum peak height. d and $h_{\min}$ are pre-set thresholds. In the next step, the exterior boundaries are separated into contour segments by concave points. Note that if initial segmentation generates interior boundaries, *convex* points can be extracted by finding local minima of $\theta(p_c)$ in a similar way, then the interior boundaries can be separated into contour segments by convex points, which are crucial to separate a highly compact clump of cells.

The contour segments are fitted to ellipses using the least squares criterion. We define a score measuring the fitness between contour segment(s) L and its fitted ellipse $\mathcal{E}(L)$ as follows

$$\text{fit}(L, \mathcal{E}) = \frac{\text{length}(L)}{\pi\sqrt{2(a^2 + b^2)}} \left(\frac{\text{area}(\mathcal{E} \cap \mathcal{B})}{\pi ab}\right)^3 \tag{9}$$

where a and b are the semi-major and semi-minor axes of $\mathcal{E}$, respectively. The first fraction on the right side is the ratio between the length of L and the (approximated) perimeter of $\mathcal{E}$. In case L consists of multiple contour segments, its length is the sum of those of all segments. The second fraction (in the bracket with cubic power) is the ratio of the area of the region enclosed by both $\mathcal{B}$ and $\mathcal{E}$ over the area of $\mathcal{E}$. For each connected component in $\mathcal{B}$, each single contour segment is fitted by an ellipse. If the fitness score is higher than a threshold f_{th}, then the segment matches the ellipse and such an ellipse is kept. Those unmatched segments are paired with each other to find the best fitted ellipse among all combinations, requiring fit $> f_{\text{th}}$. Let $L_i, i = 1, 2, ..., M$ be the unmatched segments from the same connected components. The procedure of segment combination is given in Algorithm 1. Figure 1 illustrates the extracted concave points and ellipses fitted.

3.2   Graph Construction and Vertex Coloring

Instead of assigning a unique level set to every cell as [1, 11], we aim to use a minimum number of level sets for the segmentation and tracking of the same number of cells. This problem can be solved by vertex coloring, a way of coloring the vertices of a graph such that no two adjacent vertices share the same color.

We construct a graph from the fitted ellipses as follows:

(1) Generate a planar graph by applying Delaunay triangulation on the centroids of all ellipses/cells.

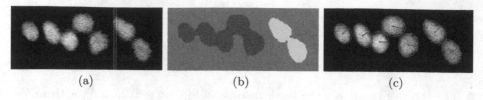

(a)   (b)   (c)

Fig. 1. (a) Original image with multiple touching cells. (b) Binary image and concave points. (c) Fitted ellipses: red ellipses are fitted to a single contour segment and blue ellipses are fitted to a pair of segments (Color figure online).

> **for** $i = 1$ *to* M **do**
>   **for** $j = i + 1$ *to* M **do**
> $L_{ij} = L_i \cup L_j$;
>   Fit an ellipse E_{ij} by using all the points on L_{ij};
> $F(i, j) = \text{fit}(L_{ij}, E_{ij})$;
>   **end**
> **end**
> $(i^*, j^*) = \arg\max_{i,j \in \{1,2,...,M\}} F(i, j)$;
> $f_{\max} = F(i^*, j^*)$;
> **while** $f_{\max} > f_{\text{th}}$ **do**
>   Keep $E_{i^* j^*}$;
> $F(i^*, j) = 0$, for $j = 1$ to M;
> $F(i, j^*) = 0$, for $i = 1$ to M;
> $(i^*, j^*) = \arg\max_{i,j \in \{1,2,...,M\}} F(i, j)$;
> $f_{\max} = F(i^*, j^*)$;
> **end**

Algorithm 1. Segment combination for ellipse fitting

(2) If the length of an edge derived from the triangulation is larger than a pre-set threshold d_e, the edge is removed from the graph.

(3) Add a vertex which represents the background and add an un-directed edge between the background vertex and every other cell vertexes (it is reasonable to assume that every cell is touching with the background).

After the graph is built, we apply Brèlaz's DSATUR algorithm [20] to assign a color tag to each vertex so that no adjacent vertices are assigned with the same color tag. The background vertex in the graph we constructed is adjacent to every cell vertices; it will be assigned a color which is different from all cell vertices. By initializing one level set function with the ellipses tagged with the same color, we need only three level set functions to represent the cells in our 2D segmentation and tracking problem.

If touching cells form a circle, the background inside the circle is assigned with another vertex and edges will be added between this vertex and the vertices of surrounding cells. Hence this vertex will be assigned with a color different from vertices of surrounding cells (but likely to be the same colors as other backgrounds).

Note that two vertexes might be adjacent in the graph even though their corresponding ellipses are not touching or overlapping. Two ellipses will be assigned to different colors if their distance is below a parameter d_e. This is to prevent them from merging in the subsequent frames. Here we assume each individual cell will overlap respectively in any two consecutive image frames. We empirically set d_e to be 1.2 times the sum of the long axes of two ellipses.

The above method for graph construction and vertex coloring can be easily extended to the representation of cell relationship for the task of 3D cell segmentation. In this case, the vertices have three coordinate elements and edges are positioned in a 3D (X, Y, Z) space instead of a 2D space. Therefore, the Delaunay triangulation and the edge length measurement need to be done in the 3D space. An example of such a graph is displayed in Fig. 2.

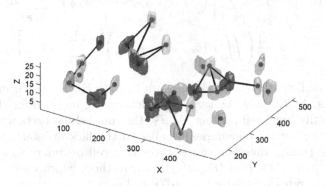

Fig. 2. A graph representing 3D cell relationship with vertices (in dots) and edges (in solid lines) (Color figure online).

3.3 Three-Color Coupled Level Sets

Our three-color coupled level sets algorithm is implemented in the nLS [1] framework to handle overlapped cells. To avoid the shrinkage or expansion on whole cell boundary caused by its VCC term, we propose an improved VCC which combines with a pair-wise coupling term. Our energy functional is defined with three level set functions:

$$E(\phi_1, \phi_2, \phi_3, c_O, c_{I,1}, c_{I,2}, c_{I,3}) = \iint_\Omega \sum_{i=1}^{3} \left[\alpha\delta(\phi_i)|\nabla\phi_i| + \lambda_I H(\phi_i)(I - c_{I,i})^2 \right.$$

$$+ \frac{\lambda_O}{3} \prod_{j=1}^{3} (1 - H(\phi_j)) (I - c_O)^2 + \gamma \sum_{j=i+1}^{3} H(\phi_i)H(\phi_j)$$

$$\left. + \frac{1}{2}\eta_i \sum_{q=1}^{N_i} \left(\left(\iint_\Omega H(\phi_{i,q})dxdy - V_{i,q}^0 \right)^2 \sum_{j=1,j\neq i}^{3} H(\phi_{i,q})H(\phi_j) \right) \right] dxdy \quad (10)$$

where N_i is the number of cells represented by $\phi_i, i = 1, 2, 3$ and $\phi_{i,q}$ is the level set function computed from the qth individual cell in ϕ_i, $q = 1, 2, ..., N_i$. N_i is determined in the vertex coloring procedure described in Sect. 3.2. As a result, the penalty of VCC (the term weighted by η_i in Eq. (10) only applies to the part of cell boundary which touches or locates inside another cell. This VCC term disappears automatically on isolated cells which do not overlap with other cells. Three evolution equations $(i = 1, 2, 3)$ can be derived by applying Euler-Lagrange equations to Eq. (10):

$$
\frac{\partial \phi_i}{\partial t} = \left[\alpha \nabla \cdot \frac{\nabla \phi_i}{|\nabla \phi_i|} - \lambda_I (I - c_{I,i})^2 + \lambda_O \prod_{j=1, j \neq i}^{3} (1 - H(\phi_j)) (I - c_O)^2 \right.
$$

$$
\left. - \gamma \sum_{j=i+1}^{3} H(\phi_j) \right] \delta(\phi_i) - \eta_i \sum_{q=1}^{N_i} \left[\left(\iint_{\Omega} H(\phi_{i,q}) dx dy - V_{i,q}^0 \right) \sum_{j=1, j \neq i}^{3} H(\phi_{i,q}) H(\phi_j) \right.
$$

$$
\left. + \frac{1}{2} \left(\iint_{\Omega} H(\phi_{i,q}) dx dy - V_{i,q}^0 \right)^2 \sum_{j=1, j \neq i}^{3} H(\phi_j) \right] \delta(\phi_{i,q}) \quad (11)
$$

In Fig. 3, we illustrate the tracking results on two consecutive frames by coupled level sets. At T_0, only two level set functions are required for the segmentation due to the small cell number. At T_1, the coupled level sets without VCC fail to track the correct boundaries because of the lack of intensity difference between cells. Dufour's method causes the whole cell boundary to shrink (purple cell) or expand (blue cell) (Fig. 3(c)). Our method, which uses an improved VCC term, generates satisfactory result (Fig. 3(e)).

3.4   Tracking Scheme

Now we describe our tracking scheme used in this work. In the first frame of a temporal sequence, the cell number and positions are determined by extracting concave points and ellipse fitting after initial segmentation. Then, the cells/ellipses are used to initialize three level set functions based on the result of vertex coloring. Three-color coupled level sets without VCC is applied to segment the cell

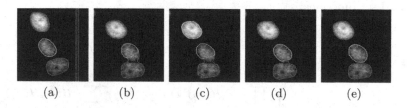

| (a) | (b) | (c) | (d) | (e) |

Fig. 3. Tracking results of coupled level sets. Contours of different color are represented by different level set functions. (a) Without VCC at T_0. (b) Without VCC at T_1. (c) Using Dufour's VCC at T_1. (d) Using Nath's explicit coupling rule without VCC at T_1. (e) Using our improved VCC at T_1 (Color figure online).

boundary. To process frames in subsequent times, the evolution result of Eq. (11) on the current frame is used to initialize the level set functions in the following frame. After each iteration, the distance between cells needs to be re-calculated. Cells within the distance threshold d_e need to change to different colors (and to re-initialize the level sets) to prevent the merge of cells of the same color.

4 Experiments

4.1 Validation Datasets

Our proposed method was tested on four publically available datasets. They are real time-lapse fluorescent microscopic image sequences, three in 2D (Hela1 [21], N2DL-Hela [22], and C2DL-MSC [22]) and one in 3D (C3DL-MDA231 [22]). The imaging acquisition setup of each dataset is listed in Table 1 [23]. Commonly used in cell population studies, the Hela1 and N2DL-Hela datasets are nuclear-stained (only nuclei are seen in the images). The two Hela datasets have high cell density and low resolution, some with very low fluorescent densities. Moreover, colliding, mitosis, entering and leaving cells are frequently present. The other two datasets, C2DL-MSC and C3DL-MDA231, are cytoplasm-stained. They are more appropriate for studies of single-cell morphology changes. The challenges in analyzing the C2DL-MSC dataset are the low signal-to-noise ratio and the presence of filament-like protrusions which often collide with each other. It is most difficult to process images in the 3D C3DL-MDA231 dataset: in addition to the colliding elongated cells, the data were acquired under high-throughput conditions (i.e., very low resolution in axial direction (difficult for segmentation) and very large time step (difficult for tracking)).

4.2 Evaluation Metrics

During ellipse fitting, the parameters were fixed: $d = 5$, $h_{min} = 3.9$, and $f_{th} = 0.5$. During evolution of the coupled level sets, the parameters were fixed to: $\alpha = 65$, $\lambda_I = 0.5$, $\lambda_O = 1$, $\gamma = 0$, $\eta = 2$, and the number of iterations for each frame is 50.

Table 1. Acquisition parameters and properties of the datasets.

Dataset	Hela1	N2DL-Hela	C2DL-MSC	C3DL-MDA231
Objective		Plan 10x/0.4	Plan-Neofluar 10x/0.3	Plan 20x/0.7
Frame size	672×512	1100×700	992×832	$512 \times 512 \times 30$
Pixel size (μm)		0.645×0.645	0.3×0.3	$1.242 \times 1.242 \times 6$
Time step	15 min	30 min	20 min	80 min
No. of frames	25	30	48	12
No. of moves	1444	760	413	331
No. of divisions	15	29	0	0

The segmentation results of the proposed three-color coupled level sets (3LS) were compared against the ground truth which is the consensus of three human experts, in terms of precision, recall, and F-score. Following the evaluation method in [23], a reference cell in ground truth and a segmented one are considered matching if their overlapping area is more than 50 % of the total area of the reference cell. Therefore, for each reference cell, there can be one matching segmented cell at most. In case there is no segmented cell matching with the reference cell, the three segmentation accuracy indices are set to zero. The segmentation accuracy is calculated as the mean of all the reference cells in the sequence, including these zeros. The percentage of matched reference cells is also computed. When we vary $d \in [1, 32]$, $h_{\min} \in [3.6, 4.2]$, $f_{th} \in [0.4, 0.7]$, the precision, recall, and F-score of the first frame of Hela1 are 0.972 ± 0.006, 0.914 ± 0.008, and 0.921 ± 0.006 respectively. The result shows that the segmentation accuracy is not sensitive to the parameters. The tracking accuracy was measured by the successful detection rate in move events and division events. A move event refers to one cell moving from one frame to the next (no division happens) or newly appears in a frame.

4.3   Numerical Results

We choose to compare the performance of our algorithm with the n-coupled level sets (nLS) [1,11], the four-coupled level sets (4LS) [16], and a publicly available software: DCellIQ [21] based on [24,25], which adopts a "detection and then linking" strategy. We use our segmentation result from the first frame to initialize the n level set functions in nLS and the four level set functions in 4LS. Examples of segmentation results are shown in Figs. 4 and 5.

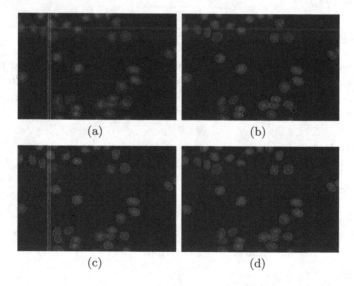

(a)   (b)

(c)   (d)

Fig. 4. Segmentation results on Hela1 dataset from (a) DCellIQ, (b) nLS, (c) 4LS, and (d) 3LS.

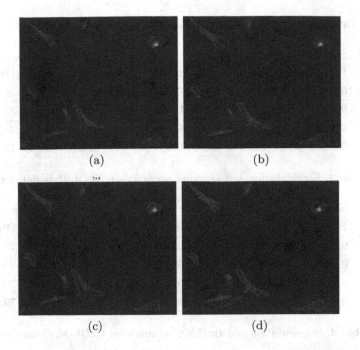

Fig. 5. Segmentation results on C2DL-MSC dataset from (a) DCellIQ, (b) nLS, (c) 4LS, and (d) 3LS.

The quantitative evaluation results are shown in Tables 2, 3, 4 and 5. 3LS's segmentation accuracy and tracking accuracy are notably higher than those of DCellIQ and nLS in all four datasets. For the Hela1 dataset, all method perform well in finding matched reference cells ('match' in Table 2) and achieve high recall of segmentation. DCellIQ and nLS perform poorer in the segmentation precision than 4LS and 3LS. 3LS is significantly better than DCellIQ, nLS and 4LS in tracking of cells in divisions. For the N2DL-Hela dataset, all accuracy measures are lower (Table 3), due to the fact that this sequence contains more nuclei of low intensity which are difficult for these two-phase level set based methods to detect. 3LS shows slight improvement of accuracy over 4LS on the two Hela datasets.

For the C2DL-MSC dataset, 3LS outperforms 4LS by around 15 % in both segmentation accuracy and tracking accuracy (Table 4). As a narrow-band approach, 4LS may be difficult to track drastically changed cell shapes across frames. Besides, its explicit topological coupling constraint can prevent false merging or absorption of neighboring cells; However, it lacks of a VCC term to handle touching cells smartly by making use of the area/volume information from the previous frame. For the C3DL-MDA231 dataset, a roughly 20 % increase in segmentation accuracy is achieved by 3LS (Table 5). Overall, 3LS is the most accurate method among the four methods under test.

The computational time per iteration of nLS and 3LS are compared in Table 6. Without VCC, i.e., the η_i term in Eqs. (1) and (10), the 3LS's computational time is only 3 % of the nLS's in the 2D image and 8 % in the 3D image. With the VCC

Table 2. Segmentation and tracking accuracy on Hela1 dataset.

Method	Segmentation				Tracking	
	Precision	Recall	F-score	Match	Move	Division
DCellIQ	0.727 ± 0.158	0.967 ± 0.167	0.825 ± 0.158	97.3%	83.9%	46.7%
nLS	0.769 ± 0.200	0.947 ± 0.179	0.838 ± 0.183	97.0%	94.9%	33.3%
4LS	0.857 ± 0.186	0.932 ± 0.162	0.885 ± 0.166	97.8%	92.7%	46.7%
3LS	0.840 ± 0.165	0.951 ± 0.162	0.887 ± 0.156	97.5%	96.9%	73.3%

Table 3. Segmentation and tracking accuracy on N2DL-Hela dataset.

Method	Segmentation				Tracking	
	Precision	Recall	F-score	Match	Move	Division
DCellIQ	0.514 ± 0.362	0.596 ± 0.408	0.543 ± 0.373	70.0%	64.1%	75.9%
nLS	0.613 ± 0.403	0.682 ± 0.415	0.635 ± 0.399	74.2%	76.1%	34.5%
4LS	0.718 ± 0.419	0.664 ± 0.387	0.684 ± 0.394	75.8%	77.0%	79.3%
3LS	0.705 ± 0.393	0.710 ± 0.399	0.700 ± 0.387	74.2%	78.0%	79.3%

Table 4. Segmentation and tracking accuracy on C2DL-MSC dataset.

Method	Segmentation				Tracking	
	Precision	Recall	F-score	Match	Move	Division
DCellIQ	0.646 ± 0.415	0.430 ± 0.313	0.505 ± 0.341	65.2%	60.1%	-
nLS	0.589 ± 0.444	0.436 ± 0.347	0.493 ± 0.377	64.3%	73.9%	-
4LS	0.584 ± 0.411	0.476 ± 0.343	0.513 ± 0.358	68.8%	79.2%	-
3LS	0.754 ± 0.340	0.604 ± 0.289	0.663 ± 0.301	83.9%	95.6%	-

Table 5. Segmentation and tracking accuracy on C3DL-MDA231 dataset.

Method	Segmentation				Tracking	
	Precision	Recall	F-score	Match	Move	Division
nLS	0.428 ± 0.354	0.572 ± 0.401	0.460 ± 0.342	70.0%	86.1%	-
4LS	0.570 ± 0.434	0.524 ± 0.380	0.528 ± 0.387	67.5%	89.1%	-
3LS	0.685 ± 0.283	0.782 ± 0.289	0.714 ± 0.267	90.0%	91.8%	-

Table 6. Computational time (sec) per iteration.

Method	2D (Hela1, 72 cells)		3D (C3DL-MDA231, 31 cells)	
	w/o VCC	with VCC	w/o VCC	with VCC
nLS	13.1	13.4	152	154
4LS	0.51	-	17.2	-
3LS	0.36	0.68	12.1	26.5

term, the 3LS's computational time is 5% of nLS's in 2D and 17% in 3D. This is because 3LS reduces the number of coupling terms from $O(N^2)$ to $O(1)$ for N objects. Comparing with the 4LS, the computational time of 3LS without VCC has also been reduced by 30%.

5 Conclusions

In this paper, a new algorithm for cell segmentation and tracking is proposed based on the coupled active contour framework. Two new solutions were presented to address the shortcomings of the original relevant algorithms. Specifically, we use only three level set functions to segment and track arbitrary number of cells in the image sequences, taking advantage of a vertex coloring approach in image graph representations. Also, we redefine the volume conservation constraint in the optimization functional. This is to reduce the undesirable shrinkage or expansion caused on the whole cell boundary. In addition, we develop an algorithm for touching cell separation in image segmentation, based on concave points and ellipse fitting. Experimental results show improved segmentation performance of our new algorithm, as well as tracking performance in terms of successful detection rates in move events and division events. Finally, the computational time of the new algorithm is notably reduced compared with the original n-coupled level set algorithm.

References

1. Dufour, A., Shinin, V., Tajbakhsh, S., Guillen, N., Olivo-Marin, J.C., Zimmer, C.: Segmenting and tracking fluorescent cells in dynamic 3-D microscopy with coupled active surfaces. IEEE Trans. Image Process. **14**, 1396–1410 (2005)
2. Zimmer, C., Zhang, B., Dufour, A., Thebaud, A., Berlemont, S., Meas-Yedid, V., Marin, J.C.O.: On the digital trail of mobile cells. IEEE Signal Process. Mag. **23**, 54–62 (2006)
3. Zhou, X., Yang, J., Wang, M., Wong, S.T.C.: A novel cell tracking algorithm and continuous hidden markov model for cell phase identification. In: IEEE/NLM Life Science Systems and Applications Workshop, Bethesda, MD, pp. 1–2 (2006)
4. Chen, X., Zhou, X., Wong, S.: Automated segmentation, classification, and tracking of cancer cell nuclei in time-lapse microscopy. IEEE Trans. Biomed. Eng. **53**, 762–766 (2006)
5. Zhou, X., Li, F., Yan, J., Wong, S.T.C.: A novel cell segmentation method and cell phase identification using markov model. IEEE Trans. Inf. Technol. Biomed. **13**, 152–157 (2009)
6. Li, F., Zhou, X., Ma, J., Wong, S.T.C.: Multiple nuclei tracking using integer programming for quantitative cancer cell cycle analysis. IEEE Trans. Med. Imaging **29**, 96–105 (2010)
7. Hu, Y., Osuna-Highley, E., Hua, J., Nowicki, T.S., Stolz, R., McKayle, C., Murphy, R.F.: Automated analysis of protein subcellular location in time series images. Bioinformatics **26**, 1630–1636 (2010)

8. Harder, N., Mora-Bermúdez, F., Godinez, W.J., Ellenberg, J., Eils, R., Rohr, K.: Automated analysis of the mitotic phases of human cells in 3D fluorescence microscopy image sequences. In: Larsen, R., Nielsen, M., Sporring, J. (eds.) MIC-CAI 2006. LNCS, vol. 4190, pp. 840–848. Springer, Heidelberg (2006)
9. Yang, X., Li, H., Zhou, X.: Nuclei segmentation using marker-controlled watershed, tracking using mean-shift, and kalman filter in time-lapse microscopy. IEEE Trans. Circ. Syst. I53, 2405–2414 (2006)
10. Zimmer, C., Labruyere, E., Meas-Yedid, V., Guillen, N., Olivo-Marin, J.C.: Segmentation and tracking of migrating cells in videomicroscopy with parametric active contours: a tool for cell-based drug testing. IEEE Trans. Med. Imaging 21, 1212–1221 (2002)
11. Zhang, B., Zimmer, C., Olivo-Marin, J.C.: Tracking fluorescent cells with coupled geometric active contours. In: Proceedings IEEE International Symposium on Biomedical Imaging (ISBI), pp. 476–479 (2004)
12. Mukherjee, D., Ray, N., Acton, S.: Level set analysis of leukocyte detection and tracking. IEEE Trans. Image Process. 13, 562–572 (2004)
13. Yang, F., Mackey, M.A., Ianzini, F., Gallardo, G., Sonka, M.: Cell segmentation, tracking, and mitosis detection using temporal context. In: Duncan, J.S., Gerig, G. (eds.) MICCAI 2005. LNCS, vol. 3749, pp. 302–309. Springer, Heidelberg (2005)
14. Padfield, D., Rittscher, J., Thomas, N., Roysam, B.: Spatio-temporal cell cycle phase analysis using level sets and fast marching methods. Med. Image Anal. 13, 143–155 (2009)
15. Dzyubachyk, O., Van Cappellen, W.A., Essers, J., Niessen, W.J., Meijering, E.: Advanced level-set based cell tracking in time-lapse fluorescence microscopy. IEEE Trans. Med. Imaging 29, 852–867 (2010)
16. Nath, S.K., Palaniappan, K., Bunyak, F.: Cell segmentation using coupled level sets and graph-vertex coloring. In: Larsen, R., Nielsen, M., Sporring, J. (eds.) MICCAI 2006. LNCS, vol. 4190, pp. 101–108. Springer, Heidelberg (2006)
17. Chan, T.F., Vese, L.A.: Active contours without edges. IEEE Trans. Image Process. 10, 266–277 (2001)
18. Thomas, R.: An update on the four-color theorem. Not. AMS 45, 848–859 (1998)
19. Bai, X., Sun, C., Zhou, F.: Splitting touching cells based on concave points and ellipse fitting. Pattern Recogn. 42, 2434–2446 (2009)
20. Brélaz, D.: New methods to color the vertices of a graph. Commun. ACM 22, 251–256 (1979)
21. DCellIQ: The Dynamic Cell Image Quantitator software package. http://www.cbi-tmhs.org/Dcelliq/index.html
22. ISBI: The First Cell Tracking Challenge. http://www.codesolorzano.com/celltrackingchallenge
23. Maška, M., Ulman, V., Svoboda, D., Matula, P., Matula, P., Ederra, C., Urbiola, A., España, T., Venkatesan, S., Balak, D.M., Karas, P., Bolcková, T., Štreitová, M., Carthel, C., Coraluppi, S., Harder, N., Rohr, K., Magnusson, K.E., Jaldén, J., Blau, H.M., Dzyubachyk, O., Krízek, P., Hagen, G.M., Pastor-Escuredo, D., Jimenez-Carretero, D., Ledesma-Carbayo, M.J., Muñoz-Barrutia, A., Meijering, E., Kozubek, M., Ortiz-de Solorzano, C.: A benchmark for comparison of cell tracking algorithms. Bioinformatics 30, 1609–1617 (2014)

24. Li, F., Zhou, X., Zhu, J., Ma, J., Huang, X., Wong, S.T.: High content image analysis for human h4 neuroglioma cells exposed to cuo nanoparticles. BMC Biotechnol. **7**, (2007). Article ID 66
25. Wang, M., Zhou, X., Li, F., Huckins, J., King, R.W., Wong, S.T.C.: Novel cell segmentation and online svm for cell cycle phase identification in automated microscopy. Bioinformatics **24**, 94–101 (2008)

OR-PCA with MRF for Robust Foreground Detection in Highly Dynamic Backgrounds

Sajid Javed[1], Seon Ho Oh[1], Andrews Sobral[2],
Thierry Bouwmans[2], and Soon Ki Jung[1][(✉)]

[1] School of Computer Science and Engineering, Kyungpook National University,
80 Daehak-ro, Buk-gu, Daegu 702-701, Republic of Korea
{sajid,shoh}@vr.knu.ac.kr, skjung@knu.ac.kr
[2] Laboratoire MIA (Mathematiques, Image et Applications),
Université de La Rochelle, 17000 La Rochelle, France
{andrews.sobral,thierry.bouwmans}@univ-lr.fr

Abstract. Accurate and efficient foreground detection is an important task in video surveillance system. The task becomes more critical when the background scene shows more variations, such as water surface, waving trees, varying illumination conditions, etc. Recently, *Robust Principal Components Analysis* (RPCA) shows a very nice framework for moving object detection. The background sequence is modeled by a low-dimensional subspace called *low-rank* matrix and *sparse error* constitutes the foreground objects. But RPCA presents the limitations of computational complexity and memory storage due to batch optimization methods, as a result it is difficult to apply for real-time system. To handle these challenges, this paper presents a robust foreground detection algorithm via *Online Robust PCA* (OR-PCA) using image decomposition along with continuous constraint such as *Markov Random Field* (MRF). OR-PCA with good initialization scheme using image decomposition approach improves the accuracy of foreground detection and the computation time as well. Moreover, solving MRF with graph-cuts exploits structural information using spatial neighborhood system and similarities to further improve the foreground segmentation in highly dynamic backgrounds. Experimental results on challenging datasets such as Wallflower, I2R, BMC 2012 and Change Detection 2014 dataset demonstrate that our proposed scheme significantly outperforms the state of the art approaches and works effectively on a wide range of complex background scenes.

1 Introduction

Foreground detection (also known as background subtraction) is one of the most important preprocessing step in many computer vision applications. Typically, the foreground detection process forms the first stage in automated visual surveillance systems, as well as other applications such as motion capture, object tracking and augmented reality.

Many algorithms have been developed to handle the problem of foreground detection in videos [1–3]. In recent years, *Robust Principal Component Analysis*

© Springer International Publishing Switzerland 2015
D. Cremers et al. (Eds.): ACCV 2014, Part III, LNCS 9005, pp. 284–299, 2015.
DOI: 10.1007/978-3-319-16811-1_19

(RPCA) based *low-rank* matrix decomposition algorithms have been used for foreground detection [4]. RPCA decomposes the original data matrix A as a sum of low-dimensional subspace called *low-rank* matrix L and correlated *sparse outliers* S. Figure 1 shows an example of foreground detection using RPCA of original images taken from i-LIDS dataset [5].

As RPCA based approaches provide a nice framework for foreground detection, but it currently faces two major difficulties. Traditional RPCA based approaches use batch optimization, e.g. in order to decompose *low-rank* and *sparse* components, a number of samples are required to store. Therefore, it suffers from high memory cost and computational complexity.

In order to tackle these issues, this paper presents a robust foreground detection algorithm via *Online Robust PCA* (OR-PCA) on decomposed images from input image. We briefly explain our methodology here: First, input image is decomposed into Gaussian and Laplacian images. Then, OR-PCA is applied to each Gaussian and Laplacian images for background modeling. Since Gaussian image is robust against noise of small pixel variations and Laplacian image preserves edge features. Therefore, our methodology improves the quality of foreground as well as computational time using alternative initialization scheme in OR-PCA. Finally, an MRF is utilized to exploit structural information and similarities to improve the foreground segmentation.

The rest of this paper is organized as follows. In Sect. 2, the related work is reviewed. Section 3 describes our methodology in detail. Experimental results are discussed in Sect. 4. Finally, conclusions are drawn in Sect. 5.

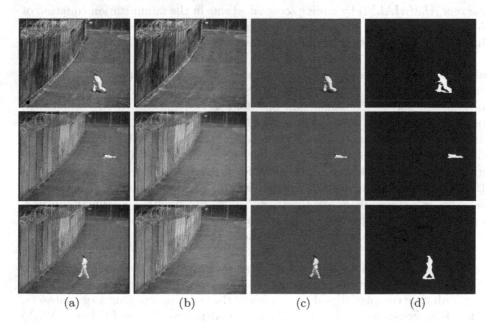

(a)   (b)   (c)   (d)

Fig. 1. An example of moving object detection using RPCA. From left to right: (a) input, (b) low-rank, (c) sparse component, and (d) foreground mask.

2   Related Work

Over the past few years, excellent methods have been proposed for foreground object detection and tracking. Among them, RPCA [6] shows promising results for background modeling. Excellent surveys on background modeling using RPCA can be found in [4,7]. All these RPCA approaches, such as *Augmented Lagrangian Multiplier* (ALM), *Singular Value Thresholding* (SVT) and *Linearized Alternating Direction Method with an Adaptive Penalty* (LADMAP) discussed in [4], solve the sub-optimization problem in each iteration under defined convergence criteria in order to separate the *low-rank* matrix and *sparse error*. All these methods work in a batch optimization manner, as a result memory storage and time complexity problems occur. Therefore *Principal Component Pursuit* (PCP) via batch optimization is not acceptable for real-time system.

Many noticeable improvements have been found in the literature to accelerate the PCP algorithms [8]. For example, Zhou *et al.* [9] proposed *Go Decomposition* (GoDec) which accelerates RPCA algorithm via PCP using *Bilateral Random Projections* (BRP) scheme to separate the *low-rank* and *sparse* matrix. Semi-Soft GoDec [9] method is an extension of GoDec which is four times faster than GoDec. It imposes hard thresholding scheme in *low-rank* and *sparse* matrix entries. In [10], Zhou *et al.* proposed *Detecting Contiguous Outliers in the low-rank Representation* (DECOLOR) method, which accelerates PCP algorithm by integrating the object detection and background learning into a single process of optimization. It also adds continuity constraints on *low-rank* and *sparse* components. In [11], a fast PCP algorithm is proposed, which reduces the SVD computational time in *inexact ALM* (IALM) by adding some constants in the minimization equation of *low-rank* and *sparse*. The results in background modeling case are very encouraging, but it is due to the base of PCP not desirable for real-time processing.

Incremental and *online robust* PCA methods are also developed for PCP algorithms. Fore example, in [12], He *et al.* proposed *Grassmanian Robust Adaptive Subspace Tracking Algorithm* (GRASTA), which is an incremental gradient descent method on Grassmannian manifold for solving the RPCA problem in online manner. In its each iteration, GRASTA uses the gradient of the updated augmented Lagrangian function after revealing a new sample to perform the gradient descent. Results are encouraging for background modeling, but no theoretic guarantee of the algorithm convergence for GRASTA is provided. Therefore, in [13], an online learning method for sparse coding and dictionary learning is proposed which efficiently solves the smooth non convex objective function over a convex set. A real-time processing is achieved, but it does not require learning rate tunning like regular stochastic gradient descents.

In [14], Guan *et al.* proposed *non-negative matrix factorization* (NMF) method which receives one chunk of samples per step and updates the basis accordingly. NMF converges faster in each step of basis update. But, using a buffering strategy both time complexity and space remain the issue for handling large datasets. Therefore, Feng and Xu [15] recently proposed *Online Robust-PCA* (OR-PCA) algorithm which processes one sample per time instance using stochastic approximations. In this approach, a nuclear norm objective function is reformulated and therefore all the samples are decoupled in optimization process for sparse error separation. In this work, we develop a background/foreground separation method based on the OR-PCA which is modified to be adapted for this application.

3   Methodology

In this section, we discuss our scheme for foreground detection in detail. Our methodology consists of several components which are described as a system diagram in Fig. 2.

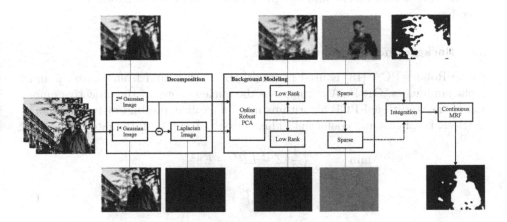

Fig. 2. Overview of our background modeling scheme.

Our methodology consists of four main stages: decomposition, background modeling, integration and continuous MRF. Initially, the input video frames are decomposed into Gaussian and Laplacian images using a set of two Gaussian kernels. Then, OR-PCA is applied to each of Gaussian and Laplacian images with different parameters to model the background, separately. In the background modeling stage, we have proposed an alternative initialization scheme to speed up the stochastic optimization process. Finally, the integration stage, which combines *low-rank* and *sparse* components obtained via OR-PCA to recover the background model and foreground image, is performed. The reconstructed sparse matrix is then thresholded to get the binary foreground mask. In order to improve the foreground segmentation, a MRF is applied which exploits structural information and similarities continuously. In the following sections, we will describe each module in detail.

3.1   Decomposition

In the first stage, two separate spatial Gaussian kernels are designed to decompose the input image into Gaussian and Laplacian images. First, Gaussian kernels are applied on the input image to get the Gaussian images. In the first case, we choose the standard deviation σ on the Gaussian kernel as 2 with a filter size of 5×5 to get the first Gaussian image. In the second case, we apply Gaussian kernel with a same σ value on the first blurred image due to its enough smoothing properties. Since the difference of Gaussians is approximately same as Laplacian of Gaussian, therefore Laplacian image is obtained by the difference of two Gaussian images.

Every input video frame is decomposed into Gaussian and Laplacian images using the method discussed above. As Gaussian image is robust against background variations and Laplacian image provides enough edge features for small pixels variations. Therefore, the false alarms are reduced from foreground region to some extent as a result, and our methodology provides accurate foreground detection.

3.2   Background Modeling

Online Robust PCA [15] is used to model the background from Gaussian and Laplacian images. OR-PCA decomposes the nuclear norm of the objective function of the traditional PCP algorithms into an explicit product of two *low-rank* matrices, i.e., basis and coefficient. Thus, OR-PCA can be formulated as

$$\min_{L \in \Re^{p \times n}, R \in \Re^{n \times r}, E} \left\{ \frac{1}{2} \| Z - LR^T - E \|_F^2 \right.$$

$$\left. + \frac{\lambda_1}{2} (\|L\|_F^2 + \|R\|_F^2) + \lambda_2 \|E\|_1 \right\}, \qquad (1)$$

where Z is an input data, L is a basis, R is a coefficient, and E is a sparse error. λ_1 controls the basis and coefficients for *low-rank* matrix, whereas λ_2 controls the sparsity pattern, which can be tunned according to video analysis. In addition, *basis* and *coefficient* depend on the value of *rank*.

In particular, the OR-PCA optimization consists of two iterative updating components. Firstly, the input video frame is projected onto current initialized basis and we separate the sparse noise component, which includes the outliers contamination. Then, the basis is updated with a new input video frame. More details can be found in [15].

The background sequence for each image is then modeled by a multiple of basis L and its coefficient R, whereas the sparse component E for each image constitutes the foreground objects.

Initialization. The number of subspace basis is randomly determined using improper value of *rank*, and no initialization method is considered for OR-PCA in [15]. The rank value R is 20 and $\lambda_1 = \lambda_2 = 0.01$ in Eq. (1). As a result, the algorithm converges slowly to the optimal solution and outliers appear in the *low-rank* matrix, which effects the *sparse* component as well as foreground mask for background modeling case, as shown in Fig. 3.

In order to meet the time complexity, the basis for low-dimensional subspace is initialized using first N video frames with a good selection of *rank*. Since we

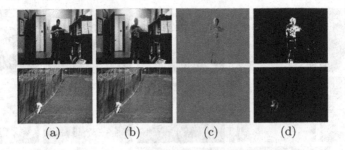

Fig. 3. OR-PCA failure using $r = 20$ and $\lambda_1 = \lambda_2 = 0.01$. From left to right: (a) input, (b) low-rank, (c) sparse component, and (d) foreground mask.

are applying OR-PCA on two images in our scheme, the basis for each image is initialized according to this scheme. In this case, the *rank* is a tunable parameter for each image, that will be discussed in the later section.

By this technique, the OR-PCA converges to the low-dimensional subspace faster than original one. The outliers are also reduced and good computational time is achieved without sacrificing the quality of foreground in surveillance case.

3.3   Integration

The *low-rank* and *sparse* components are obtained from each decomposed image after applying OR-PCA. Gaussian and Laplacian *low-rank* and *sparse* components are integrated in this step. We use different parameters setting for OR-PCA in Eq. (1) on each decomposed image. λ_1 is considered as a constant 0.01 for both images. λ_2 and rank r for Laplacian, whereas λ_2' and rank r' for Gaussian image are selected according to background scene, for obtaining enough sparsity pattern for each decomposed image.

Since Laplacian image provides enough edge features for small variations in background scene, therefore λ_2 must be smaller than λ_2'. After integrating both components of each image, the binary foreground mask f is then obtained by thresholding the integrated sparse component.

At this stage, the background subtraction scheme is good enough to deal with static and some small background dynamics such as slightly illumination changes, but it fails to handle highly dynamic backgrounds, where most part of the background pixels have high variations such as waving trees, water surface, rapid illumination changes, etc. For example, in Fig. 4 (a), (b) and (c) show the results of static and some small dynamic backgrounds. However, moving curtain and waving trees where most part of the background pixels are moving are shown in (d) and (e), respectively. We use the best parameters as $r = 1$ and $\lambda_2 = 0.03$ for both images in (a). Whereas in (b) and (c), $r = 1$, $r' = 3$, $\lambda_2 = 0.02$ and $\lambda_2' = 0.04$ are used for each decomposed images. Similarly, the best parameters are also considered for (d) and (e) as $r = 1$, $r' = 10$, $\lambda_2 = 0.02$ and $\lambda_2' = 0.06$, respectively.

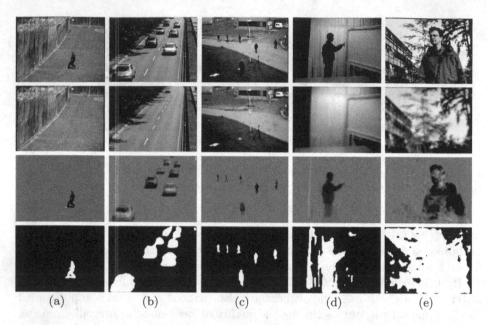

(a)   (b)   (c)   (d)   (e)

Fig. 4. OR-PCA via image decomposition. Input, low rank, sparse and foreground mask images are shown in each of rows.

OR-PCA on decomposed images without a continuous constraint is not robust to handle highly dynamic background scenes as mentioned above. As a result a large number of false alarms are generated, which is not useful for visual surveillance system. Therefore, we have employed a continuous constraint in the foreground mask such as MRF, which improves the quality of foreground segmentation in static as well as in highly dynamic backgrounds.

3.4 Improving Foreground Segmentation with MRF

The foreground labels can be not optimal, and therefore it can be improved with spatio-temporal constraints. In this paper, we utilize an MRF to optimize the labeling field. The MRF is a set of random variables having a Markov property described by an undirected graph.

Let us consider the foreground image f as a set of pixels $\mathcal{P}$ and a set of labels $\mathcal{L} = \{0, 1\}$, such that

$$f_p = \begin{cases} 0, & \text{if } p \text{ belongs to background,} \\ 1, & \text{if } p \text{ belongs to foreground.} \end{cases} \tag{2}$$

The goal is to find a labeling f which minimizes the energy function:

$$E(f) = \sum_{p \in P} D_p(f_p) + \sum_{p,q \in \mathcal{N}} V_{p,q}(f_p, f_q), \tag{3}$$

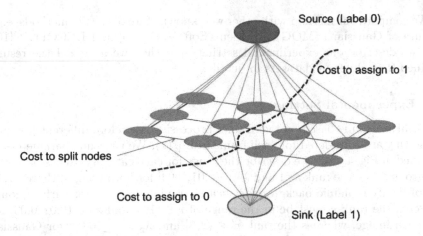

Fig. 5. Overview of solving MRF with graph cuts algorithm.

where $\mathcal{N} \subset \mathcal{P} \times \mathcal{P}$ is a neighborhood system on pixels. $D_p(f_p)$ is a function derived from the observed data that measures the cost of assigning the label f_p to the pixel p. $V_{p,q}(f_p, f_q)$ measures the cost of assigning the labels f_p, f_q to the adjacent pixels p, q. The energy functions like E are extremely difficult to minimize, however, as they are nonconvex functions in a space with many thousands of dimensions. In the last few years, however, efficient algorithms have been developed for these problems based on graph cuts.

The basic idea of graph cuts is to construct a directed graph $\mathcal{G} = (\mathcal{V}, \mathcal{E})$, where the vertices V stands for all pixels in image and edges E denotes spatially neighboring pixels having nonnegative weights that has two special vertices (terminals), namely, the source s and the sink t.

MRF that has such type of s-t graph is called graph-representable as shown in Fig. 5 and can be solved in polynomial time using graph cuts [16].

In this work, we have used the gco-v3.0 library[1] for optimizing multi-label energies via the α-expansion and α-β-swap algorithms. It supports energies with any combination of unary, pairwise, and label cost terms.

4   Experimental Results

In this section we present a set of both qualitative and quantitative experiments on four challenging datasets namely Change Detection[2] 2014 [17], Wallflower[3] [18], I2R[4] [19] and Background Models Challenge[5] (BMC) 2012 [20] dataset.

---

[1] http://vision.csd.uwo.ca/code/.

[2] http://www.changedetection.net/.

[3] http://research.microsoft.com/en-us/um/people/jckrumm/wallflower/testimages.htm.

[4] http://perception.i2r.a-star.edu.sg/bk_model/bk_index.html.

[5] http://bmc.univ-bpclermont.fr/.

We compare our method with other well known state of the art methods, e.g., Mixture of Gaussians (MOG) [21], Semi Soft GoDec [9] and DECOLOR [10]. First we describe our experimental settings and then we analyzed the results obtained from different datasets in detail.

4.1   Experimental Settings

As our algorithm is based on two frames processing, therefore different parameters setting are considered for each frame in Eq. (1). We use same parameters as described in Fig. 4. Here we describe the range for each category. In case of static backgrounds, we use rank as 1 and $\lambda_2 \in (0.01, 0.04]$ for both images. However, in case of highly dynamic backgrounds such as waving trees, water surface, fountain, etc., the rank r must be in the range of $r \in (1, 3]$ and $\lambda_2 \in (0.01, 0.03]$ for Laplacian image, whereas the rank $r' \in (r, 8]$ and $\lambda_2' \in (\lambda_2, 0.09]$ for Gaussian image, respectively. Similarly, for Bootstraping case, the rank $r \in (1, 5]$ and $\lambda_2 \in (0.01, 0.05)$ for Laplacian image and rank $r' \in (5, 10)$ and $\lambda_2' \in (0.03, 0.06]$ for Gaussian image.

4.2   Qualitative Analysis

Qualitative results are presented on selected video sequences from each dataset. Our algorithm is implemented in Matlab R2013a with 3.40 GHz Intel core i5 processor with 4 GB RAM. Additionally, 5×5 median filtering is applied as a post-processing step on binary foreground mask.

Change Detection 2014 Dataset. From Change Detection 2014 dataset [17], five sequences namely, office and pedestrains from category *baseline*, whereas canoe, fountain2 and overpass from category *dynamic backgrounds* are selected. The image size of each sequence is 320×240. Figure 6 shows the visual results of change detection dataset.

I2R Dataset. Five sequences namely, moving curtain, water surface, fountain, lobby and hall sequences are selected out of nine from I2R dataset [19]. Each sequence contains a 160×128 of frame size. Figure 7 shows results of I2R dataset.

Wallflower Dataset. Four sequences namely, waving trees, camouflage, foreground aperture (FA) and light switch (LS) sequences are taken out of seven from Wallflower dataset [18]. Each frame contains a frame size of 160×120. Figure 8 shows the qualitative results of wallflower dataset.

Background Models Challenge Dataset. Six sequences namely, Video 001, Video 002, Video 004, Video 005, Video 006 and Video 007 are tested out of nine from BMC 2012 dataset [20]. Each video sequence contains a frame size of 320×240. Figure 9 shows the qualitative results of BMC dataset with other state-of-the-art methods.

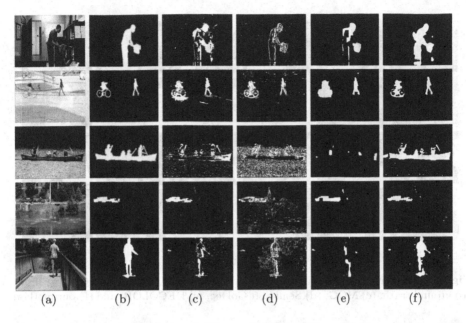

Fig. 6. Qualitative comparisons of Change Detection Dataset. From left to right: (a) input, (b) ground truth, (c) MOG, (d) Semi Soft GoDec, (e) DECOLOR, and (f) our method.

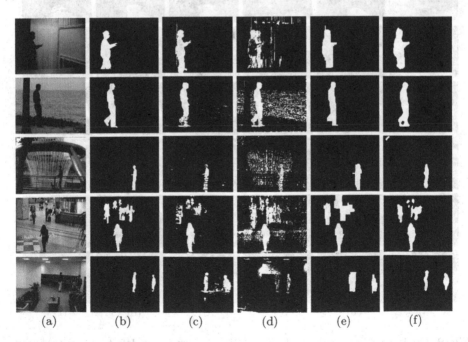

Fig. 7. Qualitative comparisons of I2R Dataset. From left to right: (a) input, (b) ground truth, (c) MOG, (d) Semi Soft GoDec, (e) DECOLOR, and (f) our method.

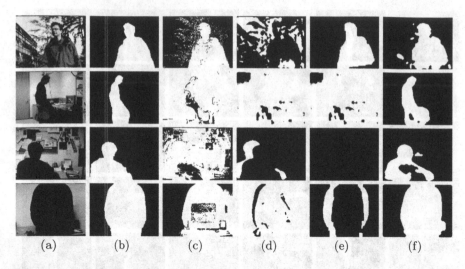

Fig. 8. Qualitative comparisons of Wallflower Dataset. From left to right: (a) input, (b) ground truth, (c) MOG, (d) Semi Soft GoDec, (e) DECOLOR, and (f) our method.

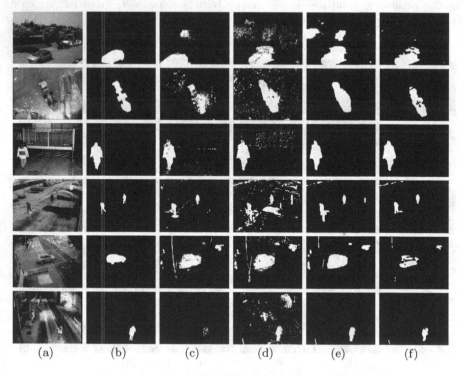

Fig. 9. Qualitative comparisons of BMC 2012 Dataset. From left to right: (a) input, (b) ground truth, (c) MOG, (d) Semi Soft GoDec, (e) DECOLOR, and (f) our method.

4.3   Quantitative Analysis

We also evaluate our algorithm quantitatively with other methods. *F-measure* score is computed for all sequences, by comparing our results with their available corresponding ground truth data. The *F-measure* is given as

$$F_{measure} = \frac{2 \times Recall \times Precision}{Recall + Precision},$$ (4)

where *Recall* and *Precision* are computed based on true positives, false positives and false negatives respectively. Wallflower, Change Detection and I2R datasets are quantitatively evaluated according to this criteria. But BMC 2012 is evaluated according to their provided procedural tool[6].

Table 1. Change Detection Dataset: *Comparison of F-measure score in % (direct one-to-one correspondence with Fig. 6).*

Method	Office	Pedestrians	Canoe	Fountain2	Overpass	Avg.
MOG	60.48	54.56	51.14	79.68	50.95	59.36
SemiSoft GoDec	56.02	70.31	30.91	31.38	55.17	48.75
DECOLOR	57.30	78.93	16.03	82.41	35.73	54.08
Ours	**88.30**	**86.43**	**85.34**	**85.17**	**82.72**	**85.59**

Table 2. I2R Dataset: *Comparison of F-measure score in % (direct one-to-one correspondence with Fig. 7).*

Method	Curtain	Water surface	Fountain	Hall	Lobby	Avg.
MOG	77.09	77.23	77.66	68.02	58.98	71.79
SemiSoft GoDec	43.44	44.73	25.74	57.13	36.02	41.45
DECOLOR	87.00	90.22	20.75	**81.69**	64.60	68.85
Ours	**89.20**	**91.66**	**82.83**	78.44	**80.81**	**84.58**

Table 3. Wallflower Dataset: *Comparison of F-measure score in % (direct one-to-one correspondence with Fig. 8).*

Method	Waving trees	LS	FA	Camouflage	Avg.
MOG	66.39	16.86	32.91	74.21	47.59
SemiSoft GoDec	18.29	26.71	24.51	66.31	33.95
DECOLOR	**88.45**	-	-	38.56	31.00
Ours	86.89	**85.17**	**69.10**	**91.18**	**83.08**

Tables 1, 2, 3 and 4 show the achieved performance on each dataset. In each case, our algorithm outperforms with other state of art methods, on average *F-measure* of 85.59 %, 84.58 %, 83.08 % and 86.19 % in each dataset, respectively.

---

[6] http://bmc.univ-bpclermont.fr/?q=node/7.

Table 4. BMC Dataset: *Comparison of PSNR/F-measure score in % (direct one-to-one correspondence with Fig.* 9).

Video	MOG	SemiSoft GoDec	DECOLOR	Ours
1	24.71/69.45	22.78/78.65	24.32/70.20	**35.06/89.16**
2	25.98/75.57	23.64/80.35	33.70/84.67	**34.11/86.18**
4	37.44/90.65	33.11/87.55	**46.35/95.52**	44.15/94.68
5	35.10/73.42	21.42/69.54	32.20/75.81	**40.38/79.17**
6	27.28/77.93	24.16/75.50	**28.12/78.89**	32.69/76.80
7	43.67/76.10	26.19/72.27	**53.71/93.51**	51.69/91.19
Avg.	32.36/77.18	25.21/77.31	36.40/83.10	**39.68/86.19**

Time Complexity. The computational time is also investigated during our experiments. The computational time is recorded frame by frame in seconds and the average time of first hundred frames is computed of different frame size. In our method, time is proportional to the value of rank. Table 5 shows the comparison of computational time.

Time is computed for each case according to our experimental settings discussed above. Since traditional RPCA via PCP based algorithms, either gets fail to load large amount of input video frames or take longer time for optimization which is not useful for real time processing. However in our approach, we have achieved a real time processing using initialization scheme with OR-PCA, moreover image decomposition together with continuous contraint improves the quality of foreground. These good experimental both qualitative and quantitative evaluations are the consequences of our proposed OR-PCA based scheme.

Discussion. We also apply OR-PCA including MRF on input images to compare our performance with decomposed images. As discussed above, decomposed images accurately detect the foreground mask and increase the *F-measure* score. Therefore we visually analyze some sequences such as WT and pedestrians as shown in Fig. 10 to show that OR-PCA using decomposed images along with MRF provides good segmentation results and best *F-measure* as compare to apply it on input images. In each case, our algorithm gives best *F-measure*

Table 5. Comparison of computational time in *seconds*.

Cases	Frame size	OR-PCA	Ours
Static	576 × 720	0.5120	**0.0512**
	288 × 360	0.1226	**0.0140**
Dynamic	240 × 320	0.130	**0.0281**
	120 × 160	0.0260	**0.0074**
Bootstrap	256 × 320	0.1166	**0.0468**
	128 × 160	0.0213	**0.0149**

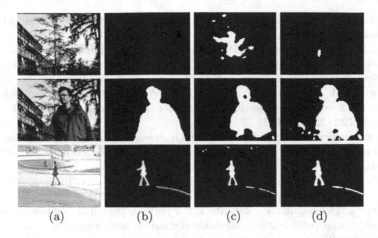

(a)   (b)   (c)   (d)

Fig. 10. From left to right: (a) input, (b) groundtruth, (c) OR-PCA with MRF on input image, and (d) ORPCA with MRF on decomposed images.

score, e.g., 95.65 %, 86.89 % and 96.25 %, respectively, whereas 78.65 %, 79.10 %, and 89.50 % are observed in case of input image.

5 Conclusion

In this paper, a robust background modeling method against challenging background scenes is presented using OR-PCA via image decomposition with continuous MRF. Our methodology is robust against different background dynamics. We first decompose the input image then OR-PCA with initialization scheme including continuous constraint is applied with parameters tuning. As a result, computational complexity is reduced as compare to other PCP methods, and foreground segmentation is improved significantly, due to spatial Gaussian kernels and structural information in MRF. Experimental evaluations and comparisons with other state of the art methods show the effectiveness and robustness of our proposed scheme.

However, we just applied OR-PCA on two decomposed images and parameters are tuned manually. Therefore, our future work will focus more on brief analysis of each layer of hierarchical image decomposition with dynamical parameters setting, which adapts changes according to background dynamics.

Acknowledgments. This work is supported by the World Class 300 project, Development of HD video/network-based video surveillance system(10040370), funded by the Ministry of Trade, Industry, and Energy (MOTIE), Korea.

References

1. Bouwmans, T., El Baf, F., Vachon, B., et al.: Statistical background modeling for foreground detection: a survey. In: Handbook of Pattern Recognition and Computer Vision, pp. 181–199 (2010)

2. Bouwmans, T.: Traditional and recent approaches in background modeling for foreground detection: an overview. Comput. Sci. Rev. **11**, 31–66 (2014)
3. Oh, S.H., Javed, S., Jung, S.K.: Foreground object detection and tracking for visual surveillance system: a hybrid approach. In: 2013 11th International Conference on Frontiers of Information Technology (FIT), pp. 13–18 (2013)
4. Bouwmans, T., Zahzah, E.H.: Robust PCA via principal component pursuit: a review for a comparative evaluation in video surveillance. Comput. Vis. Image Underst. **122**, 22–34 (2014)
5. Home Office Scientific Development Branch: Imagery library for intelligent detection systems I-LIDS. In: The Institution of Engineering and Technology Conference on Crime and Security, pp. 445–448 (2006)
6. Candès, E.J., Li, X., Ma, Y., Wright, J.: Robust principal component analysis? J. ACM (JACM) **58**, 11–37 (2011)
7. Guyon, C., Bouwmans, T., Zahzah, E.H.: Robust principal component analysis for background subtraction: systematic evaluation and comparative analysis, pp. 223–228 (2012)
8. Javed, S., Oh, S.H., Heo, J., Jung, S.K.: Robust background subtraction via online robust PCA using image decomposition. In: Proceedings of the 2014 Research in Adaptive and Convergent Systems, pp. 90–96 (2014)
9. Zhou, T., Tao, D.: Godec: randomized low-rank & sparse matrix decomposition in noisy case. In: Proceedings of the 28th International Conference on Machine Learning (ICML 2011), pp. 33–40 (2011)
10. Zhou, X., Yang, C., Yu, W.: Moving object detection by detecting contiguous outliers in the low-rank representation. IEEE Trans. Pattern Anal. Mach. Intell. **35**, 597–610 (2013)
11. Rodriguez, P., Wohlberg, B.: Fast principal component pursuit via alternating minimization. In: 20th IEEE International Conference on Image Processing (ICIP), pp. 69–73 (2013)
12. He, J., Balzano, L., Lui, J.: Online robust subspace tracking from partial information. http://arxiv.org/abs/1109.3827 (2011)
13. Mairal, J., Bach, F., Ponce, J., Sapiro, G.: Online learning for matrix factorization and sparse coding. J. Mach. Learn. Res. **11**, 19–60 (2010)
14. Guan, N., Tao, D., Luo, Z., Yuan, B.: Online nonnegative matrix factorization with robust stochastic approximation. IEEE Trans. Neural Netw. Learn. Syst. **23**, 1087–1099 (2012)
15. Feng, J., Xu, H., Yan, S.: Online robust PCA via stochastic optimization. In: Advances in Neural Information Processing Systems, pp. 404–412 (2013)
16. Kolmogorov, V., Zabin, R.: What energy functions can be minimized via graph cuts? IEEE Trans. Pattern Anal. Mach. Intell. **26**, 147–159 (2004)
17. Goyette, N., Jodoin, P., Porikli, F., Konrad, J., Ishwar, P.: Changedetection.net: a new change detection benchmark dataset. In: IEEE Computer Society Conference on Computer Vision and Pattern Recognition Workshops (CVPRW), pp. 1–8 (2012)
18. Toyama, K., Krumm, J., Brumitt, B., Meyers, B.: Wallflower: principles and practice of background maintenance. In: The Proceedings of the Seventh IEEE International Conference on Computer Vision, pp. 255–261 (1999)
19. Li, L., Huang, W., Gu, I.H., Tian, Q.: Statistical modeling of complex backgrounds for foreground object detection. IEEE Trans. Image Process. **13**, 1459–1472 (2004)

20. Vacavant, A., Chateau, T., Wilhelm, A., Lequièvre, L.: A benchmark dataset for outdoor foreground/background extraction. In: Park, J.-I., Kim, J. (eds.) ACCV Workshops 2012, Part I. LNCS, vol. 7728, pp. 291–300. Springer, Heidelberg (2013)
21. Stauffer, C., Grimson, W.E.L.: Adaptive background mixture models for real-time tracking. In: IEEE Computer Society Conference on Computer Vision and Pattern Recognition, vol. 2. IEEE (1999)

Segmentation of Cells from Spinning Disk Confocal Images Using a Multi-stage Approach

Saad Ullah Akram[1,2]([✉]), Juho Kannala[1], Mika Kaakinen[2,3], Lauri Eklund[2,3],
and Janne Heikkilä[1]

[1] Center for Machine Vision Research, University of Oulu, Oulu, Finland
{sakram,jkannala,jth}@ee.oulu.fi
[2] Biocenter Oulu, University of Oulu, Oulu, Finland
[3] Faculty of Biochemistry and Molecular Medicine, University of Oulu, Oulu, Finland
{mika.kaakinen,lauri.eklund}@oulu.fi

Abstract. Live cell imaging in 3D platforms is a highly informative approach to visualize cell function and it is becoming more commonly used for understanding cell behavior. Since these experiments typically generate large data sets their analysis manually would be very laborious and error prone. This has led to the necessity of automatic image analysis tools. Cell segmentation is an essential initial step for any detailed automatic quantitative analysis. When the images are captured from the 3D culture containing proliferating and moving cells, cell-cell interactions and collisions cannot be avoided. In these conditions the segmentation of individual cells becomes very challenging. Here we present a method which utilizes the edge probability map and graph cuts to detect and segment individual cells from cell clusters. The main advantage of our method is that it is capable of handling complex cell shapes because it does not make any assumptions about the cell shape.

1 Introduction

Imaging of living cells in 3D environments is becoming more and more essential tool to experimentally approach the fundamental questions about cell dynamics, molecular regulation of cell migration, cell invasion and cell fates. 3D scaffolds provide more realistic platform for cell cultures with respect to the physical and biochemical properties of the micro-environment compared to 2D models. This aspect is especially important in tumor cell cultures in which the composition of the micro-environment contributes to the cell behavior and drug response [1]. As in 2D cultures the cells can be labeled with fluorescent dyes to help resolve them from the background. However, in order to get statistically meaningful results especially for high-throughput screening the cell density should be considerably high. In addition many cell types, such as epithelial and endothelial cells preferentially form cell-cell contacts. In such conditions the incidences of cell collisions and cell clustering increase. Many existing solutions for segmenting individual cells from cell clusters in 3D environments have been applied to cell nuclei, which, unlike the cells themselves, retain rather constant shape over

D. Cremers et al. (Eds.): ACCV 2014, Part III, LNCS 9005, pp. 300–314, 2015.
DOI: 10.1007/978-3-319-16811-1_20

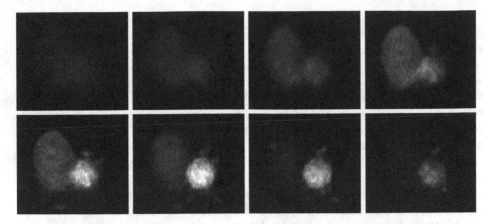

Fig. 1. Optical slices of cells expressing green fluorescent protein (GFP) captured using spinning-disk confocal microscope. From left to right: Slice # 1, 5, 9, 13, 17, 21, 25 and 29 of a cell cluster. Slices towards cluster extremities are very blurred.

time [2–4]. Shortcoming in nuclear labeling is that only a small fraction of cell is made visible and no conclusion on cell shape or extremities that mediate cell-cell interactions can be made. Moreover, use of nuclear dyes, which are typically excited with high energy low wavelength light, may adversely affect cell viability. Due to these factors, we decided to develop a segmentation method which can efficiently detect individual cells from cell clusters in 3D time-lapse image sequences without using nuclear labeling.

Confocal microscopy techniques have become a standard method for 3D imaging of fluorescently labeled cells, however, they have lower resolution in z-direction compared to resolution within a slice. Spinning disk confocal system allow lower photo toxicity and fluorophore bleaching, and faster image acquisition rates than laser scanning confocal microscopes, thus advancing long term live cell imaging in 3D. However, spinning disk provides lower confocality resulting in some blurring in z-direction due to light emitted by out of focus fluorescently labeled structures. Deconvolution can reduce this type of blurring but does not always completely eliminate it. This blurring as shown in Fig. 1 makes it more challenging to find accurate boundaries between cells.

2 Related Work

Cell segmentation is a very broad research area due to wide variability in imaging modalities, cell lines, stains, cell densities, acceptable level of manual oversight, etc. We restrict ourselves to only fluorescent microscopy case. The initial cell segmentation approaches used intensity thresholding, which is still popular [5] and common in general purpose software due to its simplicity, acceptable quality in many restricted situations and lack of any other general user-friendly method.

In dense samples, cells often come in contact with each other and form clusters. To separate individual cells from these clusters is one of the major challenges in cell segmentation. Difficulty of this task is due to lack of strong edges between cells (in case their intensity is similar), presence of strong edges within cells (due to non-homogeneous staining) and ability of cells to take wide variety of shapes. One common approach [2, 6] to solve this issue is to assume that cells have a convex shape and when they form a cluster it results in creation of concave regions. Points in these concave regions on cell boundaries are detected and then lines are drawn between these points that minimize some cost function. This approach [2] has been used to segment 3D cells by processing image stack slice by slice and considering split lines in neighboring slices to maintain spatial coherence in z-direction. These methods usually require setting multiple parameters, which is difficult for many challenging sequences.

Another common approach is to detect some key-points or regions, one for each cell, and use them to initialize level sets, watershed, or graph-cuts, for instance to obtain cell segmentation. The performance of these methods depends heavily on detection of seeds, which control where and how many cells will be detected. Some simpler methods use local peaks of intensity and distance transform [7] for seed detection. These methods suffer from over segmentation as they are sensitive to cell texture and small shape distortions. Most popular methods for detecting seeds use multi-scale blob detectors based on LoG (laplacian of gaussian) [8,9] or Hessian of gaussian [10]. They either use same scale along all axes [8] or in more general case [9] allow blobs to have different sizes along different dimensions in addition to allowing them to rotate.

Another promising method [11] creates a tree of cell candidate regions using MSER, which are scored based on a learnt cell appearance model. Then dynamic programming is used to pick non-overlapping candidates which maximize the total score. This approach unlike other methods does not make any assumption about cell shapes and learns them from training data and as a result has the potential of handling more challenging sequences.

Graph cuts have been used in the past for nuclei segmentation. Both [7,8] first used graph cuts to find the binary labeling, then they detected seeds and found initial rough segmentation. Finally they refined the segmentation boundary by using the initial segmentation and seeds to create a new multi-label graph, which they solved using α-*expansion* and α-β-*swap* algorithms [12]. Our method has similar structure but differs from them in details of how binary labeling, cell seeds and final segmentation are found. Since we use edge probabilities instead of blob detection [8] and distance transform [7] for cluster splitting, our method can cope with more challenging shapes.

3   Method

This section outlines our cell segmentation method, which is also shown in Fig. 2. Our method consists of four (for 2D images) or five (for 3D image stacks) stages. First, image is pre-processed using median filtering and edge detector is used to

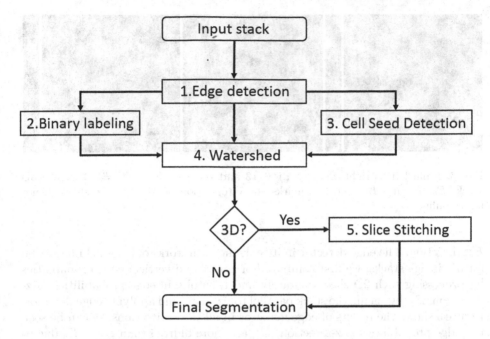

Fig. 2. Flow chart showing the overview of our method.

compute edge probability at each pixel. Next, cells are separated from background using graph cuts, in which the intensity in local neighborhood of a pixel is used to set terminal edge weights. In the third stage, seeds for individual cells are found using another graph cuts stage, in which edge probability map is used to adjust terminal edge weights. This is our main contribution as we propose a new method for locating seeds for individual cells within a cell cluster without making any assumption about cell shape. In the fourth stage, marker-controlled watershed is used to find boundaries of individual cells. Since we are working with an-isotropic 3D data, with low z-direction resolution and some blurring, direct extension of this method to 3D faces some additional challenges. To overcome them, we first segment all 2D slices in a 3D stack and then in the fifth stage 3D cell segmentation is obtained by connecting segmented objects within adjacent segmented slices.

3.1 Edge Probability Map

We have used a state of the art edge detector [13] to generate an edge probability map. This edge detector computes a large set of features from image gradients within a small patch around a pixel at multiple scales and uses structured random trees to output edge mask in a small section of input patch. The contribution of multiple trees and output patches which overlap a given pixels are averaged to obtain edge probability at that pixel. We train it to output edge probabilities at each pixel, E, as well as edge probability in both horizontal, E_h, and vertical,

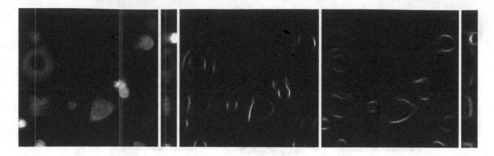

Fig. 3. From left to right: Slice (XY) # 13 and vertical slice (YZ) # 60 from a 3D stack, E_h, E_v and E_z. Red line marks the intersection of XY and YZ slices (Color figure online).

E_v, direction. The edge detector in its current form works only on 2D images. So for 3D image stacks, we first compute horizontal and vertical edge probabilities by processing each 2D slice separately and then obtain edge probabilities in z-direction, E_z, by slicing the stack parallel to yz-plane and applying edge detector. Figure 3 shows the results of edge detector in all three directions, as can be seen the edge probabilities in z-direction, E_z, are more blurred than E_h or E_v due to factors mentioned in Sect. 1.

3.2 Graph Structure

We use two separate graphs for binary labeling and cell seed detection. This section details the common elements of these graphs. We represent a 2D image (slice in the case of 3D image stack) by a two terminal grid based graph. Every pixel in the image is represented by a node, referred to as grid node in the text. Each grid node is connected to its neighboring grid nodes, we have used 4-connected neighborhood. Each grid node is also connected to two terminal nodes, source node is labeled cell/foreground and the sink node is labeled background. The details of how the costs of edges between grid nodes and terminal nodes are selected are provided in Sects. 3.3 and 3.4.

The cost of edge between neighboring grid nodes is used to enforce spatial smoothness. It is the cost which has to be paid for assigning different labels to two neighboring pixels. If both neighboring pixels are assigned same label then no cost is paid. At the boundary between multiple touching cells and between cells and background, this cost has to be low so that these pixels are not over-penalized. Everywhere else this cost has to be high. We have used the difference of edge probabilities at neighboring grid nodes to set this cost according to:

$$edge(p, q) = C * \exp(\frac{-|E_d(p) - E_d(q)|}{\sigma}) \tag{1}$$

where $edge(p, q)$ is the cost of edge between two neighboring grid nodes, p and q, $E_d \in \{E_h, E_v\}$ is the edge probability value at p and q in the direction, d, of edge

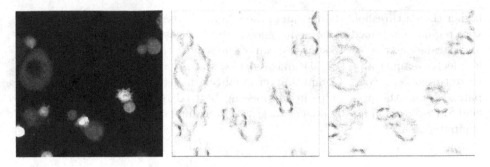

Fig. 4. Edge costs. From left to right: Slice from a 3D stack, $edge_h(p,q)$ and $edge_v(p,q)$.

between them. C is the maximum cost that a grid edge can take and it is used to adjust the relative importance of terminal edges and neighborhood edges. σ controls how quickly cost decreases as edge probability difference increases. Figure 4 shows the costs of edges between grid nodes which are neighbors in horizontal and vertical direction. Bright values indicate high cost edges which can not be easily cut and dark values indicate low cost edges, which can be easily cut to assign different label to neighboring nodes.

3.3   Binary Labeling

Binary labeling, which separates cell pixels from background pixels, is needed to ensure that cell seeds do not expand into background regions when watershed is applied to obtain cell boundaries. This stage is relatively easy but it still involves some challenges due to photo bleaching and in-homogeneous absorption of fluorescent dyes. There are cells which are very dark and can only be spotted by a human observer when carefully going through the image. Attempting to detect these cells has a trade-off, as any attempt to detect these dim cells results in inclusion of blurred regions around cells, especially in z-direction, in the final cell segmentation. This effect can be seen in Fig. 3, where blurred region above a bright cell (top left corner in XY slice) has higher intensity than one darker cell (above bottom right corner in XY slice).

Cell density and intensity profiles of individual cells differ significantly both between sequences and within any particular sequence and the distribution of image stack intensities has a very large peak at the beginning (dark background pixels) which gradually dies as intensity increases and a second much smaller peak at the highest intensity (due to overexposure). These issues make it difficult to automatically select a good cell intensity model, which is needed to set the cost of terminal edges of graphs. Otsu thresholding and clustering based solutions usually resulted in much higher threshold and they were only able to detect bright cells. To ensure that we are able to detect dim cells, we have computed terminal edge costs using a small window (larger than most cells) around each pixel. At each pixel, contrast in the window is computed. If the contrast is higher than a threshold then mean of the window is used as parameter, τ, otherwise region is assumed to be homogeneous (and consisting only of background) and parameter, τ, is set to sum of mean of the window and a parameter γ, which is selected empirically. For 3D image stacks, we use a 3D window to compute the terminal edge costs. Computing terminal cost using intensities within a local patch around the pixel helps in suppressing blurred regions around cells especially in z-direction for 3D image stacks. The terminal edge cost for this step are computed using:

$$edge(BG, p) = \exp(\frac{-I(p)}{\tau(p)}) \tag{2}$$

$$edge(FG, p) = 1 - \exp(\frac{-I(p)}{\tau(p)}) \tag{3}$$

where $edge(FG, p)$ is the cost of edge connecting the grid node p to *source* (*cell/foreground*) node, $edge(BG, p)$ is the cost of edge connecting the grid node p to *sink(background)* node, $I(p)$ is the intensity at grid node p and $\tau(p)$ is the parameter value at p, which incorporates neighborhood information.

The edge cost between neighboring grid nodes is computed using Eq. (1) but a low value of C is chosen so that fine structures at cell boundaries are preserved. The overall function which has to be minimized by min-cut in this stage is:

$$E = \sum_{p \in P}(edge(L_p, p) + \sum_{q \in N(p)} edge(p, q) * (L_p \neq L_q)) \tag{4}$$

where P contains all pixels in the image, L_p and $L_q \in \{FG, BG\}$ are the labels for pixels at location p and q. $N(p)$ is the set of all 4-connected neighbors of node p. The first term, data term, in the above energy function forces bright pixels to be labeled as cell and dark pixels as background, while the second term, boundary term, ensures that there is spatial continuity in the labels of pixels by penalizing neighboring pixels which have different labels. Min-cut of this graph which minimizes Eq. (4), separates pixels into two classes, cell and background (cell matrix). Figure 5 shows the costs of terminal edges and final labeling for one slice from a 3D stack.

Since we are using a two terminal graph, its minimal cut can be computed quickly. However for large image stacks, minimum cut solvers can still take significant memory so we have used Grid Cut [14], a fast multi-core max-flow/min-cut solver with a low memory footprint, to find the min-cut of our graphs.

3.4 Cell Seed Detection

In this section, we describe how we use edge probability map to create a barrier between touching cells within a cell cluster and use it to find cell seeds. We create a second grid graph as described in Sect. 3.2. The cost of edges between neighboring grid nodes is computed using Eq. (1) but for this graph we choose a higher value of C so that high edge probabilities within cell body due to inhomogeneous staining do not result in detection of multiple seeds. To separate

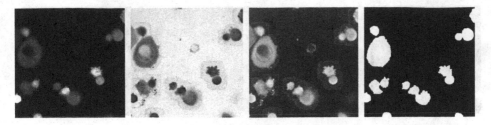

Fig. 5. Binary segmentation. From left to right: Slice from a 3D stack, edge(BG,p), edge(FG,p), binary labeling.

touching cells, we need to create a barrier between them. We create this barrier by using the edge probability map, which has high values at boundaries between cells and between cells and background. We increase the cost of edge between a grid node and background terminal node where edge probability is high. Similarly we decrease the cost of edge between a grid node and foreground terminal node where edge probability is high. This modification in terminal edge costs compensates for extra cost that has to be paid for assigning background labels to boundary pixels between cells. The cost of edges between terminal nodes and grid nodes for this graph are computed using:

$$edge(BG, p) = \exp(\frac{-I(p)}{\tau(p)}) + D * E(p) \qquad (5)$$

$$edge(FG, p) = 1 - \exp(\frac{-I(p)}{\tau(p)}) - D * E(p) \qquad (6)$$

$E(p)$ is the edge probability at pixel p obtained from edge detector, D is the parameter which controls how much adjustment is needed to terminal edge costs and is selected experimentally. If the edge probability map is very accurate and sharp then a low value suffices but when the edges are blurred and their probability is not very high, then a higher value has to be set to counteract the influence of high intensity at boundary pixels between cells and force the pixels to belong to background. The overall energy function which has to be minimized is:

$$E = \sum_{p \in P}((\exp(\frac{-I(p)}{\tau}) + D * E(p)) * (L_p == FG)$$

$$+(1 - \exp(\frac{-I(p)}{\tau}) - D * E(p)) * (L_p == BG) + \sum_{q \in N(p)} edge(p, q) * (L_p \neq L_q))$$

$$(7)$$

This function is minimized by the labeling which assigns pixels with low intensity and pixels with high edge probabilities, the background label and pixels with high intensity and low edge probability, the foreground (cell) label. We find the connected components within pixels labeled as cell and use them as cell seeds.

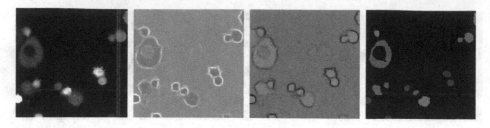

Fig. 6. Cell seed detection. From left to right: Slice from a 3D stack, edge(BG,p), edge(FG,p) and labeled cell seeds.

Figure 6 depicts the costs of terminal nodes for one slice from a 3D stack in addition to the final detected seeds, which are labeled by seven repeating colors.

3.5 Watershed

Once we have obtained cell seeds, we can use multi-label graph cuts or watershed for finding the cell region/boundaries. Multi-label graph cuts have been used in the past [8] for this task but they require a cell intensity and shape model to compute the cost of assigning a pixel to each of the terminal nodes. When cells intensity profiles and shapes vary significantly, then use of simple model like Gaussian model, especially for shape modeling, results in poor performance. This is why we have decided to use watershed for this task. There are two obvious candidates for topographic relief images, edge probability map and intensity image, which can be used by watershed but they both have their weaknesses. There is not always enough difference between the intensity of touching cells to prevent expansion of one cell into another. There are also sometimes holes in the edge probability map, which allow one cell to expand into another. We have therefore decided to combine these two images according to $R = E - I$ and use the resulting image, R, as the topographic relief for watershed. Figure 7 shows these three different topographic reliefs. This results in better performance by combining the strengths of both intensity (good barrier when intensity of touching cells is different) and edge probability map (good barrier where edge probability map is accurate). We also use the binary labeling from Sect. 3.3 to create a fence (by setting high value to boundary pixels) around foreground pixels to restrict cells from expanding into background region. Then local minima are created at cell seed locations and watershed transform is used to find the cell boundary within a cell cluster.

3.6 Slice Stitching

The method described so far can be extended to 3D and used for isotropic 3D stacks. However, we are working with an-isotropic 3D stacks, with lower z-direction resolution and blurring as mentioned in Sect. 1 and shown in Figs. 1 and 3. This often results in either significant distortion in shape of some cells

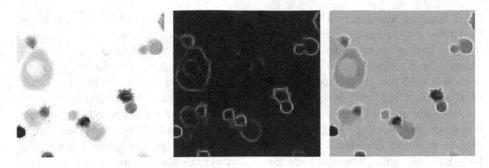

Fig. 7. Watershed relief. From left to right: Negative intensity image, edge probability image and combination of edge and intensity image, R.

or failure to separate individual cells from a cell cluster. In order to solve these problems we have decided to process 3D stacks slice by slice in 2D to obtain initial 3D segmented stack and then merging the segmented objects in adjacent slices to obtain final 3D segmentation of cells.

When computing edge probability map for each optical slice independently, there arise situations, due to local variations in intensities, in which boundary between cells within a cluster in some slices do not have high probabilities. In addition to that near the extremities of cell clusters boundaries are also much less pronounced due to blurring. These factors result in segmentation errors in few slices. We deal with these errors by using segmentation of maximum intensity image to guide slice merging process. For each detected cell in maximum intensity projection, the best match based on overlap, ratio of area of their intersection and union, is found in slice M of initial 3D segmented stack. This best matched object is usually one of the sharpest slice of that cell. This cell is then expanded in both z-directions by searching for best matching object, based on overlap and chi-squared distance of their intensity histograms, in neighboring slice on each side, slice $M + 1$ and $M - 1$. If a match is found on any side then it is assigned the same label as that of current cell and placed in final segmented stack. The cell template on that side is also updated for further search. If no good match is found then search is performed in next couple of slices. If a match is found then previous cell template is used to fill in the missing slices, otherwise search is terminated in that direction. Once all the objects in maximum intensity projected image are processed, then search is performed for leftover connected objects in initial 3D segmented stack. If any object persists, has good overlap with objects in neighboring slices and they have similar intensity profile, for multiple slices then it is also included in the final segmented 3D stack.

4   Results

We have used two sequences, $S1$ and $S2$, for evaluating our segmentation method. Both contain squamous cell carcinoma cells (HSC3) genetically labeled with

GFP. Imaging was done with EC Plan NeoFluar 40x/0.75 air objective and Zeiss Cell Observer spinning disc confocal microscope equipped with CO_2, humidity and temperature controlled top stage incubator. Sequence $S1$ contains 59 image stacks, consisting of 30 slices of 512×512 resolution with voxel size of $0.3 \times 0.3 \times 0.6$ μm. Whereas sequence $S2$ contains 156 image stacks, consisting of 47 slices of 512×512 resolution with voxel size of $0.3 \times 0.3 \times 1.5$ μm.

We have performed quantitative analysis only for sequence $S1$ because it has sparser cell density and more rigid cell shapes. Since it is very labor intensive to generate detailed (pixel level labeling) good quality ground truth, we have used bounding boxes of cells for evaluating our segmentation method. The ground truth was generated by marking a rectangle on the maximum intensity image from the top view, then two side views (maximum intensity projections) of the selected volume were displayed and the cell's bounds in z-direction were marked in the view which best separated it from other cells and background. The bounding boxes accurately marked the bounds of most cells but there were instances in which better bounding boxes could have been drawn by inspection of all slices at the expense of lot more manual effort. We have excluded cells which were mostly outside the volume being imaged or that were on the boundary but below a certain size from evaluation.

A cell detection is considered a potential true detection (true positive) if overlap of its bounding box, D, with bounding box of any cell in ground truth data, GT, is above a threshold, 0.5. Munkres assignment algorithm [15] with cost $1 - overlap(D, GT)$ is used to find bipartite matching between detected cells and ground truth cells. The overlap is computed using:

$$overlap(D, GT) = \frac{|D \cap GT|}{|D \cup GT|} \tag{8}$$

We evaluate the performance of segmentation using precision and recall. Precision measures the proportion of detected cells that are also present in ground truth data, while recall measures the proportion of cells in the ground truth that are correctly detected. To get a single number for comparing different segmentation methods and selecting parameters, we have used F-measure:

$$F = 2 * \frac{Precision * Recall}{Precision + Recall} \tag{9}$$

There are neither many openly available cell segmentation methods nor commonly used datasets, which makes it difficult to compare different methods. We have used segmentation method [8] provided in Farsight toolkit as a baseline because its code is openly available and it uses a method from a popular line of research for separating individual cells from cell clusters (detecting individual cells using blob detection). This method can automatically tune its parameters but on our sequences automatic parameters resulted in poor performance, it suffered from over-segmentation, so we manually adjusted its parameters. We have quantitatively analyzed the performance of direct extension of our approach to 3D (using 3D grid graph with 6-connected neighborhood and without slice merging stage), referred to as "3D Graph Cuts". We also provide results of two other

Table 1. Comparison of our method with Farsight, 3D Graph Cuts, MINS and 3D MLS.

	TP	FP	FN	Precision	Recall	F-measure	Time (s)
Our method	442	37	52	0.92	0.89	0.91	17.63
3D graph cuts	361	203	133	0.64	0.73	0.68	31.82
Farsight [8]	373	176	121	0.68	0.76	0.72	97.43
MINS [10]	391	226	103	0.63	0.79	0.70	86.47
3D MLS [16]	335	273	159	0.55	0.68	0.61	27.90

segmentation methods, MINS (Modular Interactive Nuclear Segmentation) [10] and 3D MLS (3D Multiple Level Sets) [16].

Table 1 presents the quantitative results for sequence $S1$ and Fig. 8 shows the segmentation for two image stacks from the same sequence. Our segmentation method outperforms other methods in terms of both recall and precision with a clear margin. Farsight and MINS resulted in over segmentation in cases where a structure within a cell appeared very dim and in under-segmentation sometimes when cells within a cluster did not have very spherical shape. 3D MLS often failed to separate cells when their intensity difference was not very high and it often produced false positive detections in cell regions with somewhat distinct intensities. 3D graph cuts resulted in slightly worse performance compared to Farsight and MINS. It sometimes produced false detection above/below very bright cells in the blurred regions as can be seen in the third column of Fig. 8, where most of the false positive detections (red bounding boxes) are partly due to this issue. It also sometimes resulted in under-segmentation in situations similar to those shown in Fig. 1. Our method was able to cope with these issues better by ignoring blurred joint objects in slices near extremities of cell clusters. However there were still situations where our method failed to prevent cells from

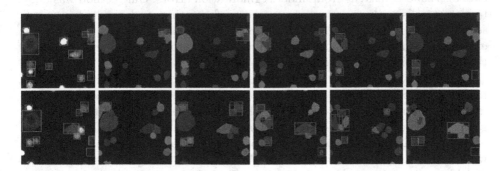

Fig. 8. Maximum intensity projection (view from top) for sequence $S1$. From left to right: Original stack, our method, 3D Graph Cuts, Farsight, MINS and 3D MLC. Bounding boxes showing the ground truth (yellow), false negatives (green) and false positives (red) are marked (Color figure online).

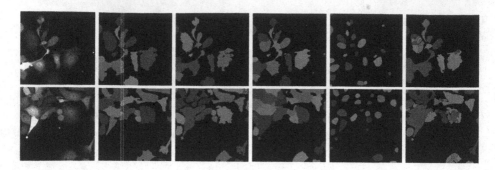

Fig. 9. Maximum intensity projection (view from top) for sequence $S2$. From left to right: Original stack, our method, 3D Graph Cuts, Farsight, MINS and 3D MLC.

expanding into blurred regions above/below them and resulted in errors (upper left corner of images in second column of Fig. 8). One drawback of our approach was that it produced rough surfaces of cells in z-direction compared to other methods.

We also tested our segmentation method on sequence $S2$, which was more challenging as cells had very flexible shape. For this sequence our segmentation method produced far better results compared to other methods. Figure 9 shows the maximum intensity projection (top view) of couple of 3D image stacks along with results from our method, 3D Graph Cuts, Farsight, MINS and 3D MLS. Farsight and MINS were able to detect many cells correctly but were not able to obtain accurate segmentations. MINS produced very compact segmentations even when cells had very non-compact shapes and Farsight often failed to prevent cell segmentations from encroaching into other cells and background despite the presence of strong boundary in many instances. 3D MLS failed to detect many actual cells (under-segmentation) and produced many false detections (over-segmentation), so its performance was worst among all the methods. 3D graph cuts also suffered heavily from under-segmentation errors. Our method was able to detect cells with decent accuracy most of the time and resulted in good segmentation of most cells. However, in situations where cells had formed long extensions, our method sometimes resulted in over segmentation or segmenting those extensions as part of other nearby cells.

We also compared the running times of our method with other methods for sequence $S1$ and Table 1 lists the average time required to process one 3D image stack on Intel Core i7-3632QM with 8 GB RAM. Both our method and 3D graph cuts were written in Matlab and used C++ packages for finding min-cut of graphs. MINS was also written in Matlab while both Farsight and 3D MLS were written in C++. MINS and Farsight had similar range of running times, which was more than 3 times slower than 3D MLS. Our method was faster than all these methods.

The performance of our method depends heavily on edge detector's performance. We could not directly evaluate the performance of edge detector due to difficulty of obtaining ground truth data but we replaced this edge detector with conventional gradient detectors (sobel, prewitt) and they resulted in significant decrease, 13 % decrease in F-measure, in performance of segmentation. Most of the additional errors were under-segmentation errors, which occurred when touching cells had a small intensity difference.

Our method was able to handle challenging (in terms of shape variability) sequences better than other methods that we tested. However there were some situations in which it produced errors. It usually resulted in under-segmentation in situations where cells had a very weak boundary between them and edge detector could not produce strong response at those boundaries. It also occasionally resulted in over-segmentation of cells, which were in-homogeneously stained and contained multiple regions of significantly different intensities and as a result caused the edge detector to produce high edge probabilities within cells.

5 Discussion and Conclusion

We have proposed a novel cell detection and segmentation method, which is able to robustly separate touching cells in confocal microscopy image sequences. Experimental evaluation has shown that our method is able to cope with sequences with very flexible cell shapes. We will in future explore the possibility of incorporating prior knowledge of cell shape within this processing pipeline which can boost performance for sequences with rigid cell shapes. Another possible extension of our work, which can result in some performance boost is to adapt the edge detector to microscopy data by extracting better features for edge detection and using training data consisting only of fluorescent microscopy images.

References

1. Kimlin, L., Kassis, J., Virador, V.: 3d in vitro tissue models and their potential for drug screening. Expert Opin. Drug Discov. **8**, 1455–1466 (2013). PMID:24144315
2. Indhumathi, C., Cai, Y., Guan, Y., Opas, M.: An automatic segmentation algorithm for 3d cell cluster splitting using volumetric confocal images. J. Microsc. **243**, 60–76 (2011)
3. Lin, G., Chawla, M.K., Olson, K., Guzowski, J.F., Barnes, C.A., Roysam, B.: Hierarchical, model-based merging of multiple fragments for improved three-dimensional segmentation of nuclei. Cytometry Part A **63A**, 20–33 (2005)
4. Ortiz de Solórzano, C., García Rodriguez, E., Jones, A., Pinkel, D., Gray, J.W., Sudar, D., Lockett, S.J.: Segmentation of confocal microscope images of cell nuclei in thick tissue sections. J. Microsc. **193**, 212–226 (1999)
5. Meijering, E.: Cell segmentation: 50 years down the road [life sciences]. IEEE Sig. Process. Mag. **29**, 140–145 (2012)
6. Farhan, M., Yli-Harja, O., Niemist, A.: A novel method for splitting clumps of convex objects incorporating image intensity and using rectangular window-based concavity point-pair search. Pattern Recogn. **46**, 741–751 (2013)

7. Daněk, O., Matula, P., Ortiz-de-Solórzano, C., Muñoz-Barrutia, A., Maška, M., Kozubek, M.: Segmentation of touching cell nuclei using a two-stage graph cut model. In: Salberg, A.-B., Hardeberg, J.Y., Jenssen, R. (eds.) SCIA 2009. LNCS, vol. 5575, pp. 410–419. Springer, Heidelberg (2009)
8. Al-Kofahi, Y., Lassoued, W., Lee, W., Roysam, B.: Improved automatic detection and segmentation of cell nuclei in histopathology images. IEEE Trans. Biomed. Eng. 57, 841–852 (2010)
9. Kong, H., Akakin, H., Sarma, S.: A generalized laplacian of gaussian filter for blob detection and its applications. IEEE Trans. Cybern. 43, 1719–1733 (2013)
10. Lou, X., Kang, M., Xenopoulos, P., Muoz-Descalzo, S., Hadjantonakis, A.K.: A rapid and efficient 2d/3d nuclear segmentation method for analysis of early mouse embryo and stem cell image data. Stem Cell Rep. 2, 382–397 (2014)
11. Arteta, C., Lempitsky, V., Noble, J.A., Zisserman, A.: Learning to detect cells using non-overlapping extremal regions. In: Ayache, N., Delingette, H., Golland, P., Mori, K. (eds.) MICCAI 2012, Part I. LNCS, vol. 7510, pp. 348–356. Springer, Berlin Heidelberg (2012)
12. Boykov, Y., Veksler, O., Zabih, R.: Fast approximate energy minimization via graph cuts. IEEE Trans. Pattern Anal. Mach. Intell. 23, 1222–1239 (2001)
13. Dollár, P., Zitnick, C.L.: Structured forests for fast edge detection. In: ICCV (2013)
14. Jamriska, O., Sykora, D., Hornung, A.: Cache-efficient graph cuts on structured grids. In: 2012 IEEE Conference on Computer Vision and Pattern Recognition (CVPR), pp. 3673–3680 (2012)
15. Munkres, J.: Algorithms for the assignment and transportation problems. J. Soc. Ind. Appl. Math. 5, 32–38 (1957)
16. Chinta, R., Wasser, M.: Three-dimensional segmentation of nuclei and mitotic chromosomes for the study of cell divisions in live drosophila embryos. Cytometry Part A 81A, 52–64 (2012)

Head Motion Signatures from Egocentric Videos

Yair Poleg[1], Chetan Arora[2], and Shmuel Peleg[1]([✉])

[1] The Hebrew University of Jerusalem, Jerusalem, Israel
peleg@mail.huji.ac.il
[2] IIIT, Delhi, India

Abstract. The proliferation of surveillance cameras has created new privacy concerns as people are captured daily without explicit consent, and the video is kept in databases for a very long time. With the increasing popularity of wearable cameras like Google Glass the problem is set to increase substantially. An important computer vision task is to enable a person ("subject") to query the video database ("observer") whether he/she has been captured on the video. Following a positive answer, the subject may request a copy of the video, or ask to be "forgotten" by erasing this video from the database. Two properties such queries should possess are: (i) The query should not reveal more information about the subject, further breaching his privacy. (ii) The query should certify that the subject is indeed the captured person before sending him the video or erasing it. This paper presents a possible solution when the subject has a head mounted camera, e.g. Google Glass. We propose to create a unique signature, based on pattern of head motion, that could identify that the subject is indeed the person seen in a video. Unlike traditional biometric methods (face, gait recognition etc.), the proposed signature is temporally volatile, and can identify the subject only at a particular time. It is of no use for any other place or time.

1 Introduction

Most people are captured on security cameras many times every day. In addition to high security places like airports, train, and bus stations, cameras are also installed in most shops. Most recorded video is kept in databases for a long time. With the increasing popularity of wearable cameras, the number of times each person is recorded on a video by complete strangers is going to increase substantially. In many countries it is a basic right of people to learn what information about them is kept in databases, and in some cases even to request removal of such information. While this issue has been approached extensively in text based databases, the case of video recordings is yet to be resolved (Fig. 1).

Consider the case where a pedestrian is possibly captured by a static security camera, or a moving wearable camera. For the purpose of this paper we refer to the pedestrian as *subject* and the entity holding the video of the subject as *observer*. The subject would like to query if he has been captured in observer's video. The subject can provide an identity signature to the observer for matching in his video. Since the subject and the observer do not trust each other, the signature should not reveal more information about the subject than what

© Springer International Publishing Switzerland 2015
D. Cremers et al. (Eds.): ACCV 2014, Part III, LNCS 9005, pp. 315–329, 2015.
DOI: 10.1007/978-3-319-16811-1_21

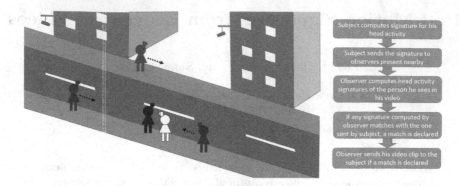

Fig. 1. With the advancement of technology, there is a growing possibility to get captured by surveillance and wearable cameras. In the schematic above, the *subject* (in white) might be captured on video by several *observers*: surveillance cameras, the person he is interacting with him (red) and multiple people around him with wearable cameras. All these observers might have captured the subject on their video. The observers can share their video with the subject or may be asked to erase it from their storage (Color figure online).

is already being held by the observer. For example, subject giving observer an image of his face is ruled out, since even if the observer has never captured the subject, he will know following the query the identity of the subject, and he could even use the face he received and search for the subject in other videos. Similar argument hold against most biometric signatures like Gait patterns etc. [1]. Another important consideration is to ensure that the subject is the owner of the claimed identity. For example, the subject may try to impersonate any other person in order to extract videos from innocent observers. Therefore even if the subject provides a face classifier which matches against a person the observer sees, it does not prove that the subject is indeed the person being watched. After all, anybody can create a face classifier of President Obama or Shakira!

An additional potential application of such privacy preserving authentication scheme is video sharing. Video sharing is particularly necessary since a wearable camera can not capture the wearer. If the wearer would like to see himself in video, the video must be taken by other people's cameras. Consider again the scenario where a pedestrian is being captured by an observer's camera. The subject should be able to prove to the observer that he has been captured in the video, and request to share his video with him. The observer may not be willing to share his entire video, but might agree to share the portion of the video where the subject appears. Such arrangement preserves the privacy of all parties involved: subject, observer and other persons appearing in observer's video.

The problem of video based authentication scheme which does not violate privacy lies in the general framework of privacy preserving secure multiparty communication (SMC) [2]. In a general SMC problem, the two parties hold a portion of data and want to evaluate a function on the union of the data without revealing their data to each other. In our problem, the function to be evaluated is whether the subject appears in a video clip and the data held by the two parties is the video held by the observer and the identification information held by the subject. Secure multiparty communication techniques are known to be computationally intensive with large communication overhead. This makes their application hard for large data sets such as images or videos. On the other hand, domain specific constraints applicable to these large data sets allow to devise new strategies which are not generic but are efficient for targeted problems. Avidan and Butman [3] address several techniques and applications of privacy preserving computation protocols within computer vision context. Privacy preserving content based image retrieval is addressed by [4]. While both methods provide means against leaking private information, they do not address our requirement of verification of ownership of data, which leaves them vulnerable to impersonation attacks in the scenarios we present.

The focus of the paper is to suggest a novel protocol and an algorithm for privacy preserving signatures for querying and certifying the identity of a person captured in a video. We propose a novel use of videos from head mounted camera (a.k.a. egocentric videos) to generate a temporally volatile personal signature of the wearer based upon his head motion. Most importantly, this signature does not contain any private information of the wearer. Intuitively the instantaneous optical flow in egocentric video is dominated by the motion of wearer's head. e.g., if a wearer moves his head to the left the optical flow for most parts of the frame is to the right and vice-versa. The optical flow over a set of frames therefore provide a compact representation of wearer's *head activity* (a sequence of instantaneous head motions) over a short period of time. We show that the head activity at a resolution of 1/30 of a second along with coarse location and time information is discriminative enough to differentiate one person from another. The signature consists of relative motions of the face with respect to the torso. When the observer's face has enough pixels to be recognizable, there is enough resolution for computing the signature as well. Older low resolution cameras, where people appear as blobs, may not have enough resolution to work with the proposed techniques. However, such low resolution videos have no use in the context of privacy preservation and video sharing application anyway.

The organization of the paper is as follows. We begin with describing the first step in our algorithm, which is to compute the signature of the subject's head activity. Section 2 describes how to compute these signatures from subject's egocentric video. Section 3 describes how to compute head activity signatures from observer's point of view. In Sect. 4 we propose a method for matching the two signatures and present theoretical bounds for the uniqueness of the signatures. Section 5 details results on various experiments conducted by us to ascertain the accuracy of the proposed matching scheme. We conclude with our thoughts on future work in Sect. 6.

2   Head Activity Signature from Subject's Camera

An ideal way of computing subject's head activity from the subject's egocentric video is to estimate the camera's egomotion and pose at each frame. Computing

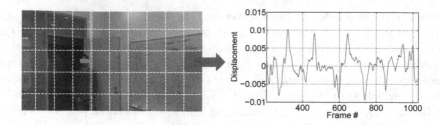

Fig. 2. Optical flow is computed at fixed image locations in the egocentric video. The optical flow is mostly proportional to the angular velocity of the wearer's head. The left image shows the fixed image locations (blocks) in which the optical flow is computed. The graph on the right shows an example of optical flow for one specific block. We estimate the optical flow in 50 such blocks and average them to compute a single global motion vector. Concatenation of the x and y components of this motion vector over a period of time is used as a signature of wearer's head activity.

egomotion is a well studied area in computer vision [5,6] with various commercial and research software available [7–9]. However, egomotion computation becomes difficult in the case of egocentric videos due to large and rapid changes in the viewing direction caused by the wearer's natural head motion. Unstructured environment coupled with lack of constraints on lighting and moving objects in the scene make the problem further challenging. Our experiments with various egomotion computation software [7–9] did not yield much success.

Computing instantaneous optical flow between two consecutive frames is a more robust estimation procedure [10]. While it doesn't yield exact camera location and pose, it provides us with enough information for our needs, as we explain next. We note that optical flow observed in an egocentric video consists of two main components. The first component is in radially outwards direction due to forward motion of the camera wearer. The second and more dominant component is due to the head motion (rotation) of the wearer. Neglecting the first component, the optical flow observed in the egocentric video is proportional to the angular velocity of the wearer's head and can be considered as a signature of wearer's head activity. The change from egomotion to optical flow allows the head activity signatures to be computed in a robust and efficient manner, making it attractive for mobile devices with relatively low compute power.[1]

Ignoring perspective effects in the instantaneous optical flow, we seek to estimate frame to frame homography using a translation only model. It would have sufficed to estimate a single homography in the ideal case. However, given the likelihood of moving objects in the scene, we divide the frame into non-overlapping tiles and compute the translation independently for each tile

---

[1] We note that inertial devices (as used by [11]) could have been used for computing head activity signatures as well. However, our experiments with such inertial devices have yielded a very noisy signal which is not useful for our case. In any case, the requirement of additional hardware restricts the potential application areas, while using image based solution widens the scope of application.

(see Fig. 2). In our experiments we divide the frame to 10×5 non-overlapping tiles and compute the optical flow using our own implementation of LK [12], similar to [10]. We chose LK due to its efficiency, simplicity and robustness. Other methods for optical flow estimation can be used as well [13].

Each tile in the frame gives an independent optical flow estimation. We average the x and y components independently to arrive at single two dimensional motion vector for every two consecutive frames. There are more robust methods than averaging, but our experiments show that simple averaging is sufficient. Concatenating these motion vectors over a period of time gives a signature of wearer's activity over the duration. Formally, let $(u_t^{i,j}, v_t^{i,j})$ be the (x, y) optical flow computed for tile $(i, j) \in (M \times N)$ at frame t. The average motion vector for frame t is defined as $(\bar{u}_t, \bar{v}_t) = (\frac{1}{MN} \sum_{i,j} u_t^{i,j}, \frac{1}{MN} \sum_{i,j} v_t^{i,j})$. The *subject's signature* for time period $[a, b]$ is then:

$$S_{[a,b]} = ((\bar{u}_a, \bar{v}_a), (\bar{u}_{a+1}, \bar{v}_{a+1}), \ldots, (\bar{u}_b, \bar{v}_b))^T. \tag{1}$$

In the context of our problem, the subject computes the signature $S_{[a,b]}$ whenever he'd like to query observers whether he appears on their video or not. The signature is then sent to the observer who then computes another signature, the *observer's signature* using a procedure we describe in next section. The observer then matches the two signatures to verify that the subject is visible in his video. It may be noted that although we call the signatures "subject's" and "observer's" signature, they both describe the activity of subject's head. The notation is only to disambiguate who computes the signature.

It may be noted that in the proposed protocol, the subject need not have seen the observer to obtain his own head activity signature. However, the observer must see the subject to be able to obtain a signature of the subject's head activity. Therefore, the requirement of having seen each other in the protocol is asymmetric and is reflective of the prevailing situation in surveillance as well as video sharing applications where the subject might not have seen the observer.

3   Head Activity Signature from Observer's Camera

The observer is willing to share (or erase) parts of his video with subjects who can provide evidence that they appear in the observer's video. In the previous section we presented the subject's signature, which can serve as an evidence for the subject's appearance in the observer's video. In order for the observer to verify the signature, he first needs to find candidate subjects within his video. Therefore, the observer first checks if there are any candidate subjects visible in his video clip. We assume the availability of off-the-shelf person/pedestrian detector for this purpose [14]. We then detect and track feature points on the head and torso of the candidate subjects separately. Any human parts based model can be used for detecting head and torso [15]. We note that the instantaneous displacement of a feature point on the head of a candidate subject (as seen from the observer's camera) has three major components. The first component is due to the walking of the candidate subject. As the candidate subject walks

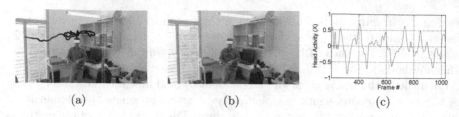

(a)   (b)   (c)

Fig. 3. Signature from observer's camera. (a) The original feature point locations on the subject (in blue) and in other frames (in red). The observed displacement is due to the combination of movement of candidate subject's head, torso as well as motion of the observer. (b) Tracked feature point after warping by the homography (shown in red). All the points on the torso are mapped to their original location. However, the feature point on the head is mapped to a different location due to change in the subject's head pose. (c) Curve showing the subject's head activity computed as concatenation of displacement of warped point on the head, over a period of time (Color figure online).

towards or away from the observer, there is a displacement in the feature point. This is true even when the head of the candidate subject was perfectly stationary with respect to his torso. The second component is due to the observer's camera motion. The third component is due to the relative motion of candidate subject's head with respect to torso. For computing observer's signatures we are interested in finding a function measuring the third component and invariant to first and second components (see Fig. 3).

Let us assume that the observer is sufficiently far from the candidate subjects he captures on the video, such that the body of a candidate subject (face as well as torso) could be treated as a plane. This makes it possible to express the displacement of feature points on the candidate subject's body by finding a planar homography. We detect and track multiple points on the torso and head of each of the candidate subjects appearing in the observer's video. We fit a homography (with respect to some reference frame r) using only the points on torso. Ideally, transforming the points using the computed homography should cancel the displacement in the feature points due to the motion of the torso. Any remaining displacement (x as well as y) observed in the feature points on the head of the candidate subject is entirely due to the change in the candidate subject's head pose with respect to his torso. The concatenation of the remaining displacement computed as described above over a time duration gives the signature of head activity of the candidate subject from observer's point of view (see Fig. 3).

Formally, let $\mathcal{C}_t^i$ be the ith candidate subject detected in the observer's video at time $t \in [a, b]$ and let $\mathcal{P}_{i,t}^{torso}$ be the sets of feature points tracked on the torso of $\mathcal{C}^i$. For simplicity, let us have a single feature point $p_{i,t}^{head} = (x, y)$ tracked on the head of $\mathcal{C}^i$ at time t and let $r \in [a, b]$ be a reference frame of our choice, in which $\mathcal{C}^i$ appears. For each frame t, we find an homography $\mathcal{H}_{t \to r}$ using $\mathcal{P}_{i,r}^{torso}$ and $\mathcal{P}_{i,t}^{torso}$. We then calculate the warped point $w_{i,r}^{head} = \mathcal{H}_{t \to r} \cdot p_{i,t}^{head}$. The displacement $\delta_{i,t} = (\delta_{i,t}^x, \delta_{i,t}^y) = w_{i,r}^{head} - p_{i,t}^{head}$ is proportional to the head pose of $\mathcal{C}^i$ relative to his torso. We concatenate the displacements for all $t \in [a, b]$ to get: $\widetilde{\mathcal{O}}_{i,[a,b]} = \left((\delta^x_{i,a}, \delta^y_{i,a}), (\delta^x_{i,a+1}, \delta^y_{i,a+1}), \ldots, (\delta^x_{i,b}, \delta^y_{i,b}) \right)^T$. Note that while the subject's signature $\mathcal{S}$ is proportional to the subject's head angular velocity, $\widetilde{\mathcal{O}}$ is proportional to the change in head displacement with respect to frame r. We therefore temporally derive $\widetilde{\mathcal{O}}$ to get the *observer's signature*: $\mathcal{O} = \frac{d\widetilde{\mathcal{O}}}{dt}$.

In our implementation we manually select one feature point on the head and at least 10 feature points on the torso of each candidate subject in the first frame of the sequence. In case of multiple feature points on a candidate subject's head, the average of the $\delta_{i,t}$ displacements per frame can be used as the elements of $\widetilde{\mathcal{O}}$.

It may be noted that, while the subject's signature indeed describes the angular velocity of the head, observer's signature describes it as observed after projecting it on the observer's image plane. The two signals are therefore not identical. However, the projection can only change the magnitude of instantaneous displacement but not the sign of the displacement. The matching strategy as we describe in the next section should therefore ignore the magnitude and focus on the sign of instantaneous displacement.

4   Matching Head Activity Signatures

Once a subject has presented his signature $\mathcal{S}$, the observer would like to verify if the subject's signature matches the observer's signatures corresponding to any of the candidate subjects that appear in the observer's video. It may be noted that the subject's and the observer's signatures have been produced from two videos which may have very little in common (looking to opposite sides, different cameras/resolution/FPS etc.). Even the derivation process of the signatures is not the same and therefore one might consider the signatures as originating from different modalities. While there are various methods available for matching signals obtained from different modalities [16], we believe that problem in our case is much simpler. Most importantly, both signatures have the same dimension and are measured in pixels. We observe that for our case the scale of the two signatures can be very different but they should agree in their phase for a correct match. We propose using Pearson Correlation Coefficient as a score for signature match. The Pearson's correlation coefficient ρ between two variables X and Y is defined as:

$$\rho(X, Y) = \frac{\text{Cov}(X, Y)}{\sigma_X \sigma_Y} = \frac{\mathbb{E}\left[(X - \mu_X)(Y - \mu_Y) \right]}{\sigma_X \sigma_Y}, \tag{2}$$

where Cov is the covariance between X and Y, σ_X is the standard deviation of X, μ_X is the mean of X and $\mathbb{E}$ is the expectation. We denote the x and y components of the subject's signature as $\mathcal{S}_x, \mathcal{S}_y$. Similarly, the components of the observer's signature is denoted by $\mathcal{O}_x, \mathcal{O}_y$. We compute independently $\rho_x = \rho(\mathcal{S}_x, \mathcal{O}_x)$ and $\rho_y = \rho(\mathcal{S}_y, \mathcal{O}_y)$. Recall that $\rho \in [-1, +1]$. We add $|\rho_x|$ and

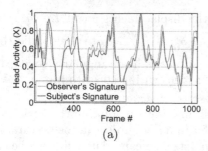
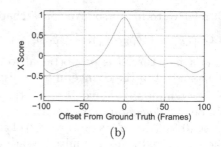

(a)   (b)

Fig. 4. (a) The curves showing subject's (in green) and observer's (in blue) signatures. (b) Correlation between observer's and subject's signatures at various temporal alignments. The zero offset implies the ground truth alignment. We show the correlation scores with various alignments in the range of ± 100. The score is significantly higher at the time instance of correct match (offset $= 0$) (Color figure online).

$|\rho_y|$ to obtain a total score for the match.[2] In an abuse of notation, we call the total score *correlation* and denote ρ_x as x-correlation and ρ_y as y-correlation.

Figure 4 shows the matching between signatures for an indicative experiment. The subject provides his signature with an indication of time where he claims to be present in observer's video. Observer computes observer's signature and tries matching it with various alignments around the time claimed by subject. This is to allow synchronization errors between subject and observer. In our implementation, we have empirically chosen a threshold of $T = 1.1$ (which is just above the half way mark) and declare that the signatures match if the total score is greater than this threshold. Note that we claim and show in the experiments section that the signatures are unique and even if observer would have chosen to match over the entire range for which subject's signature was available, he would have found a match only in case of valid subject at the correct time. The decision to search only in the search window around the claimed time is due to efficiency.

4.1   Signature Uniqueness

An important consideration at this stage is to quantitatively evaluate uniqueness of the signatures. The question we seek to answer is: How hard is it for a malicious attacker to fool the observer into sharing his video clip by 'guessing' another subject's signature? For the discussion in this section we consider each of the $\mathcal{S}_x, \mathcal{S}_y, \mathcal{O}_x$ and $\mathcal{O}_y$ as vectors in a d-dimensional space, where d is the duration of the signatures in frames. Note that correlation score is invariant to scale and shift. Therefore, we assume each vector to be normalized to unit norm and zero mean. The question we are asking now is: How easy it is for a malicious attacker

---

[2] The observed displacement in observer's signature could be opposite or in phase with subjects's signature depending upon whether the subject is seen from front or back by the observer.

to 'guess' signature vectors $\mathcal{S}_x, \mathcal{S}_y$ such that the correlation with the observer's vectors $\mathcal{O}_x$, $\mathcal{O}_y$ comes out to be more than $\frac{T}{2} = 0.55$ per vector (x and y).[3]

Geometric interpretation of the correlation coefficient views it as the cosine of the angle between the two vectors [17, 18]. A correlation score of $\frac{T}{2} = 0.55$ corresponds to an angle of about $60°$ between the vectors. With this interpretation it is easy to observe that the probability of getting another vector within $60°$ of the first one is practically zero for a large enough d. In other words, for large enough dimensions, two random vectors sampled uniformly are almost orthogonal with probability 1.[4] In our context it implies that if the values of the signature at different time instance are $i.i.d$ (identically independent distributed), then the chances of hitting a correlation of $\frac{T}{2} = 0.55$ (or for that matter any non-zero correlation) by random guessing the vector is practically zero.

The above argument is naïve in the sense that we assume the values are i.i.d. In our case, the value of the signature at a particular time instance represents the velocity of the head at that time instance. Therefore, the velocities at two consecutive time instances are strongly dependent. The head of a human being never becomes still immediately after moving at some other velocity or the other way around. A more reasonable approach would be to bound the acceleration of the head motion. Let us assume that the difference of values of the signature (head velocity) at two consecutive time instances can not be more than ϵ. Assume the signature value is ϵ at a time instance t. With the bound on acceleration, the possibilities for the next value are 2ϵ, ϵ or 0. We restrict the possibilities further and say that the next value can only be ϵ or 0. Note that this is equivalent to providing additional information to the malicious subject. We show that even with this additional information it is not possible for the malicious observer to guess the signature vector. Observe that with the additional restriction, the vector can be treated as a binary vector. It is easy to see that for sufficiently high dimension, the chance of hitting non-zero correlation, even for binary vector, is practically zero.

The above theoretical analysis is still naïve in the sense that we do not account for patterns that may arise from unique individual behaviour observed over a long time (i.e. collecting millions of signatures of the same subject). We are not aware of any work that attempts to deal with such long term patterns from egocentric videos. However, the possibility of such pattern-based attacks cannot be ruled out. We validate the theoretical analysis in this section with empirical evidence in Sect. 5.

5   Experiments

We have conducted our experiments using both self shot videos and a publicly available dataset [10, 19]. We have used GoPro Hero3+ cameras in narrow view

---

[3] Any unequal division of the total score requirement would be more difficult to meet.

[4] In our implementation, the dimension of the vectors (length of the signature) is usually more than 200 frames (corresponding to 3–4 s of video at 60 frames per second). This is a sufficiently large dimension for the proposed probabilistic analysis.

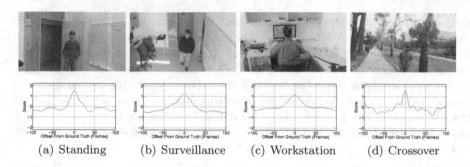

(a) Standing   (b) Surveillance   (c) Workstation   (d) Crossover

Fig. 5. Matching scores between subject's and observer's signature at different temporal offsets as described in Fig. 4. First row shows a sample frame for each sequence. (a) In this experiment subject and observer are standing in place and talking. Note that the two are not exactly stationary and there is a bit of walking by observer towards the subject. (b) Matching scores for the case when the subject is captured walking towards a surveillance camera hanged from a room's ceiling. (c) The proposed scheme also works in the scenario when observer haven't seen the 'face' of the subject. In this case, subject is working on the computer and observer is watching his back. The matching score can still accurately find the match at correct time instance. (d) The proposed scheme can also handle cases where the subject and/or observer are moving. In this scenario, the subject and observer are walking towards each other. The original video clips corresponding to results shown here can be found at the project page.

mode for shooting our videos. The videos are in full HD resolution at 60 FPS and are available at the project page: http://www.vision.huji.ac.il/egosig/. We use our own implementation of LK for computing the subject's signature. We divide each frame to a 10×5 grid and compute optical flow independently in each grid region. This grid size proved to be quite robust against moving objects in the scene and other sources of optical flow failure. Other choices of grid size did not yield much improvement in the results. For computing the observer's signature we detect GFTT features and track them using the LK. Both implementations are available in OpenCV [20]. The points are detected and tracked separately in head and torso regions. For the head region, we choose one point visible for longest duration, whereas for torso region we use all the points visible during entire length of the video. The homography between the torso points is computed using Matlab's geometric transformation estimator. The homography estimation is done by using RANSAC with outlier removal options set. We observe that homography estimation is not stable between frames separated by a long time duration. We therefore choose a new *hop-over* frame after every 60 frames (1 s in our videos). The homography is computed between the current and the hop-over frame and then multiplied by the homography between the hop-over and the reference frame to find the overall transformation. The time duration for the observer's signature is chosen to be at-least 200 frames to ensure low false-positive rates. The signatures are declared as a match if there is a correlation score (sum of x and y correlations) of more than $T = 1.1$ observed at any point. The time of match is declared at the point of maximum correlation score.

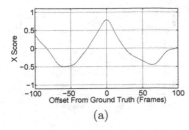 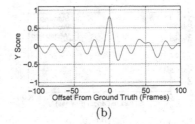

(a)   (b)

Fig. 6. (a) In case of walking there is a periodicity in subject's head activity due to natural head motion associated with walking steps. This leads to weak periodicity in the x-correlation scores. However, the head activity is not exactly same and there is still a significant peak in the correlation score at correct time instance. (b) The y-correlation scores are not affected.

We conducted experiments under various interaction scenarios between the observer and the subject. Figure 5 shows the correlation scores for indicative experiments. As described in the previous section, we compute the observer's signature and then find the correlation score with subject's signature in a window of ±100 frames around the time claimed by subject. Note that in our self-shot experiments the videos are approximately synchronized and therefore we should see a peak at origin. The proposed scheme correctly recognizes the subject while standing, talking or walking. The signatures can be successfully matched even when the observer sees the back of the subject. This exposes the strength and novelty of the proposed method with respect to face pose estimation approaches. Not only the face pose estimation is much harder to infer compared to proposed tracking based approach, but by definition face pose estimation can be applied only if the observer sees the 'face' of the subject.

We notice that there is some periodicity in the matching score in the walking sequence. The reason for this could be understood from the fact that there is a natural head motion associated with the stepping during walking. Since the stepping speed doesn't change too much over a period of few seconds there is a gross similarity in the head activity in x direction (see Fig. 6). The periodicity is limited to x direction only and is not visible in y-correlation score. Even for x correlation, although the head motion is periodic at gross level, the activity doesn't match precisely between two (walking) steps. Therefore, the peak in the score is still observed at correct time instance.

In Sect. 4.1, we presented theoretical analysis on the uniqueness of the proposed matching technique. We showed that the probability of a subject to randomly 'guess' a signature which can match observer's signature with a correlation score of more than $T = 1.1$ ($\frac{T}{2} = 0.55$ for each x and y-correlation) is practically 0. The results holds for sufficiently large dimension and we claimed that the dimension of 200 in our implementation is sufficiently large. We validate our claim with experimental evidence here. We created a repository of more than a million subject's signatures based on the videos from GeogiaTech's First-Person Social Interactions Dataset [19]. In all, the repository is based on more than 30 h

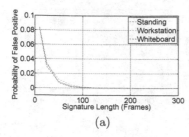
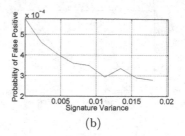

(a)   (b)

Fig. 7. (a) Average probability of false positive for various signature length corresponding to observer's signature obtained from different sequences. The false positive probability is non-zero for short signatures but quickly goes to 0 for signatures longer than 100 frames. In our implementation we use signatures of length more than 200. (b) Probability of false positive with respect to signatures of different variance. The length of the signature chosen in this case is 100. The probability is practically zero even for signatures with low variance.

of egocentric videos. For the observer's signatures, we used the signatures from the workstation, standing and whiteboard sequences that were shot by us. We evaluated the matching score between each observer signature and the entire subject's signatures repository. The probability of a false match is the number of instances where the correlation of more than 1.1 is observed against the number of evaluations. We repeat this experiment for various signature lengths. Figure 7(a) shows the results. Expectedly, the probability of false positive is non-zero for shorter signatures, but goes to 0 quickly for signatures longer than 100 frames. We also confirmed this by choosing observer's signature having different variance. Figure 7(b) shows the results. The probability of a false match is practically 0 even for signatures with low variance. To further verify the above findings, we repeated this experiment with a slight change. Instead of matching the observer's signatures (which are based on our self shot videos) with the subject's signature repository, we randomly picked signatures from the same repository and matched them against the rest of the repository. This process yielded similar results, which proves the uniqueness of the signatures.

One can think of special cases where even long signatures of more than 100 frames can be guessed. One such example is a subject's signature that represents no head activity at all (signature is a 'flat line'). e.g, the subject's camera is placed on a statue's head. It is clear that if the observer is presented with multiple such signatures from multiple statue-like subjects, there is no way of telling who produced which signature. A simple way to overcome this case is to require the signature to contain a minimal amount of information, measured as variance or entropy.

The experiments conducted as above merely serve the purpose of showing that it is practically impossible to randomly guess the signature. The question of whether it is possible or not to make an 'educated' guess of a subject's signature (based on long-term observation of the specific subject) remains open.

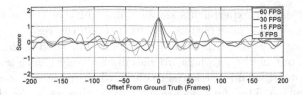

Fig. 8. Comparison of correlation scores for videos at various frames per second (FPS) corresponding to whiteboard sequence with signature length of 200 frames. We observe that although the best correlation score is similar at all FPS, the signal to noise ratio, measured as the ratio of highest peak to second highest is best at 60 FPS.

It may be noted that the correlation scores are not strongly dependent upon the frame rate of input videos. Although we use videos at 60 frames per second (FPS), the results do not change much at lower FPS. Figure 8 shows the score comparison at various FPS corresponding to the whiteboard sequence. The length of the signature is chosen to be same for all videos. Note that the correlation peak is at the correct place and of similar strength at all FPS. However, the signal to noise ratio measured as ratio of highest peak to second highest peak is best for 60 FPS. We therefore, recommend videos at 60 FPS for the problem. The 60 FPS videos have additional advantage that the observer has to keep the subject in view for a shorter amount of time (for same signature length) thereby implying more flexibility.

Using head activity signature from egocentric video as proposed in the paper is simple, efficient and robust enough for the problem we are considering. However, more sophisticated approaches for the signatures could have been used. For example, face pose estimation has been a well studied problem in the computer vision community and various algorithms have been proposed recently for the same [21,22]. We have experimented with [21] for which the source code was

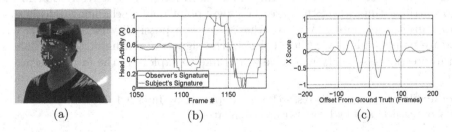

(a)   (b)   (c)

Fig. 9. (a) Face features and pose estimated by [21]. (b) Observer's signature generated using pose estimation. Also shown is the subject's signature for visual comparison. Note that [21] gives coarse pose estimation in step size of 15° only. The same is visible in observer's signature which can only take few discrete values now. (c) Matching score at various offset. While the peak is at the correct location, there is another high correlation at an offset of 60 frames from ground truth. This is corresponding to matching with next head turn as visible in (b).

publicly available. Our experiments showed ambiguity in the matching due to quantized nature of face pose output. Figure 9 shows the result. It is important to note that using face pose estimation from the said method to infer head activity will restrict our method to forward moving sequences with x head motion only. Furthermore, it would restrict us to cases when the face is seen clearly and at enough resolution. Therefore, we are not advocating its use in the context of our method.

6   Conclusion

A novel method for privacy aware sharing of egocentric videos has been presented. The proposed method paves the way for exciting applications by enabling a camera wearer to access the video clips which may have captured him. The focus of the paper is not new technology for tracking or pose detection but to use simple existing techniques to offer a practical solution for the privacy concerns associated with video capture and sharing. There is no personal information disclosure by either parties other than sharing of the requested video clip in which the subject appears. The head activity signatures are temporally volatile and can not be easily used to recognize the subject at any other time or place. Yet, the computed signatures are unique enough to distinguish the correct signature amongst the various signatures presented. The technique relies on simple steps of detecting and tracking features for which many efficient algorithms are available. This broadens the scope of application by making it attractive for mobile devices. The robustness of the tracking algorithms enables the algorithm to be applied from a distant or low resolution cameras as well. The signatures do not depend upon the visibility of a 'face' and can be computed even when the observer see the subject from the back.

A possible weakness of the current algorithm is the requirement to see the head for the duration of the signature. The duration required is not large (typically a few seconds) but even this small duration can be a restriction in an egocentric setting, where the observer's view point may be changing quickly due to natural head motion. We note that there is a possibility of reacquiring the feature points and allowing for 'holes' in the signature during matching. This is an interesting possibility which we would like to explore in the future research.

Acknowledgement. This research was supported by Intel ICRC-CI, by Israel Ministry of Science, and by Israel Science Foundation.

References

1. Shiraga, K., Trung, N.T., Mitsugami, I., Mukaigawa, Y., Yagi, Y.: Gait-based person authentication by wearable cameras. In: International Conference on Networked Sensing Systems, pp. 1–7 (2012)
2. Yao, A.C.C.: How to generate and exchange secrets. In: FOCS, pp. 162–167 (1986)

3. Avidan, S., Butman, M.: Blind vision. In: Leonardis, A., Bischof, H., Pinz, A. (eds.) ECCV 2006. LNCS, vol. 3953, pp. 1–13. Springer, Heidelberg (2006)
4. Upmanyu, M., Namboodiri, A., Srinathan, K., Jawahar, C.: Efficient privacy preserving video surveillance. In: ICCV, pp. 1639–1646 (2009)
5. Hartley, R., Zisserman, A.: Multiple View Geometry in Computer Vision, 2nd edn. Cambridge University Press, New York (2003)
6. Raudies, F., Neumann, H.: A review and evaluation of methods estimating ego-motion. CVIU 116, 606–633 (2012)
7. Castle, R.O., Klein, G., Murray, D.W.: Video-rate localization in multiple maps for wearable augmented reality. In: IEEE ISWC (2008)
8. Wu, C.: VisualSFM: A visual structure from motion system. http://ccwu.me/vsfm/
9. VISCODA: Voodoo camera tracker. http://www.digilab.uni-hannover.de/
10. Poleg, Y., Arora, C., Peleg, S.: Temporal segmentation of egocentric videos. In: CVPR (2014)
11. Spriggs, E., Torre, F.D.L., Hebert, M.: Temporal segmentation and activity classification from first-person sensing. In: CVPRW (2009)
12. Lucas, B.D., Kanade, T.: An iterative image registration technique with an application to stereo vision. In: IJCAI, pp. 674–679 (1981)
13. Baker, S., Scharstein, D., Lewis, J.P., Roth, S., Black, M.J., Szeliski, R.: A database and evaluation methodology for optical flow. IJCV 92, 1–31 (2011)
14. Enzweiler, M., Gavrila, D.: Monocular pedestrian detection: survey and experiments. TPAMI 31, 2179–2195 (2009)
15. Ramanan, D.: Part-based models for finding people and estimating their pose. In: Moeslund, T.B., Hilton, A., Krüger, V., Sigal, L. (eds.) Visual Analysis of Humans, pp. 199–223. Springer, London (2011)
16. Kidron, E., Schechner, Y.Y., Elad, M.: Pixels that sound. In: CVPR, pp. 88–95 (2005)
17. Schmid Jr, J.: The relationship between the coefficient of correlation and the angle included between regression lines. J. Educ. Res. 41, 311–313 (1947)
18. Wikipedia: Pearson product-moment correlation coefficient. http://en.wikipedia.org/wiki/Pearson_product-moment_correlation_coefficient
19. Fathi, A., Hodgins, J.K., Rehg, J.M.: Social interactions: a first-person perspective. In: CVPR (2012)
20. Bradski, G.: Opencv ver 2.4.3. (2013)
21. Ramanan, D., Zhu, X.: Face detection, pose estimation, and landmark localization in the wild. In: IEEE Conference on Computer Vision and Pattern Recognition, pp. 2879–2886 (2012)
22. Ho, H.T., Chellappa, R.: Automatic head pose estimation using randomly projected dense sift descriptors. In: ICIP, pp. 153–156 (2012)

Improving Saliency Models by Predicting Human Fixation Patches

Rachit Dubey[1], Akshat Dave[2], and Bernard Ghanem[1(✉)]

[1] King Abdullah University of Science and Technology, Thuwal, Saudi Arabia
bernard.ghanem@kaust.edu.sa
[2] University of California San Diego, San Diego, USA

Abstract. There is growing interest in studying the Human Visual System (HVS) to supplement and improve the performance of computer vision tasks. A major challenge for current visual saliency models is predicting saliency in cluttered scenes (i.e. high false positive rate). In this paper, we propose a fixation patch detector that predicts image patches that contain human fixations with high probability. Our proposed model detects sparse fixation patches with an accuracy of 84 % and eliminates non-fixation patches with an accuracy of 84 % demonstrating that low-level image features can indeed be used to short-list and identify human fixation patches. We then show how these detected fixation patches can be used as saliency priors for popular saliency models, thus, reducing false positives while maintaining true positives. Extensive experimental results show that our proposed approach allows state-of-the-art saliency methods to achieve better prediction performance on benchmark datasets.

1 Introduction

Visual attention is an integral function of the Human Visual System (HVS). By focusing on a limited set of locations in the field of vision, the HVS prioritizes the distribution of perceptual resources to various locations in the visual field, making them more salient than others. There is substantial evidence of this non-uniform distribution in eye-fixation data [1], i.e. of parsimonious fixation on certain visual regions. Given a stimulus image, fixation points generally occupy a very small percentage of the overall number of image pixels. The thrifty allocation of processing resources is a result of *visual attention*. This process makes the recognition of patterns in the visual input computationally feasible. The phenomenon of visual attention in the HVS has received consideration in recent decades, particularly in the field of psychology and neuroscience [2]. These studies help understand the HVS better and are useful for a myriad of vision tasks including object recognition [3,4], object detection [5] and action recognition [6].

Since eye fixations play an important role in object recognition/detection, a signicant amount of work has been done to automatically detect such fixations in images. Interest point detectors [7] output a particular set of points that are considered "interesting" and are extensively used in many computer vision systems. However, recent work [8] suggests that these detectors may have low

© Springer International Publishing Switzerland 2015
D. Cremers et al. (Eds.): ACCV 2014, Part III, LNCS 9005, pp. 330–345, 2015.
DOI: 10.1007/978-3-319-16811-1_22

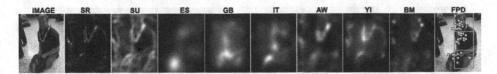

Fig. 1. Elements in the background distract saliency models. Example image showing saliency methods performing poorly due to background clutter. The last image shows human fixations in yellow and the detections of our proposed model in green. Our model is not significantly affected by background clutter, so it can be used to reduce false positives in various saliency methods (Color figure online).

perceptual relevance and are very weakly correlated to the HVS. In contrast to interest point detectors, computational saliency models create pixel-level probability maps with the goal of predicting locations that have a high chance of attracting human attention. A wide variety of models have been proposed to compute visual saliency and have been shown to be useful in several vision tasks, such as object recognition [9] and image thumbnailing [10] among others.

Most saliency models generally perform well when applied to images containing a few salient regions. However, as recently reported in [11], a major challenge for these methods is predicting human attention in scenes containing various objects and distractors. Figure 1 shows an example of such a case wherein popularly used saliency methods tend to get distracted by background clutter resulting in poor prediction performance.

In this work, we propose a system that addresses this issue and improves the performance of popularly used saliency methods by reducing false positives. Our proposed system learns directly from human fixation data and utilizes biologically plausible low-level features to automatically and reliably identify image patches where humans might fixate in a free-viewing setting. We then use the detected patches as saliency priors to improve the performance of several state-of-the-art saliency models [12–20]. Through extensive experiments, we demonstrate the effectiveness of our method in improving the performance of these models on benchmark eye-tracking datasets. The models used in our experiments include some of the most recent and top performing saliency models in current literature.

Related Work: Following the classical algorithm of Itti and Koch [15], a number of researchers have worked to study visual saliency and the mechanism of eye fixations in the HVS. Itti and Baldi [21] studied bayesian surprise quantitatively to measure the extent to which humans direct their gaze to surprising items. A spectral residual approach for saliency detection was described in [12]. Zhang et al. [13] proposed a bayesian framework for saliency using natural statistics. Harel et al. [14] proposed a bottom-up graph based saliency model. Judd et al. [22] employed machine learning techniques to develop a saliency model based on low, mid and high-level image features. More recently, a saliency method based on forward whitening of low-level features was proposed [16,17] and been shown to outperform various other methods across several datasets in [11,23]. We refer the reader to [24] for a recent survey on visual saliency modelling.

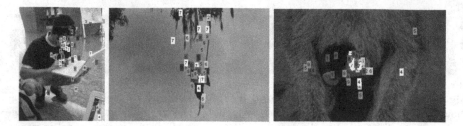

Fig. 2. Humans tend to look at the same region but not the same locations.
Sample images with fixation points from different human observers plotted in different
colors. Note the varying spatial distribution of fixations between observers (Color figure
online).

Most of the above described methods aim to predict the exact locations of
human fixations yet it is unclear whether human fixations are deterministically
repeatable locations in the visual field. As evident from data in [22], empirical
evidence points to the conclusion that no two humans fixate on the *same* points
while freely viewing the same image (refer to Fig. 2 for an example). Nonetheless,
these fixation points tend to lie in close proximity to each other and fixations from
different humans do share similar spatial neighborhoods in the same image, thus,
comprising an image region that we coin a *fixation region*. For simplicity and
computational convenience, this spatial neighborhood can simply be modeled as
a rectangular image patch.

As the main contribution of our work, we train a discriminative model to
automatically identify *fixation patches* in an image. We then use the fixation
patches as priors to reduce false positives in an effort to bridge the gap between
current saliency models and human performance. This follows from our previous
argument that saliency models tend to perform poorly on cluttered scenes.

The paper is organized as follows. Section 2 describes the feature extraction
and training stages of our patch detector. Section 3 describes our proposed approach in the context of saliency model improvement. Experimental results are
reported in Sect. 4 followed by discussion and analysis in Sect. 5.

2   Proposed Method: Fixation Patch Detector (FPD)

In this section, we give a detailed description of our learning based approach,
which is is illustrated in Fig. 3. Given an input image, we first divide the image
into a set of non-overlapping patches. Patch extraction is followed by feature
extraction wherein the extracted patches are represented by low-level and biologically inspired image features. Finally, a classifier is trained to identify image
patches that attract human attention. These regions are denoted as *fixation
patches*. In the rest of the paper, we refer to our proposed method as the Fixation Patch Detector (FPD). Next, we provide a detailed description of the steps
involved in learning the FPD, namely feature extraction, and classifier learning.

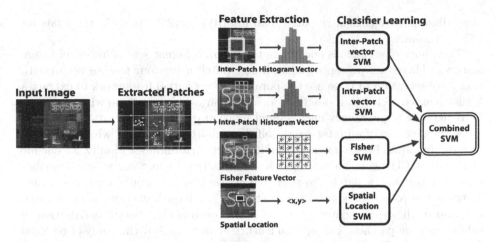

Fig. 3. Overall framework for our proposed fixation patch detector. (1) patch extraction, (2) feature extraction and (3) classifier learning.

2.1 Feature Representation

Although it is well known that human attention (even in the free-viewing case) is driven by both low-level (e.g. image intensity and gradients) and high-level features (e.g. familiar objects in the image), we focus on the former in this paper for simplicity. Our approach sheds light on how low-level features might influence human visual perception and discernibility. In this work, we propose a model that allows the prediction of image patches that have a high probability of attracting human fixations. We develop this model with the following three observations in mind.

(1) A viewer will fixate on a patch of the current image if he has fixated upon a similar patch before.
(2) A viewer will fixate on a patch that differs significantly from the patches in its local neighbourhood.
(3) A viewer will fixate on a patch within which there is a high degree of dissimilarity among pixels.

The basis for **(1)** is "familiarity", whereby humans are notoriously well equipped to recognize familiar objects, i.e. objects similar to those seen before. As such, we extend findings from previous studies [25,26] and propose that humans also recognize and fixate on familiar salient regions in an image, i.e. previously seen salient patches. In other words, a human, who has fixated on a salient patch in one image, tends to fixate on a similar looking patch in another image. The basis for **(2)** is "surprise". As suggested by [21,27], humans tend to fixate upon surprising items within the context of a scene. As such, patches in an image that significantly differ from their surroundings are expected to cause visual surprise in human viewers. Finally, observation **(3)** indicates that the content of an image patch plays a major role in attracting visual attention to this patch. In fact, humans tend to fixate *more* on image patches with heterogenous content than patches with a low pixel dissimilarity (i.e. intra-patch dissimilarity) [28,29]. As such, the basis for (3) is "variance".

The above observations encourage the use of different sets of low-level image features. Therefore, we represent an image patch using four feature vectors. To encode observation (1), we use the popular Fisher kernel framework to extract a Fisher feature vector that describes local appearance information within a patch by relating it to previously encountered fixation patches. Observation (2) motivates the creation of an inter-patch self dissimilarity histogram, which describes how dissimilar an image patch is from its direct surroundings. Finally, we encode observation (3) using an intra-patch dissimilarity histogram, which describes how heterogenous a patch's appearance content is. To supplement these three features and to encode spatial information in our model, we use the normalized location of the patch center in the image to encode the spatial distribution of salient fixation patches. This spatial feature is motivated by the study of regional focus in the HVS, which is deemed independent of image properties, as well as, the work presented in [22,30], which indicate that eye tracking datasets have a strong bias towards human fixations near the center of the image (the so-called *center bias*). As such, we divide each image $\mathbf{I}$ into a set of patches $P_{\mathbf{I}}$, each of which is represented by the four features described above and use them to train and test a fixation patch detector (FPD). This learned FPD will ultimately predict the likelihood of a patch attracting human visual attention.

Fisher Feature (F): Based on observation (1), we represent each patch $\rho \in P_{\mathbf{I}}$ according to how similar it is to fixation and non-fixation patches observed in the training images. We describe how these ground truth patches are detected during training in Sect. 2.2. In this work, we choose to represent ρ using the Fisher kernel framework [31]. Here, a set of pixels in ρ (e.g. pixels with largest gradient energy) is selected as representative instances of a patch of an image. These instances are described by the conventional SIFT descriptor (spatially localized histograms of oriented gradients). To account for the variability of these SIFT vectors in the training set, a universal Gaussian Mixture Model (GMM) is constructed on the set of all training patches [32]. Using this universal GMM, the Fisher kernel feature of ρ is computed. If a patch $\rho \in \mathbf{I}$ has a set of representative instances Ω, its corresponding Fisher vector (**F**) is computed as in Eq. (1).

$$\mathbf{F}(\rho) = \frac{1}{|\Omega|} \sum_{j \in \Omega} \nabla_{\gamma} \ln p(j|\gamma) \tag{1}$$

Here, ∇_{γ} is the gradient operator with respect to the Gaussian model parameter set γ (i.e. mean vector and variances). The Fisher feature is selected for its convenience in representing patches with different sized Ω using the same sized feature vector. In fact, our use of this type of feature is motivated by the noteworthy performance of Fisher features in other vision tasks including image classification [33]. Note that this Fisher-GMM framework is used in [34] for saliency detection, where it is assumed that images sharing global visual appearance are likely to share similar salient regions. Inspired by this work, we extend the framework on the principle that salient patches themselves are sampled from similar distributions that govern their local appearance. In that sense, our proposed method is a patch-based detector of human fixation.

Inter-Patch Dissimilarity Feature (D_1): Motivated by observation (2), we measure the dissimilarity of a patch $\rho \in P_I$ with its direct neighbors. This dissimilarity can be computed in several ways, since it is highly dependent the features used to describe each of the patches. In this paper, we define the dissimilarity of ρ to its neighbors as the average difference in internal heterogeneity of the patches. In this case, a patch that is reasonably homogenous (i.e. whose appearance has minimal variation) is quite dissimilar from a patch that is heterogenous (i.e. whose appearance has significant variation). Therefore, patch ρ is represented by a self-dissimilarity descriptor, which is computed from the self-similarity descriptor in [35]. This self-dissimilarity descriptor is a matrix that is measured densely throughout the patch and serves as a measure of how heterogenous the patch's interior is. One of the main purposes for using self-similarity is that it captures the internal layout of a patch efficiently by unifying color, texture and edge patterns. It is noteworthy to mention that self-similarity has been shown to be an effective feature in several vision tasks and has been recently made computationally efficient for large resolution images [36]. To the best of our knowledge, this work is the first to apply self-similarity to the study of human fixations.

To compute the inter-patch dissimilarity feature D_1 for ρ, we compute the histogram of the pair-wise Euclidean distances between the self-dissimilarity descriptor of ρ to those of its neighbours. This is the second ingredient of our FPD and it encodes "surprise".

Intra-Patch Dissimilarity Feature (D_2): Based on observation (3), we represent the inner content of patch ρ using a self-dissimilarity descriptor, as described before. The intra-patch dissimilarity feature D_2 is then computed by constructing a histogram of the self-dissimilarity descriptors within patch ρ. This is the third patch feature and it encodes "variance".

Spatial Location Feature (C): Since the saliency of a patch might also be affected by its spatial location in the image, we represent each patch with a fourth feature C, which is simply the normalized 2D coordinates of its center. This feature encodes "locality".

2.2 Classifier Training

This section describes how we train the classifier that will be used in FPD. Specifically, we discuss the details of preparing a fixation patch training dataset and subsequently the patch classification method.

Training Set Preparation: To train a fixation patch classifier, we require ground truth samples (positive and negative) of fixation patches. These patch samples are not readily available and manually annotating them is quite tedious, so we propose an automated way of inferring them using a dataset D_{all} of images and their corresponding human fixations from multiple observers. First, each image $\mathbf{I} \in D_{all}$ is divided into a set of non-overlapping square patches P_I, where the size of each patch is taken to be $M \times M$ pixels. We score each patch in P_I based on the probability that a human fixation falls inside it. To compute this score, we construct an RBF kernel density estimate of the spatial distribution of all human fixation locations in image $\mathbf{I}$, denoted by $p_F(\mathbf{x}|\mathbf{I})$ where $\mathbf{x}$ is an individual pixel in $\mathbf{I}$. The score of patch $\rho \in P_{\mathbf{I}}$, denoted as $r(\rho)$, is computed as the pixelwise average probability of all pixels in ρ. Mathematically, we have $r(\rho) = \frac{1}{|\rho|} \sum_{\mathbf{x} \in \rho} p_F(\mathbf{x}|\mathbf{I})$. After scoring all patches in $\mathbf{I}$, we define ground truth fixation patches (labelled $+1$) as those with a score greater than a predefined threshold τ. Patches with scores less than τ are defined as non-fixation patches (labelled -1). Selecting a suitable τ for each image is not trivial. In our experiments, we take τ to be a predefined multiple of the peak value of $p_F(\mathbf{x}|\mathbf{I})$. Examples of $p_F(\mathbf{x}|\mathbf{I})$ and ground truth fixation patches are shown in Fig. 4.

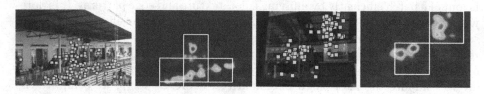

Fig. 4. Ground truth fixation patches. In each image, human fixations are plotted in *yellow*. The spatial density estimate of these fixations and the ground truth fixation patches (in *white*) are also shown. Non-fixation patches are patches whose average probability of containing a human fixation is below $\tau = 8\%$ of the peak probability (Color figure online).

Patch Classification: We apply PCA on the training set to reduce the dimensionality of the Fisher feature vector $\mathbf{F}$. Then, a standard RBF-SVM is trained on each of the four feature vectors separately: $\mathbf{F}$, $\mathbf{D}_1$, $\mathbf{D}_2$ and $\mathbf{C}$. Another SVM is then trained on the confidence values generated by the four individual SVMs. Learning is performed in this manner to *isolate* the effect of each feature type individually. This serves as the patch classifier for the FPD.

An important property of this fixation patch training set is that it is strongly unbalanced towards negative patches, i.e. non-fixation patches. This is primarily due to the sparsity of human fixations in an image. To overcome this significant data bias, conventional undersampling is incorporated in learning the classifier. In Fig. 5, we show detection results using each of the individual SVMs as well as the combined classifier. Clearly, the latter classifier is able to effectively combine the individual SVM responses to accurately predict the fixation patches.

3 Saliency Enhancement

The patches predicted as non-fixations by our FPD method suggest that they are of little value to human observers. Therefore, giving less importance to such

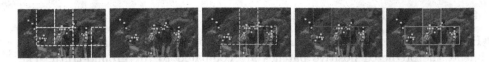

Fig. 5. Patch Classification. Detection results of SVMs using individual features (left to right): Fisher $\mathbf{F}$, inter-patch dissimilary $\mathbf{D}_1$, intra-patch dissimilarity $\mathbf{D}_2$, and location $\mathbf{C}$. The rightmost is the result of their combination and the proposed FPD.

regions in saliency maps generated by popular visual saliency methods may improve the performance of these methods. Consider a set $\{s_k\}_{k=1}^{\Sigma}$, where s_k is the kth saliency model in a set Σ. Given an input image $\mathbf{I}$, the kth model produces a saliency map $s_k(\mathbf{I})$. In an effort to improve saliency map prediction, we update $s_k(\mathbf{I})$ by combining the pixelwise saliency values with the corresponding pixelwise decision values returned by the FPD. This process effectively reduces the saliency of pixels inside predicted non-fixation patches. An added advantage of this strategy is that our FPD can also help to increase the saliency of pixels within fixation patches in case a saliency method misses strongly salient locations within these patch. In fact, we will show empirical evidence that verifies that our FPD allows popular saliency models to achieve better prediction performance on benchmark fixation datasets by reducing false positives, while maintaining true positives.

4   Experiments and Results

This section provides a quantitative analysis of our proposed FPD and empirical evidence showing that combining FPD with state-of-the-art saliency models improves their overall performance.

4.1   Dataset Description

To train the FPD, we use the MIT dataset [22] due to the diverse topical content of its images. This dataset contains 1003 high resolution images with human fixation data from 15 users per image. Maintaining the aspect ratio, each image is downsampled to no more than 2^{16} pixels. These images form our dataset D_{all}, which is randomly divided into D_{train} (903 images) and D_{test} (100 images) using K-fold cross validation (K = 10).

4.2   Parameter Settings

We use the same parameter settings in all our experiments. Based on cross validation results, each patch is taken to be $M \times M$ pixels with $M = 64$. Note that the FPD can be scaled to any patch size to suit application needs with adherence to runtime constraints. Of course, our proposed approach can be easily extended to multiple scales for more fine grained detection, accompanied by a linear increase in runtime. The value of the ground truth labeling threshold τ is set to 8 % of the peak probability estimated using kernel density estimation.

4.3   FPD Performance Evaluation

Before evaluating the performance of the proposed FPD for saliency improvement, the predicted positive patches are compared to the ground-truth. The performance of the model is represented by its average positive accuracy p and average negative accuracy rate n. Using 10-fold cross validation, the FPD performs significantly well with $p = 84\%$ and $n = 84\%$ showing that the learned FPD can indeed be used to short-list and identify human fixation patches.

To evaluate the FPD's ability to enhance popular saliency methods, we compare the accuracy of each saliency method with and without our prior. We show results on D_{all} for 8 recent and state-of-the-art saliency models, namely **SR** [12], **SU** [13], **ES** [18], **GB** [14], **IT**[1] [15], **AW** [16,17], **YI** [19] and **BM** [20].

Out of the many evaluation measures that have been used for comparing saliency models, ROC is the most widely used. The ROC curve is a measure of how well a saliency map can distinguish fixation and non-fixation points for different binary saliency thresholds. However, recent studies suggest that ROC is not always an ideal metric for comparison [11,37,38], since it only depends on the ordering of the fixations. As shown/argued in [37,38], as long as the true positive rate is high, the area under the ROC curve (AUC) is always high regardless of the false positive rate. On the other hand, the main aim of our framework is to reduce false positives generated by a particular saliency model, while keeping this method's hit rate the same. Since ROC is affected more by the hit rate rather than false alarm rate, it is not suitable for a comprehensive evaluation of our proposed framework. Instead, we use two other popular evaluation measures, namely the Linear Correlation Coefficient (CC) [11,24] and Normalized Scanpath Saliency (NSS) [39]. CC measures the strength of the linear relationship between a saliency map and the ground truth map, with an absolute value close to 1 indicating an almost perfectly linear relationship between the two. The NSS measures the average distance between the fixation saliency and zero with a larger NSS implying a greater correspondence between fixation locations and the saliency predictions [37].

Figure 6 shows the average CC and NSS scores across all images in D_{all} for each saliency method before and after applying the FPD to the resulting saliency map.[2] Clearly, there is a significant improvement in both CC and NSS scores, which verifies the ability of the FPD to benefit each saliency model. Interestingly, our saliency prior is even able to enhance the performance of **BM** and **AW**, the top performing saliency models according to current literature [11,20,23].

Table 1 reports the percentage of images for which the CC and NSS scores were increased for each method. On average, we increase the CC score for over 75 % of images and increase the NSS score for over 78 % of images across all methods. In particular, our proposed FPD increases both scores for **SR**, **SU**

---

[1] Note that there are different versions of Itti's model. Here, we used the best performing version in [14].

[2] Due to differences in image resolution, the reported scores of the saliency models are slightly different from those reported in [11,23]. However, the relative performance of the models is not significantly affected.

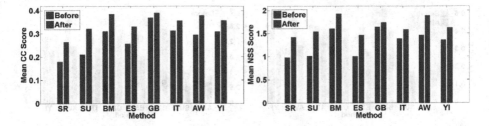

Fig. 6. Performance evaluation on MIT dataset. Average CC and NSS scores before and after applying the FPD on 8 state-of-the art saliency models. The FPD improves each score significantly for all tested methods.

Table 1. Percentage of images for which CC and NSS is increased. For each saliency method, we report the percentage of images for which the scores were increased after using the FPD.

Saliency method	SR	SU	BM	ES	GB	IT	AW	YI
CC	81%	82%	81%	73%	67%	71%	76%	72%
NSS	86%	85%	80%	82%	67%	71%	80%	76%

and **BM** on over 80% of the images. Table 1 along with Fig. 6 clearly show that higher performance is achieved when any of the saliency methods is simply combined with our proposed FPD.

Next, we test the performance of our FPD on another popular image dataset widely used for saliency evaluation. We use the FPD trained on D_{train} from the MIT dataset (refer to Sect. 4.1) and test it on the dataset in [40]. Since the training and test sets are different, this evaluates the generality of our method and its ability to transcend dataset specificities. Figure 7 shows mean scores across all images for each saliency method before and after using our method. The FPD is successful in improving the performance of all the saliency methods for this dataset as well. Interestingly, we once again observe a significant increase in performance for the top performing methods (**AW** and **BM**). Since combining these two models with our FPD significantly outperforms all other models, we recommend using this combination for future applications.

4.4 Center Bias

Even though the location feature in our model does not introduce any explicit center bias to the saliency maps (as our method focuses mainly on decreasing the false positives), it is still important to verify that the improvement in saliency performance reported in the previous section is not merely due to the location feature. It has often been pointed out in the literature that the issue of center bias is a major challenge for comparing saliency models. Several solutions have been proposed to eliminate center-bias effects, with the shuffled AUC metric being the most popularly used solution [13,20,23]. However, as discussed in Sect. 4.3,

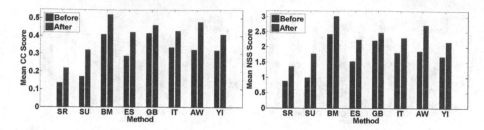

Fig. 7. Performance evaluation on Bruce-Tsotsos dataset. Average CC and NSS scores before and after applying the FPD on 8 state-of-the art saliency methods on the Bruce-Tsotsos dataset [40]. The FPD improves each score significantly for all tested methods for this dataset as well.

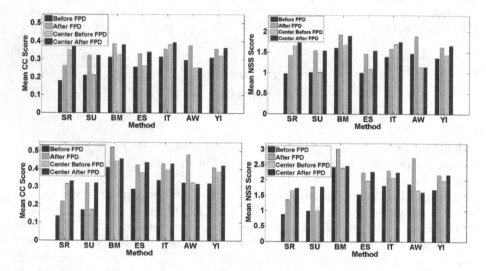

Fig. 8. Comparison of FPD with explicit center bias. Top row - performance of the FPD on center-biased saliency maps on the MIT dataset [22]. Bottom row - FPD performance on the Bruce-Tsotsos dataset [40].

AUC is not an ideal metric for evaluating FPD. Moreover, shuffled AUC comes with the drawback of de-emphasizing genuine human fixations around the image center. For a more comprehensive evaluation, we explicitly introduce center bias to all the saliency methods as suggested in [11] by applying Gaussian blobs of varying sizes to each saliency map (centered at the image center and by increasing the size of the Gaussian by varying the sigma parameter, σ from 10 to 30 units). Our FPD is then applied to these center-biased saliency maps. This helps us evaluate the effectiveness of the FPD when the effect of the location feature is nullified due to the explicit addition of center bias. Since **GB** inherently adds a center bias and since we already showed an improvement in its performance, we exclude **GB** from this comparison.

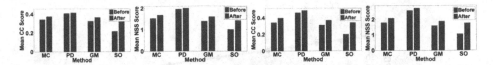

Fig. 9. Performance evaluation of the FPD on salient object methods. Average CC and NSS scores before and after applying the FPD on 4 salient object detectors on the MIT (first two plots) and Bruce-Tsotsos (last two plots) datasets.

Figure 8 shows the average CC and NSS scores after adding the center-bias and the performance of the FPD on both the original and center-biased saliency maps for both the MIT and Bruce-Tsotsos datasets when $\sigma = 20$ (as in the previous section, no training was performed on the Bruce-Tsotsos dataset). As expected, adding explicit center bias increases both the CC and NSS scores for most of the saliency methods. However, it is encouraging to see that the performance of the FPD on the original saliency maps significantly outperforms the center-biased saliency maps for the top performing models, e.g. **BM**, **AW**, and **YI**. In addition, for the majority of the methods, the FPD increases the performance of the center-biased saliency maps as well. This is due to the fact that the center bias merely increases the saliency at the center. Our method, on the other hand, reduces the saliency of pixels within non-fixation patches, which could exist around the image center as well. A similar trend was also observed for all the different Gaussian sizes, i.e. when the σ value was 10 and 30 with the FPD increasing the performance in these cases as well. These results strongly suggest that the increase in the performance of saliency methods in the previous section is *not* simply due to the spatial feature **C** and that our proposed method plays a genuine role in enhancing the saliency methods themselves.

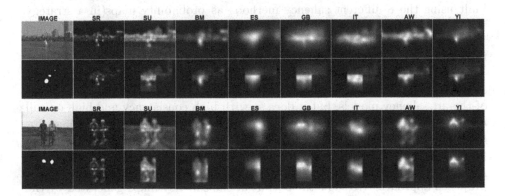

Fig. 10. Qualitative results of our proposed approach. Top and third row (left to right): Shows the input image and the saliency maps generated by 8 methods before applying the FPD. Second and last row (left to right): Shows the ground truth followed by our proposed FPD's saliency maps for each of the methods in the upper row.

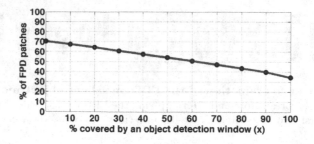

Fig. 11. Experiments on the PASCAL VOC dataset. Figure showing the percentage of patches that are covered by an object bounding box by more than x %. An object bounding box tends to have 60 % or more coverage with roughly half the fixation patches showing the potential of the detected patches to capture salient object parts.

4.5   Improvement of Salient Object Detection Methods

Motivated by the work in [41] that showed that objects are highly effective in predicting human fixations, we also test our FPD's performance with 4 state-of-art salient object detectors, namely **SO** [42], **MC** [43], **PD** [44], and **GM** [45]. Figure 9 shows the performance of these methods before and after applying the FPD for fixation prediction on the MIT and Bruce-Tsotsos datasets. Consistent with our previous findings, the FPD improves the performance of the salient object methods as well.

5   Discussion

The experimental results in Sect. 4.3 show that the FPD is able to short-list a set of fixation patches in an image with high accuracy and a reasonably low false positive rate. We also compare of the performance of our FPD against FPDs built using the 8 different saliency methods as probability maps(in a strategy similar to that in Sect. 2.2). The accuracy of our proposed FPD was greater than 12 % with respect to p accuracy and 14 % with respect to n accuracy on average from these FPDs.

To summarize the results of Sect. 4.3, the performance of our FPD demonstrates significant promise. Not only does it improve the performance of state-of-the-art saliency models, but it does so with high consistency and high overall magnitude. In particular, our method registers a significant improvement for top performing saliency methods **AW** and **BM**. This suggests that our proposed FPD can be used as a post processing step with saliency methods for pertinent vision applications. Figure 10 presents some qualitative results of our proposed approach. We show the output of the saliency maps generated by the eight different models, before and after applying FPD. The FPD benefits the saliency models by reducing the saliency of irrelevant background clutter, while maintaining the saliency of locations with high perceptual value.

Since humans fixate on objects of interest, the patches returned by the FPD have the potential of covering objects and being useful in higher level tasks. With this is in mind, we apply the FPD on the PASCAL VOC 2007 object detection dataset [46], which consists of 5011 images. Since ground-truth bounding boxes are provided for objects in all images in the dataset, we can evaluate how likely our predicted fixation patches overlap with these objects. In our experiments, we train on the entire MIT dataset D_{all} and use the VOC 2007 Trainval dataset (containing 5011 images) as the test set. We evaluate the performance of the FPD by first taking the union of all ground truth object detection windows in each image $\mathbf{I}$ of the test set to generate mask $\mathbf{M}_1$. We then take the union of all the salient fixation patches predicted by the FPD in $\mathbf{I}$ to form mask $\mathbf{M}_2$. Next, we find the intersection of all the predicted fixation patches with all the object detection windows, i.e. compute $|\mathbf{M}_1 \cap \mathbf{M}_2|$, and divide the intersection by the size of $\mathbf{M}_2$ to obtain the overall percentage overlap, i.e. compute $\frac{|\mathbf{M}_1 \cap \mathbf{M}_2|}{|\mathbf{M}_2|}$.

We repeat this process for all images in the test set and obtain an average overlap percentage of 59.6%. This implies that the predicted fixation patches are not only perceptually relevant in general but they also overlap reasonably well with object windows. For each fixation patch, we also calculate the highest percentage of the patch that is covered by a single object window. This tells us the relevance of each fixation patch in covering a single object part. Figure 11 plots the percentage of predicted fixation patches that are overlapped by more than $x\%$ by an object window. For $x = 50$, this percentage is approximately 55%. This signifies that more than half of the predicted fixation patches are significantly covered by an object window. Interestingly, roughly 35% of these fixation patches overlap with the object windows completely and reside inside an object window. Since our patch size is much smaller than the average object window size, this could possibly suggest that FPD patches have the *potential* to find object parts.

6   Conclusion

In this paper, we propose a fixation patch detector (FPD) that predicts image regions where human fixations reside. We use these fixation patches as saliency priors to reduce the saliency of pixels within non-fixation patches leading to a consistent improvement in the prediction performance of several state-of-the-art saliency methods. The FPD significantly improves the performance of the top performing saliency methods, thereby suggesting that it can be used as a post processing step with state-of-the-art methods for future vision applications like object detection, image thumbnailing, etc.

Acknowledgement. Research reported in this publication was supported by competitive research funding from King Abdullah University of Science and Technology (KAUST).

References

1. Ross, J., Burr, D., Morrone, C.: Suppression of the magnocellular pathway during saccades. (Behavioural Brain Research)

2. Itti, L., Koch, C.: Computational modelling of visual attention. Nat. Rev. Neurosci. **2**, 194–203 (2001)
3. Rutishauser, U., Walther, D., Koch, C., Perona, P.: Is bottom-up attention useful for object recognition. In: CVPR (2004)
4. Walther, D., Itti, L., Riesenhuber, M., Poggio, T.A., Koch, C.: Attentional selection for object recognition - a gentle way. In: Bülthoff, H.H., Lee, S.-W., Poggio, T.A., Wallraven, C. (eds.) BMCV 2002. LNCS, vol. 2525, pp. 472–479. Springer, Heidelberg (2002)
5. Endres, I., Hoiem, D.: Category independent object proposals. In: Daniilidis, K., Maragos, P., Paragios, N. (eds.) ECCV 2010, Part V. LNCS, vol. 6315, pp. 575–588. Springer, Heidelberg (2010)
6. Shapovalova, N., Raptis, M., Sigal, L., Mori, G.: Action is in the eye of the beholder: eye-gaze driven model for spatio-temporal action localization. In: NIPS (2013)
7. Mikolajczyk, K., Schmid, C.: Scale & affine invariant interest point detectors. Int. J. comput. vis. **60**, 63–86 (2004)
8. Dave, A., Dubey, R., Ghanem, B.: Do humans fixate on interest points? In: ICPR (2012)
9. Yang, L., Zheng, N., Yang, J., Chen, M., Chen, H.: A biased sampling strategy for object categorization. In: CVPR (2009)
10. Marchesotti, L., Cifarelli, C., Csurka, G.: A framework for visual saliency detection with applications to image thumbnailing. In: ICCV (2009)
11. Borji, A., Sihite, D., Itti, L.: Quantitative analysis of human-model agreement in visual saliency modeling: a comparative study. IEEE Trans. Image Process. **22**, 55–69 (2013)
12. Hou, X., Zhang, L.: Saliency detection: a spectral residual approach. In: CVPR (2007)
13. Zhang, L., Tong, M.H., Marks, T.K., Shan, H., Cottrell, G.W.: Sun: a bayesian framework for saliency using natural statistics. J. Vis. **8**(7), 1–20 (2008)
14. Harel, J., Koch, C., Perona, P.: Graph-based visual saliency. In: NIPS (2007)
15. Itti, L., Koch, C., Niebur, E.: A model of saliency-based visual attention for rapid scene analysis. IEEE Trans. Pattern Anal. Mach. Intell. **20**, 1254–1259 (1998)
16. Garcia-Diaz, A., Fdez-Vidal, X.R., Pardo, X.M., Dosil, R.: Saliency from hierarchical adaptation through decorrelation and variance normalization. Image Vis. Comput. **30**, 51–64 (2012)
17. Garcia-Diaz, A., Leborán, V., Fdez-Vidal, X.R., Pardo, X.M.: On the relationship between optical variability, visual saliency, and eye fixations: a computational approach. J. Vis. **12**(6), 1–22 (2012)
18. Avraham, T., Lindenbaum, M.: Esaliency (extended saliency): meaningful attention using stochastic image modeling. IEEE Trans. Pattern Anal. Mach. Intell. **32**, 693–708 (2010)
19. Li, Y., Zhou, Y., Yan, J., Niu, Z., Yang, J.: Visual saliency based on conditional entropy. In: Maybank, S., Taniguchi, R., Zha, H. (eds.) ACCV 2009, Part I. LNCS, vol. 5994, pp. 246–257. Springer, Heidelberg (2010)
20. Zhang, J., Stan, S.: Saliency detection: a boolean map approach. In: ICCV (2013)
21. Itti, L., Baldi, P.: Bayesian surprise attracts human attention. In: NIPS (2006)
22. Judd, T., Ehinger, K., Durand, F., Torralba, A.: Learning to predict where humans look. In: ICCV (2009)
23. Borji, A., Tavakoli, H., Sihite, D., Itti, L.: Analysis of scores, datasets, and models in visual saliency prediction. In: ICCV (2013)
24. Borji, A., Itti, L.: State-of-the-art in visual attention modeling. IEEE Trans. Pattern Anal. Mach. Intell. **35**, 185–207 (2012)

25. Soto, D., Humphreys, G.W., Heinke, D.: Working memory can guide pop-out search. Vis. Res. **46**, 1010–1018 (2006)
26. Sheinberg, D.L., Logothetis, N.K.: Noticing familiar objects in real world scenes: the role of temporal cortical neurons in natural vision. J. Neurosci. **21**, 1340–1350 (2001)
27. Yang, Y., Song, M., Li, N., Bu, J., Chen, C.: What is the chance of happening: a new way to predict where people look. In: Daniilidis, K., Maragos, P., Paragios, N. (eds.) ECCV 2010, Part V. LNCS, vol. 6315, pp. 631–643. Springer, Heidelberg (2010)
28. Poirier, F.J., Gosselin, F., Arguin, M.: Perceptive fields of saliency. J. Vis. **8**, 14 (2008)
29. Scharfenberger, C., Wong, A., Fergani, K., Zelek, J.S., Clausi, D.A.: Statistical textural distinctiveness for salient region detection in natural images. In: CVPR (2013)
30. Le Meur, O., Le Callet, P., Barba, D.: Predicting visual fixations on video based on low-level visual features. Vis. Res. **47**, 2483–2498 (2007)
31. Jaakkola, T., Haussler, D.: Exploiting generative models in discriminative classifiers. In: NIPS (1998)
32. Dempster, A.P., Laird, N.M., Rubin, D.B.: Maximum likelihood from incomplete data via the em algorithm. J. R. Stat. Soc. Ser. B **39**, 1–38 (1977)
33. Perronnin, F., Sánchez, J., Mensink, T.: Improving the fisher kernel for large-scale image classification. In: Daniilidis, K., Maragos, P., Paragios, N. (eds.) ECCV 2010, Part IV. LNCS, vol. 6314, pp. 143–156. Springer, Heidelberg (2010)
34. Marchesotti, L., Cifarelli, C., Csurka, G.: A framework for visual saliency detection with applications to image thumbnailing. In: ICCV (2009)
35. Shechtman, E., Irani, M.: Matching local self-similarities across images and videos. In: CVPR (2007)
36. Deselaers, T., Ferrari, V.: Global and efficient self-similarity for object classification and detection. In: CVPR (2010)
37. Zhao, Q., Koch, C.: Learning a saliency map using fixated locations in natural scenes. J. Vis. **11**, 1–15 (2011)
38. Judd, T., Durand, F., Torralba, A.: A benchmark of computational models of saliency to predict human fixations. Technical report (2012)
39. Peters, R.J., Iyer, A., Itti, L., Koch, C.: Components of bottom-up gaze allocation in natural images. Vis. Res. **45**, 2397–2416 (2005)
40. Bruce, N., Tsotsos, J.: Saliency based on information maximization. In: NIPS (2006)
41. Einhäuser, W., Spain, M., Perona, P.: Objects predict fixations better than early saliency. J. Vis. **8**, 18 (2008)
42. Rahtu, E., Kannala, J., Salo, M., Heikkilä, J.: Segmenting salient objects from images and videos. In: Daniilidis, K., Maragos, P., Paragios, N. (eds.) ECCV 2010, Part V. LNCS, vol. 6315, pp. 366–379. Springer, Heidelberg (2010)
43. Jiang, B., Zhang, L., Lu, H., Yang, C., Yang, M.H.: Saliency detection via absorbing markov chain. In: ICCV (2013)
44. Margolin, R., Tal, A., Zelnik-Manor, L.: What makes a patch distinct? In: CVPR (2013)
45. Yang, C., Zhang, L., Lu, H., Ruan, X., Yang, M.H.: Saliency detection via graph-based manifold ranking. In: CVPR (2013)
46. Everingham, M., Van Gool, L., Williams, C., Winn, J., Zisserman, A.: The pascal visual object classes challenge 2007 (voc 2007) results (2007). In: URL http://www.pascal-network.org/challenges/VOC/voc2007/workshop/index.html. (2008)

Fast Super-Resolution via Dense Local Training and Inverse Regressor Search

Eduardo Pérez-Pellitero[1,2]($\boxtimes$), Jordi Salvador[1], Iban Torres-Xirau[1],
Javier Ruiz-Hidalgo[3], and Bodo Rosenhahn[2]

[1] Technicolor R&I Hannover, Hannover, Germany
eduardo.perezpellitero@technicolor.com
[2] TNT Lab, Leibniz Universität Hannover, Hannover, Germany
[3] Image Processing Group, Universitat Politècnica de Catalunya, Barcelona, Spain

Abstract. Regression-based Super-Resolution (SR) addresses the upscaling problem by learning a mapping function (i.e. regressor) from the low-resolution to the high-resolution manifold. Under the locally linear assumption, this complex non-linear mapping can be properly modeled by a set of linear regressors distributed across the manifold. In such methods, most of the testing time is spent searching for the right regressor within this trained set. In this paper we propose a novel inverse-search approach for regression-based SR. Instead of performing a search from the image to the dictionary of regressors, the search is done inversely from the regressors' dictionary to the image patches. We approximate this framework by applying spherical hashing to both image and regressors, which reduces the inverse search into computing a trained function. Additionally, we propose an improved training scheme for SR linear regressors which improves perceived and objective quality. By merging both contributions we improve speed and quality compared to the state-of-the-art.

1 Introduction

Super resolution (SR) comprises any reconstruction technique capable of extending the resolution of a discrete signal beyond the limits of the corresponding capture device. The SR problem is by nature ill-posed, so the definition of suitable priors is critical. Over more than two decades, many of them have been proposed.

Originally, image SR methods were based on piecewise linear and smooth priors (i.e. bilinear and bicubic interpolation, respectively), resulting in fast interpolation-based algorithms. Tsai and Huang [1] showed that it was possible to reconstruct higher-resolution images by registering and fusing multiple images, thus pioneering a vast amount of approaches on multi-image SR, often called reconstruction-based SR. This idea was further refined, among others, with the introduction of iterative back-projection for improved registration by Irani and Peleg [2], although further analysis by Baker and Kanade [3] and Lin and Shum [4] showed fundamental limits on this type of SR, mainly conditioned by registration accuracy. Learning-based SR, also known as example-based, overcame

© Springer International Publishing Switzerland 2015
D. Cremers et al. (Eds.): ACCV 2014, Part III, LNCS 9005, pp. 346–359, 2015.
DOI: 10.1007/978-3-319-16811-1_23

some of the aforementioned limitations by avoiding the necessity of a registration process and by building the priors from image statistics. The original work by Freeman et al. [5] aims to *learn* from patch- or feature-based examples to produce effective magnification well beyond the practical limits of multi-image SR.

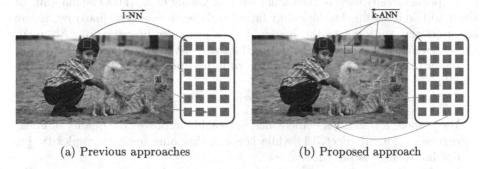

(a) Previous approaches   (b) Proposed approach

Fig. 1. Overview of the proposed inverse-search SR: (a) Previous approaches search the 1st nearest dictionary atom for each image patch. (b) Our Proposed approach searches the k-nearest image patches for each dictionary atom.

Example-based SR approaches using dictionaries are usually divided into two categories: internal and external dictionary-based SR. The first exploits the strong self-similarity prior. This prior is learnt directly from the relationship of image patches across different scales of the input image. The opening work on this subcategory was introduced by Glasner et al. [6], presenting a powerful framework for fusing reconstruction-based and example-based SR. Further research on this category by Freedman and Fattal [7] introduced a mechanism for high-frequency transfer based on examples from a small area around each patch, thus better localizing the cross-scale self-similarity prior to the spatial neighborhood. The recent work of Yang et al. [8] further develops the idea of localizing the cross-scale self-similarity prior arriving to the in-place prior, i.e. the best match across scales is located exactly in the same position if the scale is similar enough.

External dictionary-based SR methods use other images to build their dictionaries. A representative widely used approach is the one based on sparse decomposition. The main idea behind this approach is the decomposition of each patch in the input image into a combination of a sparse subset of entries in a compact dictionary. The work of Yang et al. [9] uses an external database composed of related low and high-resolution patches to jointly learn a compact dictionary pair. During testing, each image patch is decomposed into a sparse linear combination of the entries in the low-resolution (LR) dictionary and the same weights are used to generate the high-resolution (HR) patch as a linear combination of the HR entries. Both the dictionary training and testing are costly due to the L_1 regularization term enforcing sparsity. The work of Zeyde et al. [10] extends sparse SR by proposing several algorithmic speed-ups which also improves performance. However, the bottleneck of sparsity methods still remains in the sparse decomposition.

More recently, regression-based SR has received a great deal of attention by the research community. In this case, the goal is to learn a certain mapping from the manifold of the LR patches to that of HR patches, following the manifold assumption already used in the earlier work of Chang et al. [11]. The mapping of the manifold is assumed to be locally linear and therefore several linear regressors are used and anchored to the manifold as a piecewise linearization. Although these methods are among the fastest in the state-of-the-art, searching the proper regressor takes a significant quota of the running time from within the whole SR pipeline.

In this paper we introduce the following contributions:

1. We propose a training scheme which noticeably improves the quality of linear regression for SR (Sect. 3.1) while keeping the same testing complexity, i.e. not increasing testing time.
2. We formulate an inverse-search approach where for every regressor in the dictionary its k-Nearest Neighbors (k-NN) input image features are found (Fig. 1). Also, we provide a suitable and efficient spherical hashing framework to exploit this scheme, which greatly improves speed at little quality cost. (Section 3.2).

By merging the two contributions, we improve both in speed and quality to both the fastest and the best-performing state-of-the-art methods, as shown in the experimental results.

2   Regression-Based SR

In this section we introduce the SR problem and how example-based approaches tackle it, followed by a review of the recent state-of-the-art regression work of Timofte et al. [12] as it is closely related with the work presented in this paper. The contributions of this paper follow in Sect. 3.

2.1   Problem Statement

Super-Resolution aims to upscale images which have an unsatisfactory pixel resolution while preserving the same visual sharpness, more formally

$$X = \uparrow (Y) \ s.t. \ \mathcal{X} \approx \mathcal{Y}, \tag{1}$$

where Y is the input image, X is the output upscaled image, $\uparrow (\cdot)$ is an upsampling operator and calligraphic font denotes the spectrum of an image.

In the literature this transformation has usually been modeled backwards as the restoration of an original image that has suffered several degradations [9]

$$Y = \downarrow (B(X)), \tag{2}$$

where $B(\cdot)$ is a blurring filter and $\downarrow (\cdot)$ is a downsampling operator. The problem is usually addressed at a patch level, denoted with lower case (e.g. y, x).

The example-based SR family tackles the super-resolution problem by finding meaningful examples from which a HR counterpart is already known, namely the couple of dictionaries D_l and D_h:

$$\min_{\beta} \|y - D_l \beta\|_2^2 + \lambda \|\beta\|_p, \tag{3}$$

where β selects and weights the elements in the dictionary and λ weights a possible L_p-norm regularization term. The L_p-norm selection and the dictionary-building process depend on the chosen priors and they further define the SR algorithm.

2.2 Anchored Neighborhood Regression

The recent work of Timofte et al. [12] is especially remarkable for its low-complexity nature which achieves orders of magnitude speed-ups while having competitive quality results compared to the state-of-the-art. They proposed a relaxation of the L_1-norm regularization commonly used in most of the Neighbor Embedding (NE) and Sparse Coding (SC) approaches, reformulating the problem as a least squares (LS) L_2-norm regularized regression, also known as Ridge Regression. While solving L_1-norm constrained minimization problems is computationally demanding, when relaxing it to a L_2-norm, a closed-form solution can be used. Their proposed minimization problem reads

$$\min_{\beta} \|y_F - N_l \beta\|_2^2 + \lambda \|\beta\|_2, \tag{4}$$

where N_l is the LR neighborhood chosen to solve the problem and y_F is a feature extracted from a LR patch. The algebraic solution is

$$\beta = (N_l^T N_l + \lambda I)^{-1} N_l^T y_F. \tag{5}$$

The coefficients of β are applied to the corresponding HR neighborhood N_h to reconstruct the HR patch, i.e. $x = N_h \beta$. This can also be written as the matrix multiplication $x = R \, y_F$, where the projection matrix (i.e. regressor) is calculated as

$$R = N_h (N_l^T N_l + \lambda I)^{-1} N_l^T \tag{6}$$

and can be computed offline, therefore moving the minimization problem from testing to training time.

They propose to use sparse dictionaries of d_s atoms size, trained with the K-SVD algorithm [13]. A regressor R_j is anchored to each atom d_j in D_l, and the neighborhood N_l in Eq. (6) is selected from a k-NN subset of D_l:

$$N_{l_j} = \text{kNN}(d_j, D_l). \tag{7}$$

The SR problem can be addressed by finding the NN atom d_j of every input patch feature y_{iF} and applying the associated R_j to it. In the specific case of a neighborhood size $k = d_s$, only one general regressor is obtained whose neighborhood comprises all the atoms of the dictionary and consequently does not require a NN search. This case is referred in the original paper as Global Regression (GR).

2.3   Linear Regression Framework

Once the closest anchor point is found, the regression is usually applied to certain input features and aims to recover certain components of the patch. We model the linear regression framework in a general way as

$$x = \tilde{x} + R\, y_F, \tag{8}$$

where $\tilde{x}$ is a coarse first approximation of the HR patch x. The choice of how to obtain $\tilde{x}$ requires selecting a prior on how to better approximate x. In the work of Yang et al. [8] they use the in-place prior as this first-approximation and Timofte et al. [12] use the bicubic interpolation assuming a smooth prior. The regressors are trained to improve the reconstruction whenever the coarse prior is not sufficient. Intuitively, for an optimal performance, the selected feature representation has to be related with the chosen first approximation $\tilde{x}$. Supporting this, [8] uses as input feature the subtraction of the low-pass filtered in-place example to the bicubic interpolation, intuitively modeling the errors of the in-place prior for the low-frequency band; and [12] uses gradient-based features, representing the high-frequency components which are likely not going to be well-reconstructed with bicubic interpolation.

3   Fast Hashing-Based Super-Resolution

In this section we present our super-resolution algorithm based on an inverse-search scheme. The section is divided into two parts representing the contributions of the paper: We first discuss the optimal training stage for linear super-resolution regressors and then introduce our hashing-based regressor selection scheme.

3.1   Training

In regression-based SR the objective of training a given regressor R is to obtain a certain mapping function from LR to HR patches. From a more general perspective, LR patches form an input manifold M of dimension m and HR patches form a target manifold N of dimension n. Formally, for training pairs (y_{Fi}, x_i) with $y_F \in M$ and $x_i \in N$, we would like to infer a mapping $\Psi : M \subseteq \mathbb{R}^m \rightarrow N \subseteq \mathbb{R}^n$.

As we have previously seen, recent regression-based SR use linear regressors because they can be easily computed in closed form and applied as a matrix

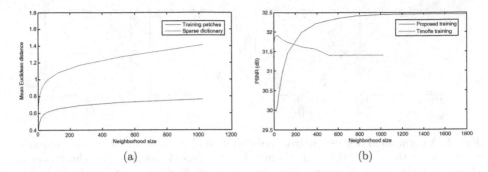

Fig. 2. (a) Mean euclidean distance between atoms and its neighborhood for different neighborhood sizes. (b) Quality improvement measured in PSNR (dB) for a reconstruction using ANR [12] together with our proposed training. 1024 anchor points were used for this experiment.

multiplication. However, the mapping Ψ is highly complex and non-linear [14]. To model the non-linearity nature of the mapping, an ensemble of regressors $\{R_i\}$ is trained, representing a locally linear parametrization of Ψ, under the assumption that both manifolds M and N have a similar local geometry. We analyze the effect on the distribution of those regressors in the manifold (i.e. the anchor points) and the importance of properly choosing the N_l in Eq. (6), concluding on a new training approach.

In the work of Timofte et al. [12], an overcomplete sparse representation is obtained from the initial LR training patches using K-SVD [13]. This new reduced dictionary D_l is used both as anchor points to the manifold and datapoints for the regression training. In their GR, a unique regressor R_G is trained with all elements of the dictionary, therefore accepting higher regression errors due to the single linearization of the manifold. For a more fine-tuned regression reconstruction they also propose the Anchored Neighborhood Regression (ANR), they use as anchor points $\{A_1, \ldots, A_{d_s}\}$ the dictionary points $\{D_1, \ldots, D_{d_s}\}$ and they build for each one of those atoms a neighborhood of k-NN within the same sparse dictionary D_l.

Performing a sparse decomposition of a high number of patches efficiently compresses data in a much smaller dictionary, yielding atoms which are representative of the whole training dataset, i.e. the whole manifold. For this reason they are suitable to be used as anchor points, but also sub-optimal for the neighborhood embedding. They are sub-optimal since the necessary local condition for the linearity assumption is likely to be violated. Due to the L_1-norm reconstruction minimization imposed in sparse dictionaries, atoms in the dictionary are not close in the Euclidean space, as shown in Fig. 2(a).

This observation leads us to propose a different approach when training linear regressors for SR: Using sparse representations as anchor points to the manifold, but forming the neighborhoods with raw manifold samples (e.g. features, patches). In Fig. 2(a) we show how, by doing so, we find closer nearest neighbors

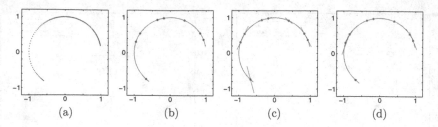

(a)   (b)   (c)   (d)

Fig. 3. A normalized degree 3 polynomial manifold illustrating the proposed approach compared to the one in [12]. (a) Bidimensional manifold samples. (b) The manifold (blue) and the sparse representation obtained with K-SVD algorithm (green) of 8 atoms. (c) Linear regressors (red) trained with the neighborhoods ($k = 1$) obtained within the sparse dictionary, as in [12]. (d) Linear regressors (red) obtained using our proposed approach: The neighborhoods are obtained within the samples from the manifold ($k = 10$) (Color figure online).

and, therefore, fulfill better the local condition. Additionally, a higher number of local independent measurements is available (e.g. mean distance for 1000 neighbors in the raw-patch approach is comparable to a 40 atom neighborhood in the sparse approach) and we can control the number of k-NN selected, i.e. it is not upper-bounded by the dictionary size. We show a low-dimensional example of our proposed training scheme in Fig. 3.

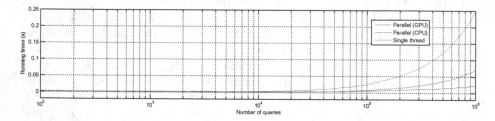

Fig. 4. Running times measured when computing 6-bit hash codes (6 hyperspheres) for increasing number of queries (in logarithmic axis and without re-ranking) for single-threaded (CPU) and parallel (CPU and GPU) implementations.

In Fig. 2(b) we show the comparison of ANR [12] with both training approaches in terms of resulting image PSNR. We use the same training dataset of the original paper, and for our neighbor embedding we use the L_2-normalized raw features which are introduced in the K-SVD algorithm. We fix the dictionary size (only used as anchor points in our scheme) to 1024. By applying our training scheme we achieve substantial quality improvements, both qualitatively and quantitatively.

3.2   Inverse Search via Spherical Hashing

When aiming at a fine modeling of the mapping between LR and HR manifolds, several linear regressors have to be trained to better represent the non-linear problem. Although state-of-the art regression-based SR has already pushed forward the computational speed with regard to other dictionary-based SR [9,10], finding the right regressor for each patch is still consuming most of the execution time. In the work of [12], most of the *encoding time* (i.e. time left after subtracting shared processing time, including bicubic interpolations, patch extractions, etc.) is spent in this task (i.e. ∼96 % of the time).

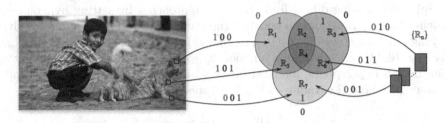

Fig. 5. Spherical hashing applied for the inverse search super-resolution problem. Certain hashing functions are optimized on feature patch statistics creating a set of hyperspheres intersections that are directly labeled with a hash code. In training time, regressors fill this intersections (i.e. bins) and in testing time the hashing function is applied to each patch, which will directly map it to a regressor.

The second contribution of this paper is a novel search strategy designed to benefit from the training outcome presented in Sect. 3.1, i.e. anchor points of the dictionary and their neighborhoods are obtained independently and ahead from the search structure.

In order to improve the search efficiency, search structures of sublinear complexity are often built, usually in the form of binary splits, e.g. trees, hashing schemes [15–18]. One might consider determining the search partitions with the set of anchor points, since those are the elements to retrieve. However, the small cardinality of this set leads to an imprecise partitioning due to a shortage of sampling density. We propose an inverse search scheme which consists in finding the k-ANN (Approximate Nearest Neighbor) patches within the image for every anchor point, as shown in Fig. 1. By doing so, we have a dense sampling (i.e. all training patches) at our disposal, which results in meaningful partitions.

We choose hashing techniques over tree-based methods. Hashing schemes provide low memory usage (the number of splitting functions in hashing-based structures is $O(\log_2(n))$ while in tree-based structures is $O(n)$, where n represents the number of clusters) and are highly parallelizable.

Binary hashing techniques aim to embed high-dimensional points in binary codes, providing a compact representation of high-dimensional data. Among their vast range of applications, they can be used for efficient similarity search, including approximate nearest neighbor retrieval, since hashing codes preserve relative distances. There has recently been active research in data-dependent hashing functions opposed to hashing methods such as [17] which are data-independent. Data-dependent methods intend to better fit the hashing function to the data distribution [18,19] through an off-line training stage.

Among the data-dependent state-of-the-arts methods, we select the Spherical Hashing algorithm of Heo et al. [16], which is able to define closed regions in $\mathbb{R}^m$ with as few as one splitting function. This hashing framework is useful to model the inverse search scheme and enables to benefit from substantial speed-ups by reducing the NN search into applying a precomputed function, which conveniently scales with parallel implementations, as shown in Fig. 4.

Spherical hashing differs from previous approaches by setting hyperspheres to define hashing functions on behalf of the previously used hyperplanes. A given hashing function $H(y_F) = (h_1(y_F), \ldots, h_c(y_F))$ maps points from $\mathbb{R}^m$ to a base $2\ \mathbb{N}^c$, i.e. $\{0,1\}^c$. Every hashing function $h_k(y_F)$ indicates whether the point y_F is inside kth hypersphere, modeled for this purpose as a *pivot* $p_k \in \mathbb{R}^m$ and a distance threshold (i.e. radius of the hypersphere) $t_k \in \mathbb{R}^+$ as:

$$h_k(y_F) = \begin{cases} 0 & when\ d(p_k, y_F) > t_k \\ 1 & when\ d(d_k, y_F) \leq t_k \end{cases}, \tag{9}$$

where $d(p_k, y_F)$ denotes a distance metric (e.g. Euclidean distance) between two points in $\mathbb{R}^m$. The advantages of using hyperspheres instead of hyperplanes is the ability to define closed tighter sub-spaces in $\mathbb{R}^m$ as intersection of hyperspheres. An iterative optimization training process is proposed in [16] to obtain the set $\{p_k, t_k\}$, aiming a balanced partitioning of the training data and independence between hashing functions.

We perform this mentioned iterative hashing-function optimization in a set of input patch features from training images, so that $H(y_F)$ adapts to the natural image distribution in the feature space. Our proposed spherical hashing search scheme becomes symmetrical as we can see in Fig. 5, i.e. both image and anchor points have to be labeled with binary codes. This can be intuitively understood as creating NN subspace groups (we refer them as *bins*), which we label with a regressor by applying the same hashing functions to the anchor points. Relating a hash code with a regressor can be done during training time.

The inverse search approach returns k-NN for each anchor point, thus not ensuring that all the input image patches have a related regressor (i.e. whenever the patch is not within the k-NN of any of the anchor points). Two solutions are proposed: (a) use a general regressor for the patches which are not in the k-NN of any anchor point or (b) use the regressor of the closest labeled hash code calculated with the spherical Hamming distance, defined by [16] as $d_{SH}(a, b) = \frac{\sum(a \oplus b)}{\sum(a \wedge b)}$, where $\oplus$ is the XOR bit operation and $\wedge$ is the AND bit operation. Note that although not being guaranteed, it rarely happens that a patch is not within any of the k-NN regressors (e.g. for the selected parameter of 6 hyperspheres it never occurs). Since we have not observed significant differences in performance, we select (a) as the lowest complexity solution, although more testing on (b) is due.

In a similar way, an inverse search might also assign two or more regressors to a single patch. It is common in the literature to do a re-ranking strategy to deal with this issue [20].

Table 1. Performance of ×3 and ×4 magnification in terms of averaged PSNR (dB) and averaged execution time (s) on datasets Set14, Kodak and 2k.

	MF	Bicubic		Sparse [10]		GR [12]		ANR [12]		NE+LS		NE+NNLS		NE+LLE		Proposed	
		PSNR	Time	PSNR	Time	PSNR	Time	PSNR	Time	PSNR	Time	PSNR	Time	PSNR	Time	PSNR	Time
Set14	3	27.54	0.002	28.67	2.981	28.31	0.528	28.65	0.771	28.59	2.854	28.44	25.372	28.60	4.356	**28.93**	**0.188**
	4	26.00	0.003	26.88	1.862	26.60	0.458	26.85	0.584	26.81	1.716	26.72	14.146	26.81	2.623	**27.04**	**0.184**
Kodak	3	28.43	0.003	29.22	5.126	28.98	0.921	29.21	1.335	29.17	4.829	29.04	44.102	29.17	7.353	**29.42**	**0.314**
	4	27.23	0.003	27.83	3.194	27.64	0.757	27.80	1.022	27.77	3.003	27.71	24.428	27.77	4.678	**27.92**	**0.309**
2k	3	31.73	0.007	32.63	27.622	32.45	4.860	32.68	7.123	32.62	26.194	32.51	242.875	32.65	40.389	**32.88**	**1.652**
	4	30.28	0.006	30.97	17.225	30.81	3.968	30.99	5.344	30.94	16.363	30.87	136.058	30.96	25.967	**31.04**	**1.578**

4 Results

In this section we show experimental results of our proposed method and we compare its performance in terms of quality and execution time to other state-of-the-art recent methods. We perform extensive experiments with image resolutions ranging from 2.5 Kpixels to 2 Mpixels, showing the performance for classic literature testing images but additionally demonstrating how these algorithms would perform in current upscaling scenarios. We further extend the benchmark in [12] by adding to *Set5* and *Set14* two more datasets: the 24 image *kodak* dataset and *2k*, which is a image set of 9 sharp images obtained from the internet with a pixel resolution of 1920 × 1080.

Table 2. Performance of ×3 and ×4 magnification in terms of PSNR (dB) and execution time (s) on the Set5 dataset.

Set5 images	MF	Bicubic		Sparse [10]		GR [12]		ANR [12]		NE+LS		NE+NNLS		NE+LLE		Proposed	
		PSNR	Time	PSNR	Time	PSNR	Time	PSNR	Time	PSNR	Time	PSNR	Time	PSNR	Time	PSNR	Time
baby	3	33.9	0.000	35.1	3.490	34.9	0.662	35.1	0.905	35.0	3.179	34.8	29.377	35.1	5.042	35.1	0.214
bird	3	32.6	0.000	34.6	1.087	33.9	0.242	34.6	0.293	34.4	1.011	34.3	9.449	34.6	1.533	34.9	0.070
butterfly	3	24.0	0.000	25.9	0.839	25.0	0.152	25.9	0.201	25.8	0.766	25.6	6.947	25.8	1.200	26.6	0.058
head	3	32.9	0.000	33.6	1.011	33.5	0.218	33.6	0.270	33.5	0.908	33.5	8.411	33.6	1.395	33.7	0.068
woman	3	28.6	0.000	30.4	0.972	29.7	0.187	30.3	0.249	30.2	0.909	29.9	8.437	30.2	1.390	30.06	0.067
average	3	30.39	0.000	31.90	1.480	31.41	0.292	31.92	0.384	31.78	1.354	31.60	12.524	31.84	2.112	**32.22**	0.095
baby	4	31.8	0.000	33.1	2.136	32.8	0.525	33.0	0.652	32.9	2.033	32.8	15.535	33.0	3.128	32.9	0.256
bird	4	30.2	0.000	31.7	0.660	31.3	0.184	31.8	0.226	31.6	0.611	31.5	4.995	31.7	0.955	31.7	0.066
butterfly	4	22.1	0.000	23.6	0.536	23.1	0.138	23.5	0.165	23.4	0.456	23.3	3.882	23.4	0.730	23.7	0.052
head	4	31.6	0.000	32.2	0.582	32.1	0.135	32.3	0.212	32.2	0.567	32.1	4.587	32.2	0.882	32.3	0.061
woman	4	26.5	0.000	27.9	0.576	27.4	0.174	27.8	0.191	27.6	0.583	27.6	4.455	27.7	0.894	28.0	0.063
average	4	28.42	0.000	29.69	0.898	29.34	0.231	29.69	0.289	29.55	0.850	29.47	6,691	29,61	1.318	**29.73**	0.100

All the experiments were run on a Intel Xeon W3690@3.47 GHz and the code of the compared methods was obtained from [12] and used with their recommended parameters. The methods compared are the sparse coding SR of

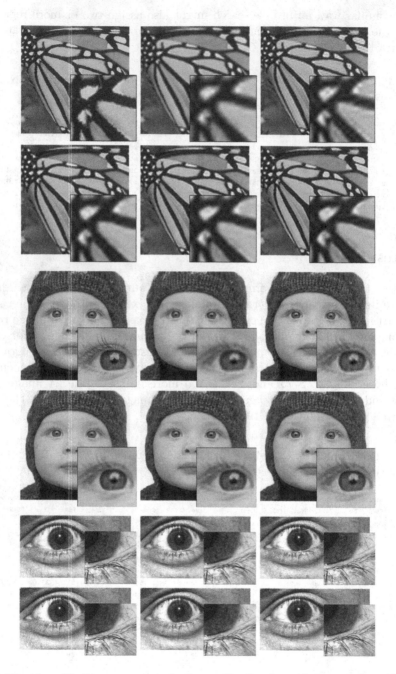

Fig. 6. Visual qualitative assessment of ×3 magnification factor for images from different datasets. From left to right and top to bottom: Original, bicubic interpolation, Global Regressor [12], Zeyde et al. [10], ANR [12] and Proposed SR. Better viewed zoomed in.

Zeyde et al. [10], an implementation of the LS regressions used by Chang et al. [11] (NE + LLE), and the Non-Negative Least Squares (NE + NNLS) method of Bevilaqcua et al. [21].

The proposed algorithm is written in MATLAB with the most time-consuming stages implemented in OpenCL without further emphasis in optimization, and runs in the same CPU platform used for all methods. Our experiments use the same K-SVD sparse dictionary of 1024 used for the compared methods.

We selected bicubic as our coarse approximation $\tilde{x}$ since it does not limit the upscaling steps for super-resolution (e.g. in-place examples are only meaningful for very small magnification factors) and also the features used by Zeyde et al. [10,12] composed by 1st and 2nd order derivative filters compressed with PCA and truncating when the feature still conserves 99.9 % of its energy. We also use a L_2-norm regularized linear regressor illustrated in Eq. (4). We build therefore on top of the regressor scheme proposed by Timofte et al. [12]. We used 6-bit spherical hashing (6 hyperspheres) and the chosen neighborhood is of 1300 k-NN. The selection of number of spheres is a trade-off between quality and speed, since when we decrease the number of hyperspheres we have more collision of regressors (i.e. more than one regressor arrives to the same bin) and due to the re-ranking process we get closer to an exact nearest neighbor search. This can be seen in Fig. 7.

In Tables 1 and 2 we show objective results of the performance in terms of PSNR (dB) and execution time (s). For both measures, our proposed algorithm is the best performing. The improvement in PSNR is more noticeable for magnification factors of 3, where we reach improvements of up to 0.3 dB when compared to the second best-performer. In terms of running time, our algorithm has consistent speed-ups in all datasets and all scales. When compared to GR (which is the fastest of the compared methods), the speed-ups are ranging from ×2 to ×3, additionally with a gap in quality reconstruction. The speed-ups for ANR range from ×3 to ×4 and for the rest of the methods, the running times are several orders of magnitudes slower. Note that the theoretical complexity

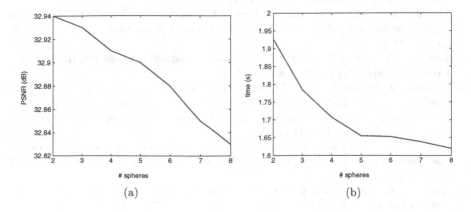

Fig. 7. Effect of the number of spheres selected in terms of PSNR (a) and time (b).

of GR is lower than that of our method since it does not perform a NN search (i.e. for similar implementations, GR should be slightly faster). Nevertheless, our parallel implementation is more efficient than the one provided by their authors [12], which mostly relies on optimized MATLAB matrix multiplication.

In Fig. 6 a visual qualitative assessment can be performed. Our method obtains more natural and sharp edges, and strongly reduces ringing. A good example of that is shown in the *butterfly* image.

5 Conclusions

In this paper we have presented two main contributions: An improved training stage and an efficient inverse-search approach for regression-based and, more generally, dictionary-based SR. Spherical hashing techniques have been applied in order to exploit the benefits of the inverse-search scheme. We obtain both quality improvements due to the optimal training stage and also substantial speed-ups from the low-complexity spherical hashing similarity algorithm used in the regressor selection. An exhaustive testing has been performed comparing our method with four datasets of several pixel resolutions, with different upscaling factors and with several state-of-the-art methods. Our experimental results show consistent improvements in PSNR and running times over the state-of-the-art methods included in the benchmark, positioning as the first in both measures.

References

1. Tsai, R., Huang, T.: Multiple frame image restoration and registration. In: Proceedings of the Advances in Computer Vision and Image Processing, vol. 1, pp. 317–339 (1984)
2. Irani, M., Peleg, S.: Improving resolution by image registration. CVGIP Graph. Models Image Process. **53**, 231–239 (1991)
3. Baker, S., Kanade, T.: Limits on super-resolution and how to break them. IEEE Trans. Pattern Anal. Mach. Intell. **24**, 1167–1183 (2002)
4. Lin, Z., Shum, H.Y.: Fundamental limits of reconstruction-based superresolution algorithms under local translation. IEEE Trans. Pattern Anal. Mach. Intell. **26**, 83–97 (2004)
5. Freeman, W., Jones, T., Pasztor, E.: Example-based super-resolution. IEEE Trans. Comput. Graph. Appl. **22**, 56–65 (2002)
6. Glasner, D., Bagon, S., Irani, M.: Super-resolution from a single image. In: Proceedings of the IEEE International Conference on Computer Vision (2009)
7. Freedman, G., Fattal, R.: Image and video upscaling from local self-examples. ACM Trans. Graph. **30**, 12:1–12:11 (2011)
8. Yang, J., Lin, Z., Cohen, S.: Fast image super-resolution based on in-place example regression. In: Proceedings of the IEEE Conference on Computer Vision and Pattern Recognition (2013)
9. Yang, J., Wright, J., Huang, T.S., Ma, Y.: Image super-resolution via sparse representation. IEEE Trans. Image Process. **19**, 2861–2873 (2010)

10. Zeyde, R., Elad, M., Protter, M.: On single image scale-up using sparserepresen-
    tations. In: Proceedings of the International Conference on Curves and Surfaces
    (2012)
11. Chang, H., Yeung, D.Y., Xiong, Y.: Super-resolution through neighbor embedding.
    (2004)
12. Timofte, R., Smet, V.D., Goool, L.V.: Anchored neighborhood regression for fast
    example-based super-resolution. In: Proceedings of the IEEE International Con-
    ference on Computer Vision (2013)
13. Aharon, M., Elad, M., Bruckstein, A.: K-SVD: an algorithm for designing overcom-
    plete dictionaries for sparse representation. IEEE Trans. Sig. Process. **54**, 4311–
    4322 (2006)
14. Peyré, G.: Manifold models for signals and images. Comput. Vis. Image Underst.
    113, 249–260 (2009)
15. Breiman, L.: Random forests. Mach. Learn. **45**, 5–32 (2001)
16. Heo, J.P., Lee, Y., He, J., Chang, S.F., Yoon, S.E.: Spherical hashing. In: Pro-
    ceedings of the IEEE Conference on Computer Vision and Pattern Recognition
    (2012)
17. Indyk, P., Motwani, R.: Approximate nearest neighbors: towards removing the
    curse of dimensionality. In: Proceedings of the Thirtieth Annual ACM Symposium
    on Theory of Computing, STOC 1998, pp. 604–613 (1998)
18. Wang, J., Kumar, S., Chang, S.F.: Semi-supervised hashing for scalable image
    retrieval (2010)
19. Weiss, Y., Torralba, A., Fergus, R.: Spectral hashing (2008)
20. He, K., Sun, J.: Computing nearest-neighbor fields via propagation-assisted kd-
    trees. In: Proceedings of the IEEE Conference on Computer Vision and Pattern
    Recognition (2012)
21. Bevilacqua, M., Roumy, A., Guillemot, C., Alberi-Morel, M.L.: Low-complexity
    single-image super-resolution based on nonnegative neighbor embedding. In: Pro-
    ceedings of the British Machine Vision Conference, pp. 1–10 (2012)

PSPGC: Part-Based Seeds for Parametric Graph-Cuts

Bharat Singh[✉], Xintong Han, Zhe Wu, and Larry S. Davis

University of Maryland, College Park, USA
{bharat,xintong,zhewu,lsd}@umiacs.umd.edu

Abstract. PSPGC is a detection-based parametric graph-cut method for accurate image segmentation. Experiments show that seed positioning plays an important role in graph-cut based methods, so, we propose three seed generation strategies which incorporate information about location and color of object parts, along with size and shape. Combined with low-level regular grid seeds, PSPGC can leverage both low-level and high-level cues about objects present in the image. Multiple-parametric graph-cuts using these seeding strategies are solved to obtain a pool of segments, which have a high rate of producing the ground truth segments. Experiments on the challenging PASCAL2010 and 2012 segmentation datasets show that the accuracy of the segmentation hypotheses generated by PSPGC outperforms other state-of-the-art methods when measured by three different metrics(average overlap, recall and covering) by up to 3.5 %. We also obtain the best average overlap score in 15 out of 20 categories on PASCAL2010. Further, we provide a quantitative evaluation of the efficacy of each seed generation strategy introduced.

1 Introduction

From the perspective of image labeling - accurately segmenting and labeling a set of known objects in an image - the goal of image segmentation is to discover a set of image regions that correspond to those objects. Since the appearance of an object may be based on a combination of color, texture and shape and is also a function of apparent size (scale), classic segmentation algorithms that construct a single partition of the image typically fail to recover segments that correspond to objects. So, vision systems have utilized families of segmentations - scale space representations and/or alternative segmentations constructed by varying parameters of bottom-up segmentation algorithms [1–3]. For example, by varying the merging parameter of multi-parametric graph-cuts (MPGC) [4–6] one can construct a pool of image segmentations. Additionally, over the past several years image segmentation has been augmented through data-driven methods. These methods can be based, for example, on examining how segmentation algorithms fragment object regions and then learning how to merge [7], or on using shape priors to bias segments selected from parametrically varied segmentation algorithms [5].

© Springer International Publishing Switzerland 2015
D. Cremers et al. (Eds.): ACCV 2014, Part III, LNCS 9005, pp. 360–375, 2015.
DOI: 10.1007/978-3-319-16811-1_24

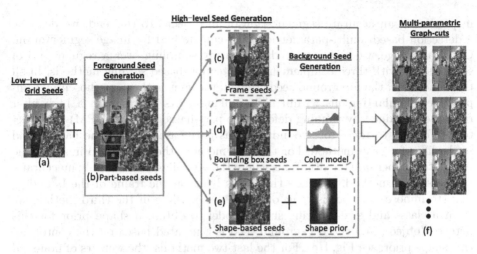

Fig. 1. Overview of PSPGC. (a) Low-level regular grid seeds are generated. (b-e) High-level seeds are generated using three different strategies. (b) Part-based foreground seeds: we apply DPM to detect parts with high filter responses (marked as yellow boxes) in a detected object, and a rectangular seed region (marked as a green rectangle) is generated inside each part. These seeds are used in all three strategies as foreground seeds. (c) Frame background seeds: the frame pixels are chosen as background seeds (marked in red). (d) Bounding box background seeds + Color model: pixels lying on the frame of the bounding box (marked as red) are set as background seeds. The weight of non-seed pixels belonging to the foreground or background depends on the color distribution of pixels lying on the bounding box frame and the foreground seed pixels. (e) Shape Prior + Shape-based background seeds: a shape prior for the detected object is selected and shape-based seeds are generated depending on this prior (marked as a red curve). The weight of non-seed pixels belonging to the foreground depends on the shape prior. (f) Segmentation hypotheses are generated by multi-parametric graph-cuts (Color figure online).

The MPGC algorithm is based on generating many seed regions - for example by sampling pixels on a rectangular grid. Enlarging the pool of seed regions increases the chance of "hitting" ground-truth objects, but at the expense of increasing the complexity of subsequent image labeling. However, the main challenge methods like these face is that the segmentations they produce depend critically on how well the seed regions sample the statistics of the object. If the seed regions are too small, they cannot provide sufficient information (e.g., color distribution) about the foreground and background, so objects will be over- or under-segmented, and when they are too large, object and background statistics are merged in the seed and again segmentation fails.

These problems can be ameliorated if some seeds are chosen using data-driven methods that capture high-level priors about the object. Good seeds should capture the location of parts, color, size and shape of an object to generate a good prior about the foreground. As a function of imaging conditions, (for example: different scales), each of these characteristics have differential utility in producing an accurate segmentation of an object. To this end, we describe a detection-based, multi-parametric graph-cut method for image segmentation. Given an image, we augment seeds chosen by sampling over a regular grid of square seeds with three complementary detection-based seeding methods. In all three methods, the foreground seeds remain the same - they are chosen by sampling rectangular regions within high ranking parts (parts with a high filter response) obtained by running deformable part-based models (DPM) [8] detectors. We refer to these foreground seeds as part based seeds. The background seeds differ for each method. For the first method, they are set to image frame pixels, to compensate for situations where the bounding box is highly inaccurate. In the second method, they are the pixels lying on the frame of the bounding box (to impose a size constraint on the object), while in the third method we train a class- and size- specific shape model to obtain a shape prior for this detected object, and the background seed is generated based on the contour of this shape prior; see Fig. 1(e). For the last two methods, the weights of non-seed pixels belonging to the foreground/background depend on the color distribution of part-based seeds (the green rectangles in Fig. 1 (b–e)) and the background seed pixels, while no such bias is used in the first method. While using shape priors, the weights of pixels belonging to the foreground also depend on the shape (along with the color distribution of seeds) projected onto the detection box. Finally, we solve multi-parametric graph-cuts to generate segmentation proposals based on these seeds.. An overview of our approach is shown in Fig. 1.

Experimental results on the PASCAL2010, 2012 datasets [9,10] show that our approach outperforms state-of-the-art methods. Furthermore, we show how the three different seeding methods (shown in Fig. 1 (b–d)) improve segmentation accuracy in a complementary way. Finally, we illustrate the effect of the number of part-based seeds on the quality of segmentation.

The contributions of our approach are as follows:

1. We combine grid based seeds with high level detection based seeds by adding information obtained from high scoring parts in DPM. Therefore, our method leverages both low-level and high-level cues.
2. Using detection-based seeds, we can capture the multi-modal color distribution of the object and enforce a spatial constraint on the size and pose of the segmentation hypothesis. A category dependent shape prior further enhances segmentation. A statistical evaluation quantifying the efficacy of each of the priors introduced is presented.
3. Experimental results on challenging image segmentation datasets show that the proposed method is superior to the state-of-the-art methods as measured by three different evaluation metrics.

2   Related Work

Current algorithms providing a single bottom-up segmentation [11–14] are not reliable. A common and highly successful approach that offers improvement over them is to generate a large set of segmentation hypotheses by using multi-parametric graph-cuts [4,6]. CPMC [4] generates segmentation hypotheses by sampling points on a grid using a rectangular basis which are used to seed the foreground color model for segmentation. The border of the image is used to seed the background, and a pixel-wise segmentation is generated with graph-cuts over simple color cues. Object proposals [6] uses a similar pipeline, but chooses seeds from a hierarchical segmentation, and learns an affinity measure between super-pixels. However, these methods rely heavily on local bottom-up cues (e.g. color, texture, contour strength). As a result, their performance deteriorates in situations where color consistency, contour information, etc. are insufficient to form a good segment. Moreover, seed positioning plays an important role in graph-cut based methods, but their seed generation schemes are not informed by high-level information. They often result in mixed or under-sampled color and texture distributions for the foreground and background. In contrast, we propose detection-based seed generation strategies based on deformable part-based models (DPM), which improve the segmentation accuracy by incorporating high-level cues in the seed generation process.

Several recent methods have attempted to obtain more accurate segmentation given detection bounding boxes [7,15–19]. However, they [15–17] trust the class assignments of detection, which makes them inaccurate in situations where the detection is inaccurate. In contrast, PSPGC uses detection priors along with low-level grid based seeds, so even when the detector fails, the performance of PSPGC does not drop significantly. Further, most of these approaches [7,15,18,19] assume the detection bounding boxes are accurate. Therefore, when the detection bounding box is inaccurate, for example, the bounding box only covers a portion of the object, these methods only segment parts of the object inside the bounding box. Unlike these methods, PSPGC not only uses the bounding box to generate background seeds, but also takes advantages of the part-based model from DPM to generate foreground seeds. These foreground seeds provide a partial spatial and color distribution of the foreground, which results in a more accurate segmentation than just using the bounding box.

Also, our work is related to methods leveraging shape priors by transfer-based approaches. These approaches match regions in the test image with similar regions in the training examples using k Nearest Neighbors or SVM, and project a shape mask over the object. Some transfer-based methods [7,20] first detect objects and then project an average mask of the training examples onto the detected object using a linear/non-linear transformation. Transferring category independent shape masks by matching regions in an image with training examples has proved effective in generating a pool of segments [5]. In addition to the above methods, category-specific shape priors from a mixture model of deformable parts have been combined with bottom-up cues [17] for segmenting objects. Inspired by SCALPEL [7], we use a class- and size-specific method to form the shape priors, which affect the probability of a pixel belonging to the foreground. We should also note that part-based seeds play a complementary role to shape priors, since when using a global shape prior it is hard to account for

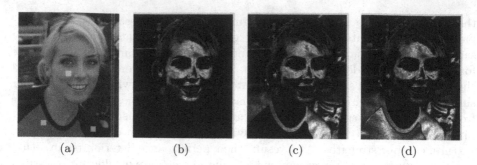

(a)   (b)   (c)   (d)

Fig. 2. In Image (a), the foreground seeds chosen by the ranker are displayed in green. The foreground unary potentials when 1, 2 and 3 seeds are selected as foreground are shown in figure (b), (c) and (d) respectively.

articulations and deformations present in an object class. However, in PSPGC, seeds generated using part scores from DPM are robust to such changes, hence can handle situations where global shape priors fail.

3   PSPGC

Given an image and a set of object categories for which DPM models have been trained, our goal is to generate a set of segmentation hypotheses such that the overlap between one of the hypothesis and each of the objects present in the image is high. To this end, we extend the existing framework of Constrained Parametric Min-Cuts (CPMC) [4] by incorporating seeds based on detections from DPM and shape priors. In order to explain our framework, we give a brief overview of CPMC.

3.1   Constrained Parametric Min-Cuts

CPMC solves multiple min cut problems with different seeds and unary terms. The selection of foreground seeds is done by placing a rectangular grid over the image and sampling pixels around the points on the grid using a rectangular basis. Frame pixels are set as background seeds. The unary cost for seed pixels is set to infinity while the unary cost for non-seed pixels is based on the color distributions of the foreground and background seeds. The pairwise potential depends on the contours obtained from the multi-cue contour detector globalPb [21]. Multiple min-cut problems are solved by varying the degree of foreground bias to generate different segmentation hypotheses. Once the segmentation hypotheses are generated, segments of very small size and those which have a high degree of similarity are discarded in a fast rejection step. Finally, the segments are ranked by graph, region and Gestalt properties.

Although CPMC is quite successful in generating a good pool of segments, the final set of segmentation hypotheses is biased towards the initial seeds. Due to its bottom up category independent approach, it is not able to utilize higher level features (for example, location of parts or shape of an object) present in the image. To this end, we augment CPMC with detection-based seeds that capture the multi-modal color distribution of the objects in the image, enforce a spatial constraint on the size of the segmentation hypothesis and a category dependent shape prior for better localization.

3.2 Segmentation Prior Using Detection Based Seeds

Given an image $I(\mathcal{V}) \rightarrow R^3$, defined over a set of pixels $\mathcal{V}$, a 4 connected weighted grid graph $G = (\mathcal{V}, \mathcal{E})$ is constructed, where edge weights quantify the similarity between neighboring pixels. In order to generate a binary partition of the image, two nodes s and t are added to $\mathcal{V}$. These nodes represent the foreground and background labels respectively, which are connected to all other nodes in the graph. The weights corresponding to these edges represent the unary cost of assigning each pixel as a foreground or a background pixel. Given foreground and background seed pixels $\mathcal{V}_f$ and $\mathcal{V}_b$, the aim is to make a label assignment $\{x_1, ..., x_n\}$, $x_i \in \{0, 1\}$, where n is the total number of pixels in the image, such that the following energy function is minimized,

$$E^\lambda(X) = \sum_{u \in \mathcal{V}} D_\lambda(x_u) + \sum_{(u,v) \in \mathcal{E}} V_{uv}(x_u, x_v)$$

where $\lambda \in \mathbb{R}$. The unary potential is defined as follows:

$$D_\lambda(x_u) = \begin{cases} 0 & \text{if } x_u = 1, u \notin \mathcal{V}_b \\ \infty & \text{if } x_u = 1, u \in \mathcal{V}_b \\ \infty & \text{if } x_u = 0, u \in \mathcal{V}_f \\ f(x_u) + \lambda & \text{if } x_u = 0, u \notin \mathcal{V}_f \end{cases}$$

The function $f(x_u)$ is either set to 0 or is computed as $\ln p_f(x_u) - \ln p_b(x_u)$, where p_f and p_b are estimates of the RGB color distributions of the foreground and background respectively. The pairwise term, V_{uv}, is set to zero if the labels are same otherwise the cost is defined as $\exp\left[-\frac{max(gPb(u),gPb(v))}{\sigma^2}\right]$, where gPb is the response of the contour detector globalPb at each pixel, while σ is a constant.

The result of graph-cut based segmentation as formulated above heavily depends on the placement of seeds. The color distribution of the seeds directly affects the unary cost throughout the graph. As is evident in Fig. 2, the unary cost which is computed using multiple seeds placed over different parts of an object results in a much better prior about the foreground object.

Part-Based Seeds: In order to localize objects, we run discriminatively trained part-based models (DPM) [8] for each class in the training set. DPM not only provides us a bounding box on the detected objects, but also scores corresponding to parts of an object. Since the distributions of the positioning of parts are learned while training, the model accounts for deformation and articulation which may be present in the test image. In our framework, we rank the part scores based on the filter response. Finally, the top k non-overlapping parts lying inside the image are selected and a rectangular basis around the center of these parts is used to sample the foreground seed pixels. Below, we describe three different strategies adopted to select the background seeds and determine weights for non-seed pixels.

Frame Seeds (FS): In the first method, the frame pixels are set as background seeds. No information about the bounding box or the color distribution of the foreground or the background is used, i.e., $f(x_u)$ is set to 0 resulting in a uniform foreground bias. The part based seeds provide a spatial prior about the location of different parts of an object. Even though the detection bounding box may be inaccurate (e.g., covering a portion of the object), they are likely to cover a reasonable portion of the foreground, which can result in an accurate segmentation.

Bounding Box Seeds + Color Model (BBSC): In the second method, pixels lying on the frame of the detection bounding box are used as background seeds. Here, we do add a foreground bias for non-seed pixels and $f(x_u)$ is computed as $\ln p_f(x_u) - \ln p_b(x_u)$. Since the background seeds are hard, the detection bounding box also enforces a size constraint on the object. Whenever detection is more accurate or the color distribution of the object is multi-modal (as in Fig. 2), these seeds provide a better segmentation than the previous ones.

Shape Prior + Shape-Based Seeds: In the final method, the average shape mask is projected on the bounding box and is first thresholdeded to create a silhouette. Finally, pixels which lie at a constant distance d from the silhouette are assigned as background seeds. An additional term depending on the intensity of the average mask projected on the image is added to the unary cost for non-seed pixels, i.e., $f(x_u)$ is computed as $\ln p_f(x_u) - \ln p_b(x_u) + c * (S(x_u))$, where S is the shape mask projected onto the image and c is a positive constant. The process for creating shape masks and predicting the correct mask for a detection bounding box is described in the next section.

3.3 Shape Prior

For the creation of shape masks, we build on SCALPEL [7]. First, for each category, silhouettes obtained from the training data are clustered based on the aspect ratio of their bounding boxes using k-means clustering. Silhouettes in each aspect ratio are further clustered again to account for pose variability present in each class. An average mask of all images within a cluster is constructed for use as a shape prior. Clusters below a certain cardinality are discarded. We employ a different strategy than SCALPEL to project the shape masks. Once we have a mapping between images and cluster ids, the bounding boxes corresponding to the silhouettes are extracted and HoG is computed over the window. We learn an SVM on these HoG features with cluster ids as labels. Given a detection box in a test image, HoG is computed over the detection window. The nearest aspect ratio is chosen and the shape prior to be used is predicted by the SVM learnt for that aspect ratio.

4   Experiments

The experiments have three goals: (1) to demonstrate the effectiveness of our approach by comparison with other state-of-the-art approaches, (2) to evaluate the impact of each seed generation strategy in our method by showing the accuracy gain for each strategy for objects of different sizes, and (3) to study the performance of our method when different numbers of parts are used.

Dataset: We use the PASCAL2010 segmentation training dataset to train our method. This training dataset has pixel-level annotations for 2,075 objects in 964 images from 20 classes. Our approach is evaluated on the PASCAL2010 segmentation validation dataset, which contains 2,128 objects in 964 images. A comparison of the proposed approach with other algorithms which have presented results on the validation set of PASCAL2010 is shown. Additionally, we also test our method on the PASCAL2012 dataset (3,422 objects in 1,449 images), and compare the results with other methods. Note that for both datasets, we use the PASCAL2010 training dataset to train our method.

Implementation Details: In our implementation, we use Version 5 (Sept. 5, 2012) of discriminatively trained deformable part models (DPM) [22], to train a detector for every class on the train set of the detection challenge in the PASCAL 2010 dataset. We sample part-based seed regions with 3 values of k - 1, 2 and 3. For the maximum k (3 in our case), we also add one seed by sampling pixels on the clique connecting the center of the parts, which improves segmentation for small objects. The detection threshold in DPM for each class is chosen such that 1.75 times the total number of objects present in the training images are detected. For clustering of shapes, we choose 4 aspect ratios and the number of clusters for each aspect ratio is set to 8. Our method takes about 4 min to generate segmentation proposals per image: 1 min for detection + 3 min for graph-cuts with an unoptimized MATLAB code running on a 64-bit 2.2 Ghz single core Linux machine. The running time for detection can be reduced to 10 s by running detectors in parallel on a 6 core processor. So the runtime of PSPGC is comparable with CPMC which takes 3 min. SCALPEL's runtime was reported as 2.5–4.5 min on a 2.8 GHz machine. Shape sharing takes 7–8 min on our 2.2 GHz machine. Moreover, all methods use the globalPb contour detector as a preprocessing step which takes 4–5 min to run. In short, every method takes around 7–12 min in total and we believe that addition of 1 min (or 10 s in parallel) would not be a large computational overhead.

Evaluation: To evaluate segmentation quality, we use three metrics: IoU [7], *covering* [4,5,21], and *recall as a function of overlap* [6].

- IoU: For each proposed segment and ground truth object, the overlap score is computed, which is the sum of the intersection of the two masks divided by their union (IoU). To evaluate a pool of segments with respect to a given object, we report the best IoU across all segments.
- Covering: For a given pool of segments and objects, the covering metric is the average best overlapping score between ground-truth and proposed segments,

Table 1. Segmentation results on PASCAL2010 validation set. Recall is computed at 50 percent overlap. The last column presents average number of segments generated per image. The first three rows show the results obtained by different strategies of PSPGC. * Results reported in SCALPEL [7].

Method	Covering (%)	IoU (%)	Recall (%)	Num Segments
FS	84.20	74.51	83.88	707
FS + BBSC	84.97	75.35	84.16	756
PSPGC	**85.21**	**75.70**	**84.67**	788
Object Proposals* [6]	82.8	71.2	82.5	650
CPMC [4]	83.01	72.37	81.39	643
Shape Sharing [5]	83.69	70.9	78.26	1132
Shape Sharing* [5]	84.3	–	–	1448
SCALPEL [7]	83.09	73.77	83.46	658
SCALPEL* [7]	84.4	–	–	1456

weighted by the size of each object. Since covering penalizes incorrect segmentation of large objects greater than small objects, it is a good complementary metric to IoU for evaluation of segmentation methods.

- Recall as a function of overlap: We calculate the percentage of objects recalled at a given overlap score in order to evaluate the overall quality of proposals.

4.1 Segmentation Pool Quality

To compare our approach with existing approaches, we run the publicly available implementation of CPMC [4], Shape Sharing [5], and SCALPEL [7] with their default parameters on the PASCAL2010 validation dataset. We also provide a comparison with the published results of Object proposals [6] mentioned in SCALPEL [7]. Table 1 shows that our approach outperforms all existing methods in all 3 metrics. Note that to study the effect of different seed generation strategies in PSPGC, we list the results when only using parts of PSPGC: FS (frame seeds), FS + BBSC (bounding box background seeds + color model), along with the full model, i.e., PSPGC. From Table 1, we make the following observations:

1. PSPGC outperforms other state-of-the-art approaches on IoU, covering, and recall. Since it is based on CPMC, we find that we improve the accuracy of segmentation of CPMC significantly by only adding a small number of hypotheses. Shape sharing has reported a covering of 84.3 %, however the number of segments generated were 1448. Similarly, SCALPEL has reported a covering score of 84.4 % with 1456 segments. It is to be noted that PSPGC generates a comparable number of segmentation proposals to CPMC, and much fewer than several methods like SCALPEL and Shape Sharing, while

Table 2. Segmentation results on PASCAL2010 validation set. The average IoU for each class is reported. The increase in percentage (by PSPGC) is measured over CPMC.

	CPMC (%)	SCALPEL (%)	Shape Sharing (%)	PSPGC (%)	Increase (%)
Aeroplane	83.04	80.86	78.64	**83.90**	0.86
Bicycle	48.29	**50.93**	42.71	50.53	2.24
Bird	85.64	83.601	84.65	**86.46**	0.82
Boat	73.30	76.06	72.26	**76.15**	2.85
Bottle	73.09	78.08	69.05	**79.06**	5.97
Bus	77.14	**82.39**	79.08	79.64	2.50
Car	54.75	62.71	51.66	**63.48**	8.53
Cat	89.72	87.94	90.16	**90.46**	0.74
Chair	69.34	66.13	66.18	**69.97**	0.63
Cow	85.22	84.54	86.19	**87.11**	1.89
Table	76.90	76.98	**82.04**	76.56	−0.34
Dog	87.66	87.63	86.59	**88.26**	0.6
Horse	79.39	78.67	79.44	**80.94**	1.55
Mobike	73.96	76.93	76.71	**77.98**	4.02
Person	64.11	66.65	62.36	**70.14**	6.03
Plant	66.32	67.18	66.87	**69.42**	3.10
Sheep	68.33	**74.45**	66.87	71.64	3.31
Sofa	85.44	80.50	**86.80**	85.69	0.25
Train	83.07	82.76	84.84	**85.24**	2.17
Monitor	82.04	80.61	80.79	**84.09**	2.05

providing a better covering score with only half the segments. Further, PSPGC provides a better overlap than CPMC for 870 out of 2128 segments in the dataset, which implies that more that 40 % of the time, the best segment in the generated pool comes from the seeds added by PSPGC.

2. PSPGC, to the best of our knowledge, is the first method after CPMC which improves the state of the art in segment pool generation significantly and consistently over all metrics. SCALPEL reported an increase in IoU, however covering improved only by 0.1 %; Shape Sharing improved covering, while IoU and recall dropped. We show an improvement of 3.3 % in IoU, 3.3 % in recall and 2.2 % in covering over CPMC on the same dataset (PASCAL2010).

3. While comparing the accuracy when utilizing different strategies of PSPGC (i.e., the results in the first three rows in Table 1), we find that by only adding 50 more segmentation hypotheses, the location information of part-based seeds can improve the segmentation accuracy significantly. Furthermore, adding almost the same number of hypotheses, by leveraging the bounding

Table 3. Segmentation results on PASCAL2012 validation set. Recall is computed at 50 percent overlap. The last column presents average number of segments generated per image.

Method	Covering (%)	IoU (%)	Recall (%)	Num Segments
PSPGC	84.74	74.12	82.74	791
CPMC [4]	82.51	70.48	78.82	646

box and color model, we obtain a considerable improvement in all three metrics. However, with the addition of the shape prior, accuracy does not improve significantly. It is to be noted that small errors in the positioning of the seeds does not affect the unary cost of non-seed pixels; however using a global prior like the shape of an object is sensitive to translation and its projection needs to be accurate. We will further discuss the effects of these parts of the algorithm in Sect. 4.3 for objects of different sizes.

Additionally, Table 2 shows IoU for different methods for each category in the dataset. PSPGC obtains the best score in 15 out of the 20 categories. It is evident that we obtain high gains for categories in which clear distinctions can be made about parts of an object. PSPGC obtains significant improvement (>6 %) for humans over CPMC, in which there is intraclass variation in the form of deformation and articulation between parts. Further, the color distribution in the case of humans is multi-modal, which can be captured by placing multiple seeds at appropriate positions. It also outperforms every other method for animals, which are likely to have significant deformation and intraclass color variations. We also obtain a noticable improvement in the case of rigid objects in which parts can be distinctly identified like bikes, bottle, bus, car, motorbike, potted plant.

It is likely that the detector might get confused because many groups of categories like animals or vehicles share significant visual properties with each other. However, in our method, even though the detection category is inaccurate, the positioning of the detected parts can provide sufficient information about the foreground. For example, in the sixth row of Fig. 5, even though the sofa was detected as a chair, the positioning and color distribution of the seeds provided significant information to improve segmentation.

In order to prove the robustness of PSPGC, we also show results on the PASCAL2012 validation dataset. The results are summarized in Table 3. PSPGC was run with the same parameters on the PASCAL2012 dataset as used in PASCAL2010. We note that the improvement in performance is 3.6 % in average overlap, 3.9 % in recall and 2.25 % in covering.

4.2 Impact of Different Seed Generation Strategies in PSPGC

In Fig. 3 (a), we present a graph to analyze the effectiveness of different seed generation strategies of PSPGC. This figure shows the gain over CPMC when

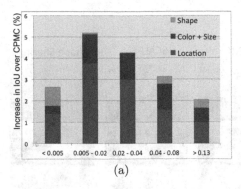
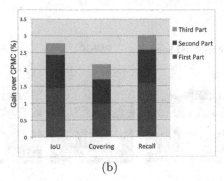

(a)   (b)

Fig. 3. (a) Gain in IoU (in percentage) due to part localization, color + size and shape for objects of different sizes is shown. The x-axis denotes the size of the object relative to the image size. The range of different sizes was chosen such that each bin contains approximately the same number of objects. (b) Gain in accuracy (in percentage) over CPMC on different metrics as we increase number of parts. No shape information is used when we calculate these metrics.

different seed generation strategies of our algorithm are applied. Additionally, it can be seen that correct localization of seeds plays a very important role in segmentation, irrespective of the size of the object. For very small objects (< 800 pixels), the improvement by estimating the color distribution from the seeds for the foreground and background is not very substantial, because these objects are very small and there are not sufficient statistics available to estimate the foreground color distribution. However, shape is quite useful in improving the quality of segmentation for very small objects. As the size of the object increases, the color distribution about the foreground/background object helps significantly to improve the segmentation accuracy. Moreover, detection accuracy improves when objects are of reasonable size and the size constraint enforced by the bounding box becomes more reliable. We observe that the improvement due to addition of part-based seeds is largest in the case of mid-sized objects, where there is

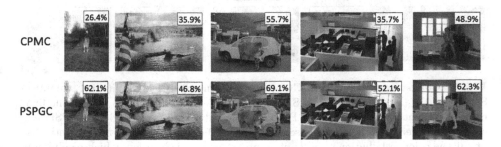

Fig. 4. Failure cases of CPMC (first row) and PSPGC (second row). We can observe that even though PSPGC is better than CPMC, there is still a scope of improvement when objects are occluded, or when they are near to each other.

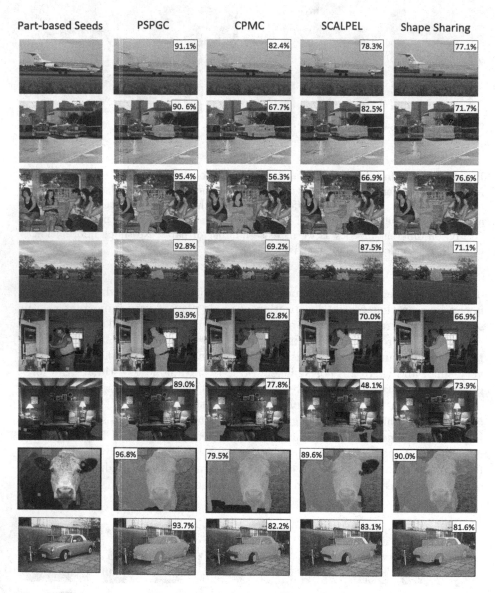

Fig. 5. Comparison among PSPGC (second column), CPMC [4](third column), SCALPEL [7] (forth column), and Shape Sharing [5] (fifth column) is shown, the first column presents the seeds used by PSPGC (marked as green rectangles). In PSPGC, since the placement of foreground seeds is appropriate, they provide a good estimate about the color distribution of parts of an object and their location, which results in a better segmentation (Color figure online).

maximum scope of improvement. We attribute this to the fact that there is not much part information in small objects, while CPMC is reasonably successful in computing the correct segmentation of large objects. Since FS and BBSC also add a spatial prior about the object and performance is measured after their addition, the effect of shape is not very evident in the combined results presented. However, only using the seeds generated by shape priors (without FS and BBSC), gives the following results: 84.4 % covering (+1.4 %), 74.1 % IoU (+1.7 %) and 82.9 % recall (+1.5 %) with 692 segments, which is a noticeable improvement over CPMC. Moreover, the number of objects in articulated and deformable classes outnumber objects in rigid classes in PASCAL (person alone comprising of 40 % of all segments). It can be seen in the results shown in the supplementary material, that shape prior helps significantly in rigid classes like Monitor, Plant, Sofa, Sheep, Motorbike, Boat and Car.

4.3   Effect of Number of Part-Based Seeds Used

We also analyze the effect of the number of part-based seeds used in PSPGC on different metrics. In this study, we do not use any prior shape information, since we aim to evaluate the effect of part-based information. From Fig. 3(b), it can be observed that we get a big improvement for the first added part because new detection based background and foreground seeds are added for the first part, while in the other two cases, only the foreground seeds are changed. We notice that although the improvement in IoU is not significant for the third added part, it helps more in improving covering. This demonstrates that more part-based seeds are helpful in segmenting larger objects.

5   Discussion

PSPGC combines grid based seeds with three higher level detection-based seed generation strategies, which help to capture more information about the location, color, size and shape of an object. Quantitative and qualitative results on challenging datasets show that these seed generation methods improve the quality of segmentation when measured by IoU, covering, and recall.

Among three seed generation strategies, the positioning of seeds plays the most important role in improving the segmentation accuracy regardless of the size of objects. Color information helps when sufficient statistics are available. Shape prior is helpful in segmenting rigid objects. Since we observe that seeds play an important role in the segmentation process, a promising step would be to incorporate relationships between objects in the seed generation process so that segmentation is more accurate in occluded situations (Fig. 4).

Acknowledgement. This work was partially supported by the US Government ONR MURI Grant N000141010934.

References

1. Arbeláez, P., Hariharan, B., Gu, C., Gupta, S., Bourdev, L., Malik, J.: Semantic segmentation using regions and parts. In: IEEE Conference on Computer Vision and Pattern Recognition (CVPR), pp. 3378–3385 (2012)
2. Carreira, J., Caseiro, R., Batista, J., Sminchisescu, C.: Semantic segmentation with second-order pooling. In: Fitzgibbon, A., Lazebnik, S., Perona, P., Sato, Y., Schmid, C. (eds.) ECCV 2012, Part VII. LNCS, vol. 7578, pp. 430–443. Springer, Heidelberg (2012)
3. Girshick, R., Donahue, J., Darrell, T., Malik, J.: Rich feature hierarchies for accurate object detection and semantic segmentation. arXiv preprint (2013). arXiv:1311.2524
4. Carreira, J., Sminchisescu, C.: Cpmc: Automatic object segmentation using constrained parametric min-cuts. IEEE Trans. Pattern Anal. Mach. Intell. **34**, 1312–1328 (2012)
5. Kim, J., Grauman, K.: Shape sharing for object segmentation. In: Fitzgibbon, A., Lazebnik, S., Perona, P., Sato, Y., Schmid, C. (eds.) ECCV 2012, Part VII. LNCS, vol. 7578, pp. 444–458. Springer, Heidelberg (2012)
6. Endres, I., Hoiem, D.: Category independent object proposals. In: Daniilidis, K., Maragos, P., Paragios, N. (eds.) ECCV 2010, Part V. LNCS, vol. 6315, pp. 575–588. Springer, Heidelberg (2010)
7. Weiss, D., Taskar, B.: Scalpel: Segmentation cascades with localized priors and efficient learning. In: IEEE Conference on Computer Vision and Pattern Recognition (CVPR), pp. 2035–2042 (2013)
8. Felzenszwalb, P.F., Girshick, R.B., McAllester, D., Ramanan, D.: Object detection with discriminatively trained part-based models. IEEE Trans. Pattern Anal. Mach. Intell. **32**, 1627–1645 (2010)
9. Everingham, M., Van Gool, L., Williams, C.K.I., Winn, J., Zisserman, A.: The PASCAL Visual Object Classes Challenge. In: VOC2010 Results. (2010). http://www.pascal-network.org/challenges/VOC/voc2010/workshop/index.html
10. Everingham, M., Van Gool, L., Williams, C.K.I., Winn, J., Zisserman, A.: The PASCAL Visual Object Classes Challenge. In: VOC2012 Results (2012). http://www.pascal-network.org/challenges/VOC/voc2012/workshop/index.html
11. Shi, J., Malik, J.: Normalized cuts and image segmentation. IEEE Trans. Pattern Anal. Mach. Intell. **22**, 888–905 (2000)
12. Felzenszwalb, P.F., Huttenlocher, D.P.: Efficient graph-based image segmentation. Int. J. Comput. Vis. **59**, 167–181 (2004)
13. Boykov, Y.Y., Jolly, M.P.: Interactive graph cuts for optimal boundary & region segmentation of objects in nd images. In: Proceedings of the Eighth IEEE International Conference on Computer Vision, 2001. ICCV 2001. vol. 1, pp. 105–112. IEEE (2001)
14. Rother, C., Kolmogorov, V., Blake, A.: Grabcut: Interactive foreground extraction using iterated graph cuts. In: ACM Transactions on Graphics (TOG). vol. 23, pp. 309–314. ACM (2004)
15. Xia, W., Song, Z., Feng, J., Cheong, L.-F., Yan, S.: Segmentation over detection by coupled global and local sparse representations. In: Fitzgibbon, A., Lazebnik, S., Perona, P., Sato, Y., Schmid, C. (eds.) ECCV 2012, Part V. LNCS, vol. 7576, pp. 662–675. Springer, Heidelberg (2012)
16. Dai, Q., Hoiem, D.: Learning to localize detected objects. In: IEEE Conference on Computer Vision and Pattern Recognition (CVPR), pp. 3322–3329 (2012)

17. Yang, Y., Hallman, S., Ramanan, D., Fowlkes, C.C.: Layered object models for image segmentation. IEEE Trans. Pattern Anal. Mach. Intell. **34**, 1731–1743 (2012)
18. Brox, T., Bourdev, L., Maji, S., Malik, J.: Object segmentation by alignment of poselet activations to image contours. In: IEEE Conference on Computer Vision and Pattern Recognition (CVPR), pp. 2225–2232 (2011)
19. Lempitsky, V., Kohli, P., Rother, C., Sharp, T.: Image segmentation with a bounding box prior. In: IEEE 12th International Conference on Computer Vision, pp. 277–284 (2009)
20. Gu, C., Arbeláez, P., Lin, Y., Yu, K., Malik, J.: Multi-component models for object detection. In: Fitzgibbon, A., Lazebnik, S., Perona, P., Sato, Y., Schmid, C. (eds.) ECCV 2012, Part IV. LNCS, vol. 7575, pp. 445–458. Springer, Heidelberg (2012)
21. Arbelaez, P., Maire, M., Fowlkes, C., Malik, J.: Contour detection and hierarchical image segmentation. IEEE Trans. Pattern Anal. Mach. Intell. **33**, 898–916 (2011)
22. Girshick, R.B., Felzenszwalb, P.F., McAllester, D.: Discriminatively trained deformable part models, release 5. http://people.cs.uchicago.edu/~rbg/latent-release5/

Multi-cue Mid-level Grouping

Tom Lee[✉], Sanja Fidler, and Sven Dickinson

University of Toronto, Toronto, Canada
{tshlee,fidler,sven}@cs.toronto.edu

Abstract. Region proposal methods provide richer object hypotheses than sliding windows with dramatically fewer proposals, yet they still number in the thousands. This large quantity of proposals typically results from a diversification step that propagates bottom-up ambiguity in the form of proposals to the next processing stage. In this paper, we take a complementary approach in which mid-level knowledge is used to resolve bottom-up ambiguity at an earlier stage to allow a further reduction in the number of proposals. We present a method for generating regions using the mid-level grouping cues of closure and symmetry. In doing so, we combine mid-level cues that are typically used only in isolation, and leverage them to produce fewer but higher quality proposals. We emphasize that our model is mid-level by learning it on a limited number of objects while applying it to different objects, thus demonstrating that it is transferable to other objects. In our quantitative evaluation, we (1) establish the usefulness of each grouping cue by demonstrating incremental improvement, and (2) demonstrate improvement on two leading region proposal methods with a limited budget of proposals.

1   Introduction

Casting object recognition as object detection diminishes the need for bottom-up grouping: a high-level model does not need the help of weaker mid-level and low-level cues to locate the object. However, as the level of ambiguity rises with the number of possible objects, the more prohibitive it becomes to exhaustively search over object detectors in a cluttered scene. This motivates the role of bottom-up cues for achieving a reduction in search complexity.

Bottom-up grouping has re-emerged in the form of class-independent *region proposals* [1,2] which are increasingly combined with object detectors and have been shown to improve performance on competitive challenges [3]. Region proposal methods typically start with a generation stage that uses a bottom-up grouping algorithm to output a diverse set of proposals, which are then passed to a ranking stage where they are evaluated by a trained scoring function. The ranked proposals have richer structure than sliding windows, which are typically fixed in aspect ratio, and have higher precision than sliding windows, whose proposals number in the millions. In contrast, region proposal methods achieve state-of-the-art results with only thousands of proposals.

Region proposal methods forward bottom-up ambiguity from the generation stage to the ranking stage in the form of proposals, at which point stronger cues

© Springer International Publishing Switzerland 2015
D. Cremers et al. (Eds.): ACCV 2014, Part III, LNCS 9005, pp. 376–390, 2015.
DOI: 10.1007/978-3-319-16811-1_25

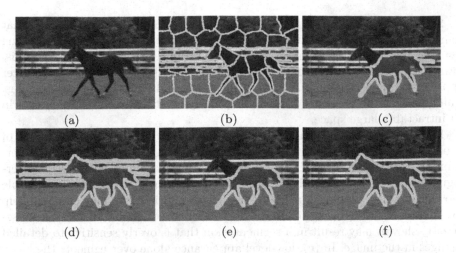

(a)   (b)   (c)

(d)   (e)   (f)

Fig. 1. Given an input image as shown in (a), our method first oversegments into superpixels in (b), which are to be grouped into regions based on a combination of perceptual grouping cues. In this example, both the horse and the fence are relatively homogeneous in color and exhibit contrasting boundaries, however the horse's neck is slightly darker than its torso. As shown in (c), low level appearance alone oversegments the horse at the neck where a large gap in contour is attempted. When including contour closure in (d), the boundary correctly encloses the head, but elsewhere strays along the fence. Conversely in (e), including symmetry without closure separates the fence from the horse, but fails to enclose the head. With closure and symmetry together in (f), the entire horse is correctly segmented.

are available to reduce the ambiguity. Unlike hierarchy-based models [4], proposals are often explicitly isolated from object class labels. Typical methods like [1,2], however, rely on only low-level appearance and contour cues to generate proposals, and as a result must diversify their proposals in large quantities to preserve recall. In this paper, we present a complementary approach to diversification that uses mid-level grouping cues to resolve ambiguity at an early stage to avoid the need to generate proposals in excessive quantities.

By approaching the problem as figure-ground separation, we draw on a large body of work in perceptual grouping. Mid-level cues capture non-accidental relations between image elements that are exhibited by all objects. They are less specific than a high-level object model, yet more discriminative than low-level cues like appearance similarity and contour continuity. Here we highlight two mid-level cues of interest:

Closure [5,6] is a regularity that favors regions that are enclosed by strong contour evidence along the boundary. Bottom-up approaches to finding closure vary in the types of cues used, and may include continuity and convexity. The problem is often cast as finding a cycle of graph edges in a very large space, and is exacerbated when allowing for gaps in the closure (an illustrative example being the Kanizsa triangle).

Symmetry [7–9] is a ubiquitous and powerful regularity with scope that spans entire objects or their parts. Since the early days, perceptual grouping research has produced such varied representations as the medial axis transform [10], generalized cylinders [11], superquadrics [12], and geons [13]. Later approaches applied symmetry toward cluttered and occluded image domains, which present the challenge of searching for symmetrically related elements in an intractably large space.

Like other bottom-up cues, closure and symmetry govern the perception of figure and ground. Our method, as illustrated in Fig. 1, groups regions by leveraging mid-level and low-level cues in combination. An input image (a), is oversegmented into superpixels (b), to be grouped together into regions. The example shown contains a horse as foreground, for which multiple grouping cues will help to separate from the background. Relying on a limited number of cues, as subsequently shown, may result in a segmentation that is overly sensitive to detailed changes in the image. In (c), low-level appearance alone oversegments the horse at the slightly darker neck, while jumping a large gap in contour. Including contour closure in (d), attracts the boundary to pixels with strong contour evidence and encloses the head, but elsewhere strays along the fence. Symmetry is a regularity that groups objects, such as the fence, into its coherent parts, but as shown in (e), does not group the head with the horse. In (f), closure and symmetry combine their strengths to correctly segment the horse.

Mid-level cues extend beyond any particular object, and symmetry and closure, in particular, are ubiquitous over all objects. Since our model is aware of objects only at the mid-level and unaware of their specific appearance, the model can easily transfer from one object to another. In this paper, as a case in point, we learn our model on the Weizmann Horse Dataset (WHD) [14], and then apply it to diverse non-horse objects from the Weizmann Segmentation Dataset (WSD) [15]. Quantitative experiments are performed on WHD to (1) establish the usefulness of each cue by demonstrating improvement as they are incrementally added, and to (2) demonstrate improvement on two leading region proposal methods with a limited budget of proposals. The contributions of our paper are summarized as follows:

1. **Perceptual search.** We focus on the front-end stage where the generation of region proposals is driven by bottom-up grouping. We argue that stronger mid-level cues play an important role in reducing the number of proposals.
2. **Mid-level cue combination.** We improve upon previous approaches that lack mid-level knowledge or combine only one mid-level cue with low-level cues, by leveraging the combination of mid-level closure and mid-level symmetry to group regions together.
3. **Trained cue combination.** While perceptual grouping methods often make ad hoc grouping decisions, we capture all cues in a single energy function and jointly learn their weighted combination.

2   Related Work

Viewing region proposals as object hypotheses for recognition, we begin by broadening our scope to include methods designed for sliding window detectors. Among these, the *objectness* detector of Alexe *et al.* [16] computes low-level features on superpixels [17] to score sampled image boxes. *Selective search* of Uijlings *et al.* [2] outputs boxes that bound regions generated from agglomerative clustering of superpixels [17]. The method accumulates a pool of regions over each step of region-merging until all regions are merged together, and ensures diversity by pooling results over multiple color and texture feature spaces. The method is very fast, yet is based on low-level appearance alone.

Arbelaez *et al.* [18] produces regions by merging superpixels of [19] over multiple scales. The method considers a limited number of all pairs, triples, and quadruples of adjacent superpixels. Our approach is different in that we operate on a single layer of compact superpixels, and define a set of low-level and mid-level cues that quantify the likelihood of grouping.

The *shape sharing* method of Kim & Grauman [20] matches part-level regions in a given image to a bank of exemplars, which project object-level information back into the image to help with segmentation. The *category-independent proposals* of Endres & Hoiem [21] develops a CRF model to label superpixels based on segment seeds. The resulting region proposals are ranked using structured learning on grouping cues. The energy potentials are pairwise and submodular, and inference is done by graph cuts. While we use a similar procedure to generate regions, we combine mid-level cues at the front-end without seeding from a fixed hierarchical segmentation.

The *CPMC* method of Carreira & Sminchisescu [1] generates regions directly from the image rather than deriving them from a fixed segmentation. The method solves multiple parametric min-cut instances over color seeds. Regions are re-ranked by regressing on overlap with region-scoped features, including mid-level features such as convexity and eccentricity. The emphasis is on ranking rather than the front-end grouping, which samples color seed models over millions of pixels. Our approach is qualitatively different from the above methods as we focus on bottom-up grouping, however our mid-level front-end is complementary to the ranking stage.

Viewing region proposals as figure-ground labeling calls on a large literature covering low-level and mid-level Gestalt cues. Rather than covering methods on individual mid-level cues like symmetry [7–9] and closure [5,6], we consider holistic approaches that combine low- and/or mid-level cues. The *region competition* approach of Zhu & Yuille [22] combines the objectives of snakes and region growing into a single Bayes criterion, effectively integrating the relative strengths of contour-based and region-based cues. An algorithm for optimizing the new criterion was introduced, however only guaranteed convergence to a local minimum. Our approach differs in using superpixels which, providing access to both contours and regions, serves as a convenient basis for combining their respective cues, independently from the optimization approach.

Cue combination is alternately formulated as a linear combination of terms that make up a cost or scoring function. Graph-based image partitioning [17, 23] requires an affinity function to be specified between pairs of pixels and therefore falls under this category. For example, the *intervening contour* method of Leung & Malik [24] includes a contour-based term into the appearance-based affinity and solves the normalized cut problem. Like [24], we combine cues in a linear combination of terms, but differ in the overall grouping approach and use different cues on superpixels.

Inspired by random field models, the *cue integration* method of Ren et al. [25] develops an energy function that integrates appearance similarity, contour continuity, contour closure, and object familiarity on triangular tokens. The model was trained and solved using loopy belief propagation. Like [25], we combine multiple grouping cues over adjacent regions, but we take the approach of expressing the energy potentials in a form that allows efficient and exact solutions.

Our approach is most similar to Levinshtein et al. [26], which elegantly formulated contour closure as finding minimum energy labelings, and used parametric min-cut to find globally optimal solutions. A gap cost was trained on superpixel boundary features and incorporated into a gap-to-area ratio cost. We differ from [26] by combining multiple cues, among which contour closure counts as only one, and furthermore we learn to combine cues in a random field energy model.

3   Approach Overview

We develop an energy function over superpixel labelings that captures a combination of low-level and mid-level grouping cues. In Sect. 4, we motivate the cues of low-level appearance, mid-level closure, and mid-level symmetry from perceptual grouping principles and define their corresponding energy potentials. We use a mathematical form that is flexible enough to accommodate additional cues, yet conforms to a structure that can be exploited to obtain efficient and exact solutions. In Sect. 5, we introduce a scaling term in the energy that represents ambiguity in scale, and use it to obtain multiple solutions. Section 6 formulates the loss-based framework with which we train the weights of the energy function. We present and discuss results in Sect. 7 and conclude in Sect. 8.

4   Grouping Cues

Our method operates on superpixels as grouping primitives from which regions are composed. Superpixels provide a rich topology of regions and boundaries on which a diverse set of cues can be defined to capture different grouping relations. Specifically, an input image $\mathbf{x}$ is oversegmented into P superpixels, where each superpixel p is assigned a binary label $y_p \in \{1 = \text{figure}, 0 = \text{ground}\}$. The labeling space $\mathcal{Y} = \{1, 0\}^P$ contains all possible vectors $\mathbf{y} = \{y_1, \ldots, y_P\}$ of superpixel labels and thus represents all possible groupings. An energy function $E(\mathbf{y}; \mathbf{x})$ is defined on $\mathcal{Y}$ that favors labelings based on a combination of cues observed on the image $\mathbf{x}$, and captures this combination as a decomposition into potentials corresponding to different cues:

$$E(\mathbf{y};\mathbf{x}) = \sum_{cue} \sum_{I \in \mathcal{N}^{cue}} E_I^{cue}(\mathbf{y}_I;\mathbf{x}_I) \tag{1}$$

In (1), *cue* varies over low-level appearance (*app*), mid-level closure (*clo*), and mid-level symmetry (*sym*). The set $\mathcal{N}^{cue}$ of neighborhoods for a particular cue defines the local subsets of superpixels on which the cue is repeatedly observed. Potentials in our model are restricted to pairwise order. By finding a labeling that globally minimizes the energy, we obtain a region that exhibits strong grouping relations. In this section, we discuss the contributions of the cues of symmetry, closure, and appearance and define their corresponding energy potentials.

4.1   Appearance Similarity

Similarity is a basic perceptual grouping cue that we capture in the form of color and texture similarity. We note that even objects of heterogeneous appearance are often composed of homogeneous parts. For each superpixel p, we compute a d-dimensional normalized histogram descriptor $\mathbf{h}^p$ that summarizes its appearance. We then compute the similarity between a pair p, q of adjacent superpixels using the histogram intersection kernel:

$$s^{pq} = \sum_{i=1}^{d} \min(h_i^p, h_i^q).$$

Color and texture are captured with different histograms $\mathbf{h}_c, \mathbf{h}_t$ which are computed in the manner of Uijlings *et al.* [2] using multiple color channels and SIFT-like features. Similarity is computed for both histograms to obtain the two-dimensional feature:

$$\phi_{pq}^{app}(\mathbf{x}) = (s_c^{pq}, s_t^{pq}).$$

The pairwise appearance potential for each adjacent pair p, q combines the cues and is defined as follows:

$$E_{pq}^{app}(\mathbf{y}_{pq};\mathbf{x}) = \begin{cases} \mathbf{w}_{app}^T \phi_{pq}^{app}(\mathbf{x}) & y_p \neq y_q \\ 0 & y_p = y_q \end{cases} \tag{2}$$

4.2   Contour Closure

Contour closure is a key challenge of perceptual grouping. One of the key ingredients of closure is strong contour evidence along the boundary that separates figure from ground. Since we prefer boundaries that avoid large gaps of contour (weak evidence), we define for any given labeling $\mathbf{y}$ the gap cost $G(\mathbf{y})$ in terms of the corresponding region's boundary $\partial(\mathbf{y})$:

$$G(\mathbf{y};\mathbf{x}) = \sum_{x \in \partial(\mathbf{y})} g(x).$$

This cost accumulates a positive gap $g(x)$ over all boundary pixels $x \in \partial(\mathbf{y})$. We compute $g(x) \in [0,1]$ at every boundary pixel using the trained measure of [26], which accounts for discrepancy between contour map and superpixel boundaries in location and orientation.

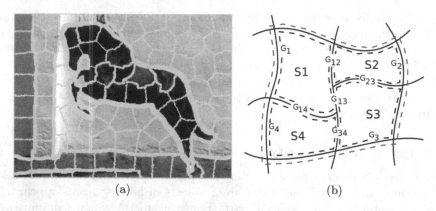

(a)   (b)

Fig. 2. To support the cue of mid-level closure, contour evidence is computed along superpixel boundaries as shown in (a), where thickness indicates the degree of contour evidence (lack of gap) [26]. In (b), the gap cost $G(\mathbf{y})$ for a hypothetical labeling $\mathbf{y}$ over the corresponding region's boundary $\partial(\mathbf{y})$ is shown in dashed red and consists of superpixels S1-S4. Unary potentials sum gap along the corresponding boundaries G1-G4, and pairwise potentials sum gap along the shared boundaries G12-G34. The total gap $G(\mathbf{y})$ along the dashed red is obtained by subtracting twice the pairwise potentials from the unary potentials. (We thank the authors of [26] for permission to reproduce figure (b)).

We directly incorporate $G(\mathbf{y})$ into our energy function by expressing it in terms of unary and pairwise potentials over $\mathbf{y}$. We encode the potentials as in [26], for which a schematic example is provided in Fig. 2. Unary potentials are defined to sum gap along the corresponding superpixel's boundary $\partial(p)$ when $y_p = 1$. Pairwise potentials between p and q sum gap only along the boundary $\partial(p, q)$ shared by *both* superpixels, when $y_p = y_q = 1$:

$$E_p^{clo}(y_p) = \begin{cases} \sum_{x \in \partial(p)} g(x) & y_p = 1 \\ 0 & y_p = 0 \end{cases} \quad E_{pq}^{clo}(\mathbf{y}_{pq}) = \begin{cases} \sum_{x \in \bar{\partial}(p,q)} g(x) & y_p = y_q = 1 \\ 0 & \text{otherwise} \end{cases}$$

$$(3)$$

As illustrated in Fig. 2(b), unary potentials sum gap along their superpixel boundaries. For a region consisting of a single superpixel, the unary potential reflects the correct gap cost. However, for a region consisting of multiple superpixels, simply summing the corresponding unary potentials will double count the gaps along the boundaries shared by adjacent superpixels in the region, which are exactly those counted by the pairwise potentials. The gap $G(\mathbf{y})$ along the

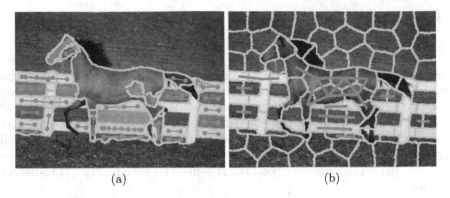

$$(a) \qquad\qquad\qquad\qquad (b)$$

Fig. 3. Symmetric parts detected by [27] as sequences of medial points represented as region masks, as shown in (a). In (b), straight lines indicate strong pairwise affinities between superpixels that belong to the same symmetric part.

true boundary of the region can thus be easily expressed as the sum of the unary potentials, minus twice the pairwise potentials:

$$E^{clo}(\mathbf{y};\mathbf{x}) = w_{clo} \cdot \left(\sum_p E_p^{clo}(y_p;\mathbf{x}) - 2 \sum_{p,q} E_{pq}^{clo}(\mathbf{y}_{pq};\mathbf{x}) \right) \tag{4}$$

4.3   Symmetry

Symmetry relates together local features that span the entire object or its parts and, as such, is a powerful mid-level cue. Its large spatial scope, however, makes the associated grouping problem combinatorially hard. In the context of our representation in the labeling space $\mathcal{Y}$, the region corresponding to an object or its part can be composed from any number of superpixels, and thus induces dependencies of arbitrarily high order.

Our method draws on the approach of Lee *et al.* [27] for finding symmetrically related features, which circumvents the above difficulty by leveraging the scope of large superpixels. By operating on successively coarser superpixels, pairwise combinations are able to cover successively larger regions, effectively achieving higher orders of dependency. This allows local sections of symmetry of the same object part to be composed from a *sequence* of pairwise superpixels at the correct scale. Furthermore, [27] finds optimal sequences of superpixels that lie along the symmetry axes of object parts, as shown in Fig. 3.

We incorporate the symmetry cue in the above form into our method by favoring the grouping of superpixels that belong, with high likelihood, to the same symmetric part. In practice, we run the sequence optimization of [27] independently on multiscale superpixels to obtain a set S of symmetric parts, as shown in Fig. 3(a), and define pairwise potentials that favor grouping of superpixels that belong to the same symmetric part, as shown in Fig. 3(b).

For each pair of adjacent superpixels p, q, we define the feature:

$$\phi_{pq}^{sym}(\mathbf{x}) = \max_{s \in S(p,q)} \text{score}(s),$$

which takes on the score of the best scoring symmetric part $s \in S(p,q)$, where $S(p,q) \subseteq S$ is the subset of symmetric parts for which the overlap with p and q both exceed $\tau = 0.75$. When $S(p,q)$ is empty, the feature takes on a value of zero. The value $\text{score}(s) \in [0,1]$ is the part's detection score, which we interpret as positive grouping evidence. We perform non-maximum suppression over all superpixels pairs so that each pairwise relation is influenced by at most one symmetric part. The symmetry potential is defined for each pair (p,q) of adjacent superpixels as:

$$E_{pq}^{sym}(\mathbf{y}_{pq}; \mathbf{x}) = \begin{cases} \mathbf{w}_{sym}^T \phi_{pq}^{sym}(\mathbf{x}) & y_p \neq y_q \\ 0 & y_p = y_q. \end{cases} \tag{5}$$

5 Figure-Ground Labeling

We incorporate the potentials corresponding to the grouping cues into our final energy function as follows:

$$E(\mathbf{y}) = \sum_{p,q} E_{pq}^{app}(\mathbf{y}) + \sum_{p} E_p^{clo}(\mathbf{y}) - 2\sum_{p,q} E_{pq}^{clo}(\mathbf{y}) + \sum_{p,q} E_{pq}^{sym}(\mathbf{y}) + \lambda \sum_{p} \phi_p(\mathbf{y}). \tag{6}$$

In (6), the grouping cues are rescaled by a scaling potential $\phi_p(\mathbf{y})$ by a factor of $\lambda > 0$ that is defined as follows:

$$\phi_p(\mathbf{y}) = \begin{cases} -\text{area}(p) & y_p = 1 \\ 0 & y_p = 0. \end{cases} \tag{7}$$

The scaling potential removes trivial solutions associated with the empty grouping with zero energy. Furthermore, as λ increases, the scaling potential favors labelings of larger area, and thus λ adjusts the energy's preference for regions of smaller or larger scale.

To minimize (6), we rewrite it as a sum of unary and pairwise potentials:

$$E(\mathbf{y}; \mathbf{x}) = \sum_{p} \mathbf{w}_1^T \phi_p^\lambda(\mathbf{y}, \mathbf{x}) + \sum_{p,q} \mathbf{w}_2^T \phi_{pq}(\mathbf{y}, \mathbf{x}), \tag{8}$$

noting that the pairwise potentials are submodular when weights are non-negative (features are non-negative). When λ is fixed, (8) can be minimized efficiently with a maxflow algorithm. In our model, λ is an unknown variable that represents the scale of an object, and so we minimize (8) for all values $\lambda \in \Lambda$, for $\Lambda \subset \mathbb{R}$. This is known as the parametric maxflow problem [28], which can be shown to yield a finite number of solutions as λ varies over Λ. The set of globally optimal solutions can be found with a linear number of calls to the maxflow algorithm. We use $\Lambda = [0,1]$ to yield a dozen solutions on average per image, thereby obtaining multiple proposals varying in scale.

6   Learning

We train the weights of the energy function (8) by incorporating it into the Structured SVM framework. The framework is instantiated with the loss function:

$$\Delta(\hat{\mathbf{y}}, \mathbf{y}) = \frac{1}{\text{area}(\mathbf{x})} \sum_p \text{area}(p) \cdot \phi_p^\Delta(\hat{y}_p, y_p) \qquad \phi_p^\Delta(\hat{y}, y) = \begin{cases} 1 - \alpha_p & \hat{y} = 1 \\ \alpha_p & \hat{y} = 0 \end{cases} \quad (9)$$

where $\alpha_p \in [0, 1]$ is the fraction of pixels inside superpixel p labeled by the ground truth pixel mask. Weights are optimized using StructSVMCP [29] and constrained to be non-negative. We note that the learning step assumes that the loss for a particular example is obtained by minimizing the corresponding energy with a particular value of λ. For simplicity, we have fixed $\lambda = 0.01$ for all training examples. During testing, however, we vary λ over Λ for each example.

7   Evaluation

A key point of our approach is that our model being mid-level enables it to directly transfer from one object class to another. To illustrate this point, we use the Weizmann Horse Dataset (WHD) [14] to build our model, while applying it on diverse non-horse objects from the Weizmann Segmentation Dataset (WSD) [15]. Section 7.2 describes the qualitative results obtained on WSD. We additionally perform quantitative experiments to study the individual contributions of our grouping cues, and to demonstrate an improvement over two leading region proposal methods. Results are presented in Sects. 7.1 and 7.3, respectively.

Contained in WHD are 328 images, each annotated with a ground truth mask. We train on the first 200 images, and hold out the remainder for test. As an evaluation metric, we compute the average best overlap [2]:

$$\mathcal{O}(\mathcal{G}, \mathcal{R}; k) = \frac{1}{|\mathcal{G}|} \sum_{(g,i) \in \mathcal{G}} \max_{r \in \mathcal{R}(i;k)} o(r; g),$$

where $\mathcal{G}$ and $\mathcal{R}$ are the ground truth and region masks, respectively, and the quantity k is the number of top-ranked proposals. Intersection-over-union overlap between a region r and the ground truth mask g is denoted by $o(r; g)$. We plot overlap against k to measure the trade-off between overlap and k.

7.1   Cue Combination

We study the effect of incrementally combining the cues of appearance, closure and symmetry, by including their respective potentials in the energy function (6). Each cue observes a different type of grouping evidence, and we expect the best result from combining the strengths of all cues. Figure 4 shows the effect of incrementally adding closure and symmetry to appearance, as well as using mid-level cues without appearance. We observe that closure and appearance work

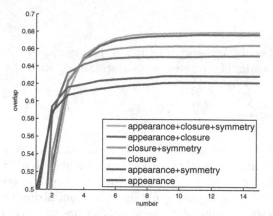

Fig. 4. Improvement in recall as grouping cues are incrementally added to the energy.

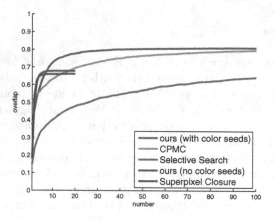

Fig. 5. Improvements over CPMC [1] and Selective Search [2] with a limited budget of proposals, and improvement over Superpixel Closure [26]. Our method is evaluated with and without color seeds. See text for details.

well together, while symmetry helps for all combinations. The results confirm our hypothesis that each cue individually contributes useful information, with the best result from combining all cues. Our symmetry cue contributed a smaller than expected improvement on WHD. We expect symmetry's contribution to be better reflected in more challenging datasets of objects whose regions cannot be as easily computed with the remaining cues alone.

7.2   Qualitative Results

We present qualitative results for a diverse set of objects in Fig. 6, where each row shows the top proposed regions produced from a given input image, along with the corresponding ground truth mask. Our method successfully separates horses from cluttered and occluded backgrounds. We observe that alternative regions

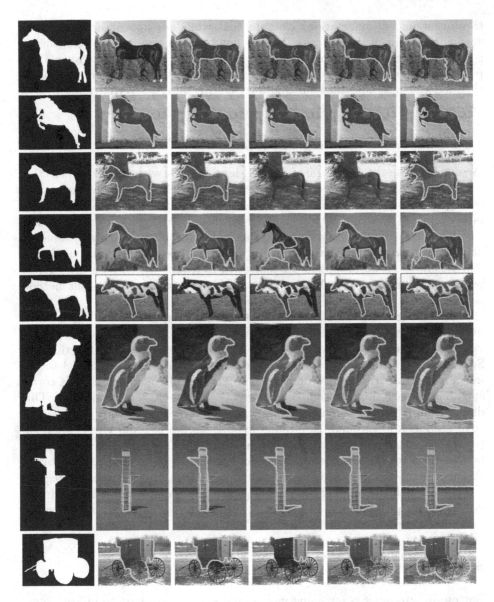

Fig. 6. Top region proposals from our method from different images. Leftmost column shows corresponding ground truth masks and remaining columns show region proposals. Rows 1–5 correspond to images from the Weizmann Horse Database (WHD), and rows 6–8 correspond to images from the Weizmann Segmentation Database (WSD). See text for details.

often arise when there are spurious contours, particularly within the horse and shadows under the horse. False negative contours, however, can cause under-segmentation, *e.g.*, in row 4. Symmetry of occluded fences is often sufficient to prevent undersegmentation. We note that while our appearance cue favors grouping regions of similar color, it does not penalize regions of heterogeneous color and correctly segments the horse in row 5. The remaining rows show results on different objects from WSD and demonstrate that our method is class-independent, and that our mid-level cues trained on WHD transfers well to objects of different classes.

7.3   Comparison with Region Proposals

We demonstrate the advantage of our mid-level method with respect to Selective Search [2] and CPMC [1] in Fig. 5. For comparison with [2], we have measured overlap with respect to the agglomerated regions (rather than their bounding boxes), pooled over color types, similarity measures, and the parameter of [17]. The quantitative comparison demonstrates an improvement on [2] with a budget of a hundred proposals. We note that our method focuses on resolving ambiguity and generates 20–30 proposals per image. In contrast, [2] relies on diversity of proposals and requires over 100 proposals to achieve the same recall. Our method is thus more effective for a limited budget of proposals.

For comparison with [1], we have measured overlap with their regions produced using color seeds, where a color seed model is fit to sampled locations. For this comparison, we have also added color seeds to our energy function (6). Specifically, for any given test image, we fit a Gaussian mixture model to the image's RGB distribution to obtain a compact set of color seed models corresponding to each mixture component (we obtain 4–6 clusters per image). This differs from [1] which densely samples color seeds over a grid. For each pair of color seed as a foreground-background hypothesis, we bias our energy function (6) with a unary potential that scores the corresponding superpixel's log likelihood ratio between the foreground seed and the background seed, as done in [1]. Parametric min-cut is solved for each pair of color seed, and the resulting regions are pooled with the original (unbiased) regions, obtaining several hundred proposals per image. Our method with color seeds improves on [1] with a budget of a hundred proposals.

8   Conclusion

Bottom-up grouping is regaining momentum as a counterpart to object detection, and is a promising area in which to explore the importance of mid-level grouping cues. Mid-level cues are ubiquitous and transcend individual object classes, yet can be leveraged effectively only in combination. We have presented a method to combine appearance, closure, and symmetry, and demonstrated the usefulness of each cue. We have also demonstrated the effectiveness of using mid-level cues to resolve ambiguity with a limited budget of proposals, and shown that our model complements diversification techniques when a large number of proposals is affordable.

References

1. Carreira, J., Sminchisescu, C.: Cpmc: Automatic object segmentation using constrained parametric min-cuts. PAMI **34**, 1312–1328 (2012)
2. Uijlings, J., van de Sande, K., Gevers, T., Smeulders, A.: Selective search for object recognition. IJCV **104**, 154–171 (2013)
3. Fidler, S., Mottaghi, R., Yuille, A., Urtasun, R.: Bottom-up segmentation for top-down detection. In: CVPR, pp. 3294–3301 (2013)
4. Fidler, S., Boben, M., Leonardis, A.: Learning a hierarchical compositional shape vocabulary for multi-class object representation. ArXiv:1408.5516 (2014)
5. Elder, J., Zucker, S.: Computing contour closure. In: Buxton, B.F., Cipolla, R. (eds.) ECCV 1996. LNCS, vol. 1064, pp. 399–412. Springer, Heidelberg (1996)
6. Jacobs, D.: Robust and efficient detection of convex groups. PAMI **18**(1), 23–37 (1996)
7. Loy, G., Eklundh, J.-O.: Detecting symmetry and symmetric constellations of features. In: Leonardis, A., Bischof, H., Pinz, A. (eds.) ECCV 2006. LNCS, vol. 3952, pp. 508–521. Springer, Heidelberg (2006)
8. Mohan, R., Nevatia, R.: Perceptual organization for scene segmentation and description. PAMI **14**, 616–635 (1992)
9. Tsogkas, S., Kokkinos, I.: Learning-based symmetry detection in natural images. In: Fitzgibbon, A., Lazebnik, S., Perona, P., Sato, Y., Schmid, C. (eds.) ECCV 2012, Part VII. LNCS, vol. 7578, pp. 41–54. Springer, Heidelberg (2012)
10. Blum, H.: A transformation for extracting new descriptors of shape. In: Wathen-Dunn, W. (ed.) Models for the Perception of Speech and Visual Form, pp. 362–380. MIT Press, Cambridge (1967)
11. Binford, T.: Visual perception by computer. In: ICSC (1971)
12. Pentland, A.: Perceptual organization and the representation of natural form. AI **28**, 293–331 (1986)
13. Biederman, I.: Human image understanding: Recent research and a theory. In: CVGIP (1985)
14. Borenstein, E., Ullman, S.: Class-specific, top-down segmentation. In: Heyden, A., Sparr, G., Nielsen, M., Johansen, P. (eds.) ECCV 2002, Part II. LNCS, vol. 2351, pp. 109–122. Springer, Heidelberg (2002)
15. Alpert, S., Galun, M., Basri, R., Brandt, A.: Image segmentation by probabilistic bottom-up aggregation and cue integration. In: CVPR (2007)
16. Alexe, B., Deselaers, T., Ferrari, V.: What is an object? In: CVPR, pp. 73–80 (2010)
17. Felzenszwalb, P., Huttenlocher, D.: Efficient graph-based image segmentation. IJCV **59**, 167–181 (2004)
18. Arbeláez, P., Pont-Tuset, J., Barron, J., Marques, F., Malik, J.: Multiscale combinatorial grouping. In: CVPR (2014)
19. Arbeláez, P., Maire, M., Fowlkes, C., Malik, J.: Contour detection and hierarchical image segmentation. PAMI **33**, 898–916 (2011)
20. Kim, J., Grauman, K.: Boundary preserving dense local regions. In: CVPR (2011)
21. Endres, I., Hoiem, D.: Category independent object proposals. In: Daniilidis, K., Maragos, P., Paragios, N. (eds.) ECCV 2010, Part V. LNCS, vol. 6315, pp. 575–588. Springer, Heidelberg (2010)
22. Zhu, S., Yuille, A.: Region competition: Unifying snakes, region growing, and bayes/mdl for multiband image segmentation. PAMI **18**, 884–900 (1996)

23. Shi, J., Malik, J.: Normalized cuts and image segmentation. PAMI **22**, 888–905 (2000)
24. Leung, T., Malik, J.: Contour continuity in region based image segmentation. In: Burkhardt, H.-J., Neumann, B. (eds.) ECCV 1998. LNCS, vol. 1406, pp. 544–559. Springer, Heidelberg (1998)
25. Ren, X., Fowlkes, C., Malik, J.: Cue integration for figure/ground labeling. In: NIPS (2005)
26. Levinshtein, A., Sminchisescu, C., Dickinson, S.J.: Optimal image and video closure by superpixel grouping. IJCV **100**, 99–119 (2012)
27. Lee, T., Fidler, S., Dickinson, S.: Detecting curved symmetric parts using a deformable disc model. In: ICCV (2013)
28. Kolmogorov, V., Boykov, Y., Rother, C.: Applications of parametric maxflow in computer vision. In: ICCV, vol. 8 (2007)
29. Schwing, A., Fidler, S., Pollefeys, M., Urtasun, R.: Box in the box: Joint 3d layout and object reasoning from single images. In: ICCV (2013)

Simple-to-Complex Discriminative Clustering for Hierarchical Image Segmentation

Haw-Shiuan Chang and Yu-Chiang Frank Wang[✉]

Research Center for Information Technology Innovation,
Academia Sinica, Taipei, Taiwan
ycwang@citi.sinica.edu.tw

Abstract. We propose a novel discriminative clustering algorithm with a hierarchical framework for solving unsupervised image segmentation problems. Our discriminative clustering process can be viewed as an EM algorithm, which alternates between the learning of image visual appearance models and the updates of cluster labels (i.e., segmentation outputs) for each image segment. In particular, we advance a simple-to-complex strategy during the above process, which allows the learning of a series of classifiers with different generalization capabilities from the input image, so that consecutive image segments can be well separated. With the proposed hierarchical framework, improved image segmentation can be achieved even if the shapes of the segments are complex, or the boundaries between them are ambiguous. Our work is different from existing region or contour-based approaches, which typically focus on either separating local image regions or determining the associated contours. Our experiments verify that we outperform state-of-the-art approaches on unsupervised image segmentation.

1 Introduction

With the goal of partitioning an image into several spatially coherent regions, image segmentation has been a fundamental computer vision task, which benefits a variety of applications such as object recognition [1–3] and video object segmentation/tracking [4–6]. Generally, challenges of image segmentation lie in the diversity and ambiguity of visual patterns presented in images. Therefore, without any prior knowledge or user interaction, *optimal* image partition might not be easily determined in an *unsupervised* way.

As suggested in [7,8], one can divide existing unsupervised segmentation algorithms into two categories: *region* [9–13] and *contour*-based [8,14–16] approaches. The former considers the input image as a graph, in which each node represents a pixel or an image segment, while the edges connecting each node pair indicate the associated similarity. Thus, the problem of image segmentation turns into a

Electronic supplementary material The online version of this chapter (doi:10.1007/978-3-319-16811-1_26) contains supplementary material, which is available to authorized users.

© Springer International Publishing Switzerland 2015
D. Cremers et al. (Eds.): ACCV 2014, Part III, LNCS 9005, pp. 391–407, 2015.
DOI: 10.1007/978-3-319-16811-1_26

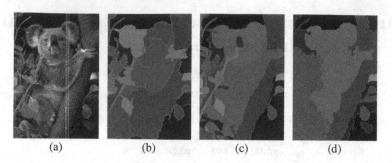

(a)   (b)   (c)   (d)

Fig. 1. Illustration of region and contour-based approaches. (a) Input image, (b) region-based output by SAS [12], (c) contour-based output by gPb [8], and (d) ours by advancing both region and contour information with a hierarchical segmentation framework.

clustering task, which can be solved by techniques like normalized cut (NCut) [9]. To better deal with image segments at different scales, more advanced graph representations have been proposed for improved segmentation (e.g., MNCut [10], correlation clustering [11], SAS [12], FNCut [13]).

Instead of merging local image regions into segments, contour-based approaches aim at exploring local image regions for determining the object boundaries [8,14–16]. This type of methods design classifiers for identifying image contours using feature cues like color or texture (e.g., gPb [8]), and thus image segments can be estimated accordingly (e.g., OWT-UCM [8] or Multicut [15]). However, contour-based approaches might not generalize well if there exist large scale changes for the objects presented in the input image [8]. In addition, contour detection might fail in determining object edges for blurry or articulated regions. Therefore, recent approaches like SWA [17,18], gPb-OWT-UCM [8], or ISCRA [16] advocate an agglomerative clustering (bottom-up) strategy for alleviating the above problems by performing segmentation from finer to coarser image scales. However, as pointed out in [16], if one cannot properly update the contour information during the above hierarchical process (e.g., contour probability of gPb-OWT-UCM only determined at the bottom level), the resulting segmentation performance would still be limited.

As noted in [19,20], successful image segmentation would benefit from feature cues extracted beyond local regions. For local image regions with sufficient and distinct feature information, although promising results have been reported by state-of-the-art methods like gPb-OWT-UCM, human segmentation still achieves much better performance due to the consideration of information extracted beyond local contours. As studied in [20], this is because that human tends to consider feature cues from *non-local* regions (e.g., those farther away from the detected contours) when performing segmentation, even he/she does not recognize the object presented in the input image.

Motivated by the above observations, we propose a novel framework for unsupervised hierarchical image segmentation. Our approach utilizes contour detection at different image scales as initialization, and unsupervised image

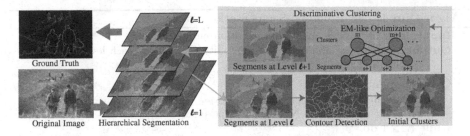

Fig. 2. Our proposed hierarchical image segmentation framework.

segmentation is achieved by an EM-like iterative algorithm, which essentially performs discriminative clustering and maximizes the separation between consecutive image regions. The proposed hierarchical segmentation process is able to integrate both local and global (non-local) statistics for improved segmentation. As depicted in Fig. 1, improved segmentation can be expected by our proposed approach.

In our discriminative clustering process, we advocate a *simple-to-complex* strategy for learning a series of classifiers with different generalization capabilities at each image scale. This unique technique allows us to adaptively separate consecutive object regions by maximizing the differences between the associated feature distributions.

1.1 Our Contributions

- Starting from contour detection, our hierarchical segmentation framework advances graph-based clustering which exploits and integrates local and non-local feature cues for unsupervised segmentation.
- The proposed simple-to-complex discriminative clustering strategy allows automatic learning of a series of classifiers, which exhibit different generalization capabilities for discriminating between image segments, while no additional training process or data are needed.

2 Our Proposed Method

2.1 Hierarchical Image Segmentation

As illustrated in Fig. 2, we advance a hierarchical (i.e., bottom-up) framework for unsupervised image segmentation, in which we consider the clustering outputs at each image scale as the input segments for its upper (coarser) level in the hierarchy. For the interest of computation efficiency, instead of performing pixel-level segmentation at the starting bottom level $l = 1$, we over-segment the input image and start the hierarchical process using superpixels. We apply Turbopixel [21] for performing over-segmentation, which is able to produce compact superpixels with similar sizes (we fix the number of superpixels N as 1200 in our

---

Algorithm 1. Our Proposed Segmentation Framework

Input: Image $\mathbf{I}$, ratio r, maximum iteration number k_{max}
Output: Segments s^l and contour probability $P^l_{contour}$ for each level l in the
hierarchy

Over-segmentation step:
    Over-segment $\mathbf{I}$ and produce superpixels $s^l_{1,...,K}$,
    where level $l \leftarrow 1$, $K \leftarrow$ Number of superpixels N
while $K > 1$ **do**
 | **Discriminative clustering step**:
 | $P^l_{contour} \leftarrow$ Detect contours between $s^l_{1,...,K}$
 | $s^{l+1}_{1,...,\lceil K \times r \rceil} \leftarrow$ Initially cluster $s^l_{1,...,K}$ by NCut
 | **for** *Iteration* $k = 1$ **to** k_{max} **do**
 | | **M-step**:
 | | Construct probability models for each cluster m
 | | $P^k_c(i|m)$ (1), $P^k_t(i|m)$ (3), $P^k(p_s|m)$ (5)
 | | **E-step**:
 | | $\mathbf{m}^l_{1,...,K} \leftarrow$ Classify $s^l_{1,...,K}$ by minimizing E^l in (8)
 | | $s^{l+1}_{1,...,\lceil K \times r \rceil} \leftarrow$ Merge $s^l_{1,...,K}$ by $\mathbf{m}^l_{1,...,K}$
 | **Simple-to-complex step**:
 | Updating σ (1), $w_{t,k}$ (4), w_k (7) for classifier models in each feature
 | space
 |_ $K \leftarrow \lceil K \times r \rceil$ and $l \leftarrow l + 1$

---

work). Since we do not assume the number of clusters known at each level l, we fix the ratio of the numbers of clusters K in consecutive scales as $r = 1/2$, and this hierarchical segmentation process would terminate once the minimum number of clusters allowed is reached. Our proposed segmentation process is summarized in Algorithm 1. In the following subsections, we will detail how we observe multiple feature cues for performing unsupervised segmentation in each level of our hierarchical framework.

2.2 Discriminative Clustering via EM Optimization

As noted above, we view the segmentation output of a lower level in the hierarchy as the input of the current level. We now discuss how the segmentation at each level can be viewed as solving a graph-based optimization task.

Take level l in the hierarchy for example, we start from determining the probability $P^l_{Contour}$ for the edges between image segments being object contours, as depicted in Fig. 2. These probabilities are calculated by the differences of texture and color distributions between consecutive image segments using χ^2 and Earth Mover Distances (EMD) [22,23], respectively. Different from mPb [8,14], we do not consider the use of any training data for estimating such probabilities. With image segments and the associated contour probabilities are obtained, we apply NCut [9] for performing graph-based optimization. This would separate the input segments from K into $K \times r$ clusters, which will be viewed as initial segmentation results as shown in Figs. 2 and 3.

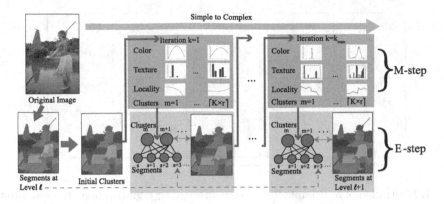

Fig. 3. Our discriminative clustering process with a simple-to-complex strategy at level l in the hierarchy (K is the number of segments).

Since graph-based segmentation techniques like NCut are known to produce clusters (i.e., image segments) with similar sizes [12], complex or ambiguous image regions might not be properly separated. This is why we advance discriminative clustering in our proposed framework, aiming at the refinement of the clustering/labeling outputs at each level in our hierarchy. For the task of unsupervised segmentation, separation between clusters needs to be automatically achieved by observing the features/classifiers from consecutive image segments.

For discriminative clustering in our proposed segmentation method, we propose to learn of a series of classifiers with different generalization capabilities for refined image segmentation. More precisely, each image cluster (i.e., a set of image segments with the same label) will be recognized by a particular classifier, which will be automatically learned from the input image data using multiple types of features. Essentially, our discriminative clustering strategy can be considered as an EM-like process, which is summarized as follows:

- M-step: Given the clustering outputs, construct the probability model of each image cluster in different feature spaces
- E-step: Given the observed cluster models, classify each image segment into the corresponding cluster based on the estimated probabilities

Although prior works on foreground object segmentation like GrabCut also utilized similar iterative clustering techniques [4–6,24,25], they typically required additional efforts or information for annotating foreground/background regions (e.g., user interaction or use of temporal features), otherwise the associated classifiers cannot be easily derived. On the other hand, while EM-based image segmentation has been previously explored in [26–28], such methods still require proper selection of parameters (e.g., the number of segments) for performing segmentation.

In our work, we focus on *unsupervised* image segmentation. At each scale in the hierarchy, our proposed segmentation algorithm is able to discriminate between consecutive segments using classifiers with different generalization capabilities. These classifier models will first be observed at the M-step of each iteration, and

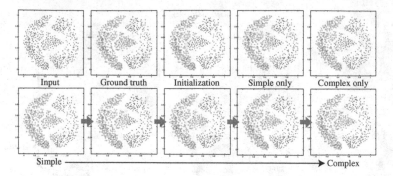

Fig. 4. Illustration of our simple-to-complex strategy for segmentation. Top row (from left to right): input instances, those with ground truth labels, initial clustering output by NCut, and clustering outputs by Gaussian kernel density estimation (KDE) classifiers with $\sigma = 0.35$ and 0.1, respectively. Bottom row: refined clustering outputs obtained by our simple-to-complex strategy (i.e., decreasing σ from 0.35 to 0.1). Note that different colors denote the resulting cluster labels (Color figure online).

they will be applied to separate image segments at the following E-step. In Sect. 2.3, we will detail how we apply a simple-to-complex strategy for discriminative clustering in our hierarchical segmentation framework.

2.3   Simple-to-Complex Classification and Segmentation

As depicted in Fig. 3, our simple-to-complex strategy for discriminative clustering first observes *simpler* classifiers (e.g., kernel density estimation based classifier with larger σ) at the M-step of each iteration. This results in *coarser* separation between image segments at the E-step by updating the cluster labels. With this simple-to-complex strategy, it will be less likely for segmentation outputs to overfit the initial contour detection results in the beginning of the segmentation process. For the subsequent iterations, we treat the newly-predicted segment pairs as updated training data, and we re-design the classifiers with increased complexities (e.g., smaller σ for Gaussian kernels). Figure 4 illustrates our proposed simple-to-complex strategy. It is clear that, our simple-to-complex strategy effectively performs a coarse-to-fine separation between the observed features.

We note that, the use of our simple-to-complex discriminative clustering strategy is to handle objects regions with complex or ambiguous patterns at each image scale. This is very different from existing work like [29,30], which either chose to discriminate between image clusters using predetermined SVMs, and only considered global image statistics for segment discrimination. In our work, the series of classifiers derived by multiple types of features not only make the separation between complex/ambiguous object regions more feasible, the resulting outputs (i.e., clustering results) would also reflect the flexibility of the way human discriminates between different object regions (which is consistent with the observations [31]). In the following subsections, we discuss how we automatically learn the classifiers (or image visual appearance models) with different complexities in each feature space for performing simple-to-complex classification and segmentation.

Multiple Feature Cues

Color Cues. Color information is among the most representative feature cues for image segmentation. As suggested in [8,14], we use CIE Lab color space for representing each image segment, and each channel is represented by a histogram of n bins with equal widths (we set $n = 50$). Using such features, we apply Naive Bayes classifiers based on kernel density estimation (KDE) [25,32] for separating consecutive image segments.

At iteration k of discriminative clustering, we derive the probability distribution of color histograms for each cluster m (i.e., segment label) using Gaussian kernels by:

$$P_c^k(i|m) \propto \sum_{j=1}^{n} \left(\exp \left(-\frac{(j-i)^2}{\sigma^2} \right) h_m^c(j) \right), \tag{1}$$

where c indicates the color channel of interest, and i is the bin index of the associated histogram. From (1), we see that $h_m^c(j)$ returns the pixel number observed in the jth bin of color channel c, and this number is weighted by a Gaussian kernel with width σ. Note that we do not use the equality sign for (1), since the derived probability for each bin will be normalized for ensuring $\sum_i P_c^k(i|m) = 1$.

As noted in Sect. 2.2 and depicted in Fig. 3, the derivation of (1) can be viewed as the M-step for modeling the cluster information at each iteration in our discriminative clustering process. At the E-step, with the equal prior assumption of the clusters (i.e., same $P(m)$ for each cluster), we classify each image segment s to cluster m (at the E-step) by updating the following probability output:

$$P_{Color}^k(m|s) \propto P_{Color}^k(s|m)P(m) = \left(\prod_{p=1}^{|s|} \prod_{c=1}^{3} P_c^k(i_p|m) \right), \tag{2}$$

where i_p denotes the bin which the pixel p (in segment s) belongs to, and $|s|$ represents the size of segment s. Similar to (1), the calculated probability for each cluster will be normalized for ensuring $\sum_m P_{Color}^k(m|s) = 1$. It is worth noting that, we view each pixel as an independent observation for fulfilling Naive Bayes assumptions.

Based on our simple-to-complex strategy, we start our KDE-based classification using *larger* σ values, which perform *coarser* separation between image segments and alleviate potential overfitting problems. As the iteration continues, we reduce σ (which increases the complexity of KDE) and thus introduce additional classification capabilities based on the separation determined at previous iterations.

Texture Cues. In addition to color, we consider texture information as feature cues for segmentation. As did in [33,34], we also apply 17 Gaussian/Laplacian-type filters and their derivatives in the CIE Lab color space, and we calculate their responses as textural features. In order to describe and summarize such textural responses in each image segment, we perform GMM to construct the textons for computing the associated bag-of-words (BoW) models [34,35].

We note that the number of textons would be a tradeoff between the representation and generalization capabilities for the resulting BoW models. While a smaller number of textons produces a simpler/coarser BoW model for describing the texture information, a larger one would exhibit a better representation ability (but more possible for overfitting the texture cues). Therefore, based on our proposed simple-to-complex strategy, we will adjust this parameter during the discriminative clustering process. In our work, we consider 9 different BoW models with different numbers (2 to 32, according to an equal logarithm scale) of textons as discussed below.

For the M-stage at iteration k, we estimate the probability distribution of the tth BoW model ($t = 1$ to 9) for segmentation cluster m. Based on the law of total probability, we calculate $P_t^k(i|m)$ as follows:

$$P_t^k(i|m) = \sum_{p \in m} P^k(i|p) P^k(p|m),\tag{3}$$

where i is the bin (i.e., texton) index of the tth BoW model, $P^k(p|m)$ is that of pixel p presented in cluster m [18], and $P^k(i|p)$ calculates the probability of pixel p assigned to bin i (by GMM).

At the E-step for re-determining the cluster output for each segment, we need to calculate the probability of assigning each segment s to cluster m (i.e., $P_{Text}^k(m|s)$). Similar to the use of color cues, we define $P_{Text}^k(m|s)$ as follows:

$$P_{Text}^k(m|s) \propto \prod_{t=1}^{9} \left(\prod_{i=1}^{H_t} P_t^k(i|m)^{P(i|s)} \right)^{w_{t,k}}\tag{4}$$

where $P(i|s) = \sum_p P(i|p) P(p|s)$. H_t indicates the number of textons/bins considered for the tth BoW model ($t = 1 \sim 9$), which ranges from 2 to 32 in a descending order.

It is worth noting that, $w_{t,k}$ in (4) controls the weight for each BoW model, and it is a function of the iteration number (for simple-to-complex purposes). More specifically, we determine $w_{t,k} = P(s) \exp(-\beta(\frac{k}{k_{max}} - 0.5)t)$, where k_{max} is the maximum iteration number allowed (we set $\beta = 0.1$), and $P(s) = \sum_p P(s|p)$ is the total number of pixels belonging to segment s. Similar to (2), the calculated probability of (4) will be normalized for ensuring $\sum_m P_{Text}^k(m|s) = 1$. It can be seen that we impose a *larger* weight $w_{t,k}$ on BoW models with *fewer* number of textons (i.e., *simpler* models) in the beginning stages of our discriminative clustering process. As the iteration increases, a finer separation will be achieved by higher $w_{t,k}$ for the BoW models with *larger* H_t texton numbers (i.e., *finer* models). This is how we apply our simple-to-complex strategy for performing textural-based clustering process for segmentation.

Locality Cues. For image segmentation, since the object regions are typically compact and locally connected, spatial information is often considered as another important cue [4,5,36]. In our work, we consider Gaussian and shape prior classifiers. The Gaussian classifiers utilize the x and y coordinates of superpixel centers (extracted at the bottom level in the hierarchy) as features, and thus the observed 2D Gaussian distributions $P_G^k(m|s)$ can be applied to discriminate between image segments s of different clusters m. On the other hand, inspired by [4], our shape prior classifier aims at deriving the probability $P(p_s|m)$ that a superpixel p_s is presented at cluster m in terms of its distance to the cluster contour. To be more precise, at the kth iteration of our discriminative clustering process, we derive $P_S^k(p_s|m)$ at the M-step by:

$$P_S^k(p_s|m) \propto S(d(p_s, m)/\bar{d}(m)), \tag{5}$$

where $d(p_s, m)$ measures the shortest distance between superpixel p_s to the contour of cluster m. The sigmoid function $S(x) = \frac{1}{1+\exp(-x)}$ is used to estimate the likelihood of assigning p_s to m, and $\bar{d}(m)$ is the average distance of d.

Assuming the pixels in p_s are i.i.d., we estimate the probability of assigning segment s to cluster m as follows:

$$P_{Shape}^k(m|s) \propto \prod_{p_s \in s} (P_S^k(p_s|m))^{|p_s|}, \tag{6}$$

where $|p_s|$ is the size of the superpixel p_s. Similar remarks can be applied to the use of Gaussian classifiers. Thus, at the E-step we update the locality cues by fusing the results of the two classifiers by:

$$P_{Local}^k(m|s) = P_G^k(m|s)^{(1-w_k)} P_{Shape}^k(m|s)^{w_k}, \tag{7}$$

where $w_k = k/k_{max}$. It can be seen that, as iteration k increases, the weight for the shape prior classifier becomes larger, allowing one to emphasize on object regions with complex shape information (i.e., for *finer* separation). This is again consistent with our simple-to-complex strategy of the proposed discriminative clustering for segmentation.

Graph-Based Optimization. At the E-step of each iteration in our discriminative clustering process, we apply multi-label Markov Random Fields (MRF) for prediction based on the observed feature cues. As discussed later in Sect. 2.4, this graph-based optimization can be viewed as fitting the observed features of superpixels at the bottom level by the clusters (i.e., image segments) determined at each level in the hierarchy.

In our work, we determine the MRF energy term $E^l(\mathbf{m})$ at level l as follows:

$$E^l(\mathbf{m}) = E_D^l(\mathbf{m}) + E_S^l(\mathbf{m})$$
$$E_D^l(\mathbf{m}) = -\sum_s w_C \cdot log(P_{Color}^k(m_s|s))$$
$$+w_T \cdot log(P_{Text}^k(m_s|s)) + w_L \cdot log(P_{Local}^k(m_s|s))$$
$$E_S^l(\mathbf{m}) = \lambda \sum_{s,q} \mathbb{1}_{(m_s \neq m_q)}(-log(P_{Contour}^l(s,q))), \tag{8}$$

where $\mathbf{m}$ is the labeling vector indicating the segmentation output, and thus its dimension K is equal to the number of the input segments at that level (i.e., its sth entry m_s indicates the corresponding output for segment s). $E_D^l(m)$ and $E_S^l(m)$ are the data and smoothness terms, respectively. While $E_D^l(m)$ integrates the probabilities observed in different feature spaces (with weights w_C, w_T, and w_L), $E_S^l(m)$ preserves the consistency of segmentation outputs of neighboring segments. Note that q is the neighboring segments of segment s, and we have m_s and m_q as cluster labels of segments s and q, respectively. The function $\mathbb{1}()$ is the indicator function, and $P_{Contour}^l(s,q)$ is the detected contour probability (see Sect. 2.2).

At iteration k in level l of the hierarchy, we apply α-β swap [37–39] to minimize (8), and update the cluster label m of each segment s accordingly. With the above MRF model, our discriminative clustering starts segmentation from initial clustering results produced by locally detected contours, and we update the segmentation results at each iteration with increasingly complex classifiers in different feature spaces.

2.4   Probabilistic Interpretation

As discussed above, our simple-to-complex discriminative clustering solves a graph-based optimization problem at each level in the hierarchy, in which each segment is viewed as an input node to be clustered. By increasing the complexities of the MRF energy terms, improved optimization can be achieved. Effectively, at level l, this process is equivalent to the fitting of features observed from superpixels at the bottom level using the clusters determined at level l.

For each level l in our hierarchy, minimizing the MRF model in (8) is effectively solving the maximum likelihood estimation (MLE) of probability $P^l(X)$:

$$P^l(X) = \prod_{p_s=1}^{N} P(x_{p_s}) \prod_{p_s,p_q} P_{Contour}^l(p_s, p_q), \qquad (9)$$

where X represents the observed image features. $P(x_{p_s})$ denotes the estimated probability of superpixel p_s at the bottom level, which is observed across $K \times r$ different clusters. In other words, we have $P(x_{p_s}) = \sum_{y=1}^{K \times r} P(m_{p_s} = y)P(x_{p_s}|m_{p_s} = y)$. The probability term $P(m_{p_s} = y)$ indicates how likely p_s belongs to cluster y, and $P(x_{p_s}|m_{p_s} = y)$ is the probability of observing x_{p_s} in that cluster. For image segmentation, since consecutive superpixels are *not* independent of each other, we have $P_{Contour}^l(p_s, p_q)$ denote the contour probability of the associated superpixel pair.

For our discriminative clustering, each E-step can be viewed as estimating $P(m_{p_s} = y)$ by minimizing E^l in (8), given $P(x_{p_s}|m_{p_s} = y)$ observed from the previous M-step (see the supplementary material for detailed derivations). On the other hand, the M-step at each iteration updates the observed feature models/classifiers, using outputs determined at the E-step. Thus, our simple-to-complex clustering process is effectively solving the above MLE problem.

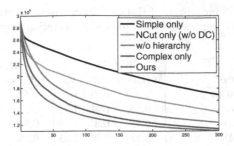

Fig. 5. Optimized energy function outputs of (8) on BSDS300. The vertical axis is the negative log-likelihood of $P^l(X)$ of different approaches, and the horizontal axis indicates the number of clusters determined at each level in our hierarchy. Note that DC denotes discriminative clustering.

In Fig. 5, we show that our discriminative clustering strategy with hierarchical segmentation achieved better and optimized energy function outputs produced at the final iteration in each level, compared with other simplified/controlled versions of our segmentation framework (see our experiments).

3 Experiments

3.1 Unsupervised Segmentation

We evaluate our proposed method on the Berkeley Segmentation Datasets (BSDS) [31], MSRC [33], and the Stanford Background Dataset (SBD) [40]. For MSRC, we apply the ground truth labels provided by [41] for evaluation (as [8,16] did). As for SBD, we choose the semantic labels (i.e., "regions" given in [40]) of images as ground truth. We consider three different metrics for evaluating the performance: SegCover [8], PRI [42], and VoI [43]. Note that *larger* SegCover/PRI and *lower* VOI numbers indicate better performance. Our code is available at http://mml.citi.sinica.edu.tw/papers/HDC_code_ACCV_2014/.

For our approach, the parameters for BSDS300 are selected based on the performance of the training data of the same dataset. On the other hand, we apply the training data of BSDS500 to determine the parameters for MSRC, SBD, and BSDS500. For evaluation, we perform quantitative evaluations based on the *optimal image scale* (OIS). That is, the final segment number of interest is determined by the optimal value of each metric based on the ground truth of each image. In order to produce all possible cluster numbers (i.e., other than K at level l, $K \times r$ at level $l + 1$, etc.), we merge the segmentation outputs at that level using the associated contour probability values, so that the intermediate cluster numbers can be obtained. We note that we do not fix the image scale over all images (i.e., *optimal dataset scale* (ODS)), since unsupervised image segmentation is typically performed prior to higher-level tasks like object recognition or retrieval (e.g. [1–3]). For such tasks, image priors of class labels or their semantic information will be provided, which can be viewed as OIS. Later our experiments on semantic segmentation in Sect. 3.2 will support this observation.

Table 1. Performance comparisons of BSDS (* indicates the methods requiring training data). Note that DC represents discriminative clustering applied in our proposed framework.

	Methods	BSDS300			BSDS500		
		SegCover	PRI	VoI	SegCover	PRI	VoI
	MNCut	0.53	0.79	1.84	0.53	0.80	1.89
	SWA	0.55	0.80	1.75	-	-	-
	FH	0.58	0.82	1.79	0.57	0.82	1.87
	MS	0.58	0.80	1.63	0.58	0.81	1.64
	SAS	0.610	0.834	1.534	0.610	0.840	1.552
	gPb-OWT-UCM*	0.646	0.852	1.466	0.647	0.856	1.475
	ISCRA*	0.66	0.86	1.40	0.66	0.85	1.42
	Ours (Full version)	0.660	0.854	1.443	0.655	0.859	1.454
	NCut only (w/o DC)	0.583	0.814	1.734	0.578	0.825	1.784
	Complex only	0.627	0.840	1.569	0.618	0.845	1.613
Ours	w/o MRF	0.633	0.843	1.536	0.634	0.849	1.548
	Color cues only	0.595	0.810	1.695	0.598	0.823	1.724
	Color + spatial cues	0.605	0.824	1.653	0.605	0.832	1.699

Table 2. Performance comparisons of MSRC and SBD datasets.

Methods	MSRC			SBD		
	SegCover	PRI	VoI	SegCover	PRI	VoI
SAS	0.712	0.823	1.052	0.649	0.856	1.474
gPb-OWT-UCM	0.745	0.850	0.989	0.642	0.858	1.527
ISCRA	0.75	0.85	1.02	0.68*	0.90*	1.50*
Ours	0.772	0.862	0.920	0.681	0.870	1.425

Tables 1 and 2 summarize and compare the segmentation results, in which we compare our method with MNCut [10], SWA [17], FH [45], MS (mean shift) [46], SAS [12], gPb-OWT-UCM [8], and ISCRA [16]. From Table 1, it is clear that our approach outperformed baseline approaches. Compared with gPb-OWT-UCM and ISCRA, we achieved comparable or slightly improved results (see examples in Fig. 6). As commented in [8], this is due to the fact that inherent photographic bias in BSDS would make images contain sufficient local information, which favors contour-based segmentation approaches like gPb-OWT-UCM or ISCRA. However, it is worth repeating that gPb-OWT-UCM and ISCRA applied pre-trained classifiers for contour detection, while ours is an unsupervised approach and does not require the collection of any training data. We note that, if the recently proposed object and part metric of F_{op} [47] is applied, we achieved a higher score of 0.389 than gPb-OWT-UCM did (0.380). In Table 2, we see that our method achieved the best performance (for ISCRA, we directly apply the results presented in [16], which utilized region-based labels (i.e., "layers" given in [40]) for SBD as ground truth, as noted by * in Table 2). Different from the ground truth of BSDS which separates an object into several regions, image

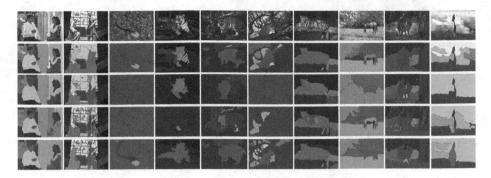

Fig. 6. Example segmentation results of BSDS300. From top to bottom: original images, results produced by Mobahi *et al.* [44], SAS [12], gPb-OWT-UCM [8], and ours. Note that the results for gPb-OWT-UCM, SAS [12] and our method are based on the largest SegCover value, while those of [44] are based on the highest PRI.

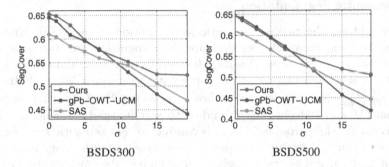

BSDS300   BSDS500

Fig. 7. Performance comparisons (in SegCover) on degraded versions of BSDS.

labels for MSRC and SBD are generally able to identify semantical objects [20]. Since our approach is able to observe multiple feature cues for discriminating between image regions, improved performance on these two datasets can be achieved.

In addition, we provide controlled experiments in Table 1, which present the contributions of each component in our proposed framework. For example, *NCut only* represents the use of our hierarchical segmentation framework without performing simple-to-complex discriminative clustering, and *complex only* indicates that the use of complex classification models in our proposed method. On the other hand, *w/o MRF* in Table 1 means the direct use of the predicted probabilities from each feature cue for determining the segmentation outputs (i.e., no smoothness term is considered in (8)).

To verify that our approach is able to consider non-local information and generalizes well for blurred image contours, we compare the performance our method with those of gPb-OWT-UCM and SAS on BSDS with degraded resolutions. We downgrade the resolution of BSDS300 and BSDS500 images using Gaussian filters with different σ, and we compare the SegCover values in Fig. 7.

Table 3. Average recognition results of different methods for semantic segmentation.

Methods	MSRC		SBD	
	Naive Bayes	SVM	Naive Bayes	SVM
SAS	0.272	0.330	0.399	0.423
gPb-OWT-UCM	0.285	0.352	0.406	0.426
Ours	0.294	0.362	0.414	0.454
Ground truth	0.366	0.474	0.502	0.570

From this figure, we outperformed SAS (region-based) and gPb-OWT-UCM (contour-based) especially when σ is large. Thus, the effectiveness of our approach on lower-resolution images can be verified.

3.2 Semantic Segmentation

We now address the task of semantic segmentation using MSRC and SBD datasets. To be more specific, we evaluate the recognition/annotation accuracy of the output segments, using classifiers learned from training data (with ground truth object label information) of the corresponding dataset. We apply the metric of $(\frac{GT_i \cap R_i}{GT_i \cup R_i})$ for each semantic class i as recent PASCAL challenges did. Note that GT and R denote the ground truth and detected segments for class i, respectively. A 5-fold cross-validation is conducted. For semantic segmentation, we extract color and texture histograms from ground truth image segments of the training data, and we train classifiers on such image segments using the associated label information (standard Naive Bayes and linear SVM are considered). For the test (validation) images of the same data, we perform image segmentation using our proposed method based on OIS, and we apply the aforementioned classifiers for predicting the class label of each image segment.

We compare the performance of ours with SAS and gPb-OWT-UCM. Table 3 compares the averaged results of different approaches. From Table 3, we can see that the average annotation accuracy based on our proposed segmentation method was higher than those using SAS and gPb-OWT-UCM. Note that the optimal performance (denoted as Ground truth in Table 3) was obtained by applying the derived classifiers on the ground truth labeled segments as shown in the last row of Table 3. As a result, we see that our method not only outperformed recent segmentation algorithms in terms of unsupervised segmentation, improved image annotation accuracy also confirms that our approach is able to achieve better semantic segmentation, which would benefit future tasks such as object retrieval and classification.

3.3 Remarks on Computation Costs

Finally, we comment on the computation time and memory requirements of our proposed method. In average, it took 230 s for processing an image in BSDS300 with image resolution around 481×321 pixels. The feature processing part (including generating superpixel and building textons) took about 78 % of the entire computation time, while our proposed hierarchical segmentation process only required the remaining 22 %. Although our method was slightly slower than gPb-OWT-UCM (increased by 5 % of the computation time), our method could be easily accelerated if feature extraction or preprocessing steps are performed offline. For example, if we build the textons in advance, our method only took about 60 s (only 27 % of computation time w.r.t. gPb-OWT-UCM), while the performance only slightly dropped (e.g., SegCover became 0.64 for BSDS500).

It is worth noting that, we do not need to solve large-scale eigen-analysis problems as gPb-OWT-UCM does. The memory requirement of our method was about 700MB for each image, which was only 12 % of that required by gPb. Note that ISCRA is based on gPb-OWT-UCM and applies more sophisticated features. Therefore, so its memory and computation costs were higher than those of gPb-OWT-UCM. From the above remarks, it can be concluded that our approach is computationally feasible. Note that the above runtime and memory estimates were obtained by Matlab on an Intel Quad Core workstation with 2.2 GHz.

4   Conclusions

This paper presented a hierarchical image segmentation framework, in which an EM-based discriminative clustering is utilized at each level for discriminating between image segments. By our proposed simple-to-complex strategy, a series of classifiers with different generalization capabilities can be learned during the clustering process, so that segmentation of different image segments at each level can be performed automatically. The deployment of our discriminative clustering process in a hierarchical framework allows us to exploit both local and non-local image statistics across image scales when performing unsupervised segmentation. Experimental results on several benchmark datasets confirmed the use of our proposed method for image segmentation, and our method was shown to achieve competitive or improved results than state-of-the-art region or contour-based approaches did.

References

1. Pantofaru, C., Schmid, C., Hebert, M.: Object recognition by integrating multiple image segmentations. In: Forsyth, D., Torr, P., Zisserman, A. (eds.) ECCV 2008, Part III. LNCS, vol. 5304, pp. 481–494. Springer, Heidelberg (2008)
2. Gu, C., Lim, J.J., Arbelaez, P., Malik, J.: Recognition using regions. In: CVPR(2009)
3. Arbelaez, P., Hariharan, B., Gu, C., Gupta, S., Bourdev, L.D., Malik, J.: Semantic segmentation using regions and parts. In: CVPR (2012)
4. Bai, X., Wang, J., Simons, D., Sapiro, G.: Video snapcut: robust video object cutout using localized classifiers. In: SIGGRAPH (2009)

5. Papoutsakis, K.E., Argyros, A.A.: Object tracking and segmentation in a closed loop. In: Bebis, G., Boyle, R., Parvin, B., Koracin, D., Chung, R., Hammoud, R., Hussain, M., Kar-Han, T., Crawfis, R., Thalmann, D., Kao, D., Avila, L. (eds.) ISVC 2010, Part I. LNCS, vol. 6453, pp. 405–416. Springer, Heidelberg (2010)

6. Chen, A.Y.C., Corso, J.J.: Temporally consistent multi-class video-object segmentation with the video graph-shifts algorithm. In: WACV (2011)

7. Freixenet, J., Muñoz, X., Raba, D., Martí, J., Cufí, X.: Yet another survey on image segmentation: region and boundary information integration. In: Heyden, A., Sparr, G., Nielsen, M., Johansen, P. (eds.) ECCV 2002, Part III. LNCS, vol. 2352, pp. 408–422. Springer, Heidelberg (2002)

8. Arbelaez, P., Maire, M., Fowlkes, C., Malik, J.: Contour detection and hierarchical image segmentation. IEEE Trans. Pattern Anal. Mach. Intell. **33**(5), 898–916 (2011)

9. Shi, J., Malik, J.: Normalized cuts and image segmentation. In: CVPR (1997)

10. Cour, T., Benezit, F., Shi, J.: Spectral segmentation with multiscale graph decomposition. In: CVPR (2005)

11. Kim, S., Nowozin, S., Kohli, P., Yoo, C.D.: Higher-order correlation clustering for image segmentation. In: NIPS (2011)

12. Li, Z., Wu, X.M., Chang, S.F.: Segmentation using superpixels: A bipartite graph partitioning approach. In: CVPR (2012)

13. Kim, T.H., Lee, K.M., Lee, S.U.: Learning full pairwise affinities for spectral segmentation. IEEE Trans. Pattern Anal. Mach. Intell. **35**(1), 171–184 (2013)

14. Martin, D.R., Fowlkes, C., Malik, J.: Learning to detect natural image boundaries using local brightness, color, and texture cues. IEEE Trans. Pattern Anal. Mach. Intell. **26**, 530–549 (2004)

15. Andres, B., Kappes, J.H., Beier, T., Kothe, U., Hamprecht, F.A.: Probabilistic image segmentation with closedness constraints. In: ICCV (2011)

16. Ren, Z., Shakhnarovich, G.: Image segmentation by cascaded region agglomeration. In: CVPR (2013)

17. Sharon, E., Galun, M., Sharon, D., Basri, R., Brandt, A.: Hierarchy and adaptivity in segmenting visual scenes. Nature **442**(7104), 810–813 (2006)

18. Alpert, S., Galun, M., Basri, R., Brandt, A.: Image segmentation by probabilistic bottom-up aggregation and cue integration. In: CVPR (2007)

19. Fowlkes, C.C., Martin, D.R., Malik, J.: Local figure-ground cues are valid for natural images. J. Vis. **7**, 1–9 (2007)

20. Zitnick, C.L., Parikh, D.: The role of image understanding in contour detection. In: CVPR (2012)

21. Levinshtein, A., Stere, A., Kutulakos, K.N., Fleet, D.J., Dickinson, S.J., Siddiqi, K.: Turbopixels: Fast superpixels using geometric flows. IEEE Trans. Pattern Anal. Mach. Intell. **2**, 416–423 (2009)

22. Pele, O., Werman, M.: A linear time histogram metric for improved SIFT matching. In: Forsyth, D., Torr, P., Zisserman, A. (eds.) ECCV 2008, Part III. LNCS, vol. 5304, pp. 495–508. Springer, Heidelberg (2008)

23. Pele, O., Werman, M.: Fast and robust earth mover's distances. In: ICCV (2009)

24. Rother, C., Kolmogorov, V., Blake, A.: "GrabCut": interactive foreground extraction using iterated graph cuts. In: SIGGRAPH (2004)

25. Pham, V.Q., Takahashi, K., Naemura, T.: Foreground-background segmentation using iterated distribution matching. In: CVPR (2011)

26. Zhu, S.C., Yuille, A.L.: Region competition: Unifying snakes, region growing, and bayes/mdl for multiband image segmentation. IEEE Trans. Pattern Anal. Mach. Intell. **18**(9), 884–900 (1996)

27. Belongie, S., Carson, C., Greenspan, H., Malik, J.: Color-and texture-based image segmentation using EM and its application to content-based image retrieval. In: Computer Vision (1998)

28. Achanta, R., Shaji, A., Smith, K., Lucchi, A., Fua, P., Ssstrunk, S.: SLIC superpixels compared to state-of-the-art superpixel methods. IEEE Trans. Pattern Anal. Mach. Intell. **34**(11), 2274–2282 (2012)

29. Xu, L., Neufeld, J., Larson, B., Schuurmans, D.: Maximum margin clustering. In: NIPS (2004)

30. Gomes, R., Krause, A., Perona, P.: Discriminative clustering by regularized information maximization. In: NIPS (2010)

31. Martin, D.R., Fowlkes, C., Tal, D., Malik, J.: A database of human segmented natural images and its application to evaluating segmentation algorithms and measuring ecological statistics. In: ICCV (2001)

32. Witten, I., Frank, E., Hall, M.: Data Mining: Practical Machine Learning Tools and Techniques. Morgan Kaufmann, San Francisco (2005)

33. Shotton, J., Winn, J., Rother, C., Criminisi, A.: Textonboost: Joint appearance, shape and context modeling for multi-class object recognition and segmentation. In: Leonardis, A., Bischof, H., Pinz, A. (eds.) Computer Vision – ECCV 2006. LNCS, vol. 3951. Springer, Berlin (2006)

34. Yu, Z., Li, A., Au, O.C., Xu, C.: Bag of textons for image segmentation via soft clustering and convex shift. In: CVPR (2012)

35. Calinon, S., Guenter, F., Billard, A.: On learning, representing and generalizing a task in a humanoid robot. IEEE Transactions on Systems, Man and Cybernetics, Part B. Special issue on robot learning by observation, demonstration and imitation (2007)

36. Carreira, J., Sminchisescu, C.: Constrained parametric min-cuts for automatic object segmentation. In: CVPR (2010)

37. Boykov, Y., Veksler, O., Zabih, R.: Fast approximate energy minimization via graph cuts. IEEE Trans. Pattern Anal. Mach. Intell. **23**(11), 1222–1239 (2001)

38. Kolmogorov, V., Zabih, R.: What energy functions can be minimized via graph cuts? IEEE Trans. Pattern Anal. Mach. Intell. **26**(11), 1521–1525 (2004)

39. Boykov, Y., Kolmogorov, V.: An experimental comparison of min-cut/max-flow algorithms for energy minimization in vision. IEEE Trans. Pattern Anal. Mach. Intell. **26**(9), 1124–1137 (2004)

40. Gould, S., Fulton, R., Koller, D.: Decomposing a scene into geometric and semantically consistent regions. In: ICCV (2009)

41. Malisiewicz, T., Efros, A.A.: Improving spatial support for objects via multiple segmentations. In: BMVC (2007)

42. Unnikrishnan, R., Pantofaru, C., Hebert, M.: Toward objective evaluation of image segmentation algorithms. IEEE Trans. Pattern Anal. Mach. Intell. **29**, 929–944 (2007)

43. Meila, M.: Comparing clusterings: an axiomatic view. In: ICML (2005)

44. Mobahi, H., Rao, S., Yang, A.Y., Sastry, S.S., Ma, Y.: Segmentation of natural images by texture and boundary compression. Int. J. Comput. Vis. **95**, 86–98 (2011)

45. Felzenszwalb, P.F., Huttenlocher, D.P.: Efficient graph-based image segmentation. Int. J. Comput. Vis. **59**, 167–181 (2004)

46. Comaniciu, D., Meer, P.: Mean shift A robust approach toward feature space analysis. IEEE Trans. Pattern Anal. Mach. Intell. **24**(5), 603–619 (2002)

47. Pont-Tuset, J., Marqus, F.: Measures and meta-measures for the supervised evaluation of image segmentation. In: CVPR (2013)

Learning One-Shot Exemplar SVM from the Web for Face Verification

Fengyi Song and Xiaoyang Tan[✉]

Department of Computer Science and Technology,
Nanjing University of Aeronautics and Astronautics, Nanjing 210016, China
{f.song,x.tan}@nuaa.edu.cn

Abstract. We investigate the problem of learning from a single instance consisting of a pair of images, often encountered in unconstrained face verification where the pair of images to be verified contain large variations and are captured from never seen subjects. Instead of constructing a separate discriminative model for each image in the couple and performing cross-checking, we learn a single Exemplar-SVM model for the pair by augmenting it with a negative couple set, and then predict whether the pair are from the same subject or not by asking an oracle whether this Exemplar-SVM is for a client or imposter in nature. The oracle by itself is learnt from the behaviors of a large number of Exemplar-SVMs based on the labeled background set. For face representation we use a number of unlabeled face sets collected from the Web to train a series of decision stumps that jointly map a given face to a discriminative and distributional representation. Experiments on the challenging Labeled Faces in the Wild (LFW) verify the effectiveness and feasibility of the proposed method.

1 Introduction

In many computer vision applications, we often encounter the problem of comparing the similarity between two images which are captured from never seen objects. For example, in the unconstrained face verification, the task is to decide whether a pair of images are from the same person or not, in which not only the images given are never seen, but the subjects behind are usually never seen as well (see Fig. 1). This problem is challenging mainly due to the following two reasons: (1) the images by themselves contain large variations which have to be dealt with. (2) since the information source (subjects which generate the images) is hidden, the known knowledge to infer them is extremely scarce (actually only one shot of sample per subject). Moreover, these two issues seem to be closely related - the task of learning good representation that well supports the one-shot similarity evaluation is much more difficult than doing that when the training samples are abundant.

To address these issues, many different "pairwise" approaches have been developed in recent years - either directly learn same person/different person decision rules, or that learn pairwise similarity metrics that can be used to produce such rules [2–5]. The key idea behind these approaches roots from the

© Springer International Publishing Switzerland 2015
D. Cremers et al. (Eds.): ACCV 2014, Part III, LNCS 9005, pp. 408–422, 2015.
DOI: 10.1007/978-3-319-16811-1_27

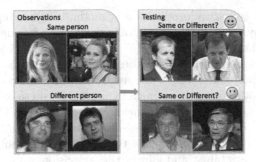

Fig. 1. Illustration of the two key problems in face verification, i.e., the pair of images to be verified contain *large variations* and are captured from *never seen subjects*. Images from the LFW face database [1].

attempt to learn a suitable distance measure that compares pair of examples in spite of large appearance variations existed. For example, in [2] a logistic discriminant approach (LDML) was introduced to learn the metric from a set of labelled face pairs, while [4] propose to use an ensemble of extremely randomized binary trees to quantize the differences between pairs of "same" and "different" images. However, due to the complicated distribution of facial appearance, formulating an appropriate distance function is still very difficult.

Many recent works hence turn to mine domain-specific knowledge or to disentangle various explanatory factors of variation from a large amount of background data [3,5]. One successful approach of this type is the attribute-based method [3], where the domain-specific knowledge is encoded as a bunch of attribute extractors (gender, race, hair color, etc.) which effectively facilitate similarity measuring. This method is extended in [5] by focusing more on automatically detecting such attribute-like features without human labeling. Their idea is based on the observation that the evidence about how two faces are different is much easier to be identified than how they are similar, and therefore, a large number of so-called "Tom-vs-Peter" classifiers are learned from images of two persons, while these training data are collected from the Web according to their identities. This method achieves state-of-the-art results on the challenging LFW face database [5].

However, there are some limitations in [5]. First, although the "Tom-vs-Peter" classifier significantly alleviates the burden of manual labeling of attributes, one does need to know his/her name before collecting his/her face images. Such a supervised way for data collecting would be less practical than an unsupervised one. Second, the collected data tends to be biased towards celebrated people since they are the people who are most likely to have lots of images per person while images from less familiar people might be ignored. Finally, the collected data may become too complex to be properly handled, since each subject may have a large number of images with large variations. Actually, to deal with such variations, a complicated face alignment algorithm has to be adopted to ensure very good correspondence for the "Tom-vs-Peter" classifier.

To address these issues, we propose a new method for face representation that does not require any manual labeling efforts during or after data collection and is less sensitive to the "celebrated people" problem. The key idea of our method is to collect the background data from the Web using the appearance of a query face instead of his/her name, due to the availability of numerous internet image search engines. In other words, we may utilize such "meta-learners" to model the local variability of the face space near each centre. For this we adopt the same method as [5] by constructing decision stumps between two face groups, and each provides us a 'view' about how two faces are different to each other in terms of their local variability, and jointly these decision stumps give a mapping from the image space to a discriminative and distributional representation space.

Another problem in face verification is that the subjects to be verified may be never seen by the system, which means that a fixed pre-trained same person/ different person decision rule may be inappropriate since in this case samples from the test subjects may not be regarded as i.i.d ones with those in the training set any more. To address this issue, in this paper we propose a new strategy that essentially allows the verifier adaptive to the specific test sample. Actually the idea of training test-sample-specific model at the testing phase is not new. One of a successful early attempt in this regard is the SVM-KNN classifier [6], which built a new model for each test sample by finding the training data in the region around it. Another idea is to treat each image in a test couple as a single training example and the other one as a test example (hereafter the SVM trained with only one single positive sample and a large number of negative background samples is called Exemplar-SVM following [7]), and this is adopted in the so called One-Shot Similarity (OSS) method [8].

However, the above strategies somehow cut off the connection between the two images in a couple, and this could prevent the utilization of domain specific knowledge which characterizes how two images can be jointly similar (or dissimilar) to each other. Inspired by this, we treat the test couple as a whole as the single training example, and encode the similarity/dissimilarity relationship contained in the couple with an Exemplar-SVM. As a result, the problem of face verification boils down to decide whether this Exemplar-SVM is in nature client-biased or imposter-biased[1].

To this end, we construct an oracle which gains knowledge from client and imposter pairs of the same generic category (i.e., human face) (see Fig. 4). In implementation, it is just a classifier of classier which learns information from the behaviors of a large number of background Exemplar-SVMs, while the latter are trained respectively using a single client instance or a single imposter instance as the 'Exemplar'. We call our method One-Shot Exemplar-SVM to emphasize the fact that it is used for one shot face verification with never seen persons. Hence our "one shot" is very different from many works which transfer knowledge from

---

[1] Here the terminologies 'client' and 'imposter' are used slightly different from those in the usual face verification context: a client instance means that both images in a couple are from the same person while an imposter instance means they are from different subjects.

related domains to *improve* generalization capability of the model learnt with very few training samples, e.g., Bayesian one shot learning [9].

The paper is organized as follows. Sections 2 and 3 introduces our face representation and the One-shot Exemplar-SVM scheme, respectively. Section 4 shows experimental results. The conclusion is in Sect. 5.

2 Learning Face Representation from the Web

2.1 Approach Overview

As mentioned before our face representation method is partially inspired by the attribute-based representation [3,5], which can be justified in two aspects: on one hand, there is little relationship between each individual attribute and a particular face image, and in this sense an attribute is highly invariant to various appearance variations from pose, illuminations and so on; on the other hand, combining a number of attributes can rapidly shrink the range of possible face images simultaneously satisfying these conditions. Consequently, different attributes provide us an invariant and abstract representation space, whose effectiveness has been witnessed by many recent successful applications in face verification [3] and object recognition [10].

However, among others, there are several challenges in attribute learning. First, attributes are difficult to be defined, in particular for non-experts it is very hard to define a suitable set of attributes for object representation. In addition, even the attribute set are properly defined, the task of checking the presence/absence of each attribute for a particular face is non-trivial, not to mention the additional labeling about the locations where the attribute appears. This labeling procedure involves exhaustive human labors, and can hardly guarantee high labeling quality for accurate attribute learning. Hence it is not surprising that in literatures there are many works which try to bypass these difficulties, for example, using various automatic attribute naming and discovery mechanisms [11], but unfortunately most of them are not designed for face recognition.

In our method, images in each reference set are essentially concrete instances which in all define a high level attribute template. This is possible since each of our reference set is constructed based on the criterion of visual similarity, meaning that the variations contained in the reference set can be somewhat controlled. In this sense the explored similarities can be thought of as special kind of attributes which are not necessary describable with human thesaurus[2], but might cover various types of attributes like the style of the contour of faces, the facial texture, skin color, affection states, and more complicated attributes that can be understood by human visual cognition. It is worthy mentioning that our method enjoys the same advantages as the previous attribute-based methods [3,10] such as high-level visual semantic, sharable for images with different

---

[2] Of course if needed we can still name such template with some complex attribute sentence such as "white middle-aged man with beard", although we do not have to do this considering that our ultimate goal is for classification in this work.

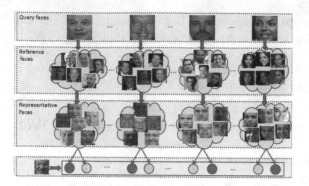

Fig. 2. An overview of the proposed method. A set of reference sets of images are collected from the Web according to their similarity to a query face in appearance. Then some representative images are selected from each of the reference set, serving as the attribute templates for a decision stump. Finally the ensemble of decision stumps maps a given face to its high-level representation.

identities and also description efficiency, and we obtain these cheaply in a pure unsupervised way without any attribute naming and labeling supervision except a query face.

The architecture of the method is shown in Fig. 2. Note that there is a key difference between our method with [5], i.e., we use appearance of the query face to collect the data while [5] uses his/her name. This results in very different reference sets between the two methods.

2.2   The Reference Sets

The reference sets are indexed by its query face and hence it is important to carefully choose diverse and representative face images as queries. To choose these queries, we run K-means (with cosine similarity measure) over the training set of the LFW face database [1] and in each cluster we select the face image that is the most similar to the cluster center as the query. Following this procedure we select 116 query face images among 7701 training images. Note that although these selected query images may appear in the test set of certain training/test set partition, the corresponding labels (information about their identification) are kept unknown to us. This is similar to the strategy adopted in the One-Shot Similarity (OSS) method [8]. All the images in the reference sets undergo the same geometric normalization (detailed in the next section) and are represented using Local Ternary Patterns (LTP) [12] prior to clustering.

Next, to model the local variability of the face space near each centre, we collected 1,000 images for each of the selected 116 faces by searching each face with an image search engine[3]. Note that the search engine we used is appearance based rather than name based. Figure 2 gives some illustration of the resulting

---

[3] We used the Baidu image search engine (http://shitu.baidu.com/) in this work.

images and their corresponding query face. One can see that these images are quite similar to the query face in appearance (such as face contour style, skin color, expression and pose) and if the person to be searched is an ordinary people, the search engine just outputs similar face images from other subjects.

One possible criticism to our method is that since the search engine uses its own notion of locality, our results are likely to be influenced by the quality of the search engine output. To reduce such an effect, in our experiment we use only first 1000 most similar faces and check the results using a face detector and a facial points detector [13]. All those images that either don't contain a face or have large appearance deformations are discarded. Finally we obtained 77,408 images in total, belonging to 116 reference sets with each about 667 images.

2.3   Face Alignment

In [5], the "Tom-vs-Peter" classifier is a local classifier in the sense that each of them works on the corresponding small patches of two faces to detect the evidence that the two faces are different. Hence it is essential to use a carefully designed face alignment mechanism to ensure its performance [5], see also [14]. Considering that the reference sets themselves may not be very coherent at the level of a single local region even after alignment and that there are so many possible combinations of patches with different sizes and locations, we take an alternative method which relies on the global representation of appearance of faces to construct the decision stumps. This means that a relatively simple alignment would be enough (actually the low-level features we adopted are tolerant to the misalignment to some extent, see below).

Specifically, for each image a Viloa and Jones detector is first used to detect the boundary of its face region, then a face region as large as 1.5 times the radius of the detected face is cropped from the original image. Then we run the congealing alignment algorithm [15] over these cropped images for coarse alignment, which helps to reduce the variations in pose and scale. The congealing method is an unsupervised alignment approach which learns a particular affine transformation for each facial image such that the entropy of a group of them is minimized.

To get better global representation of a face, instead of directly cropping the face from the resulting image of congealing, we further fine-tune it with the positions of 9 key facial landmarks (see Fig. 3) estimated using the method of [13]. Based on these landmarks, we first rotate the facial image such that the straight line connecting the centers of two eyes coincides with the horizontal line. Next we should estimate a bounding box for face cropping, which has to be robust enough to tolerate the slight errors in landmark localization. Figure 3 illustrates the measurements we use to calculate the shape parameters which define the bounding box (i.e., its center, width and length).

In particular, to estimate the face width, we first estimate the width of eyes w_{eye} by averaging the width of both eyes (w_1, w_2) and the distance between the two eyes (w_3)(from the left eye corner to the right eye corner) based on

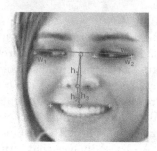

Fig. 3. Illustration of the measurements for face cropping in the final alignment, where the yellow crosses denote the nine facial landmarks estimated by [13] (Color figure online).

the positions of four eye landmarks, i.e., $w_{eye} = (w_1 + w_2 + w_3)/5$, and then empirically estimate the face width as $w_{eye} \times 4.2$.

Similarly, we estimate the face height with the eye-mouth height h_{avg}, which is estimated by averaging the following three measurements: (1) the height between the center of two eyes and nose center (h_1); (2) the height between the nose center and the mouth center (h_2); (3) the height between the center of two eyes and the mouth center (h_3). Then the final face height is empirically estimated as $h_{avg} \times \frac{5}{3}$.

Finally, we assume that the face region is centered at the mean position (indicated by the red circle in Fig. 3) of the nine landmarks.

2.4   Mapping to the Representation

As the final step for our face descriptor, we should construct a series of discriminative decision stumps which jointly map a given face to a sequence of visual bits. The 'visual bits'-type descriptor is very popular in computer vision due to its capability to capture different aspects of the image information in a distributed and compact way.

This can be simply implemented as a binary classifier (decision stump) trained using a low-level feature on images of two different reference set. Not that we use the whole face instead of a local region as the input to the decision stump, as mentioned in Sect. 2.3. For n reference set and k low-level features, we will have $D = k \cdot n(n - 1)/2$ binary classifiers. Here we use linear support vector machines which selects some most representative samples from the reference set and compares them to the test face to make a binary judgement. Denote the i-th decision stump as h_i, one can see that these decision stumps define for a test face x a map which transforms the face to a high-dimensional representation, i.e., $h(x) = (h_1(x), h_2(x), ..., h_D(x)) \in R^D$.

As for low-level features, we use a texture descriptor and a region descriptor which capture the local texture details and local shape information of the face respectively. In particular, for texture information extraction we use the Local Ternary Pattern (LTP) [12], which is a simple generalization of Local Binary Patterns (LBP) with 3-valued codes in discretization of the difference between

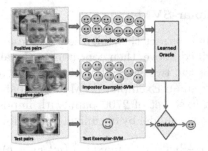

Fig. 4. Overview of the proposed One-Shot Exemplar-SVM method for face verification, where a smiling face icon denotes a client Exemplar-SVM model while an unhappy face icon denotes an imposter Exemplar-SVM. For a test Exemplar-SVM from a pair of test faces with never seen subjects, we want to know which kind of Exemplar-SVM it is, by asking the oracle learnt from the training data.

the central pixel and its surrounding pixels, tackling challenging conditions such as uneven illumination and image noise. While for local shape information we use a variant of Histogram of Oriented Gradients (HOG) [16] called Histogram of Principal Oriented Gradients (HPOG) proposed in [17]. In HPOG the gradient information at each pixel is computed using the eigenvector with the largest eigenvalue of a 2×2 covariance matrix which models the gradient distribution in a neighboring region of that pixel. We expect that such a gradient smoothing operation could help to alleviate the influence of small appearance changes due to image blur, noise, low resolution, etc.

3   One Shot Exemplar-SVM

In this section we give a detailed account on our One-Shot Exemplar-SVM method for face verification with never seen subjects. Figure 4 gives an overview of the proposed method. Here, instead of pre-training one fixed verification model, we allow our model adaptive to the test pair. For this we train an Exemplar-SVM for the test face pair with a held-out set of imposter pairs as negative instances. Note that although the images of the test pair may be either from the same person or from different persons, we always treat it as the single positive instance. As a result, the problem of face verification is transformed into a problem of deciding whether this model is a client model (i.e., trained with a matched pair) or an imposter model (i.e., trained with a unmatched pair). In other words, a problem of comparing two faces becomes now a problem of model comparison. To make the final decision, we use an oracle which is learnt from behaviors of those client/imposter Exemplar-SVMs. The motivation to adopt this strategy is based on the assumption that face verification at the model level could be easier than that at the feature level, since a model can be thought of as the generalization of samples which essentially compensates for the insufficient information of a single instance.

3.1   Learning Exemplar-SVMs

Given a face pair, we first extract their high level representation from each face using the method described above, then concatenate the absolute difference and element-wise product of the two face descriptors as the representation for the pair, following [3]. To train an Exemplar-SVM for the pair, we use it as a single positive instance and a fixed set of 2700 pairs with imposter pairs as negative instances. Then we train the model by optimizing the following convex objective,

$$\min_{w,b} \tfrac{1}{2}||w||^2 + C_1 \max(1 - (w^T x_E + b), 0)$$
$$+ C_2 \sum_{x \in \mathcal{N}_E} \max(1 - (-w^T x - b), 0) \tag{1}$$

where the x_E is the exemplar of face pair and the $\mathcal{N}_E$ is the negative pairs set. C_1 and C_2 are the loss penalty coefficients for positive and negative samples respectively. In our setting, we set $C_1 = 0.5$ and $C_2 = 0.01$ (as did in [7]) for balancing the loss penalty between the two classes. Then we calibrate the output of the exemplar-SVM by fitting them to a sigmoid function on a validation set, which contains 5400 instances with both positive and negative pairs. Then the prediction is calibrated as follows.

$$f(x|w_E, \alpha_E, \beta_E) = 1/(1 + e^{-\alpha_E(w_E^T x - \beta_E)}) \tag{2}$$

where, w_E is the parameter of the learned Exemplar-SVM, α_E and β_E are the Sigmoid parameters.

3.2   Training the Oracle

To train the oracle, we use the Exemplar-SVMs as examples, including 2700 client Exemplar-SVM and 2700 imposter ones. These are trained respectively with 2700 positive pairs and 2700 negative pairs in the training set of the LFW face dataset, with each positive pair as the single positive instance for the client Exemplar-SVM and each negative pair for the imposter Exemplar-SVM. In training both kinds of Exemplar-SVMs we share the same 2700 negative pairs as negative instances. After this we can observe the behavior of a learned Exemplar-SVM on all the 5400 training face pairs by sending each pair into this Exemplar-SVM and concatenating the responses as a 5400-D vector. These response vectors are in turn used for training the oracle, which is a linear SVM in our case. See the top of Fig. 4 for illustration.

3.3   Face Verification Using the Oracle

For a test pair of images, we first train an Exemplar-SVM for it using the same 2700 negative pairs mentioned before, then attach a 5400-D response vector for the obtained model by running it on the 5400 training pairs, which is very efficient (about 0.027 ms per pair on average). We pass this response vector to the oracle to make the same-or-different decision.

4   Experimental Results

In this section, we conduct a series experiments to validate the effectiveness and feasibility of the proposed method on the LFW face database [1], which contains 13233 face images of 5749 people collected from the Web, with large variations in pose, expression and illumination etc. These images are divided into ten folds with each containing 300 matched pairs and 300 unmatched pairs, and the identities between folds are mutually exclusive, which means that the subjects in the test fold will be never seen in the training folds. We follow the "image-restricted" evaluation protocol, in which only a same or different label is assigned to each face pair without any identity information about each face.

In what follows we first evaluate the effectiveness of the proposed method in two aspects, i.e., the face representation and the One-Shot Exemplar-SVM verification method, then we compare our method with other related state-of-the-art methods.

4.1   Effectiveness of Unsupervised Representation Learning

To demonstrate the advantage of the proposed unsupervised representation learning method, we compare its verification performance with that of the several other face descriptors. In particular, following the method of [3], we first construct those descriptors from each single face image, then represent a pair of images by concatenating the absolute difference and element-wise product of the two face descriptors. We use the standard linear SVM trained with the LIB-LINEAR package [18] as the verifier.

- Low-level features: Use the LTP [12] and the HPOG [17] for face description as described in Sect. 2.4
- Attribute-based representation: Directly use the attribute data provided by [3].
- Random Splitting: Replace the query face indexed reference sets with randomly partitioned groups of face images.

Table 1 lists the results. Although directly using our low-level feature for verification looks effective (77.6 %), its performance is much inferior to that of more high-level representation, such as the attribute based representation (84.75 %). However, if we replace the original attribute representation [3] with our representation, the verification improves to 86.7 %. In contrast to [3], our representation is constructed in a completely unsupervised way without any human supervision in terms of attribute labeling.

To further understanding our method, instead of grouping collected images according to query faces, we randomly split those data and use them for decision stumps training. One can see from Table 1 that such a random splitting degrades the performance significantly by over 20.0 %, which indicates the importance of using relative consistent faces for constructing high-level features. As shown in Fig. 2, images in each reference set are similar to each other in many aspects, including the face shape, gender, age and so on, and that's the major reason why

Table 1. Comparison of verification performance of our method with other face representation methods in the restricted setting of LFW [1], using the linear SVM as the verifier.

Method	Accuracy
Low-level features (LTP+HPOG)	0.7764 ± 0.0056
Random splitting	0.6083 ± 0.0083
Attribute-based representation [3]	0.8475 ± 0.0051
Our method	**0.8670** ± 0.0057

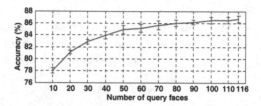

Fig. 5. The influence of the number of query faces on the verification performance in the restricted setting of LFW, using linear SVM as the verifier.

we regard them as sampling from a common (complex and unnamable) attribute template (Fig. 5).

We then investigate the influence of the different number of query faces to the performance. In particular, we conduct a series of experiments by varying the number of reference sets from 10 to 116 with the step as 10 and Fig. 5 gives the results. One can see a general tendency of increasing verification performance with the increasing of the number of reference sets. Specifically, our system reaches the performance of 78.03% with only 10 query faces, and the speed of performance improvement begins to slow down when 80 reference sets are used, with an accuracy of 86.02%, which is nearly comparable to the best performance of 86.7% achieved using 30 more query faces.

4.2 Effectiveness of the One-Shot Exemplar-SVM

To investigate the effectiveness of the proposed One-Shot Exemplar-SVM scheme, we compare it with several closely related verification methods. All these classifiers are based on our face representation method.

- KNN (feature level): Since KNN can also be regarded as a method which adjusts its model according to the test instance, we include it for comparison as well.
- KNN (model level): The same as above, but at the level where each pair is represented as an Exemplar-SVM model and the similarity between two models is measured in the same way as described in Sect. 3.2.

Table 2. Comparison of the verification performance of the proposed method with closely related methods in the restricted setting of LFW, using our face representation method.

Method	Accuracy
KNN (feature level)	0.8083 ± 0.0047
KNN (model level)	0.8442 ± 0.0061
SVM-KNN (feature level)[6]	0.8332 ± 0.0059
SVM-KNN (model level)	0.8392 ± 0.0061
One-Shot Similarity (OSS) [8]	0.8650 ± 0.0042
One-Shot Exemplar-SVM (ours)	$\mathbf{0.8805 \pm 0.0054}$

- SVM-KNN (feature level) [6]: Each time pair of images is verified by a new model trained using K nearest neighbors of the test couple.
- SVM-KNN (model level): A variant of [6] in which the K nearest neighbors are the Exemplar-SVMs on the training set, instead of a pair of images.
- One Shot Similarity (OSS) [8]: This implementation is based on the codes provided by the authors.

Table 2 gives the results. One can see from the table that our One-Shot Exemplar SVM scheme yields the best performance among the compared ones. This is mainly due to its capability to generalize beyond the test samples. Actually for both KNN and SVM-KNN [6], their model level version consistently gives better performance than the corresponding feature level version. The One Shot Similarity Kernel method [8] works better than the SVM-KNN on this dataset, but it models each image in a couple independently, while our method effectively exploits the correlation between the two images in a couple by incorporating them in a single model.

One obvious concern about our Exemplar-SVM is its performance since it is assumed to be a weak classifier trained with only one single positive instance.

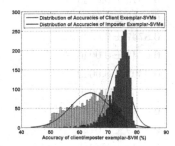

Fig. 6. Histogram of verification accuracy of Exemplar-SVMs over the training data.

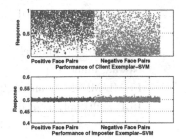

Fig. 7. Illustration of the typical behavior of the client/imposter Exemplar-SVM on labeled face pairs.

Figure 6 gives the histogram of verification accuracy of the trained Exemplar-SVMs over the training data. One can see that the accuracy of client Exemplar-SVMs tends to be distributed in a single mode at 73.3 % with a narrow support ranged from 60.0 % to 80.0 % while that of the imposter Exemplar-SVMs is distributed in a relatively flat way. Such a difference is exploited by the oracle to make a prediction for a new Exemplar-SVM trained on the test pair.

Furthermore, Fig. 7 details the behavior of two typical Exemplar-SVMs (one client and one imposter Exemplar-SVM) over the training face pairs. The figure reveals that the behavior of a client Exemplar-SVM is very different to that of an imposter one. This is reasonable since the imposter Exemplar-SVM trained with an imposter pair serves only as a background model which is almost not sure of anything.

4.3   Comparison with State-of-the-art Methods

We now compare our method with other related state-of-the-art methods on the LFW data set [1]. Table 3 lists the results. Note that each of these published results varies in its feature extraction (the first group in the table) or similarity measuring techniques (the second group), while our methods are most related to those methods in the third group in terms of methodology. It can be seen that our method outperforms most of these methods, and is comparable to [19], but loses about 2.0 % in performance compared to the Tom-Peter Classifier with affine aligned faces [5]. However in the "Tom-vs-Peter" method [5] the identity of each face collected from the Web is known to the model (note that this is a rather strong assumption and thus making it not comparable to ours directly).

Table 3. Comparison of the proposed method with other related state-of-the-art methods on the LFW [1], where the methods marked with '*' means they are evaluated in the image unrestricted setting otherwise in the restricted setting.

Method	Accuracy
LARK supervised, aligned [20]*	0.8510 ± 0.0059
CSML + SVM, aligned [19]	0.8800 ± 0.0037
Fisher vector faces [21]	0.8747 ± 0.0149
SIFT Sub-SML, funneled [22]*	0.8642 ± 0.0046
Nowak, funneled [4]	0.7393 ± 0.0049
LDML-MkNN, funneled [2]*	0.8750 ± 0.0040
LBP multishot, aligned [8]*	0.8517 ± 0.0061
Attribute and Simile classifiers [3]	0.8529 ± 0.0123
Tom-vs-Peter Classifier, **affine aligned** [5]	$0.9047 \pm \text{N/A}$
Tom-vs-Peter Classifier, **full** [5]	$0.9310 \pm \text{N/A}$
One-Shot Exemplar-SVM (ours)	$\mathbf{0.8805} \pm 0.0054$

5   Conclusions

In this paper we propose a new method to deal with two key problems in unconstrained face verification. First, to address the large variation problem, we propose an unsupervised face representation learning method from the Web, with the major advantages of effectiveness and convenience in practice since no supervision is required in terms of the attribute or the identity labeling. Another problem we addressed concerns how to verify pair of images from never seen subjects and we propose the One-shot Exemplar-SVM scheme which is characterized by making the prediction at the model level rather than that at the feature level. Experiments on the challenging LFW database show that our method achieves encouraging verification performance comparable to other related state-of-the-art algorithms. Last but not least, it is worthy mentioning that the best performer on the LFW database has achieved an accuracy as high as 99.15 % [23] based on the deep learning technique. Nevertheless, in our opinion exploring alternative methods like ours to learn feature representation from unsupervised data in a more efficient and more interpretable way is still useful.

Acknowledgement. The authors want to thank the anonymous reviewers for their helpful comments and suggestions. This work was supported by the National Science Foundation of China (61073112, 61035003, 61373060), Jiangsu Science Foundation (BK2012793), Qing Lan Project, Research Fund for the Doctoral Program (RFDP) (20123218110033).

References

1. Huang, G.B., Ramesh, M., Berg, T., Learned-Miller, E.: Labeled faces in the wild: A database for studying face recognition in unconstrained environments. Technical Report 07–49, University of Massachusetts, Amherst (2007)
2. Guillaumin, M., Verbeek, J., Schmid, C.: Is that you? metric learning approaches for face identification. In: ICCV, pp. 498–505 (2009)
3. Kumar, N., Berg, A., Belhumeur, P., Nayar, S.: Describable visual attributes for face verification and image search. PAMI **33**, 1962–1977 (2011)
4. Nowak, E., Jurie, F.: Learning visual similarity measures for comparing never seen objects. In: CVPR (2007)
5. Berg, T., Belhumeur, P.N.: Tom-vs-Pete classifiers and identity-preserving alignment for face verification. In: BMVC, Vol.1, p. 5 (2012)
6. Zhang, H., Berg, A.C., Maire, M., Malik, J.: SVM-KNN: discriminative nearest neighbor classification for visual category recognition. In: CVPR, vol. 2, pp. 2126–2136 (2006)
7. Malisiewicz, T., Gupta, A., Efros, A.A.: Ensemble of Exemplar-SVMs for object detection and beyond. In: ICCV, pp. 89–96 (2011)
8. Wolf, L., Hassner, T., Taigman, Y.: The one-shot similarity kernel. In: CVPR, pp. 897–902 (2009)
9. Fe-Fei, L., Fergus, R., Perona, P.: A Bayesian approach to unsupervised one-shot learning of object categories. In: ICCV, pp. 1134–1141 (2003)

10. Farhadi, A., Endres, I., Hoiem, D., Forsyth, D.: Describing objects by their attributes. In: CVPR (2009)
11. Berg, T.L., Berg, A.C., Shih, J.: Automatic attribute discovery and characterization from noisy web data. In: Daniilidis, K., Maragos, P., Paragios, N. (eds.) ECCV 2010, Part I. LNCS, vol. 6311, pp. 663–676. Springer, Heidelberg (2010)
12. Tan, X., Triggs, B.: Enhanced local texture feature sets for face recognition under difficult lighting conditions. TIP **19**, 1635–1650 (2010)
13. Everingham, M., Sivic, J., Zisserman, A.: "Hello! My name is... Buffy" - automatic naming of characters in TV video. In: BMVC (2006)
14. Peng, Y., Ganesh, A., Wright, J., Xu, W., Ma, Y.: RASL: Robust alignment by sparse and low-rank decomposition for linearly correlated images. IEEE Trans. Pattern Anal. Mach. Intell. **34**, 2233–2246 (2012)
15. Huang, G.B., Jain, V., Learned-Miller, E.: Unsupervised joint alignment of complex images. In: ICCV (2007)
16. Dalal, N., Triggs, B.: Histograms of oriented gradients for human detection. In: CVPR, pp. 886–893 (2005)
17. Song, F., Tan, X., Liu, X., Chen, S.: Eyes closeness detection from still images with multi-scale histograms of principal oriented gradients. Pattern Recognit. **47**, 2825–2838 (2014)
18. Fan, R.E., Chang, K.W., Hsieh, C.J., Wang, X.R., Lin, C.J.: LIBLINEAR: A library for large linear classification. JMLR **9**, 1871–1874 (2008)
19. Nguyen, H.V., Bai, L.: Cosine similarity metric learning for face verification. In: Kimmel, R., Klette, R., Sugimoto, A. (eds.) ACCV 2010, Part II. LNCS, vol. 6493, pp. 709–720. Springer, Heidelberg (2011)
20. Seo, H.J., Milanfar, P.: Face verification using the lark representation. TIFS **6**, 1275–1286 (2011)
21. Simonyan, K., Parkhi, O.M., Vedaldi, A., Zisserman, A.: Fisher vector faces in the wild. In: BMVC (2013)
22. Cao, Q., Ying, Y., Li, P.: Similarity metric learning for face recognition. In: ICCV (2013)
23. Sun, Y., Wang, X., Tang, X.: Deep learning face representation by joint identification-verification. CoRR abs/1406.4773 (2014)

Unsupervised Segmentation of RGB-D Images

Zhuo Deng[✉] and Longin Jan Latecki

Department of Computer and Information Sciences, Temple University,
Philadelphia, USA
{zhuo.deng,latecki}@temple.edu

Abstract. While unsupervised segmentation of RGB images has never led to results comparable to supervised segmentation methods, a surprising message of this paper is that unsupervised image segmentation of RGB-D images yields comparable results to supervised segmentation. We propose an unsupervised segmentation algorithm that is carefully crafted to balance the contribution of color and depth features in RGB-D images. The segmentation problem is then formulated as solving the Maximum Weight Independence Set (MWIS) problem. Given superpixels obtained from different layers of a hierarchical segmentation, the saliency of each superpixel is estimated based on balanced combination of features originating from depth, gray level intensity, and texture information. We want to stress four advantages of our method: (1) Its output is a single scale segmentation into meaningful segments of a RGB-D image; (2) The output segmentation contains large as well as small segments correctly representing the objects located in a given scene; (3) Our method does not need any prior knowledge from ground truth images, as is the case for every supervised image segmentation; (4) The computational time is much less than supervised methods. The experimental results show that our unsupervised segmentation method yields comparable results to the recently proposed, supervised segmentation methods [1,2] on challenging NYU Depth dataset v2.

1 Introduction

Unsupervised Image Segmentation (UIS) is one of the oldest and most widely researched topics in the area of computer vision, of which the goal is to partition an image into several groups of pixels that are visually meaningful using only the information provided by the single image.

In the past few decades, many great accomplishments have been made in this field from the early techniques [4,5], which usually are based on the region splitting or merging framework to more recent works which tend to either integrate global constraints into grouping task, such as intra-region consistency and inter-region dissimilarity [6–9], or formulate segmentation problem under clustering framework [10]. However, unsupervised image segmentation has remained an unsolved problem of computer vision, since RGB color information alone of a single image often does not provide sufficient information to successfully complete this task. There are many reasons for this, e.g., lack of distinctive features

© Springer International Publishing Switzerland 2015
D. Cremers et al. (Eds.): ACCV 2014, Part III, LNCS 9005, pp. 423–435, 2015.
DOI: 10.1007/978-3-319-16811-1_28

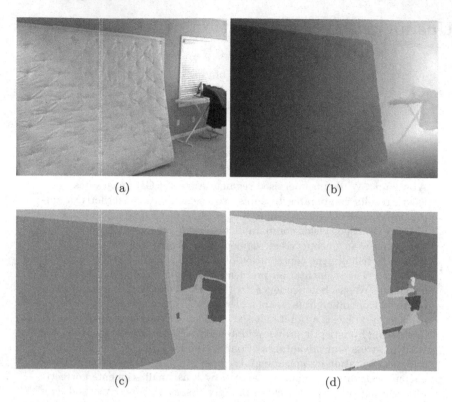

Fig. 1. A typical indoor scene and our segmentation results. (a) Original RGB image obtained from Kinect camera. (b) Depth image, the missing values of which has been filled by the approach in [3]. (c) Ground truth segmentation. (d) Final segmentation result based on the proposed method.

and instability of features due their sensitivity to illumination variation. Generally speaking, UIS is extremely difficult since incorrect segmentations (either too fine or too coarse) can be easily derived, even when employing algorithms that require the user to guess the number of segments.

Recently, with the advent of Microsoft Kinect, the landscape of various vision-related tasks has been changed. Firstly, using an active infrared structured light sensor, the Kinect can provide directly the depth information that is hard to infer from traditional RGB images. Secondly, RGB and depth information are generated synchronously and can be easily aligned, which makes their direct integration possible. A wide range of research works have demonstrated that RGB-D information is useful for improving the performance of vision tasks such as object recognition [11], scene labeling [1], body pose estimation [12], saliency detection [35] etc. The depth information itself is also very helpful for scene geometric structure estimation.

The main goal of this paper is to explore the impact of RGB-D information on improving the unsupervised image segmentation. As we will demonstrate, the improvement is dramatic to the point that for many scenes the segmentation results are comparable to the results of supervised segmentation. Both supervised and unsupervised image segmentation that return a single scale complete image segmentation face the same problem of obtaining image segments correctly representing the scene objects of varying sizes. In particular, segments belonging to a single segmentation result may differ dramatically, some segments may fill nearly the whole image, representing objects like sofas in close view, and some may have area smaller that $1/100$ of the image area. To solve this problem, we formulate the single scale segmentation as finding a maximum weight independent set (MWIS). This way we can automatically partition an RGB-D image into several salient regions with no need to specify either the number or sizes of regions in advance. A representative example is shown in Fig. 1.

The MWIS segmentation has been proposed for RGB images in [9]. It yields good segmentation results when foreground objects are very different from the background, since only then the region saliency measure is able to provide useful segment weights. Due to specific of RGB-D images, our saliency measure is very different and more informative. The main contribution of the proposed approach is a definition of region saliency measure that incorporates both RGB and depth information. As stated above such measure needs to properly balance the color and depth information, since for many objects only one of them is informative.

We test our method on the NYU depth dataset [1] and compare it to supervised hierarchical segmentation approaches in [1,2]. Silberman et al. [1] starts from an over-segmentation, and adapts the algorithm in [13] to iteratively merge regions based on boundary strength. This approach is supervised, since the boundary strength needs to be learned from labeled instances. Similarly, [2] trains oriented contour detectors based on features extracted from watershed over-segmentation contours. Finally, initial over-segmentation regions are merged based on the average strength of oriented contour detectors. Although our method is unsupervised, it obtains comparable results to [1,2]. Moreover, we also compare our approach to an unsupervised segmentation method in [14]. It extends the work of [6] by creating an extra edge on the original graph, of which the weight is measured based on the angle difference of surface normals obtained from depth information. In addition, we also use gpb-owt-ucm as a baseline where depth information is not used. We evaluate the segmentation quality based on five standard measures: Probabilistic Rand Index (PRI) [15], Variation of Information (VI) [16], Global Consistency Error (GCE) [17], Boundary Displacement Error (BDE) [18] and Jaccard Index (JI) [8]. Our approach significantly outperforms [14] in all five measures, which clearly demonstrates the superiority of the proposed combination of color and depth information.

2   Related Works

Image segmentation is a fundamental problem and has been studied extensively. Classic image segmentation approaches include normalized cuts [7], minimum spanning tree [6], meanshift [10], and gPb-OWT-UCM [8]. However, these approaches can only obtain segmentation results comparable to humans if their parameters are known in advance or in other words manually tuned. For example, the normalized cuts requires assigning a specific number of regions at the beginning. Therefore, these algorithms are usually run with different parameter settings, which yields multi-scale image segmentation results. While multi-scale results are very useful for many supervised methods for object detection, scene labeling or image segmentation, it is hard to utilize them to obtain a single segmentation result of an RGB image in unsupervised setting.

One common drawback of these unsupervised segmentation techniques is that they have no prior knowledge about the geometric structure of the scene, which leads to the segmentation to be either too coarse if two spatially separated regions have similar appearance or too fine when one planar region contains subregions with different textures. Although recent approaches that try to infer the 3D structure of the scene given only a single RGB image, e.g., [19–23], they are limited to very simple structures.

The emergence of the RGB-D technology provides a great opportunity to take advantages of merits from both RGB and depth information. Some of the recent works on unsupervised RGB-D segmentation integrate the image segmentation with plane fitting [24,25]. In [24], the RGB-D segmentation is formulated as iterative refinement of the pixel-to-plane assignment and optimized as discrete labeling in a Markov Random Field (MRF), with plane merging controlled by a threshold. Erdogan et al. [25] formulates the plane fitting as a linear least-squares problem and infers the segmentation of the scene in a Bayesian framework. The other unsupervised segmentation works are trying to adapt the classic segmentation algorithms into the RGB-D field. Taylor and Cowley [26] first detects edges on RGB images and computes triangular tessellation of images based on edge information by the Delaunay Triangulation algorithm. Then a variant of N-cut is applied to the graph constructed from the triangular regions. Finally the segments from N-cuts are used to suggest groupings of depth samples from depth image. Taylor and Cowley [27] extends the work in [26] to segment the Manhattan structure of an indoor scene from a single RGB-D frame into floor plane and walls. In contrast to these approaches, our method is not limited to planar structures in the scene. Similar to our work, in [28], image segmentation is formulated as finding high-scoring maximal weighted cliques in a graph connecting non-overlapping putative figure-ground segment hypothesis. In [36], the pylon model is proposed to find a globally optimal subset of segment pool and their labels through graph-cuts and max-margin learning. But both [28,36] are supervised whereas ours is an unsupervised method. Except for unsupervised segmentation, supervised segmentation also benefits from the RGB-D technology. One of the most recent works is [1], where regions with minimum boundary strength are iteratively merged in a hierarchical framework. The boundary is predicted by a trained boosted decision tree classifier based on labeled instances. The other one proposed in [2] utilize depth information to train several oriented contour detectors. Hierarchical segmentation is constructed by merging regions of initial over-segmentation based on the average strength of those oriented contour detectors. Unlike the above works, the proposed approach is completely unsupervised, since it does not require any parameter learning from labeled instances, nor we make any assumptions about the number of regions to be segmented.

3 General Framework

3.1 Hierarchical Image Segmentation

To partition one image into superpixels, there are several excellent algorithms such as the gPb-OWT-UCM method of [8], the minimum spanning tree segmentation [6], the multi-scale normalized cuts [29], mean shift segmentation [10], and watershed based segmentation [30]. In this paper, we adapt the method introduced in [8] to integrate both RGB and depth information for hierarchical segmentation. In [8], firstly an over-segmentation is derived based on the watershed transformation of the gradient map, which is a linear combination of brightness, color, texture gradients and spectral signal. Following the multiple cues combination framework, we integrate depth and normal gradients directly into the final gradient map. Suppose we denote an image as $I(x, y)$, the gradient map $G(x, y)$ is represented as

$$G(x, y) = w_b G_b + w_c G_c + w_d G_d + w_n G_n + w_s G_s, \tag{1}$$

where G_b and G_c are brightness and color gradient signals respectively, which are computed in the CIE-LAB color space. G_d is the gradient signal estimated based on depth image. G_n represents the normal signal where the difference of two normal vectors $\mathbf{n}_i$ and $\mathbf{n}_j$ is measured as

$$Dist(\mathbf{n}_i, \mathbf{n}_j) = sin(acos(\frac{\mathbf{n}_i \bullet \mathbf{n}_j}{|\mathbf{n}_i||\mathbf{n}_j|})), \tag{2}$$

and G_s is the spectral signal. All the gradient signals except for the spectral signal are estimated by convolving a 3×3 sobel kernel with signals themselves. Then an over-segmentation is obtained by applying the watershed transformation to $G(x, y)$. In order to present the hierarchical segmentation, Ultrametric Contour Map (UCM) is used to capture the average strength of shared boundary between two adjacent regions based on $G(x, y)$. For an input RGB-D image, we obtain 7 scales of hierarchical image segmentation by adjusting the strength threshold θ_g on the UCM. We denote with V the set of all superpixels from all scales and from both RGB and D images.

3.2 Saliency Measure of Superpixels

The goal of this section is to compute the saliency measure for each superpixel in V. For RGB-D segmentation, a critical issue is how to integrate depth information with RGB information in order to obtain a weight of each superpixel. Previous works such as [24,31] assign a fixed importance weight to RGB and depth information respectively based on parameter training or empirical setting. However, it is not the case that depth information is more important than RGB information nor vice versa. In reality, when we are trying to identify a salient object from its background, the criteria used always change. For example, based on depth it is easy to separate the surface of a desk from the floor. Whereas, to distinguish a bedsheet from a bed frame, color or texture properties are more helpful. Based on this intuition, we propose a novel weighting scheme to estimate the saliency of superpixels in RGB-D images.

We estimate the saliency by combining three kinds of information: depth, gray level intensity, and textures. Suppose we denote a superpixel as $S_i \in V$ and given depth image $I_d(x,y)$, and RGB image $I_c(x,y)$. We extract gray scale image $I_g(x,y)$ from $I_c(x,y)$. The corresponding saliency measures $C_d(S_i)$, $C_g(S_i)$, $C_t(S_i)$ are defined below. The higher their values, the more uniform is superpixel S_i. We define the saliency of superpixel S_i as their weighted average

$$w(S_i) = W_{area}(w_1 C_d(S_i) + w_2 C_g(S_i) + w_3 C_t(S_i)), \tag{3}$$

where $w_1, w_2, w_3 \geq 0$, $w_1 + w_2 + w_3 = 1$,

$$W_{area} = (1 - \exp(-\eta \frac{|S_i|}{|I(x,y)|}))$$

is used to slightly favor larger regions. The weights w_1, w_2, w_3 are dynamically assigned so that the value of most informative of the three saliency measures $C_d(S_i)$, $C_g(S_i)$, $C_t(S_i)$ has the higher weight. We have three constant values $\alpha > \beta > \gamma > 0$ for the weights and assign the largest value to the largest feature, e.g., if $C_d(S_i) > C_g(S_i) > C_t(S_i)$, then $w_1 = \alpha, w_2 = \beta, w_3 = \gamma$.

Unlike [35] where the relationship between saliency and depth is trained by fitting a GMM, we directly define the confidence from depth information $C_d(S_i)$ as

$$C_d(S_i) = \exp(\frac{-std(\{G_d(p)|p \in S_i\})}{|avg_{p\in S_i}(\{I_d(p)\}) - avg_{p\in S_{ext}^i}(\{I_d(p)\})|}) \tag{4}$$

where $p = (x,y)$ represents a pixel at position (x,y), S_{ext}^i denotes the neighboring area of S_i, and $G_d(x,y)$ represents the gradient map of $I_d(x,y)$. This term encourages the planar region that has high contrast to its surrounding area on the depth value.

The gray scale confidence is defined as

$$C_g(S_i) = \exp(\frac{-std_{p\in S_i}(\{I_g(p)\})}{std_{p\in S_{ext}^i}(\{I_g(p)\})}). \tag{5}$$

The region where pixels have similar intensity value within it and dissimilarity is high with respect to its neighbor area should be assigned a heavier weight.

In order to estimate the weight from the texture perspective, we firstly apply the Maximum Response (MR8) filter bank [32] to the gray scale image $I_g(x,y)$.

MR8 filter bank consists of 38 filters (6 orientations at 3 scales for 2 oriented filters and 2 isotropic filters) and the number of filter responses is reduced to eight. Each pixel of $I_g(x, y)$ is attached with a filter response vector $\mathbf{f}_r$. Then K-means clustering are used to extract k "vector words". Each vector $\mathbf{f}_r$ is assigned an integer label of the "vector word" which is closest. In order to measure the texture saliency, we use the J-measure proposed in [33] that is based on spatial distributions of pixels of similar properties. Suppose there are n_c different labels in S_i, C_i denotes all pixels in S_i with the same quantized label, and N_i is the number of pixels in C_i. The center of C_i is denoted as $m_i = \frac{1}{N_i} \sum_{p \in C_i} p$. We define

$$S_W = \sum_{i=1}^{n_c} \sum_{p \in C_i} ||p - m_i||^2 \tag{6}$$

and observe that S_W is small if there are compact clusters of labels in S_i while it is large if pixels with different labels are uniformly distributed in S_i. We also define the spread of all pixels in S_i as

$$S_T = \sum_{p \in S_i} ||p - m||^2 \tag{7}$$

where m is the central point of S_i. The texture salience is then defined as

$$C_t(S_i) = \exp(\frac{S_W - S_T}{S_W}) \tag{8}$$

If all the pixel labels are distributed uniformly over the entire superpixel area, the value of $C_t(S_i)$ is large. In contrast, it is small if there are compact clusters of labels in S_i.

3.3   Final Segmentation as MWIS

We first construct a graph composed of superpixels $S_i \in V$ as its nodes, where $|V| = n$ We assign to each node $S_i \in V$ a weight $w_i = w(S_i)$ defined in formula (3). We observe that all weights are nonnegative and denote with $\mathbf{w} = [w_1, w_2, ..., w_n]^\top$ the weight vector.

The adjacency matrix M is defined as follows. An edge exists between two superpixels S_i and S_j if they overlap, i.e., $M_{ij} = 0$ if $S_i \cap S_j = \emptyset$ and $M_{ij} = 1$ otherwise. We obtain an undirected graph $G = (V, M, \mathbf{w})$.

In graph theory, an *independent* set is a set of vertices in a graph where no two vertices are adjacent. The *maximal independent set* is an independent set which has the largest number of vertices. In the case we have a weight attached to each vertex, the *maximum weight independent set (MWIS)* is an independent set with the largest sum of the node weights.

An indicator vector, $\mathbf{x} = [x_1, x_2, ..., x_n]^\top \in \{0, 1\}^n$, is used to denote any subset B of the graph nodes, where $x_i = 1$ means node $S_i \in B$ and $x_i = 0$ means node $S_i \notin B$. When B is an independent set and $\mathbf{x}$ its indicator vector, we have $\forall (i, j), x_i \cdot x_j = 0$ if $M_{ij} = 1$. Hence it holds that $\mathbf{x}^\top M \mathbf{x} = 0$. Therefore,

$\mathbf{x}^*$ representing the MWIS can be obtained as the solution of the following quadratically constrained integer linear program

$$\mathbf{x}^* = \underset{\mathbf{x}}{argmax} \ \ \mathbf{w}^\top \mathbf{x}$$
$$s.t. \ \forall i \in V : x_i \in \{0, 1\}, and \ \ \mathbf{x}^\top M \mathbf{x} = 0 \tag{9}$$

We solve the program (9) with the algorithm introduced in [9]. The solution vector $\mathbf{x}^*$ selects superpixels that compose our final single scale segmentation of a given image.

4   Experiments

This section presents both qualitative and quantitative evaluation of our unsupervised segmentation algorithm on 1449 pairs of aligned RGB and depth images from the NYU Depth Dataset V2 [1]. Detailed ground truth segmentation is provided for each image. This data set is very challenging for segmentation, even with RGB-D information, because of poor illumination, often rendering RGB information useless, cluttered non-planar stuff (e.g. bedsheets, sofa, clothes etc.), which strongly limits the depth cues, large variation of scene types, and non-perfect depth measurement. In particular, depth images contain "black holes" due to missing data, and random error of depth measurements increase quadratically with the increasing distance from the sensor [34]. Also the average density of depth measurements decreases when the distance to the objects increases, since the resolution of Kinect is fixed at $480 * 640$.

In order to evaluate our algorithm quantitatively, five standard evaluation measures are employed. The first one is Probabilistic Rand Index (PRI), which estimates the ratio between pairs of pixels, whose labelings are consistent in both ground truth and estimated segmentation, and the total number of pixel pairs. Variation of Information (VI) measures the distance between two segmentations by the average conditional entropy of one segmentation given the other. Global Consistency Error (GCE) measures the extent to which one segmentation can be viewed as a refinement of the other. The Boundary Displacement Error (BDE) measures the average displacement error of boundary pixels between two segmented images. Particularly, it defines the error of one boundary pixel as the distance between the pixel and the closest pixel in the other boundary image. The Jaccard Index (JI) measures similarity between two segmentations, and is defined as the size of the intersection divided by the size of the union of the two segmentations.

We first compare our method to the two baseline UIS methods: in [8], depth information is not used and in [14], normal vector information is applied. For [8], we select the best layer from the hierarchical segmentation based on the five evaluations. As can be seen in Table 1, our method significantly outperforms both of the baseline methods on all five evaluation measures. Surprisingly, the result of [8] is slightly better than [14]. We also compare our approach to two recent RGB-D supervised segmentation methods proposed in [1,2]. Therefore, following the same dataset split setting, training set contains 795 images, and performance is evaluated on 654 test images. Since the algorithm in [1] outputs a hierarchical segmentation composed of five segmentation levels, we choose the best result based on the five standard evaluation measures out of the five levels for each image. Gupta et al. [2] similarly outputs a hierarchical segmentation of 99 segmentation levels. We use the best layer as evaluated in their paper (threshold = 0.54). Although our method is unsupervised, for fair comparison, we also evaluate it on the 654 test images. As can be seen in Table 1, the performance of our method is very close to theirs. This is very surprising for at least three reasons: (1) Our method is unsupervised, while the method in [1,2] are supervised. (2) Our method is much simpler than the methods in [1,2]. (3) Our segmentation result sometimes shows more details than the ground truth, since it is not restricted to known object classes, which incorrectly lowers our accuracy.

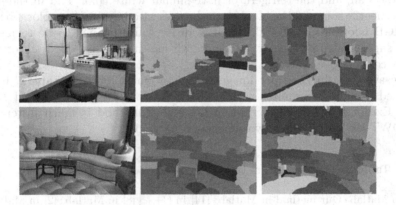

Fig. 2. Two examples to illustrate the benefits of using depth information. The first column contains two original RGB images from Kinect. The second column is the segmentations only based on RGB information. The third column contains the corresponding segmentations based on both RGB and depth information.

In order to visually compare supervised segmentation results [1,2] with our unsupervised segmentation results, we list 8 different samples in the Fig. 3. In varieties of scene categories such as bookstore, living rooms, offices, classrooms and so forth. As can be seen the segmentation of our result is very competitive. Our approach is robust to the variation of illumination, even when scenes are dark (e.g.the scene in the bathroom) or when scenes are extremely bright, e.g., the blinds of the living room in Fig. 1 and the surface of the blackboard in the conference room, or when shades are projected on objects, e.g., the shades on the floor and wall of the bedroom scene. Our approach also works well in very cluttered indoor scenes, like the scenes in the bookstore and the lady's office.

The results in Fig. 2 also demonstrate that depth information is really helpful in our framework for distinguishing objects with similar colors but different locations from each other. As can be seen in the kitchen scene, the surface of the

Table 1. Segmentation accuracy evaluated on 654 test RGB-D images in the NYU Depth Dataset V2 [1], since methods in [1,2] are supervised. The values are: PRI (larger is better), VI (smaller is better), GCE (smaller is better), BDE (smaller is better) and JI (larger is better).

Method	PRI	GCE	VI	BDE	JI
RGB [8]	0.889	0.178	2.253	9.236	0.527
RGBD [14]	0.875	0.298	2.165	11.381	0.488
RGBD [1]	**0.917**	0.122	1.706	**7.509**	0.605
RGBD [2]	0.916	0.162	**1.501**	7.808	**0.622**
Ours RGBD	0.914	**0.120**	1.891	8.488	0.583

table, the wall, and the refrigerator have similar white color, and in the living room scene, the sofa and the blanket on the floor also have similar color. So when only RGB information is used, different objects are inclined to be segmented as one superpixel. However, when the depth information is added, all of them become correctly separated.

The average run time per image segmentation is listed in Table 2. It was evaluated on a PC computer with AMD Eight-core CPU@3.1 HZ and 16 GB RAM. Except for [14] which runs in C++, our method is much faster than GPb-OWT-UCM and other two supervised methods.

Table 2. The average run time in seconds to segment a single image.

[1] in Matlab	Our method in Matlab	[14] in C++	[8] in Matlab	[2] in Matlab
122.1	68.8	7.39	301.1	>300

Parameter Setting: The input to our segmentation are superpixels obtained from hierarchical segmentations. As is mentioned in Sect. 3.1, we obtain segmentations at different levels by changing the value of the strength threshold θ_g which falls between 0 and 1. When θ_g increases, the number of regions segmented is reduced. Experimentally, we find that if the segmentation in each layer is too fine, it may produce many areas that consists of only several pixels. They are not only meaningless but also tend to increase the burden of computation. On the other hand, if the segmentation in each layer is too coarse, it also can not provide good candidate regions. Therefore, we set the θ_g to $[0.05, 0.1, 0.2, 0.3, 0.4, 0.5, 0.6]$. For the weights of different gradient signals, we simply set them as $w_b = 1.0$, $w_c = 0.5$, $w_n = 3.0$, $w_d = 2.0$ and $w_s = 3.0$ since depth information and global spectral signal are much more reliable than brightness and color. In addition, we set constants α, β, and γ to 0.5, 0.3, 0.2 respectively. The constant η is set to 10 in our experiment.

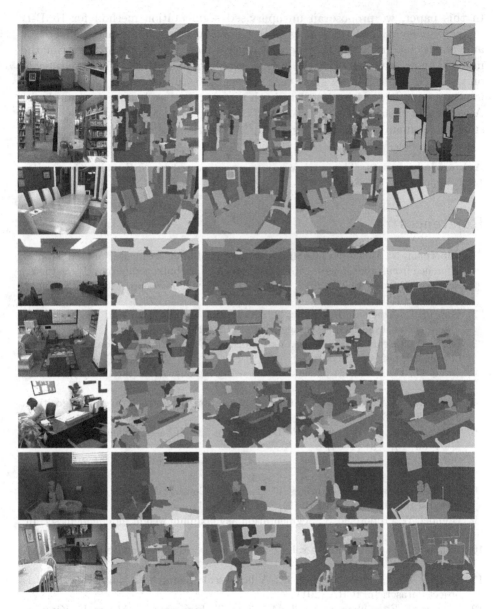

Fig. 3. Examples of unsupervised indoor scene segmentation obtained by our method and supervised methods in [1,2]. Column 1 shows the original RGB images. Column 2 shows results in [1]. Column 3 shows results in [2]. Column 4 shows our segmentations and last column shows the ground truth.

5   Conclusion

In this paper, we propose an unsupervised segmentation method for RGB-D image segmentation. It integrates both color and depth information effectively and partitions one RGB-D image into several most salient regions without the need to know the number or the size of segments in advance. Our experiments on the NYC depth dataset show that the segmentation accuracy of our method is very competitive with respect to both unsupervised and supervised methods. Also the fact that our method is very efficient due to its simplicity, makes it very suitable for many applications from object to action recognition.

Acknowledgements. This work was in part supported by NSF under Grants IIS-1302164 and OIA-1027897.

References

1. Silberman, N., Hoiem, D., Kohli, P., Fergus, R.: Indoor segmentation and support inference from rgbd images. In: Fitzgibbon, A., Lazebnik, S., Perona, P., Sato, Y., Schmid, C. (eds.) ECCV 2012, Part V. LNCS, vol. 7576, pp. 746–760. Springer, Heidelberg (2012)
2. Gupta, S., Arbelaez, P., Malik, J.: Perceptual organization and recognition of indoor scenes from RGB-D images. In: CVPR (2013)
3. Levin, A., Lischinski, D., Weiss, Y.: Colorization using optimization. ACM Trans. Graph. **23**, 689–694 (2004)
4. Brice, C., Fennema, C.: Scene analysis using regions. Artif. Intell. **1**(3), 205–226 (1970)
5. Horowitz, S., Pavlidis, T.: Picture segmentation by a tree traversal algorithm. JACM **23**, 368–388 (1976)
6. Felzenszwalb, P., Huttenlocher, D.: Efficient graph-based image segmentation. IJCV **59**, 167–181 (2004)
7. Shi, J., Malik, J.: Normalized cuts and image segmentation. PAMI **22**, 888–905 (2000)
8. Arbelaez, P., Maire, M., Fowlkes, C., Malik, J.: Contour detection and hierarchical image segmentation. PAMI **33**(5), 898–916 (2011)
9. Brendel, W., Todorovic, S.: Segmentation as maximum weight independent set. In: NIPS (2010)
10. Comaniciu, D.: Mean shift: a robust approach toward feature space analysis. PAMI **24**(5), 603–619 (2002)
11. Lai, K., Bo, L., Ren, X., Fox, D.: A large-scale hierarchical multi-view RGB-D object dataset. In: ICRA (2011)
12. Shotton, J., Fitzgibbon, A., Cook, M., Sharp, T., Finocchio, M., Moore, R., Kipman, A., Blake, A.: Real-time human pose recognition in parts from single depth images. In: CVPR (2011)
13. Hoiem, D., Efros, A., Hebert, M.: Recovering occlusion boundaries from an image. IJCV **91**(3), 328–346 (2011)
14. Strom, J., Richardson, A., Olson, E.: Graph-based segmentation for colored 3d laser point clouds. In: IROS (2010)

15. Unnikrishnan, R., Pantofaru, C., Hebert, M.: A measure for objective evaluation of image segmentation algorithms. In: CVPRW (2005)
16. Meila, M.: Comparing clusterings by the variation of information. In: Schölkopf, B., Warmuth, M.K. (eds.) Learning Theory and Kernel Machines. LNCS, vol. 2777, pp. 173–187. Springer, Heidelberg (2003)
17. Martin, D., Fowlkes, C., Tal, D., Malik, J.: A database of human segmented natural images and its application to evaluating segmentation algorithms and measuring ecological statistics. In: ICCV (2001)
18. Freixenet, J., Muñoz, X., Raba, D., Martí, J., Cufí, X.: Yet another survey on image segmentation: region and boundary information integration. In: Heyden, A., Sparr, G., Nielsen, M., Johansen, P. (eds.) ECCV 2002, Part III. LNCS, vol. 2352, pp. 408–422. Springer, Heidelberg (2002)
19. Hoiem, D., Efros, A., Hebert, M.: Geometric context from a single image. In: ICCV (2005)
20. Hedau, V., Hoiem, D., Forsyth, D.: Recovering the spatial layout of cluttered rooms. In: ICCV (2009)
21. Hedau, V., Hoiem, D., Forsyth, D.: Thinking inside the box: using appearance models and context based on room geometry. In: Daniilidis, K., Maragos, P., Paragios, N. (eds.) ECCV 2010, Part VI. LNCS, vol. 6316, pp. 224–237. Springer, Heidelberg (2010)
22. Lee, D., Hebert, M., Kanade, T.: Geometric reasoning for single image structure recovery. In: CVPR (2009)
23. Lee, D., Gupta, A., Hebert, M., Kanade, T.: Estimating spatial layout of rooms using volumetric reasoning about objects and surfaces. In: NIPS (2010)
24. Guan, L., Yu, T., Tu, P., Lim, S.: Simultaneous image segmentation and 3D plane fitting for RGB-D sensors - an iterative framework. In: CVPRW (2012)
25. Erdogan, C., Paluri, M., Dellaert, F.: Planar segmentation of RGBD images using fast linear fitting and Markov chain monte carlo. In: CRV (2012)
26. Taylor, C., Cowley, A.: Segmentation and analysis of RGB-D data. In: RSS (2011)
27. Taylor, C.J., Cowley, A.: Parsing indoor scenes using RGB-D imagery. In: Robotics (2013)
28. Ion, A., Carreira, J., Sminchisescu, C.: Image segmentation by figure-ground composition into maximal cliques. In: ICCV (2011)
29. Cour, T., Benezit, F., Shi, J.: Spectral segmentation with multiscale graph decomposition. In: CVPR (2005)
30. Meyer, F.: Color image segmentation. In: Image Processing and its Applications (1992)
31. Ren, X., Bo, L., Fox, D.: RGB-(D) scene labeling: features and algorithms. In: CVPR (2012)
32. Varma, M., Zisserman, A.: A statistical approach to texture classification from single images. IJCV 62(2), 61–81 (2005)
33. Deng, Y., Manjunath, B., Shin, H.: Color image segmentation. In: CVPR (1999)
34. Khoshelham, K.: Accuracy analysis of kinect depth data. In: ISPRS Workshop (2011)
35. Lang, C., Nguyen, T.V., Katti, H., Yadati, K., Kankanhalli, M., Yan, S.: Depth matters: influence of depth cues on visual saliency. In: Fitzgibbon, A., Lazebnik, S., Perona, P., Sato, Y., Schmid, C. (eds.) ECCV 2012, Part II. LNCS, vol. 7573, pp. 101–115. Springer, Heidelberg (2012)
36. Lempitsky, V., Vedaldi, A., Zisserman, A.: Pylon model for semantic segmentation. In: NIPS (2011)

Class-Driven Color Transformation
for Semantic Labeling

Arash Shahriari[1,2]([✉]), Jose M. Alvarez[1,2], and Antonio Robles-Kelly[1,2]

[1] Research School of Engineering, Australian National University,
Action, ACT 2601, Australia
[2] NICTA, Locked Bag 8001, Canberra, ACT 2601, Australia
arash.shahriari@nicta.com.au

Abstract. We propose a novel class-driven color transformation aimed at semantic labeling. In contrast with other approaches elsewhere in the literature, our approach is a supervised one employing class information to learn a color transformation. Our method maps image color to a target space with maximum pairwise distances between classes and minimum scattering within each of them. To compute the color transformation, we pose the problem in terms of a composition of two mappings. The first mapping employs a pairwise discriminant cost function minimized through a steepest descent optimization to map the image color data onto a space spanned by the class set. It targets better separability between distinct classes as well as less scattering within each individual class. The second mapping corresponds to subspace projection of this class data to a target space with same dimensionality of image color data. To preserve distances attained by the first of the mappings, this subspace projection is effected making use of metric multi-dimensional scaling. We report our experiments on MSRC-21 and SBD datasets, where our method consistently improves overall and average performances of well-known publicly available TextonBoost and DARWIN multiclass segmentation frameworks at a negligible computational cost. These results confirms our contribution towards reflection of higher distinction in color space by imposing better separability in a novel representation which is learned from class information of the dataset under consideration.

1 Introduction

Color has been used as a cue for numerous tasks in computer vision [1]. Due to its importance, a number of color spaces and descriptors have been formulated to address problems spanning from accurate capture and reproduction of images acquired by digital camera sensors [2] to scene and object recognition [1].

Color, as perceived by the observer, is the result of interactions between light sources, material reflectance, surface texture and other photometric effects due

National ICT Australia (NICTA) is funded by the Australian Government as represented by the Department of Broadband, Communications and the Digital Economy and the Australian Research Council through the ICT Center of Excellence program.

D. Cremers et al. (Eds.): ACCV 2014, Part III, LNCS 9005, pp. 436–451, 2015.
DOI: 10.1007/978-3-319-16811-1_29

to object shape and shadows. Photometric invariance is often achieved by use of surface reflectance as a means toward classification and recognition via a descriptor which is robust to changes in illumination, noise, geometric and photometric effects. For instance, Nayar *et al.* [3] proposed a method of object recognition based on the reflectance ratio between object regions. Dror *et al.* [4] described a vision system that learned the relationship between surface reflectance and certain statistics computed from gray-scale images. Slater *et al.* [5] used a set of Gaussian filters to derive moment invariants for recognition. Jacobs *et al.* [6] employed image ratios for comparing images under variable illumination. Lin *et al.* [7] utilized an eigen-space of chromaticity distributions to obtain illumination direction and color and specularity-invariants for three-dimensional object recognition. Lenz *et al.* [8] deployed perspective projections in canonical space of color signals to separate intensity from chromaticity and recover a three-dimensional color descriptor.

The performance of a number of computer vision methods not only depends on color descriptor used but also space or gamut in which they are defined [9]. This is why the color in an image may be adjusted and adapted using a suitable transformation [10]. The selection of an optimal transformation is not straightforward since, different color spaces may be better adapted to handle textures or complex shapes [11]. For segmentation, the CIE, LUV or Lab spaces [12] are often employed as they map each RGB pixel value in image to a point in color space for which the pairwise deviation in perceived color is equal to Euclidean distance in feature space [13].

Here, we note that color transformations found elsewhere in the literature are often derived by perceptual criteria rather by image information. Thus, we propose a novel approach to find a color transformation for semantic labeling based on class information of image dataset for the application at hand. This transformation is computed via supervised learning from dataset and could be employed as a general preprocessing before feature extraction step in standard pipeline of pixel-wise classifiers.

The core idea is to map primary color space *i.e.* RGB, to a new representation of the same dimensionality *i.e.* target space with maximum class separation. To this end, we decompose the problem into the recovery of two mappings. The former concerns mapping of the primary color space to a class space spanned by the classes in the dataset and the latter corresponds to subspace projection from the class space to above target space. Our proposal in essence follows the practice of many successful learning schemes, where a combination of two mappings could unravel desired structure of data. While our formulation for both mappings is inspired by well-known machine learning techniques, combination in this context is a novel contribution. Moreover, our choice of color space, provides fair comparisons with state-of-the-art which use color features in their experiments. It also achieves a low-cost machinery that could process large amount of images in mobile platforms.

For the mapping of the primary color to the class space, we employ a method akin to the pairwise discriminant analysis developed by Fu and Robles-Kelly [14].

Note that here, the aim is to map the color channels to a higher-dimensional space spanned by the class set using an approach devoid of matrix inversions, whereas the method in [14] is a subspace projection method. This also contrasts with approaches such as Linear Discriminant Analysis (LDA) [15], where class-specific covariance is used to define within-class scattering while between-class scatter is considered to be uniform for distinct classes. The lack of between-class scatter specificity [16] is compounded by the burden of dimensionality. To deal with high-dimensional data, a number of approaches have been proposed. These include independence rule [17], feature annealed independence rule [18] and nearest shrunken centroid classifier [19]. Nonetheless, these methods may still be potentially unstable due to matrix inversions.

As mentioned earlier, the subspace projection is tackled using metric Multi-dimensional Scaling (MDS) to preserve the distances achieved by the first of our mappings. Given a highly distinct color representation, it is feasible to utilize any sophisticated feature sets in classification process. For instance, in our experiments, TextonBoost [20] uses color, histogram of oriented gradients (HOG), and pixel location features and DARWIN [21] employs RGB color of the pixel, dense HOG, LBP-like features, and averages over image rows and columns. We validate our class-driven color transformation by applying it as a general preprocessing step of semantic labeling process. Experiments conducted on MSRC-21 [22] and Stanford Background Dataset (SBD) [23] for semantic segmentation shows that our color transformation consistently improves the overall and average precisions of both TextonBoost and DARWIN pixel-wise segmentation algorithms at the cost of a simple matrix multiplication.

The rest of paper is organized as follows. In the next section, we expose our color transformation method. In Sect. 3, we discuss the implementation of our algorithm and its initialization. Finally, in Sects. 4 and 5, we report experiments and then conclude on the work presented here respectively.

2   Class-Driven Color Transformation

To commence, let us define the generic color transformation problem as treated in this paper. Given the M image color pixels $\mathcal{X} = \{x_1, x_2, \ldots, x_M\}$ labeled into N distinct classes $\mathcal{L} = \{C_1, C_2, \ldots, C_N\}$, our goal is to recover a matrix $A \in \mathcal{R}^{3 \times 3}$ that transforms input color pixels x_i onto a 3-dimensional vector z_i in the target space such that $z_i = Ax_i$ maximizes the separation between color pixels in distinct classes and minimizes the scattering in each individual class.

Posed in this way, we formulate the problem as an optimization one where objective function depends on both, dimensions of the target space and number of classes in the dataset under consideration. As a result, we decompose the matrix A as follows

$$A = BC \tag{1}$$

where $C \in \mathcal{R}^{N \times 3}$ is a mapping matrix that transforms the input color space to the N-dimensional class space, spanned by classes in the dataset and $B \in \mathcal{R}^{3 \times N}$ is another mapping that projects the class space onto the output target space.

With above decomposition, we can introduce our objective function as a composition of the form

$$\arg \min_{\mathbf{A}=\mathbf{BC}} f(\mathbf{A}) = h(\mathbf{B}) \circ p(\mathbf{C}) \tag{2}$$

where both $h(\cdot)$ and $p(\cdot)$ are cost functions that take the matrices $\mathbf{B}$ and $\mathbf{C}$ as their arguments.

It is worth discussing implications of the formulation above. Note that Eqs. 1 and 2 are a direct consequence of properties known for decomposition of matrices and composition of functions, where the functions $p(\cdot)$ and $h(\cdot)$ have been composed into objective $f(\mathbf{A})$. Moreover, if $p(\cdot)$ is convex, the optimization in Eq. (1) can be affected by recovering the matrix $\mathbf{C}$ to later optimizing $h(\cdot)$ with respect to $\mathbf{B}$ [24]. The minimization of the cost function $h(\mathbf{B})$ can then be treated in a manner akin to that used by linear feature extraction methods such as LDA or Maximum Margin Criterion (MMC) [25] which are often employed for utilizing label information to learn a linear transformation for classification. Indeed, since the matrix $\mathbf{B}$ is effectively a subspace projection matrix that maps the class space onto the target space, such methods may be used to optimize Eq. (1) in case the matrix $\mathbf{C}$ is at hand.

Further, by minimizing $p(\mathbf{C})$ and $h(\mathbf{B})$ in consecutive steps and choosing cost functions which are convex, $f(\mathbf{A})$ can be shown to be also convex [24]. This follows from the composition of a convex function with a non-increasing one and it is valid since $p(\mathbf{C})$ does not increase once minimized. Our goal of minimizing $h(\mathbf{B})$ is to preserve the class distinctions induced by minimizing $p(\mathbf{C})$ while projecting from the class space to the target space. Our inference on not increasing $p(\mathbf{C})$ comes from the fact that $h(\mathbf{B})$ just tries to fix the class distances resulted by $p(\mathbf{C})$ and hence, we consider minimization of $h(\mathbf{B})$ as an independent optimization while $p(\mathbf{C})$ has been minimized.

Thus, in Sect. 2.1 we turn our attention to mapping the color space to the class space using a convex cost function and later on, in Sect. 2.2, we elaborate on subspace projection of the class space to the target space.

2.1 Mapping of Color Space to Class Space

In order to map color values to the space spanned by classes in the dataset under consideration, we learn the relevant mapping by using a cost function which accumulates the combination of costs for pairs of binary classes. This is consistent with the notion that any multiclass classification problem can be converted to a number of binary ones by deploying a pairwise fusion framework [26]. This can also be viewed as a process akin to training of a classifier for every two classes and making final prediction based on the combination of decisions yielded by binary classifiers. Moreover, the matrix $\mathbf{C}$ can then be interpreted as a mapping of image color values onto the N-dimensional class space.

Objective Function. We view recovery of $\mathbf{C}$ as the optimization of function $p(\mathbf{C})$ such that pairwise cluster distances are maximized. As a result, we opt for objective function presented in [14], given by

$$\arg\min_{\mathbf{C}^T\mathbf{C}=\mathbf{I}} p(\mathbf{C}) = \sum_{i=1}^{N-1} \sum_{j=i+1}^{N} \beta_{i,j} g\left(\Phi_{i,j}(\mathbf{C})\right) \tag{3}$$

where $\Phi_{i,j}(C)$ is a class-pair dependent distance function, $\beta_{i,j}$ is a weight that moderates contribution of the class pair i, j to the objective function and

$$g(\Phi_{i,j}(\mathbf{C})) = \frac{1}{1 + \exp(\gamma(\Phi_{i,j}(\mathbf{C}) - \tau))} \tag{4}$$

is a logistic regression function with parameters γ and τ which maps class separability to pairwise costs. Importantly, $g(\cdot)$ takes values in the range $(-\infty, \infty)$ to bounded interval $[0, 1]$. This choice also implies that the function is monotonically decreasing to assign lower costs to increasing class separability values.

It is consistent with the notion that the optimization problem at hand should be solved such that the matrix $\mathbf{C}$ maximizes the costs, *i.e.* separability, for every pair of classes. The target function in Eq. (4) hence aims at maximizing these costs in a cumulative fashion. This equation also reflects the fact that, to derive final target function, we require a criterion to measure separability between two classes in the class space.

Indeed, the choice here is not unique. A straightforward way would be to use the same objective function as in [16] with different definitions for intra and inter-class scatter matrices on every pair of classes. However, it involves a matrix inversion operation for each pairwise within-class scatter matrix. This is undesirable since it can incur in numerical instability when small training sets are available for any of the classes or categories under consideration. Another way would be to assume an underlying Gaussian distribution for each of the above classes and employ information theoretic divergence measures, such as Kullback-Leibler divergence or Bhattacharyya distance with closed form solutions. Unfortunately, this would still require matrix inversion operations and hence may be unstable for applications with small training sets.

In this paper, we follow [14] and employ the distance between class centroids in the color space such that

$$\Phi_{i,j}(\mathbf{C}) = d_{i,j}^{(1)} - d_{i,j}^{(2)} - d_{i,j}^{(3)} \tag{5}$$

where $d_{i,j}^{(1)}$ is the distance between centroids subtracted by $d_{i,j}^{(2)}$ and $d_{i,j}^{(3)}$ which are projections of color scatterings for classes, along direction $\mathbf{C}^T \mu_{i,j}$ given by

$$d_{i,j}^{(1)} = ||\mathbf{C}^T \mu_{i,j}||$$

$$d_{i,j}^{(2)} = \frac{\sqrt{\mu_{i,j}^T \mathbf{C}\mathbf{C}^T \mathbf{S}_i \mathbf{C}\mathbf{C}^T \mu_{i,j}}}{||\mathbf{C}^T \mu_{i,j}||}$$

$$d_{i,j}^{(3)} = \frac{\sqrt{\mu_{i,j}^T \mathbf{C}\mathbf{C}^T \mathbf{S}_j \mathbf{C}\mathbf{C}^T \mu_{i,j}}}{||\mathbf{C}^T \mu_{i,j}||} \tag{6}$$

Here, μ_i and $\mathbf{S_i}$ are the mean and scatter for the ith class of pixels in the color space and $\mu_{i,j}$ is defined as $\mu_i - \mu_j$.

Note that, we made no assumptions or constraints on standard/spherical cluster distances in our formulation. Both metrics are employed to define class-pair distance in Eq. (5) via aggregation of radial distances between centroids and angular projections of color value scatters in Eq. (6) which latter may create elliptical clusters.

Steepest Descent Optimization. At first glance, Eq. (3) appears to be a hard optimization problem. Surprisingly, it can be optimized using steepest descent optimization since it is defined on a Grassmann manifold [27]. In addition to unitary constraint, as a consequence of developments in [27], it can be shown that the objective function is invariant to any rotations in transformed feature space. It also assures that the objective function is a convex one. Thus, by building on recent advances in optimization theory, we can extend unconstrained optimization methods in Euclidean space to Grassmann manifold. Here, we use a projection-based steepest descent with backtracking line search based on [28].

The objective function above can be optimized using a steepest descent method whereby at iteration t the matrix $\mathbf{C}$ can be updated using the rule

$$\mathbf{C}^{(t+1)} = \mathbf{C}^{(t)} + \lambda \Delta \mathbf{C}^{(t)} \tag{7}$$

where λ is a step-size variable and the descent direction is given by

$$\Delta \mathbf{C}^{(t)} = -(\mathbf{I} - \mathbf{C}^{(t)T}\mathbf{C}^{(t)})\nabla_{\mathbf{C}}p(\mathbf{C}^{(t)}) \tag{8}$$

One of the main benefits of this steepest descent approach is that, in contrast to traditional subspace projection methods, the optimization of $p(\cdot)$ can be effected without any need for matrix inversions. Moreover, note that the function $\Phi_{i,j}(\mathbf{C})$ is not a metric in the sense that it can be negative. Nonetheless, this is not a problem as we are not using it directly for optimization purpose, rather it is treated as a variable in the objective function.

To appreciate this more clearly, we proceed to compute gradient of the function $p(\cdot)$ *i.e.* $\nabla_{\mathbf{C}}p(\mathbf{C})$ as gradient of the cost function $g(\cdot)$ in Eq. (3) with respect to $\mathbf{C}$. It can be expressed in closed form as follows

$$\nabla_{\mathbf{C}}p(\mathbf{C}) = -\sum_i \sum_j \gamma \beta_{i,j}(\Phi_{i,j}(\mathbf{C}) - \tau)g^2(\Phi_{i,j}(\mathbf{C}))\nabla_{\mathbf{C}}\Phi_{i,j} \tag{9}$$

where

$$\nabla_{\mathbf{C}}\Phi_{i,j}(\mathbf{C}) = \nabla_{\mathbf{C}}d_{i,j}^{(1)} - \frac{(\Gamma_i + \Gamma_j)\nabla_{\mathbf{C}}d_{i,j}^{(1)}}{d_{i,j}^{(1)^2}} - \frac{d_{i,j}^{(1)}(\nabla_{\mathbf{C}}\Gamma_i + \nabla_{\mathbf{C}}\Gamma_j)}{d_{i,j}^{(1)^2}}$$

$$\nabla_{\mathbf{C}}d_{i,j}^{(1)} = \frac{1}{d_{i,j}^{(1)}}\mu_{i,j}\mu_{i,j}^T\mathbf{C}$$

$$\nabla_{\mathbf{C}}\Gamma_i = \frac{2}{\Gamma_i}sym(\mu_{i,j}\mu_{i,j}^T\mathbf{C}\mathbf{C}^T\mathbf{S}_i)\mathbf{C}$$

$$\nabla_{\mathbf{C}}\Gamma_j = \frac{2}{\Gamma_j}sym(\mu_{i,j}\mu_{i,j}^T\mathbf{C}\mathbf{C}^T\mathbf{S}_j)\mathbf{C} \tag{10}$$

and $sym(\boldsymbol{\Theta}) = \dfrac{\boldsymbol{\Theta} + \boldsymbol{\Theta}^T}{2}$ denotes a symmetry inducing operator for matrix $\boldsymbol{\Theta}$. In the equations above, we used the shorthand $\Gamma_i = \sqrt{\mu_{i,j}^T \mathbf{C}\mathbf{C}^T \mathbf{S}_i \mathbf{C}\mathbf{C}^T \mu_{i,j}}$.

2.2   Subspace Projection of Class Space to Target Space

Once the matrix $\mathbf{C}$ is at hand, we focus our attention on recovery of the matrix $\mathbf{B}$. As mentioned earlier, this can be viewed as a subspace projection matrix which maps the class space onto the target space. This potentially allows for any convex subspace projection method to be employed for computing $\mathbf{B}$. Moreover, literature on multi-dimensional scaling and subspace projection is vast.

Here, we aim at preserving pairwise cluster distances derived from the learned matrix $\mathbf{C}$. This naturally leads to application of linear and non-linear embedding techniques for dimensionality reduction that attempt to preserve global or local properties of original data in low-dimensional representations. Here, we use metric Multi-dimensional Scaling (MDS) due to both, its capacity to preserve pairwise distances in the class space and the fact that, it is a natural generalization of classical approaches elsewhere in the literature. Moreover, metric MDS can employ a wide variety of loss functions. We employ the stress function to measure the error between the pairwise distances in the high-dimensional class space and the low-dimensional target space. Thus, the cost function $h(\mathbf{B})$ becomes

$$h(\mathbf{B}) = - \sum_{\mathbf{x}_i \in \mathcal{X}} (\|\mathbf{y}_i - \mathbf{y}_j\|^2 - \|\mathbf{B}(\mathbf{y}_i - \mathbf{y}_j)\|^2)^2 \qquad (11)$$

where $\| \cdot \|$ is vector norm and we have used shorthand $\mathbf{y}_i = \mathbf{C}\mathbf{x}_i$ to denote instances in the class space corresponding to the pixel color value $\mathbf{x}_i \in \mathcal{X}$. Note that, in the stress function above, the term $\|\mathbf{B}(\mathbf{y}_i - \mathbf{y}_j)\|$ is effectively the Euclidean distance in the target space whereas $\|\mathbf{y}_i - \mathbf{y}_j\|$ is the corresponding Euclidean distance in the class space.

As a result of the approach taken in previous section, the separation between pixel pairs belonging to different classes is maximized by $\mathbf{C}$ and hence, the matrix $\mathbf{B}$ is expected to preserve these distances. Moreover, the minimization of $h(\mathbf{B})$ can be performed using various methods such as eigen-decomposition or pseudo-Newton minimization or conjugate gradient which we employed.

3   Implementation

Following the previous sections, the training step of our algorithm becomes

1. Compute an initial estimate of matrix $\mathbf{C}$ *i.e.* $\mathbf{C}^{(0)}$.
2. Apply steepest descent of Sect. 2.1 to optimize the cost function $p(\mathbf{C})$.
3. Once $\mathbf{C}$ is at hand, compute $\mathbf{y}_i = \mathbf{C}\mathbf{x}_i$ for all $\mathbf{x}_i \in \mathcal{X}$.
4. Recover matrix $\mathbf{B}$ using MDS to compute $\mathbf{z}_i = \mathbf{B}\mathbf{y}_i$ for all $\mathbf{y}_i \in \mathcal{Y}$.
5. Train classifier of choice by the transformed training color values $\mathbf{z}_i = \mathbf{A}\mathbf{x}_i$.

whereas for a testing RGB pixel value $\mathbf{x}_i^*$ the step sequence is as follows

1. Compute $\mathbf{z}_i^* = \mathbf{A}\mathbf{x}_i^*$.
2. Feed the transformed testing color value $\mathbf{z}_i^*$ to the classifier.

In the training step sequence above, we commence by computing an initial estimate of $\mathbf{C}$ by employing Fisher's class separability criterion and properties of the matrix span. The reason for our choice hinges in both, the vast amount of work that shows effectiveness of Fisher's criterion for purposes of maximizing class separability and its ease of computation. It is worth noting that Fisher's criterion has been used extensively in LDA.

The literature on LDA is extensive, dwelling into a wide variety of variants of the method itself. For instance, Non-parametric Discriminant Analysis (NDA) incorporates boundary information into between-class scatter. Boudat *et al.* [29] have proposed a kernel version of LDA that can cope with severe non-linearity of sample set. On the numerical stability and tractability of LDA, there are also a number of methods which aim at overcoming singularity of the inverse intra-class covariance matrix inherent to sub-sampled feature spaces. In a related development, MMC employs an optimization procedure whose constraint is not dependent on the non-singularity of within-class scatter matrix. Here, we use the method of Wang *et al.* [30] which employs dual subspaces to construct LDA classifiers.

To employ Fisher's criterion, we construct the matrix $\mathbf{D}$. Making use of notation introduced in Sect. 2.1, we can define entry indexed i, j of the matrix $\mathbf{D}$ as follows

$$D_{i,j} = \frac{||\mu_{i,j}||}{||\mu_{i,j}(\mathbf{S}_i - \mathbf{S}_j)||} \tag{12}$$

which is the distance between class centroids over the projected scatters.

With the matrix $\mathbf{D}$ at hand, we employ its QR decomposition and developments to compute $\mathbf{C}^{(0)}$ by using subspace spanned by the first three columns of $\mathbf{Q}$, *i.e.* $\lfloor \mathbf{C}^{(0)} \rfloor$ as the best second order approximation to $\mathbf{C}^{(0)}$. Being more formal, given $\rho(\mathbf{C}^{(0)}) = \lfloor \mathbf{J}[\mathbf{I} \mid \mathbf{0}]^T \rfloor$, then

$$\rho(\mathbf{C}^{(0)}) = \lfloor \mathbf{C}^{(0)} \rfloor = \lfloor \arg\min_{\mathbf{J}^T\mathbf{J}=\mathbf{I}} ||\mathbf{C}^{(0)} - \mathbf{J}||^2 \rfloor . \tag{13}$$

where $\mathbf{J}$ is comprised of the first three singular vectors, computed using SVD of $\mathbf{Q}$ such that $\mathbf{D} = \mathbf{Q}\mathbf{R}$ is QR decomposition of $\mathbf{D}$ and $[\mathbf{I} \mid \mathbf{0}]^T$ is a rectangular matrix conformed by concatenation of the identity matrix $\mathbf{I}$ and the empty matrix $\mathbf{0}$.

Our choice of SVD for our initialization stems from both, the fact that singular value decomposition corresponds to the best second-order approximation to the span and there are efficient methods to compute it.

Once $\mathbf{C}^{(0)}$ has been computed, we minimize $p(\mathbf{C})$ making use of steepest descent optimization in Sect. 2.1. This is a gradient descent method which consists of two steps interleaved to find a minimum of the objective function. Here, we use interleaved steps of gradient calculation and back-tracking line search along the steepest descent direction until convergence. As a result, we iterate until $\Delta\mathbf{C}^{(t)}$ or $p(\mathbf{C}^{(t)})$ in Eq. (8) are sufficiently small, *i.e.* less than a predefined threshold ϵ.

Also, recall that our steepest descent method employs the step size λ. Here, we follow Armijo's rule and use the expression

$$\lambda = \begin{cases} 2\lambda & \text{if } p(\mathbf{C}^{(t)}) - p(\mathbf{C}^{(t)} + 2\lambda\Delta\mathbf{C}^{(t)})) \geq \lambda||\Delta\mathbf{C}^{(t)}|| \\ \frac{1}{2}\lambda & \text{if } p(\mathbf{C}^{(t)}) - p(\mathbf{C}^{(t)} + \lambda\Delta\mathbf{C}^{(t)})) < \frac{1}{2}\lambda||\Delta\mathbf{C}^{(t)}|| \end{cases} \tag{14}$$

4   Experiments

In this section, we present our experiments on semantic labeling using proposed class-driven color transformation and a number of alternatives. To illustrate the utility of our method, we consider a standard multi-class segmentation pipeline where above transformation is included as a preprocessing step.

Given an input image, we apply our color transformation and use the output as an input to a pixel-level classifier. Here, in order to analyze robustness of the transformation to different number of classes and various classifiers, we consider two publicly available frameworks *i.e.* TextonBoost [20] and DARWIN [21] implementation. The former only gives unary terms for each class as output whereas the latter delivers unary and pairwise terms provided by a post-processing step consisting of a conditional random field (CRF). By using this pipeline, our experiments are conducted on two standard datasets for semantic segmentation *i.e.* MSRC-21 [22] and Stanford Background Dataset (SBD) [23]. To our knowledge, TextonBoost and DARWIN provide competitive results on publicly available frameworks to the state-of-the-art for these datasets, respectively.

For the purposes of quantitative evaluation, we provide pixel-wise comparisons between outputs of the classifiers and ground-truth. To do this, we report global and per-class average accuracies [22]. Here, the global accuracy represents the ratio of correctly classified pixels to total number of pixels in test set. Per-class average accuracy, on the other hand, is computed as the average over all classes for the ratio of correctly classified pixels in a class to total number of pixels in the same class.

In our experiments, both pixel-level classifiers under consideration are learned using training sets of features in [20] for the MSRC-21 and [23] for the SBD. We use all training samples available to learn projection from the input color data to the classes. To apply metric MDS, we use a Markov Chain Monte Carlo (MCMC) random sampler to select a balanced distribution of samples. The class mapping matrix $\mathbf{C}$ and subspace projection matrix $\mathbf{B}$ are then multiplied to compute color transformation matrix $\mathbf{A}$.

In Fig. 1, we show the transformed color cubes for both, MSRC-21 and SBD datasets. As mentioned earlier, note that the mapping induced by $\mathbf{A}$ can potentially yield negative values in the target space. This can be appreciated in the figure, where the transformed cubes have been colored as per the original RGB value at input taken from the cube on the right-hand panel. These transformed

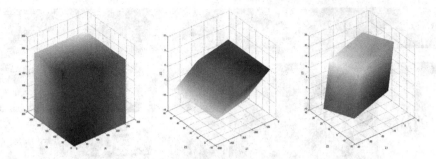

Fig. 1. RGB color cube (*left*) and transformed color cubes for MSRC-21 (*middle*) and SBD (*right*) datasets, respectively (Color figure online).

cubes do have negative values and moreover, they are consistent with the notion that our approach gives a linear transformation yielded from a convex function.

Recall that both TextonBoost and DARWIN employ positive RGB inputs. To accommodate this requirement, we bound the transformed color cubes using the matrix

$$\mathbf{A}^* = \mathbf{A} \times \mathbf{H} + \mathbf{T} \tag{15}$$

as an alternative to $\mathbf{A}$. In the equation above, $\mathbf{H}$ and $\mathbf{T}$ are diagonal scaling and translation matrices, respectively. This is a straightforward scaling-translation operation in the transformed target space and hence, we do this without any loss of generality. Further, we compute the diagonal matrices $\mathbf{H}$ and $\mathbf{T}$ deploying vertices in the color cubes as an additional training step. This is done by solving a linear equation where six vertices in the RGB color cube are used to obtain six degrees of freedom comprised by three diagonal elements of each of the above two matrices.

For a comprehensive evaluation, we compare accuracy of our method with the results obtained when our color transformation is not included. We have done this to set a baseline that can be employed as an indicator of the contribution of our color transformation to classification performance. As both TextonBoost and DARWIN employ the Lab color space, our baseline results represents this color transformation as well. Hence, for the purposes of comparison, we have employed some other widely used classic color transformations in compute vision including YCrCb, HSL, Luv [12], I1I2I3 [31] and O1O2O3 [32]. TextonBoost and DARWIN compute textons on luminance channel and so, in our experiments, it is given by the L-channels of the canonical color transformations, more specifically, I1 and O3 of the illumination invariant color spaces under study *i.e.* I1I2I3 and O1O2O3.

Finally, to further justify our choice of MDS for purposes of subspace projection throughout the Sect. 2.2, we also explore effect of various subspace projection methods as alternatives to metric MDS. The methods used here to that aim are Heteroscedastic Discriminant Analysis (HDA) [16], Maximum Margin Criterion (MMC), Singular Value Decomposition (SVD) and Kernel Principal

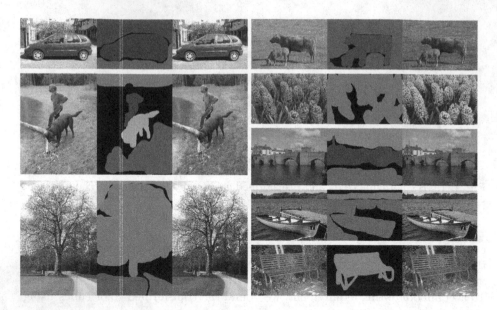

Fig. 2. Sample images for MSRC-21 dataset. In each panel, we show the RGB image on the dataset (*l*eft), corresponding labeling (*m*iddle) and transformed image (*r*ight) (Color figure online).

Component Analysis (KPCA). HDA is based on the heteroscedastic two-class technique using Chernoff criterion and MMC geometrically maximizes the average margin between classes after reducing number of dimensions.

4.1   MSRC-21 Dataset

The MSRC-21 dataset [22] consists of 591 color images of size 320×213 with corresponding ground truth labeling for 21 object classes. As mentioned above, we use the same evaluation procedure as [20] e.g. 276 images for training and 256 images for testing.

To illustrate high-distinct transformed colors in comparison to the original ones with respect to ground-truths on MSRC-21 dataset, we show the transformed color images together with corresponding labeling and RGB color inputs in Fig. 2. To produce these images, we have used the matrix $\mathbf{A}^*$ as an alternative to $\mathbf{A}$. This, in turn has the effect of portraying the images as they would be taken at input by the classifiers. Note that, the transformed colors are somewhat consistent with the labels. This is expected, since the matrix $\mathbf{C}$ is obtained based on the label information and, later on, the metric MDS used to compute $\mathbf{B}$ aims at preserving induced class distances. For instance, the chair and tree are in almost the same green spectrum in the RGB image but in the transformed one, green chair and purple tree provide higher visual separation for different classes.

We summarize our evaluation results in Table 1 for the TextonBoost and in Table 2 for the DARWIN. As shown in the tables, our color transformation

Table 1. MSRC-21: Summary of per-class results on TextonBoost [20]. Bold values indicate the highest accuracies.

	Bldg.	Grass	Tree	Cow	Sheep	Sky	Aeropl.	Water	Face	Car	Bicycle	Flower	Sign	Bird	Book	Chair	Road	Cat	Dog	Body	Boat	Avg.	Global
Baseline	68	**98**	88	85	76	92	**86**	68	84	77	87	86	57	45	92	60	87	74	36	75	22	73.9	82.0
MMC	72	**98**	90	86	81	94	83	72	87	**84**	**89**	**93**	66	45	**97**	68	88	72	**42**	80	21	76.5	84.1
HDA	**73**	**98**	**91**	85	82	92	81	71	87	77	88	91	64	48	93	68	**89**	72	41	81	24	76.0	83.9
SVD	71	**98**	**91**	**87**	81	**95**	82	70	87	81	**89**	89	**70**	48	93	65	88	73	37	80	**30**	76.4	84.0
KPCA	72	**98**	89	85	**85**	94	**86**	70	87	82	88	90	66	**53**	96	56	88	**78**	38	80	24	76.3	83.9
Ours	70	**98**	90	86	83	94	**86**	**74**	**89**	81	87	92	63	45	96	65	88	72	**42**	**84**	27	**76.8**	**84.2**

Table 2. MSRC-21: Summary of results for subspace projections (*left*) and color transformations (*right*) on DARWIN [21]. Bold values indicate the highest accuracies.

	Unary		Pairwise	
	Avg.	Gb.	Avg.	Gb.
Baseline	67.1	78.9	70.2	82.8
MMC	68.1	78.5	71.3	82.7
HDA	67.4	77.9	70.8	82.2
SVD	67.3	79.8	69.1	83.5
KPCA	68.3	79.2	71.9	83.4
Ours	**68.9**	**80.0**	**72.1**	**84.0**

	Unary		Pairwise	
	Avg.	Gb.	Avg.	Gb.
Baseline	67.1	78.9	70.2	82.8
YCrCb	65.4	77.8	69.5	81.8
HSL	65.2	77.0	70.3	82.1
Luv	65.9	78.1	70.3	82.1
I1I2I3	62.6	75.2	69.6	81.3
O1O2O3	62.3	75.1	68.9	81.2
Ours	**68.9**	**80.0**	**72.1**	**84.0**

outperforms the alternatives with respect to the baseline when applied as a preprocessing step. This improvement is consistent across a variety of subspace projection methods and color transformations. Note also that in Table 2, pattern of improvement holds when a pairwise term is applied after the classifier.

We employed publicly available code of TextonBoost to compare the classification performance with and without our color transformation but due to fine tuning of parameters, preprocessing of images or randomization functions, accuracy on different platforms/compilers were not consistent with those reported in [20]. However, our experiments still confirm the advantages of using the transformed images over original ones for classification.

4.2 Standford Background Dataset (SBD)

The Stanford Background Dataset [23] consists of 715 color images of size 320 × 240 with corresponding ground labeling over 8 classes. In this case, we use the same evaluation procedure as in [23], *i.e.* 5-fold cross validation with 572 images for training and 143 images for testing.

To present the effect of our color transformation on SBD dataset, we show sample images together with their labeling and RGB color inputs in Fig. 3. As previous section, we have used the matrix $\mathbf{A}^*$ as an alternative to $\mathbf{A}$ to produce these images. Note that, colors in the transformed images are also somewhat

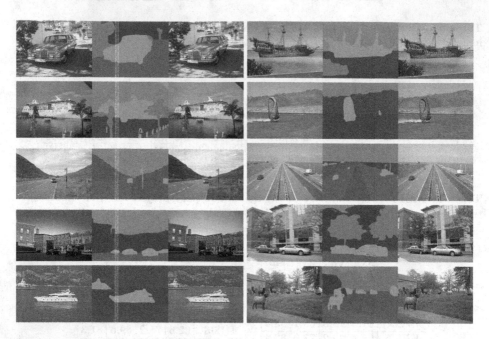

Fig. 3. Sample images for SBD dataset. In each panel, we show RGB image on the dataset (*left*), corresponding labeling (*middle*) and transformed image (*right*) (Color figure online).

Table 3. SBD: Summary of per-class results on TextonBoost [20]. Bold values indicate the highest accuracies.

	Sky	Tree	Road	Grass	Water	Bldg.	Mntn.	Forgr.	Avg.	Global
Baseline	**86**	64	89	65	65	76	03	60	63.5	74.0
MMC	**86**	**68**	90	72	62	79	01	63	65.2	76.3
HDA	**86**	66	**91**	72	65	**80**	02	**65**	65.8	76.7
SVD	**86**	67	**91**	**73**	64	**80**	06	63	66.3	76.7
KPCA	**86**	**68**	**91**	**73**	65	**80**	03	61	65.9	76.6
Ours	**86**	**68**	90	68	**67**	79	**09**	**65**	**66.5**	**76.8**

consistent with the label information. This, as mentioned earlier, is expected due to the manner in which we have computed matrix **A**.

Table 3 presents outcomes for TextonBoost and Table 4 summarize the results for DARWIN for different subspace projections and color transformations under consideration. It is clear that, by using our method as a preprocessing step, we can consistently improve both unary and pairwise classification accuracies. Moreover, using metric MDS as subspace projection method outperforms others, including the baseline.

Therefore, we can conclude that our class-driven color transformation improves classification accuracy when used as a preprocessing step within a

Table 4. SBD: Summary of results for subspace projection techniques (*left*) and color transforms (*right*) on DARWIN [21]. Bold values indicate the highest accuracies.

	Unary		Pairwise	
	Avg.	Gb.	Avg.	Gb.
Baseline	68.3	78.5	70.2	81.5
MMC	69.6	79.9	71.7	82.9
HDA	68.9	79.3	71.2	82.4
SVD	69.2	79.8	70.9	82.8
KPCA	68.5	78.8	70.7	82.0
Ours	**70.4**	**81.4**	**72.5**	**84.2**

	Unary		Pairwise	
	Avg.	Gb.	Avg.	Gb.
Baseline	68.3	78.5	70.2	81.5
YCrCb	68.7	77.1	70.7	80.2
HSL	68.0	76.9	70.0	80.1
Luv	68.3	76.9	70.5	80.1
I1I2I3	67.1	75.9	68.6	78.7
O1O2O3	66.7	75.9	68.5	79.0
Ours	**70.4**	**81.4**	**72.5**	**84.2**

multi-class segmentation framework. Importantly, the improvement is independent of dataset and number of classes. Further, this improvement is an additional gain over the classifier output, hence, not being exclusive of other common post-processing steps such as the application of CRFs. Finally, it is worth mentioning that this improvement comes at a negligible computational cost.

5   Conclusion

In this paper, we derived an image color transformation based on label information of classes in dataset under study. We did this by posing the problem in terms of a composition of two mappings. The first of these, maps the image color onto a space spanned by the class set. We computed this mapping by optimizing an objective function formulated in terms of the aggregation of pairwise distances within and between the classes using a steepest descent scheme devoid of matrix inversions. The second mapping corresponds to transforming data in the class space to a target space, which we calculated making use of metric multi-dimensional scaling. Our experiments confirm the applicability of our algorithm to enhance global and average precisions of pixel-wise classifiers when it is employed as a general preprocessing step for segmentation and labeling.

Acknowledgement. Authors would like to highly appreciate reviewers' efforts and positive feedbacks which improve the quality and readability of this work.

References

1. Van De Sande, K., Gevers, T., Snoek, C.: Evaluating color descriptors for object and scene recognition. IEEE Trans. Pattern Anal. Mach. Intell. **32**(9), 1582–1596 (2010)
2. Finlayson, G.D., Drew, M.S.: The maximum ignorance assumption with positivity. In: Society for Imaging Science and Technology Conference on Color and Imaging, pp. 202–205 (1996)

3. Nayar, S.K., Bolle, R.M.: Reflectance based object recognition. Int. J. Comput. Vis. **17**(3), 219–240 (1996)
4. Dror, R.O., Adelson, E.H., Willsky, A.S.: Recognition of surface reflectance properties from a single image under unknown real-world illumination (2001)
5. Slater, D., Healey, G.: Object recognition using invariant profiles. In: IEEE Computer Society Conference on Computer Vision and Pattern Recognition (CVPR), pp. 827–832 (1997)
6. Jacobs, D.W., Belhumeur, P.N., Basri, R.: Comparing images under variable illumination. In: IEEE Computer Society Conference on Computer Vision and Pattern Recognition (CVPR), pp. 610–617 (1998)
7. Lin, S., Lee, S.W.: Using chromaticity distributions and eigenspace analysis for pose-, illumination-, and specularity-invariant recognition of 3D objects. In: IEEE Computer Society Conference on Computer Vision and Pattern Recognition (CVPR), pp. 426–431 (1997)
8. Lenz, R., Carmona, P.L., Meer, P.: The hyperbolic geometry of illumination-induced chromaticity changes. In: IEEE Conference on Computer Vision and Pattern Recognition (CVPR), pp. 1–6 (2007)
9. Chong, H.Y., Gortler, S.J., Zickler, T.: A perception-based color space for illumination-invariant image processing. ACM Trans. Graph. **27**(3), 61 (2008)
10. Strutz, T.: Adaptive selection of colour transformations for reversible image compression. In: IEEE European Signal Processing Conference (EUSIPCO), pp. 1204–1208 (2012)
11. Hu, G., Liu, C., Chuang, K., Yu, S., Tsui, T.: General regression neural network utilized for color transformation between images on RGB color space. In: IEEE International Conference on Machine Learning and Cybernetics (ICMLC), vol. 4, pp. 1793–1799 (2011)
12. Wyszecki, G., Stiles, W.S.: Color Science. Wiley, New York (1982)
13. Meyer, G.W., Greenberg, D.P.: Perceptual color spaces for computer graphics. In: ACM SIGGRAPH Computer Graphics, vol. 14(3), pp. 254–261 (1980)
14. Fu, Z., Robles-Kelly, A.: Learning object material categories via pairwise discriminant analysis. In: IEEE Computer Society Conference on Computer Vision and Pattern Recognition (CVPR) (2007)
15. McLachlan, G.: Discriminant Analysis and Statistical Pattern Recognition. Wiley, Hoboken (2004)
16. Loog, M., Duin, R., Haeb-Umbach, R.: Multiclass linear dimension reduction by weighted pairwise Fisher criteria. IEEE Trans. Pattern Anal. Mach. Intell. **23**(7), 762–766 (2001)
17. Bickel, P.J., Levina, E.: Some theory for Fisher's linear discriminant function, 'naive Bayes', and some alternatives when there are many more variables than observations. J. Bernoulli **10**, 989–1010 (2004)
18. Fan, J., Fan, Y.: High dimensional classification using features annealed independence rules. Ann. Stat. **36**(6), 2605 (2008)
19. Tibshirani, R., Hastie, T., Narasimhan, B., Chu, G.: Diagnosis of multiple cancer types by shrunken centroids of gene expression. Proc. Nat. Acad. Sci. **99**(10), 6567–6572 (2002)
20. Krähenbühl, Ph., Koltun, V.: Efficient inference in fully connected crfs with gaussian edge potentials. arXiv preprint arXiv:1210.5644 (2012)
21. Gould, S.: DARWIN: a framework for machine learning and computer vision research and development. J. Mach. Learn. Res. **13**, 3533–3537 (2012)

22. Shotton, J., Winn, J., Rother, C., Criminisi, A.: Textonboost for image understanding: Multi-class object recognition and segmentation by jointly modeling texture, layout, and context. Int. J. Comput. Vis. **81**(1), 2–23 (2009)
23. Gould, S., Fulton, R., Koller, D.: Decomposing a scene into geometric and semantically consistent regions. In: IEEE International Conference on Computer Vision (ICCV), pp. 1–8 (2009)
24. Boyd, S., Vandenberghe, L.: Convex Optimization. Cambridge University Press, New York (2009)
25. Li, X., Jiang, T., Zhang, K.: Efficient and robust feature extraction by maximum margin criterion. IEEE Trans. Neural Netw. **17**(1), 157–165 (2006)
26. Hastie, T., Tibshirani, R.: Classification by pairwise coupling. Ann. Stat. **26**(2), 451–471 (1998)
27. Harris, C.: Tracking with rigid models. In: Blake, A., Yuille, A. (eds.) Active Vision, pp. 59–73. MIT Press, Cambridge (1993)
28. Lin, D., Yan, S., Tang, X.: Pursuing informative projection on Grassmann manifold. In: IEEE Computer Society Conference on Computer Vision and Pattern Recognition (CVPR), vol. 2, pp. 1727–1734 (2006)
29. Baudat, G., Anouar, F.: Generalized discriminant analysis using a kernel approach. Neural Comput. **12**(10), 2385–2404 (2000)
30. Wang, X., Tang, X.: Dual-space linear discriminant analysis for face recognition. In: IEEE Computer Society Conference on Computer Vision and Pattern Recognition (CVPR), vol. 2, p. 564 (2004)
31. Geusebroek, J., Van den Boomgaard, R., Smeulders, A.W.M., Geerts, H.: Color invariance. IEEE Trans. Pattern Anal. Mach. Intell. **23**(12), 1338–1350 (2001)
32. Álvarez, J.M., Gevers, T., López, A.M.: Learning photometric invariance for object detection. Int. J. Comput. Vis. **90**(1), 45–61 (2010)

Discovering Harmony: A Hierarchical Colour Harmony Model for Aesthetics Assessment

Peng Lu[1]($^{(\boxtimes)}$), Zhijie Kuang[1], Xujun Peng[2], and Ruifan Li[1]

[1] Beijing University of Posts and Telecommunications, Beijing 100876, China
lupeng@bupt.edu.cn
[2] Raytheon BBN Technologies, Cambridge, MA, USA

Abstract. Color harmony is an important factor for image aesthetics assessment. Although plenty of color harmony theories are proposed by artists and scientists, there is little firm consensus and ambiguous definition amongst them, or even contradictory between them, which causes the existing theories infeasible for image aesthetics assessment. In order to overcome the problem of conventional color harmony theories, in this paper, we propose a hierarchical unsupervised learning approach to learn the compatible color combinations from large dataset. By using this generative color harmony model, we attempt to uncover the underlying principles that generate pleasing color combinations based on natural images. The main advantage of our method is that no prior empirical knowledge of image aesthetics, color harmony or arts is needed to complete the task of color harmony assessment. The experimental results on the public dataset show that our method outperforms the conventional rule based image aesthetics assessment approach.

1 Introduction

With the pervasive use of digital cameras and cell-phones and the deluge of online multimedia sharing communities, image retrieval has drawn much attention in recent years. As revealed in [1,2], besides semantic relevance, users prefer more appealing photos retrieved by image search engines, which indicates aesthetics and quality properties of images play a more important role than semantic relevance. Also, by integrating photograph aesthetics models into hand-held devices, a real-time recommendation can be made to facilitate professional and amateur users to manipulate the captured images. Thus, to assess photographs quality automatically from the perspective of visual aesthetics is of great interest in the research of web image search [1] and multimedia processing [3,4].

Although there have been many researches focusing on the image aesthetics estimation, assessing aesthetics quality of photographs is still an extremely challenging problem because it is a subjective task and different people may have various tastes to the same image. Despite lack of firm consensus and ambiguous definition of aesthetics, there exists several simple criteria to distinguish "good" images from "bad" ones. For example, as shown in Fig. 1, most people agree that the sample photos on the bottom row have higher aesthetics attributes than

© Springer International Publishing Switzerland 2015
D. Cremers et al. (Eds.): ACCV 2014, Part III, LNCS 9005, pp. 452–467, 2015.
DOI: 10.1007/978-3-319-16811-1_30

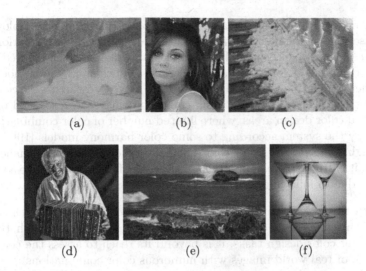

(a)   (b)   (c)

(d)   (e)   (f)

Fig. 1. Examples of low aesthetics quality photographs vs high aesthetics quality photographs. (a) Low aesthetics quality photo with blur. (b) Amateurish portrait with compression artifacts. (c) Example photo breaking the rule of thirds. (d) Portrait has professional lighting and color harmony. (e) Photo with well balanced composition. (f) Professional lighting and symmetry on a lovely colored picture (Color figure online).

the images on the top row, which have degradations due to out-of-focus blur, compression artifacts, distortion, etc. Moreover, for professional photographers, various principles (*e.g.* composition, sharpness, proper contrast and lighting as well as special photographic techniques as shown in Fig. 1(d), (e) and (f)) are taken into consideration to make a photo more attractive. Then, it is possible to design computational methods to automatically assess which image is more appealing than the others.

Many early photo quality assessment approaches attempted to formulate those commonly accepted rules empirically, such as the methods described in [5–8]. The potential problem of this type of methods is that the models are designed based on authors' intuition and only global features are selected. In order to address the shortcoming of relying on global features only, some researchers focused their studies on local features which show better performance to predict aesthetics quality, as illustrated in [9–12]. Recently, researchers explored methods to encode photographic criterion indirectly into a learning phase, which discovered the relationship between aesthetics quality and underlying features automatically [13,14].

Amongst the existing features used for photo aesthetics assessment, color harmony has been considered as one of the most important factors which has a significant influence on photo aesthetics but has been ignored for a long time. Only from the more recently, a few studies were applied on image aesthetics assessment by introducing some naive color harmony theories and models into the image quality classification/image harmonization tasks, which shows the effectiveness of the color harmony models [15–17]. However, those pioneer researches are still immature because the color harmony models employed are mostly based on the one which was found to have poor predictive performance [18], such as Moon-Spencer model used in [17], or the one which ignored partial important components for color harmony analysis, such as Matsuda model used in [15] where only Hue was used. More often, recent researches of color harmony theories in the image processing community have been focused on color selection and color design areas, where limited number of color combinations are suggested by the system according to some color harmony models [19].

Although some progresses of color harmony models have been made in the past years, it is still hard to apply them to the area of automatic image aesthetics assessment due to following reasons:

1. Most existing color harmony models are heuristically defined which can represent limited number of color harmony combinations. Although they are suitable for color design tasks, it is beyond its reach to assess the color compatibility of real world images with numerous color combinations.
2. Even plenty of color harmony models are proposed by researchers, they are defined in different color spaces and there is a lack of consensus between them. As these theories are various enough, nearly every color combination can be considered as harmonious if all models are considered [20].

In order to break through these limitations, researchers attempted to use machine learning approaches to "learn" compatible colors from large scale datasets. In [19], O'Donovan *et al.* trained a color harmony model from large datasets by using a least absolute shrinkage and selection operator (LASSO) regression approach, which can predict whether the user provided color combination is harmony or not. Inspired by this work, we applied a latent Dirichlet allocation (LDA) and Gaussian mixture model (GMM) based hierarchical learning approach to train a color harmony model dependent on large amount high quality images, and estimated the aesthetics quality of photos based on the trained color harmony model.

To the best of our knowledge, we are the first to reveal the process of how a color harmonious image is generated by learning this underlying principles from natural images. In summary, two main contributions are presented in this paper:

1. An generative, instead of empirical rule based, color harmony model is proposed by using large set of natural images to facilitate the task of image aesthetics assessment;
2. A hierarchical unsupervised learning model is proposed to learn the complex color combinations from photos. Based on this model, a principled probability based metric is also defined and applied for the aesthetics assessment task.

We organize the rest of the paper as follows. Section 2 is the review of related work, and Sect. 3 describes the details of the proposed LDA and GMM based hierarchical color harmony model, including a brief introduction of these two models, and their implementation for our tasks. The experimental setup and analysis are provided in Sect. 4. Section 5 concludes the paper.

2   Related Work

Color harmony, which is defined by Holtzschue as *"two or more colors are sensed together as a single, pleasing, collective impression"* [21], *"is one of the reputed daughters of Aphrodite, goddess of beauty, and this indicates that harmony is the province of aesthetics"*, stated by Westland in [22]. Due to the direct relationship between color harmony and image aesthetics, the exploration for the principles of color harmony has dominated the research of many artists and scientists.

Generally, most theories of color harmony follow the rule that multiple colors in neighboring areas produce a pleasing effect and thus can be roughly categorized into three types.

The first type of color harmony theories are originated from Newton's color theory, where hue circle is used to mathematically define different sets of color harmony principles. In [23], Itten suggested that a small number of colors uniform distributed on the hue wheel can be considered as harmonious. Derived from this idea, Matsuda designed a set of hue templates which defined ranges of harmony colors on the color circle [24].

The second category color harmony models are not only relied on hue information, but also introduce multiple features from color space to determine the color harmonious. In order to emphasize balance as a key factor of color harmony, Munsell [25] suggested that color harmony can be attained if colors with various saturation are in the same region of hue and value. To quantitatively represent Munsell's color harmony model, Moon and Spencer [26] proposed a model based on color difference, area and an esthetic measure, where color combination is harmonious when color difference is in the pattern of *identity*, *similarity*, or *contrast*.

The third category suggests that color harmony can be achieved when colors are similar in terms of hue or tone level. For example, in Natural Color System (NCS) which was detailed described by Hård and Sivik [27], colors are represented using the six elementary colors based on percepts of human vision, and the color combination can be classified according to *distinctness of border*, *interval kind* and *interval size*.

It should be noted that because the concepts of color harmony are highly dependent on nurture and culture, there are no obvious borderline between each type of classical color harmony theories. Many principles are shared by these theories and contradictory can also be found between them. Thus, in recent years, research interests were aroused in computer vision community to use machine learning approach to "learn" rules or patterns of color harmony from large data set based on images' statistical properties, such as method proposed in [19], where compatible color combinations were learnt from large amount rated images.

In this paper, we propose a hierarchical color harmony model to learn the underlying rules of compatible colors from high quality images, and evaluate this model by assessing the aesthetics quality of images. Our work is related to method presented in [19] in the sense of color harmony modeling and methods described in [12,17] in the sense of image aesthetics assessment.

3   Hierarchical Color Harmony Model

"Pleasing joint effect of two or more colors" [28] is a prevalently accepted definition for the color harmony theories. Originated from this definition, a hierarchical
color harmony model (HCHM) is proposed in this paper to learn those pleasing
color combinations from images, which is used to predict the degree of harmony
for unseen images. Initially, the HCHM learns the co-occurrence colors (color
groups in our scenario) in images, followed by a GMM learning phase to encode
the relations between color groups. By using this hierarchical structure, HCHM
can model the complex color combination which represents the color harmony
of the image.

3.1   Color Quantization

Prior to the color groups learning phase, each image is initially divided into
small patches and colors are averaged within each patch. By quantizing each
color patch using a color codebook, the mosaiced image can be represented by a
set of "color words". Considering that human vision perception is more sensitive
to the color with high perceived luminance, we use a non-linear quantization
approach in HSV color space, which can be expressed as Eq. 1:

$$BIN = 1 + \sum_{i=2}^{L} i \times (i-1) \times q \tag{1}$$

where BIN is the total number of code words for hue-saturation-value (HSV)
space, L means we partition the entire HSV space into L subspace evenly according to *value*, and then we divided each subspace using $(i-2) \times q$ radial lines and
i circles. In this paper, we set $L = 10$ and $q = 4$.

Under this quantization scheme, the color space is coarsely partitioned in the
region with low *value*, whilst the space is intensively separated in the region with
high *value*, as illustrated in Fig. 2(a). In Fig. 2(b), an example image along with
its corresponding mosaiced image and color words encoded image is shown.

Thus, a given image i can be represented as a set of color words $\mathbf{c} = \{c_1^{(i)}, \cdots, c_n^{(i)}\}$, where $n \in N$ and N is the total number of patches in image i.

3.2   LDA Based Color Groups Learning

In the information retrieval and data mining area, Latent Dirichlet Allocation
(LDA) is a widely used unsupervised approach to find patterns in unstructured
data, which inherently has the capability to discover the semantic coherent item
within large corpus. In the framework of LDA, each document can be represented
by a distribution over topics, where each topic is a distribution over the vocabulary. In our scenario, by considering each quantized color as a word, LDA can
be used to learn the coherent colors through topics, which correspond to color
groups in HCHM, and to represent images' color property through the topics
distribution.

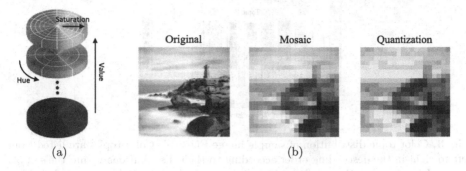

Fig. 2. An example of image mosaicing and quantization. (a) HSV cylinder is non-linearly divided into small regions. (b) A high quality image along with its mosaiced image and quantized image by using quantization codebook provided by Fig. 2(a).

By using LDA, the generative process to create an image can be formally described as below:

1. Given a set of K color topics:
   - Draw a multinomial color topic distribution over color codebook according to $\varphi_k \sim Dir(\cdot \mid \boldsymbol{\beta})$ for each color topic $k \in \{1, \cdots, K\}$, where $Dir(\cdot)$ is a Dirichlet distribution, $\boldsymbol{\beta}$ is a V-dimensional Dirichlet parameter and V is the color codebook size.
   - A color topic matrix $\boldsymbol{\Phi} = \varphi_{1:K}$ is formed, whose size is $V \times K$ and its element indicates the probability of the color word v given a topic k.
2. For each image i in the dataset:
   - Draw a parameter $\boldsymbol{\vartheta}^{(i)}$ that determines the distribution of the color topic. This is done by choosing $\boldsymbol{\vartheta}^{(i)} \sim Dir(\cdot \mid \boldsymbol{\alpha})$ for image i, where $\boldsymbol{\alpha}$ is a K-dimensional Dirichlet parameter. $\boldsymbol{\vartheta}^{(i)}$ is a K-dimensional parameter of a multinomial distribution, and $\boldsymbol{\vartheta}_k^{(i)}$ is the proportion of color topic k in image i.
   - To generate a color word (quantized image patch) $c_n^{(i)}$ in the image i:
     • Choose a color topic $z_n^{(i)} \in \{1, \cdots, K\} \sim Mult(\cdot \mid \boldsymbol{\vartheta}^{(i)})$, where $Mult(\cdot)$ is a multinomial distribution, $z_n^{(i)}$ is a color topic assignment and K is the total number of topics.
     • Choose a color $c_n^{(i)} \in \{1, \cdots, V\} \sim Mult(\cdot \mid \varphi_{z_n^{(i)}})$, where V is the size of the color codebook.

With the quantized color words from the training set, the parameter $\boldsymbol{\vartheta}^{(i)}$ for each image and φ_k for each topic can be estimated by Gibbs LDA. In Fig. 3, we illustrate the color topic distribution of sample image in Fig. 2(b), which is inferred from our trained LDA. More details of LDA's training and inference can be found in [29].

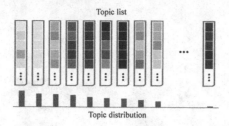

Fig. 3. Color topic distribution of sample image Fig. 2(b). Color topics are listed from left to right in the descending order according to their distributions within the sample image. In each topic, the top five color words are illustrated (Color figure online).

3.3   Applying GMM for Color Harmony Model

In order to model the dependency between topics for a given corpus, a Gaussian mixture model is learned on the top of LDA based on the color topic distribution $\vartheta^{(i)}$. Theoretically, it can be shown that by using infinite number of mixtures, GMM can approximate every general continuous probability distribution to arbitrary precision.

Given a Gaussian mixture model, the probability of a topic distribution of image i in topic space can be described as:

$$p(\vartheta^{(i)} \mid \xi) = \sum_{i=m}^{M} \omega_m \mathcal{N}(\vartheta^{(i)} \mid \boldsymbol{\mu}_m, \boldsymbol{\Sigma}_m) \qquad (2)$$

where $\mathcal{N}(\cdot)$ is a Gaussian probability density function:

$$\mathcal{N}(\vartheta^{(i)} \mid \boldsymbol{\mu}_m, \boldsymbol{\Sigma}_m) = \frac{\exp\left(-\frac{1}{2}(\vartheta^{(i)} - \boldsymbol{\mu}_m)^T \boldsymbol{\Sigma}_m^{-1}(\vartheta^{(i)} - \boldsymbol{\mu}_m)\right)}{(2\pi)^{D/2}|\boldsymbol{\Sigma}_m|^{1/2}} \qquad (3)$$

where $\vartheta^{(i)}$ is the color topic distribution in topic space, which is obtained by applying LDA on the image i, parameters $\xi = \{\omega_m, \boldsymbol{\mu}_m, \boldsymbol{\Sigma}_m\}$ denote the weight, the mean and the covariance of the mth Gaussian distribution that satisfy $\sum_{m=1}^{M} \omega_m = 1$, and M is the number of mixtures. $\mathcal{N}(\vartheta^{(i)} \mid \boldsymbol{\mu}_m, \boldsymbol{\Sigma}_m)$ reflects the probability of $\vartheta^{(i)}$ being to the mth Gaussian distribution. For the correct estimation of Gaussian mixture model, the so-called Expectation-Maximization (EM) algorithm is used.

Normally, the likelihood $p(\vartheta^{(i)} \mid \xi)$ can be used directly to measure the color harmony of unseen images. In our work, in order to fit the color harmony model into the image aesthetics assessment task, we use $\epsilon = \frac{p(\vartheta^{(i)} | \xi^+)}{p(\vartheta^{(i)} | \xi^-)}$ to represent the degree of color harmony of a given image, where GMM parameter ξ^+ is trained by using high aesthetics quality images while ξ^- is trained with low aesthetics quality images. To an unseen high quality image, it should have higher probability with $p(\vartheta^{(i)} \mid \xi^+)$, whereas its probability on low quality images trained $p(\vartheta^{(i)} \mid \xi^-)$ should be lower. Then ϵ can represent the degree of color harmony.

4   Experimental Results

4.1   Dataset

In our experiments, we created a color harmony evaluation dataset (CHE-Dataset), which was a subset of AVA dataset [30], for our training and evaluation purpose. To the aim of aesthetics assessment, AVA dataset contains more than 250,000 images which are categorized into over 60 groups. These images have plenty of meta-data, including a large number of aesthetics scores for each image, and semantic labels for groups. The quality scores of AVA dataset are based on various aesthetics aspects including color harmony, composition, subject, blur, etc. Only top ranked and bottom ranked images' scores are correlated with the degree of color harmony. So in order to meet the requirements of our color harmony model training and evaluation purpose, we followed the same method as [17] to select the top 2,000 images and the bottom 2,000 images based on their aesthetics scores for each category, respectively. All monochrome images were excluded from our dataset. To the high aesthetics and low aesthetics subsets of each category, images were evenly divided into a training set and a testing set. In this work, we collected the total number of 29,844 images from eight different categories in AVA (a single image in our corpus may have multiple category labels), whose labels are: Floral, Landscape, Architecture, Food and Drink, Animals, Cityscape, Portraiture and Still Life.

In Fig. 4, we illustrate the statistic properties of our dataset, where Fig. 4(a) shows the mean values and variances of high aesthetics quality subset and low aesthetics quality subset for each category. In Fig. 4(b), the number of individuals who provided scores for images in CHE-Dataset is shown. From this figure, we can see that most images in our dataset have plenty number of individuals (>200).

4.2   System Analysis

To evaluate the performance of the proposed model, we firstly mosaiced each image and quantized image patches using the codebook introduced in Sect. 3.1.

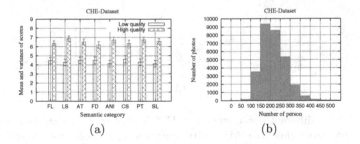

(a)   (b)

Fig. 4. Statistic properties of CHE-Dataset. (a) Box-plots of the means and variances of each category's scores. FL, LS, AT, FD, ANI, CS, PT and SL denote Floral, Landscape, Architecture, Food and Drink, Animals, Cityscape, Portraiture and Still Life, respectively. (b) The number of scores available for images in CHE-Dataset.

Then in the training phase, an LDA was trained by using 1000 high aesthetics quality images for each category. Further more, as described in Sect. 3.3, on the top of LDA we trained two GMMs with three Gaussian mixture components by using 1000 images with high aesthetics quality and 1000 images with low aesthetics quality, separately. In the testing phase, the color topic distribution $\vartheta^{(i)}$ of test image i from a given category was computed based on corresponding LDA. Then the color harmony score ϵ was obtained based on the trained GMMs and the image with high ϵ score was classified as a high aesthetics image. In our experiments, 2000 test images from each category were used for the evaluation purpose.

In this experiment, different sets of parameters of patch size, quantization codebook size and topic numbers were investigated. As the target of the color harmony modeling is to assess the images aesthetics quality, we evaluated the performance of the proposed method using the average areas under the ROC curve (AUC) for the entire test set.

In Fig. 5(a), AUCs of four sets of patch sizes were evaluated and the best classification accuracy was achieved by using 12×12 patch size. From this figure, an interesting phenomenon can be observed that smaller or larger patch sizes can provide better performance than the patch size of 16×16. The reason is that the color harmony information can be encoded by LDA when smaller patches contain pure colors. Whilst, color compatibility information in image space can also be encoded in patch level with suitable patch size, which was revealed in Fig. 5(a).

In Figs. 5(b) and (c), different values of the codebook size for quantization in HSV color space and the number of topics for LDA were examined, which showed better performance with codebook size of 1321 and topic number of 300 for aesthetics assessment. As the codebook size decreased, more colors were mapped to one code, which cannot effectively represent the color combinations before LDA and degrade the system performance. As the codebook size increased from some point, more and more similar color codes appeared in the same color topic, which cannot effectively represent the color combinations after LDA.

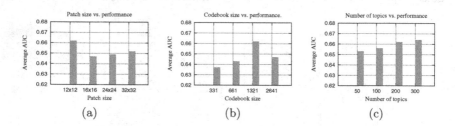

Fig. 5. AUC with different parameters. (a) AUC with various patch sizes which were used for image mosaicing. (b) AUC with different codebook size for quantization. (c) AUC with different color topic numbers for LDA (Color figure online).

To visually demonstrate the discriminate capability of the proposed color harmony model, we illustrated the top ranked images and bottom ranked images from three different categories: Animals, Floral and Architecture in Fig. 6. From this figure, we can see that although both top ranked and bottom ranked images contain rich colors, the proposed color harmony model can reveal the subtle difference between them and distinguish high quality images from low quality images.

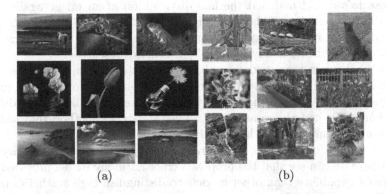

(a)   (b)

Fig. 6. High aesthetics quality images and low aesthetics quality images classified by the proposed system. (a) Top ranked images with high aesthetics scores. (b) Bottom ranked images with low aesthetics scores.

In order to discover what type of color combinations is learned by the proposed hierarchical color harmony model, we illustrated the top 10 color topics (groups) of each image category in Fig. 7, where 5 top ranked color words of each topic are shown. From this figure, we can see that the proposed model is capable to capture key color combination patterns for each category. For example, to the floral category, the flower related colors: purple, red, pink are among the top list through our system. And to the portraiture category, photographers tend to use dark colors as background, which are also revealed by the proposed system.

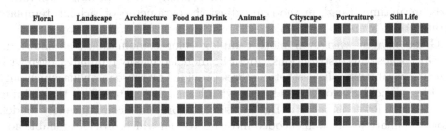

Fig. 7. Top-10 ranked color groups (topics) learned from LDA for each image category (Color figure online).

4.3   Comparison and Discussion

In our experiments, we compared the proposed unsupervised color harmony model to other three the state-of-the-art color harmony models for image aesthetics assessment task, which are briefly summarized below.

Moon and Spencer's color harmony model used a quantitative aesthetics measure $M = O/C$, where C represents complexity and O means order of a color combination. The quantitative definition of C and O can be found in [31].

Matsuda's model matched the hue distribution of an image against eight hue distribution templates, where the highest matching score was used to represent the degree of image's color harmony. In this model, the parameters of hue distributions were heuristically defined by aesthetics researchers.

Tang's color harmony model was based on Matsuda's hue template, where hue distributions of each template were learnt from a set of training images. Although the parameters of the Tang's hue template were adaptive for different type of images, it had the same drawback as Matsuda's method that only hue information was employed in the color harmony model.

In Fig. 8, the ROC curves of different approaches for each category were shown, where we can see that the proposed color harmony model provided more discriminant capability than other models to distinguish high aesthetics quality images from low aesthetics quality images.

To further analyze the performance gain of the proposed method, experimental results on different level of color complexities were illustrated in Fig. 9, where the images' aesthetics ranks of different methods were listed in corresponding tables, along with the user labeled ranks.

In Fig. 9(a), two sample images have a simple color combination (distribution) which can be modeled by hue templates (as shown by the corresponding hue wheels). To this type of images, both rule based color harmony models, such as Matsuda and M&S's models, and the learning based models, such as Tang's and the proposed methods, can effectively represent the harmony information contained in images.

To images shown in Fig. 9(b), whose color distributions cannot be accurately modeled by empirically defined hue templates, rule based methods predict relatively low aesthetics scores which causes those images had low aesthetics ranks. In the mean time, Tang's method can adjust the parameters of each hue template through the learning phase, which still provides reliable ranking score.

Given images with even more complex color combinations, as shown in Fig. 9(c), whose hue distributions cannot be modeled by any templates, even with adaptive parameters, the aesthetics scores provided by those methods which only consider particular color channel, even with learnt parameters from the training set, are much lower than truth. But by using the proposed color harmony model, color combinations are well encoded into the system which provides reliable aesthetics assessment ranking for test images.

Compared with rule based methods, the proposed color harmony model relies on the quality of the training dataset. From our experiments, we found that by using the data selection approach described in [17], the annotated scores of each

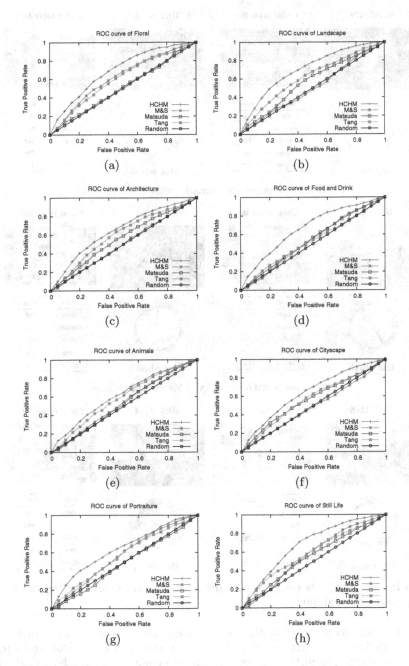

Fig. 8. ROC curves of image aesthetics assessment for each category.

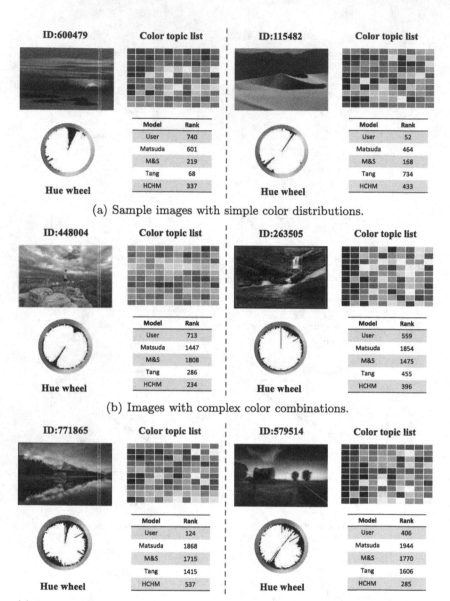

(a) Sample images with simple color distributions.

(b) Images with complex color combinations.

(c) Images with wide range of color distributions that cannot be represented by heuristic based models.

Fig. 9. Comparison of image aesthetics assessment with different color complexities. To each sub-figure, the original color image along with its top 10 color topics (color groups) are illustrated in the top row. The corresponding hue distribution, the user labeled ranks and predicted ranks by different color harmony models are shown in bottom row of each sub-figure (Color figure online).

photo still cannot precisely represent the color harmony degree for low quality images, where images with low quality scores may be harmonious but have other type of degradations, such as blur, bad composition, etc. This is the main reason for the most of misclassifications in our experiments. Thus, to build a dataset with more reliable scores measuring the color harmony degrees can overcome the problem of false alarm for the proposed color harmony model, which will be our future research focus.

5   Conclusions

In this paper, a hierarchical unsupervised learning approach is proposed to learn the compatible color combinations from large dataset. In this hierarchical framework, the LDA is adopted to learn the simple color groups, followed by the GMM training procedure to learn the combinations of color groups. By using this hierarchical structure, we can discover the harmonious colors, which facilitates the color selection for design industry. The HCHM can also encode the complex color combinations from the dataset images, which provides a feasible way to assess the aesthetics quality of natural images. Experimental results show the HCHM's capability of learning the complex color combinations.

The proposed method provides an example of learning the color harmony from natural photos, which is a promising way to increase our knowledge of color harmony.

Our future work includes to extend our method by taking the spatial relationship between colors in images and combining other features to improve the aesthetics assessment performance.

Acknowledgement. This work was supported by the National Natural Science Foundation of China (Grant No. 61273365 and No. 61100120) and the Fundamental Research Funds for the Central Universities (No. 2013RC0304).

References

1. Murray, N., Marchesotti, L., Perronnin, F.: Learning to rank images using semantic and aesthetic labels. In: 23th British Machine and Vision Conference (BMVC) (2012)
2. Geng, B., Yang, L., Xu, C., Hua, X.S., Li, S.: The role of attractiveness in web image search. In: Proceedings of the 19th ACM International Conference on Multimedia, pp. 63–72 (2011)
3. Wang, Y., Dai, Q., Feng, R., Jiang, Y.G.: Beauty is here: evaluating aesthetics in videos using multimodal features and free training data. In: Proceedings of the 21st ACM International Conference on Multimedia, pp. 369–372 (2013)
4. Bhattacharya, S., Nojavanasghari, B., Chen, T., Liu, D., Chang, S.F., Shah, M.: Towards a comprehensive computational model for aesthetic assessment of videos. In: Proceedings of the 21st ACM International Conference on Multimedia, pp. 361–364 (2013)

5. Damera-Venkata, N., Kite, T., Geisler, W., Evans, B., Bovik, A.: Image quality assessment based on a degradation model. IEEE Trans. Image Process. **9**, 636–650 (2000)
6. Li, X.: Blind image quality assessment. In: Proceedings, 2002 International Conference on Image Processing, vol. 1, pp. 449–452 (2002)
7. Datta, R., Joshi, D., Li, J., Wang, J.Z.: Studying aesthetics in photographic images using a computational approach. In: Leonardis, A., Bischof, H., Pinz, A. (eds.) ECCV 2006. LNCS, vol. 3953, pp. 288–301. Springer, Heidelberg (2006)
8. Ke, Y., Tang, X., Jing, F.: The design of high-level features for photo quality assessment. In: 2006 IEEE Computer Society Conference on Computer Vision and Pattern Recognition, vol. 1, pp. 419–426 (2006)
9. Li, C., Chen, T.: Aesthetic visual quality assessment of paintings. J. Sel. Top. Sig. Process. **3**, 236–252 (2009)
10. Luo, Y., Tang, X.: Photo and video quality evaluation: focusing on the subject. In: Forsyth, D., Torr, P., Zisserman, A. (eds.) ECCV 2008. LNCS, vol. 5304, pp. 386–399. Springer, Heidelberg (2008)
11. Luo, W., Wang, X., Tang, X.: Content-based photo quality assessment. In: 2011 IEEE International Conference on Computer Vision (ICCV), pp. 2206–2213 (2011)
12. Tang, X., Luo, W., Wang, X.: Content-based photo quality assessment. IEEE Trans. Multimedia **15**, 1930–1943 (2013)
13. Marchesotti, L., Perronnin, F., Larlus, D., Csurka, G.: Assessing the aesthetic quality of photographs using generic image descriptors. In: 2011 IEEE International Conference on Computer Vision (ICCV), pp. 1784–1791 (2011)
14. Marchesotti, L., Perronnin, F.: Learning beautiful (and ugly) attributes. In: 24th British Machine and Vision Conference (BMVC) (2013)
15. Cohen-Or, D., Sorkine, O., Gal, R., Leyvand, T., Xu, Y.Q.: Color harmonization. ACM Trans. Graph. **25**, 624–630 (2006)
16. Tang, Z., Miao, Z., Wan, Y., Wang, Z.: Color harmonization for images. J. Electron. Imaging **20**, 023001–023001–12 (2011)
17. Nishiyama, M., Okabe, T., Sato, I., Sato, Y.: Aesthetic quality classification of photographs based on color harmony. In: 2011 IEEE Conference on Computer Vision and Pattern Recognition (CVPR), pp. 33–40 (2011)
18. Pope, A.: Notes on the problem of color harmony and the geometry of color space. J. Opt. Soc. Am. **34**, 759–765 (1944)
19. O'Donovan, P., Agarwala, A., Hertzmann, A.: Color compatibility from large datasets. ACM Trans. Graph. **30**, 63:1–63:12 (2011)
20. Schloss, K., Palmer, S.: Aesthetic response to color combinations: preference, harmony, and similarity. Attention Percept. Psychophysics **73**, 551–571 (2011)
21. Holtzschue, L.: Understanding Color: An Introduction for Designers, 4th edn. Wiley, Hoboken (2011)
22. Westland, S., Laycock, K., Cheung, V., Henry, P., Mahyar, F.: Colour harmony. J. Int. Colour Assoc. **1**, 1–15 (2007)
23. Itten, J.: The Art of Color: The Subjective Experience and Objective Rationale of Color. Wiley, New York (1997)
24. Matsuda, Y.: Color Design. Asakura Shoten, Tokyo (1995)
25. Munsell, A.H.: A Grammar of Color: A Basic Treatise on the Color System. Van Nostrand Reinhold Co., New York (1969)
26. Moon, P., Spencer, D.E.: Geometric formulation of classical color harmony. J. Opt. Soc. Am. **34**, 46–50 (1944)
27. Hård, A., Sivik, L.: A theory of colors in combination descriptive model related to the NCS color-order system. Color Res. Appl. **26**, 4–28 (2001)

28. Holtzschue, L.: Understanding Color: An introduction for Designers. Wiley, New York (2011)
29. Heinrich, G.: Parameter estimation for text analysis (2005). http://www.arbylon.net/publications/text-est.pdf
30. Murray, N., Marchesotti, L., Perronnin, F.: Ava: a large-scale database for aesthetic visual analysis. In: 2012 IEEE Conference on Computer Vision and Pattern Recognition (CVPR), pp. 2408–2415 (2012)
31. O'Connor, Z.: Colour harmony revisited. Color Res. Appl. 35, 267–273 (2010)

Deconstructing Binary Classifiers
in Computer Vision

Mohsen Ali[1]([✉]) and Jeffrey Ho[2]

[1] Information Technology University, Lahore, Pakistan
mohsen.ali@itu.edu.pk
[2] University of Florida, Gainesville, USA

Abstract. This paper further develops the novel notion of deconstructive learning and proposes a practical model for deconstructing a broad class of binary classifiers commonly used in vision applications. Specifically, the problem studied in this paper is: Given an image-based binary classifier **C** as a black-box oracle, how much can we learn of its internal working by simply querying it? To formulate and answer this question computationally, we propose a novel framework that explicitly identifies and delineates the computer vision and machine learning components, and we propose an effective deconstruction algorithm for deconstructing binary classifiers with the typical two-component design that employ support vector machine or cascade of linear classifiers as their internal feature classifiers. The deconstruction algorithm simultaneously searches over a collection of candidate feature spaces by probing the spaces for the decision boundaries, using the labels provided by the given classifier. In particular, we demonstrate that it is possible to ascertain the type of kernel function used by the classifier and the number of support vectors (and the subspace spanned by the support vectors) using only image queries and ascertain the unknown feature space too. Furthermore, again using only simple image queries, we are able to completely deconstruct OpenCV's pedestrian detector, ascertain the exact feature used, the type of classifier employed and recover the (almost) exact linear classifier.

1   Introduction

This paper further develops on the notion of deconstructive learning [1] and proposes a practical model for deconstructing a broad family of binary classifiers (e.g., object detectors) in computer vision. While the ultimate objective of all types of learning in computer vision is the determination of classifiers from labeled training data, for deconstructive learning, the objects of interest are the classifiers themselves. As its name suggests, the goal of deconstructive learning is to deconstruct a given binary classifier **C** by determining and characterizing (as much as possible) the full extent of its capability, revealing all of its

---

Electronic supplementary material The online version of this chapter (doi:10.1007/978-3-319-16811-1_31) contains supplementary material, which is available to authorized users.

© Springer International Publishing Switzerland 2015
D. Cremers et al. (Eds.): ACCV 2014, Part III, LNCS 9005, pp. 468–482, 2015.
DOI: 10.1007/978-3-319-16811-1_31

power, subtlety and limitation. As an example, imagine that we are presented with a classifier of great repute, say a pedestrian (human) detector. The detector, as a binary classifier of images, is presented only as a binary executable that takes images as inputs and outputs ± 1 as its decision for each image. The classifier is laconic in the sense that except the predicted label ± 1, it does not divulge any other information such as confidence level or classification margin associated with each decision. However, we are allowed to query the detector (classifier) using images, and the problem studied in this paper is to determine the inner working of the classifier using only image queries and the classifier's laconic responses. For example, can we determine the type of features it uses? What kind of internal classifier does it deploy? Support vector machine (SVM) or cascade of linear classifiers or something else? If it uses SVM internally, what kind of kernel function does it use? How many support vectors are there and what are the support vectors?

Similar to many problems tackled in computer vision, deconstructive learning is an inverse problem; therefore, without an appropriate regularization, the problem is ill-posed and it is impossible to define desired solutions. In particular, since we are allowed to access only the laconic responses of the classifier, the scope seems almost unbounded. The appropriate notion of regularization in this context is to define a tractable domain on which solutions can be sought, and the main contribution of this paper is the proposal of a computational framework that would allow us to pose and answer the above questions as computationally tractable problems. Our proposal is based on a specific assumption on the classifier $\mathbf{C}$ that its internal structure follows the common two-component design: a feature-transform component that transforms the input image into a feature and a machine-learning component that produces the output by applying its internal classifier to the feature (see Fig. 1). Many existing binary classifiers in computer vision follow this type of design, a clear demonstration of the division of labor between practitioners in computer vision and machine learning. For example, most of the well-known detectors such as face and pedestrian detectors (e.g., [2–4]) conform to this particular design, with other lesser-known but equally-important examples in scene classification, object recognition and others (e.g., [5,6]) adopting the same design. By clearly delineating the vision and learning components, we can formulate a computational framework for deconstructing $\mathbf{C}$ as the identification problem for its two internal components from a finite collection of potential candidates.

More precisely, for a given vision classifier $\mathbf{C}$ (e.g., an object detector), the deconstruction process requires a list of features (and their associated transforms) $\mathcal{F}$ and a list of (machine learning) classifiers $\mathcal{C}$. Based on these two lists, the algorithm would either identify the components of $\mathbf{C}$ among the elements in $\mathcal{F}$ and $\mathcal{C}$ or return a void to indicate failure in identification. Computationally, the lists define the problem domain, and they constitute the required minimal prior knowledge of $\mathbf{C}$. In practice, the general outline of the feature used in a particular vision algorithm is often known and can be ascertained through various sources such as publications. However, important design parameters such as smoothing values, cell/block/bin sizes etc., are often not available and these parameters can be determined by searching over an expected range of values that made up the elements in $\mathcal{F}$. Similarly, the type of classifier used can often be narrowed down to a small number of choices (e.g., an SVM or a cascade of linear classifiers). Within this context, we introduce three novel notions, feature identifiers, classifier deconstructors and geometric feature-classifier compatibility, as the main technical components of the deconstruction process. Specifically, feature identifiers are a set of image-based operations such as image rotations and scalings that can be applied to the input images, and the different degree of sensitivity and stability of the features in $\mathcal{F}$ under these operations would allow us to exclude elements in $\mathcal{F}$, making the process more efficient. For example, suppose $\mathcal{F}$ contains both SIFT and HOG-based features. Since SIFT is in principle rotationally invariant, SIFT-based features are more stable under image rotations than HOG-based features; and therefore, if $\mathbf{C}$ uses a SIFT-based feature internally, it outputs would be expected to be more stable under image rotations. Therefore, by querying $\mathbf{C}$ with rotated images and comparing the results with un-rotated images, we can exclude features in $\mathcal{F}$ that are rotationally sensitive. The classifier deconstructors, on the other hand, are algorithms that can deconstruct classifiers in $\mathcal{C}$ using a (relatively) small number of features by recognizing certain geometric characteristics of the classifier's decision boundary (e.g., its parametric form). For example, an SVM deconstructor algorithm is able to (given sufficiently many features) determine the number of support vectors and the type of kernel used by a kernel machine by recognizing certain geometric characteristics of its decision boundary. The interaction between elements in $\mathcal{F}$ and $\mathcal{C}$ during the deconstruction process is based on the notion of geometric feature-classifier compatibility: for a pair (f, c) of feature f and classifier c, they are compatible if given sufficiently many features defined by f, the deconstructor algorithm associated to c can correctly recognize its decision boundary. More specifically, given a vision classifier $\mathbf{C}$ internally represented by a pair (f, c) of feature f and classifier c, we can query $\mathbf{C}$ using a set of images $\mathbf{I}_1, ..., \mathbf{I}_n$, and using the feature (and it associated transform) f, we can transform the images into features in the feature space specified by f. The deconstructor algorithm associated with c then determines the classifier based on these features. However, for an incorrect hypothetical pair $(\overline{f}, c)$, the difference between the transformed features specified by $\overline{f}$ and f are generally non-linear, and this non-linearity changes the geometric characteristics of the decision boundary in the feature space specified by $\overline{f}$, rendering the deconstructor algorithm c unable to identify the decision boundary (see Fig. 1). The abstract framework outlined above provides a practical and useful modularization of the deconstruction process so that the individual elements such as the formation of feature and classifier lists, feature identifiers and classifier deconstructors can be subject to independent development and study. In this paper, we realize the abstract framework in concrete terms. Specifically, we introduce two deconstructor algorithms for support vector machine (SVM) and for the cascade of linear classifiers. The former is a popular family of classifiers widely used in vision applications and the latter is often deployed in object detectors, with the face detector of Viola-Jones as perhaps the most well-known example [4]. In the experimental section, we present three preliminary experimental results demonstrating the viability of the ideas proposed in this paper. In the first experiment, we show the application of a few

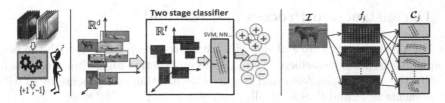

Fig. 1. Left: Schematic illustration of deconstructive learning. **Center:** Two-component design of a classifier: a feature-transform component provided by computer vision followed by a feature-classification component furnished by machine learning. **Right:** Schematic illustration of the proposed deconstruction algorithm. Internally, the algorithm searches over a set of candidate feature spaces and probes the spaces for decision boundaries. Only in the correct feature space the parametric form of the decision boundary would be recognized by the deconstructor algorithm.

simple heuristics can substantially reduce the size of feature list $\mathcal{F}$ and therefore, allow for a more efficient deconstruction process. In the second experiment, we show, using MNIST dataset, how the type of kernel functions used in a support vector machine and the number of support vectors can be determined using only image queries. In the third and final experiment, we present the result of a complete deconstruction of OpenCV's HOG-based pedestrian detector. The entire deconstruction process searches over one hundred potential features to correctly identify the linear classifier used in the detector. The normal vector of the linear classifier recovered by our algorithm has the normalized correlation of more than 0.99 with the ground truth (i.e., with an angular difference smaller than $2°$). The MATLAB implementation of the deconstruction algorithm is only around 100 lines of code and it takes no longer than an hour to correctly identify the feature, the classifier type (linear SVM) and the linear classifier itself.

Related Work. To the best of our knowledge, there is not a previous work on deconstructive learning comparable to the one outlined above. However, [7] studied the problem of deconstructing linear classifiers in a context that is quite different from ours. Since only single linear classifiers are studied and there is no explicit considerations of the interaction between feature transforms and classifiers, their scope is considerably narrower than ours. Active learning (e.g., [8–10]) shares certain similarities with deconstructive learning (**DL**) in that it also has a notion of querying a source (classifier). However, the main distinction is their specificities and outlooks: for active learning, it is general and relative while for **DL**, it is specific and absolute. More precisely, for active learning, the goal is to determine a classifier from a concept class with some prescribed (PAC-like) learning error bound using samples generated from the underlying joint distribution of feature and label. In this model, the learning target is the joint distribution and the optimal learned classifier is relative to the given concept class. On the other hand, in **DL**, the learning target is a given classifier and the classifier defines an absolute partition of the feature space into two disjoint regions of positive and negative features. In this absolute setting, geometry replaces probability as the joint feature-label distribution gives way to the geometric notion of decision boundary as the main target of learning.

2   Deconstruction Process and Method

Let $\mathcal{F}, \mathcal{C}$ denote the feature and classifier lists. Given a classifier $\mathbf{C}$ with the two-component design as described above, the deconstruction algorithm attempts to identify the feature-transform and feature-classification components of $\mathbf{C}$ with the elements in $\mathcal{F}$ and $\mathcal{C}$. Specifically, we assume that

- Each feature $f_i \in \mathcal{F}$ defines a feature transform $f_i : \mathbb{R}^d \to \mathbb{R}^{n_i}$ from the image space $\mathbb{R}^d$ to a feature space $\mathbb{R}^{n_i}$ of dimension n_i. For technical reason, the feature transform $f_i : \mathbb{R}^d \to \mathbb{R}^{n_i}$ is assumed to be Lipschitz continuous in that $\|f_i(\mathbf{I}_a) - f_i(\mathbf{I}_b)\|_2 < L_i \|\mathbf{I}_a - \mathbf{I}_b\|_2$ for some positive constant $L_i > 0$ and $\mathbf{I}_a, \mathbf{I}_b \in \mathbb{R}^d$. Furthermore, we assume that an inverse of the feature transform f_i can also be computed: for $v_i \in \mathbb{R}^{n_i}$, an image in $f_i^{-1}(v_i)$ can be computed[1].
- Each element $c_i \in \mathcal{C}$ represents a known family of classifiers (e.g., SVM and cascade of linear classifiers as two different families) and has its associated deconstructor algorithm (also denoted as c_i). For each feature space $\mathbb{R}^{n_i}$, with sufficiently many (feature) points located on a hypothetical decision boundary, c_i can determine if such decision boundary is the result of one of its member classifiers and provide other more detailed information about the specific classifier. For example, for the deconstructor associated with SVM, with enough feature points located on a hypothetical decision boundary in $\mathbb{R}^{n_i}$, it can determine if the decision boundary is the result of an SVM classifier and if so, it will return the type of kernel and the number of support vectors, etc. The number of required points on the decision boundary depends on each deconstructor algorithm.

We have assumed that the feature spaces are all continuous ($\mathbb{R}^{n_i}$) and the feature transforms f_i are surjective maps. Technically, working in continuous domains is simpler because useful differential-geometric features such as the normal vectors of the classifier's decision boundary are available. Furthermore, continuous domains allow us to locate the decision boundary within any prescribed accuracy using the simple idea of bracketing (as in root-finding [12]): given a pair of positive and negative images (PN-pair), we can produce a PN-pair of images near the decision boundary in the image space by successively halving the interval between a pair of positive and negative images, using the labels provided by $\mathbf{C}$. By Lipschitz continuity, a PN-pair (sufficiently) near the decision boundary in the image space can be transformed by a feature $f_i \in \mathcal{F}$ into a PN-pair near the decision boundary in the feature space $\mathbb{R}^{n_i}$. By sampling enough PN-pairs that are near the decision boundary in the image space, we obtain the corresponding PN-pairs near the decision boundary in each feature space $\mathbb{R}^{n_i}$ specified by the feature $f_i \in \mathcal{F}$. For these sampled PN-pairs in each feature space $\mathbb{R}^{n_i}$, we apply the deconstructor algorithm c to see if it recognizes the decision boundary from these samples. Furthermore, the inverse feature transform f_i^{-1} permits the deconstructor algorithm that operates in the (opaque) feature space $\mathbb{R}^{n_i}$ to

---

[1] For simplicity, we assume that the transform f_i is surjective and as a set (of images), $f_i^{-1}(v_i)$ is nonempty and we can compute an element (image) in $f_i^{-1}(v_i)$ (e.g., [11]).

sample additional features near the decision boundary if necessary. Essentially, each deconstructor algorithm is designed to probe a given feature space for the decision boundary and it recognizes the parametric form of the decision boundary arising from a classifier in its associated family. In particular, starting with a small number of positive features, the deconstructor algorithm proceeds to explore each feature space $\mathbb{R}^{n_i}$ by generating points near the decision boundary.

Given the two lists $\mathcal{F}, \mathcal{C}$, the deconstruction process proceeds in a direct manner: run all deconstructor algorithms in $\mathcal{C}$ in parallel over all the candidate features in $\mathcal{F}$, and for each pair (f_i, c_j) of feature (space) and deconstructor, c_i either succeeds in detecting a recognizable boundary or fails to do so. If there are no successful pairs (f_i, c_j), the algorithm then fails to deconstruct $\mathbf{C}$. Otherwise, it provides the user with all the successful pairs (f_i, c_j) as potential candidates for further investigation[2]. In this paper, the classifier list $\mathcal{C}$ contains two elements: the family of support vector machines (SVM) and the family of cascades of linear classifiers, and in the following three subsections, we provide the remaining details in the proposed deconstruction process.

2.1   Feature Identifiers

An important first step in the deconstruction process is to properly define the lists $\mathcal{F}$ and $\mathcal{C}$, with the aim of making them as short as possible. Various heuristics based on exploiting the differences between various types of features can be developed to accomplish this goal. For example, it is possible to exclude simple HOG-based features from $\mathcal{F}$ by perturbing the images slightly. In particular, because HOG (unlike SIFT) is in general not rotationally invariant, and hence, if the images are slightly rotated, we can expect less-than-stable results from the classifier $\mathbf{C}$ if it uses HOG as the main feature. In the experimental section, we study several such feature identifiers in the form of simple image operations such as rotations and scalings, and demonstrate their usefulness in excluding features in $\mathcal{F}$. On the other hand, the difference between the classifiers in $\mathcal{C}$ can also be exploited to shorten the list $\mathcal{C}$. In our case, it is straightforward to determine if the given $\mathbf{C}$ uses SVM or a cascade of linear classifiers as its internal classifier. Recall that a cascade of linear classifiers is a decision tree with a linear classifier associated with each tree node. Consequently, positive features always take longer to process than negative features and among the negative features, the running time can vary considerably depending on the depth of the tree. However, for an SVM-based $\mathbf{C}$, all features are expected to have the same or similar running times. Therefore, by checking the distribution of the running time among positive and negative features, we can determine with great certainty the type of classifier used internally by $\mathbf{C}$.

2.2   Deconstructor Methods

We summarize below prominent and important features of one the deconstructor algorithms.

---

[2] This part is beyond the scope of this paper.

Deconstructor for SVM. Given a feature space $\mathbb{R}^l$ and sufficiently many PN-pairs near the decision boundary, the deconstructor algorithm is able to

- Determine the kernel type (assuming polynomial, exponential and hyperbolic tangent kernels).
- Determine the (kernel) subspace spanned by the support vectors. If the number m of support vectors is smaller than the feature space dimension l, then the dimension of the kernel subspace also gives the number of support vectors, assuming linear independent.
- For linear SVM (i.e., one single global linear classifier), $h(\mathbf{x}) = \mathbf{n}^\top \mathbf{x} + b$, the normal vector $\mathbf{n}$ and bias b can be determined.
- In theory, the number of sampled features required is in the order of $\mathbf{O}(ml)$.

The detailed analysis of the SVM deconstructor algorithm is presented in [1] and in the remaining section, we present the simplest case of polynomial kernels, demonstrating that the kernel type and the kernel subspace can be determined by simply querying the classifier $\mathbf{C}$. Recall that the general polynomial kernel of degree d has the form: for $\mathbf{x}, \mathbf{y} \in \mathbb{R}^l$,

$$\mathbf{K}(\mathbf{x}, \mathbf{y}) = (\mathbf{x}^\top \mathbf{y} + 1)^d, \tag{1}$$

and the decision function is given as

$$\mathbf{\Psi}(\mathbf{x}) = \omega_1 \mathbf{K}(\mathbf{x}, \mathbf{y}_1) + \cdots \omega_m \mathbf{K}(\mathbf{x}, \mathbf{y}_m), \tag{2}$$

where $\mathbf{y}_i, \omega_i$ are the support vectors and their weights, respectively, and the decision boundary $\mathbf{\Sigma}$ is defined by the equation $\mathbf{\Psi}(\mathbf{x}) = b$ for some $b \geq 0$. The reason that we can determine the kernel type (in this case, the degree d) is that the locus of the intersection of the decision boundary $\mathbf{\Sigma}$ with a two-dimensional affine subspace containing a point close to the decision boundary is (generically) a polynomial curve of degree d.

More specifically, let $\mathbf{x}_+, \mathbf{x}_-$ denote a PN-pair that is sufficiently close to $\mathbf{\Sigma}$. We can randomly generate a two-dimensional subspace containing $\mathbf{x}_+, \mathbf{x}_-$ by, for example, taking the subspace $\mathbf{A}$ containing $\mathbf{x}_+, \mathbf{x}_-$ and the origin in $\mathbb{R}^l$. For a generic two-dimensional subspace $\mathbf{A}$, its intersection with $\mathbf{\Sigma}$ is an one-dimensional curve, and the parametric form of this curve is determined by the (yet unknown) kernel function. This can be easily seem as follows: take $\mathbf{x}_+$ as the origin on $\mathbf{A}$ and choose an (arbitrary) pair of orthonormal vectors $\mathbf{U}_1, \mathbf{U}_2 \in \mathbb{R}^l$ such that the triplet $\mathbf{x}_+, \mathbf{U}_1, \mathbf{U}_2$ identifies $\mathbf{A}$ with $\mathbb{R}^2$. Therefore, any point $p \in \mathbf{A}$ can be uniquely identified with a two-dimensional vector $\mathbf{p} = [\mathbf{p}_1, \mathbf{p}_2] \in \mathbb{R}^2$ as

$$p = \mathbf{x}_+ + \mathbf{p}_1 \mathbf{U}_1 + \mathbf{p}_2 \mathbf{U}_2. \tag{3}$$

If $\mathbf{p} \in \mathbf{A}$ is a point in the intersection of $\mathbf{A}$ with the decision boundary $\mathbf{\Psi}(\mathbf{p}) = \mathbf{b}$, we have

$$\sum_{i=1}^{l} w_i((\mathbf{x}_+^\top \mathbf{Y}_i + \mathbf{p}_1 \mathbf{U}_1^\top \mathbf{Y}_i + \mathbf{p}_2 \mathbf{U}_2^\top \mathbf{Y}_i) + 1)^d = \mathbf{b}, \tag{4}$$

which is a polynomial of degree d in the two variables $\mathbf{p}_1, \mathbf{p}_2$. Therefore, to ascertain the degree of the polynomial kernel, we can (assuming $d < 4$).

- Sample at least 9 points on the intersection of the Σ and $\mathbf{A}$.
- Fit a bivariate polynomial of degree d to the points. If the fitting error is sufficiently small, this gives a good indication that the polynomial kernel is indeed of degree d.

On the other hand, the reason that the kernel subspace $\mathbf{S_Y}$ spanned by the support vectors $\mathbf{y}_i$ can be recovered is the following well-known formula for the normal vector of the decision boundary at a point $\mathbf{x} \in \Sigma$:

$$\mathbf{n}(\mathbf{x}) = \nabla \Psi(\mathbf{x}) = \sum_{i=1}^{m} \alpha \, d\, \omega_i \left(\mathbf{x}^\top \mathbf{y}_i + 1\right)^{d-1} \mathbf{y}_i. \tag{5}$$

We remark that even though the support vectors $\mathbf{y}_i$ and weights ω_i are unknown, the above formula shows that the normal vectors of the decision boundary Σ span the kernel subspace $\mathbf{S_Y}$. Therefore, if sufficiently many points on Σ and their normal vectors can be determined, the kernel subspace can also be determined. For non-polynomial kernels, the corresponding formula for the normal vectors is more complicated and the algorithm to extract the kernel subspace from the sampled normal vectors requires a more elaborated convex optimization.

2.3   Geometric Compatibility Between Features and Deconstructors

In the deconstruction process, the interaction between the features in $\mathcal{F}$ and deconstructors in $\mathcal{C}$ is based on the notion of geometry compatibility, and the deconstruction algorithm selects the pair (f, c) as a solution if the deconstructor algorithm c recognizes the decision boundary from a collection of sampled points in the feature space $\mathbb{R}^n$ specified by f. The geometric picture is neatly captured by the following diagram:

$$
\begin{array}{ccc}
\mathbb{R}^d & \xrightarrow{f_2} & \mathbb{R}^{n_2} \\
\cong \downarrow & & \uparrow \pi \\
\mathbb{R}^d & \xrightarrow{f_1} & \mathbb{R}^{n_1}
\end{array}
$$

Suppose f_1, f_2 are two features in $\mathcal{F}$ with their respective feature spaces $\mathbb{R}^{n_1}, \mathbb{R}^{n_2}$, and the vision classifier $\mathbf{C}$ internally employs the pair (f_1, c). Therefore, if we reconstruct the decision boundary in the correct feature space $\mathbb{R}^{n_1}$, the deconstructor algorithm would be able to recognize the decision boundary and hence the pair (f_1, c) would be selected by the deconstruction algorithm. However, for the incorrect feature f_2, the decision boundary reconstructed in $\mathbb{R}^{n_2}$ is related to the decision boundary reconstructed in $\mathbb{R}^{n_1}$ via a map π that arises from the fact that we use the same set of images in the image space $\mathbb{R}^d$ to reconstruct the decision boundary in both $\mathbb{R}^{n_1}$ and $\mathbb{R}^{n_2}$. The important observation (or assumption) is that for different features f_1, f_2, the map π is generally nonlinear and it would map the decision boundary in $\mathbb{R}^{n_1}$ to a decision boundary $\mathbb{R}^{n_2}$ with an unknown parametric form. For example (as will be shown later), for a linear decision boundary in $\mathbb{R}^{n_1}$, the corresponding decision boundary in $\mathbb{R}^{n_2}$ would generally be nonlinear. Therefore, if c is a deconstructor for linear classifier, it would fail to recognize the decision boundary in $\mathbb{R}^{n_2}$. For SVM deconstructor, the map π essentially maps a decision boundary of a known parametric form to a boundary with unknown parametric form, i.e., the decision boundary in $\mathbb{R}^{n_2}$ is not compatible with the deconstructor c.

3   Experiments

In this section, we present three experimental results. In the first experiment, we demonstrate the idea of using simple heuristics (image operations) to shorten the feature list $\mathcal{F}$. In the second experiment, we show that with real image data how a classifier employing polynomial kernel can be deconstructed. In the third experiment, we detail the experimental result of deconstructing the pedestrian (human) detector in the OpenCV library. More experimental results are presented in the supplemental material.

Table 1. Effects of different image transforms on classification results. HOG-based features as expected produce unstable results under rotation and scale change.

	SIFT + BoW	Dense-SIFT + spatial pyramid	HOG(4)	HOG(8)
Rotation(180°)	0.8000	0.4300	0.6800	0.7450
Zoom-in	0.9950	0.9600	0.3550	0.3850
Translation (8,8)	0.9550	0.8500	0.9550	0.9350

3.1   Distinguish Between HOG and SIFT

Many vision algorithms use features derived from the well-known gradient-based features such as HOG [13] or SIFT [14]. To shorten the search list $\mathcal{F}$, we use various invariance properties of these features. For examples, with non-dense SIFT used in the bag of words model, it is generally invariant under scale, rotation and even shifting transformation. On the other hand, the dense SIFT, when used in a pyramid scheme, is generally invariant under *reasonable* amount of scale change, image flipping and small amount of translations. It is generally not invariant under rotation or flipping (unless object is symmetric). HOG as mentioned previously in not invariant under rotation, although it is invariant under small amount of translation when it is smaller than the size of its cells. In this experiment, we experimentally demonstrate the above general impression on the invariance property of the HOG and SIFT under various image transforms. We compared these properties of the four different type features (see Table 1 and supplementary materials for further details) by constructing aeroplane SVM classifiers using the images from Caltech 101 dataset [15]. We randomly selected 100 aeroplane images as positive samples and 100 images from other categories as negative samples. We used four type features extracted from these samples to

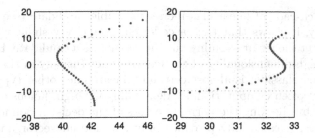

Fig. 2. Examples of the intersection of the decision boundary Σ with a 2–D subspace.

train linear SVMs. In the test phase, three simple image transforms are applied to the 200 randomly selected test images. The transformations are 180° rotation, a translation of eight pixels in both x and y directions, and a simple zoom in (achieved by scaling the by a factor of 1.2 and cropping the boundaries). The classification rates of the SVMs constructed using the four different types of features and under the three transforms are demonstrated in Table 1. As shown in the table, rotational invariance of SIFT make it relatively stable under rotation and scale transforms. We use these invariance results to decrease out feature list during our experiments.

3.2 Deconstructing a Cubic Kernel Machine

In this experiment we trained a simple SVM classifier with cubic kernel using images from the MNIST dataset [2]. These images were not subjected to feature transform and the SVM was trained directly on the vectorized images. Using the method described earlier, we perform bracketing to locate pairs of positive and negative features (PN-pairs) that are close to the decision boundary. Given a PN-pair $\mathbf{x}_+, \mathbf{x}_-$, we randomly generate a two-dimensional subspace $\mathbf{A}$ containing these two points and compute the intersection of the decision boundary Σ with the subspace. We remark that this intersection can be easily computed by randomly generating points on the subspace $\mathbf{A}$ and applying bracketing on $\mathbf{A}$. Two typical intersections are shown in Fig. 2 and both examples display the "two humps" characteristic of cubic curves. Small fitting error, when approximating each curve with bivariate cubic polynomial, is a good indication that the underlying polynomial kernel is of degree three.

3.3 Deconstructing OpenCV HOG-Based Pedestrian Detector

In this experiment, we deconstruct the pedestrian (human) detector provided in the OpenCV library [16]. This implementation is based on the algorithm proposed in [13], where histogram of oriented gradients (HOG) is used as feature with linear (SVM) classifier as internal feature classifier. The goal of this deconstruction experiment is to recover. **(a)** The three important design parameters for the HOG feature: cell size, block size and block stride. **(b)** The parameters for the linear (SVM) classifier: its weight (normal) vector and bias. For this experiment, a quick check on the running times of a few positive images immediately rules out the cascade of linear classifiers as a viable candidate (see Sect. 3.1) or more precisely, it shows that the cascade must be a very shallow tree and we simply interpret the result as ruling out the cascade as a candidate. Furthermore, because the high-dimensionality of the feature space (usually in the thousands), the SVM-based classifier is almost certainly linear, since other types of nonlinear kernels are often computationally demanding for high-dimensional features. In particular, by checking the normal vectors of the decision boundary at forty different places, it essentially provides only one normal vector, indicating the underlying linear classifier. Therefore, the classifier list C has only one element and the kernel type is assumed to be linear. For the feature list F, we define approximately 30 candidate parameter settings and accordingly, the feature list F has length 100. More specifically, the cell size can take the three integral values $\{4, 8, 16\}$, and for each cell size, the block size can equal to cell size, double the cell size or triple the cell size. Similarly, the block stride is set either to half of the block size, the full block size or twice the block size. We note that different parameters give different HOG features that typically reside in different feature spaces (in particular, with different dimension). Note that since we randomly pair positive and negative images, PN-pair set can have size equal to product of size of positive image set and negative image set. This restricts which feature dimensions we can take in consideration. We use the classifier as provided in the OpenCV without any modification and positive and negative images are obtained by running the classifier over a set of images. We remark that the positive and negative images are according to the outputs of the classifier C, not visually which class they should belong to. We randomly pair these positive and negative images and run the bracketing algorithm to locate PN-pairs (Fig. 3) close to the decision boundary in the (fixed) image space, and for each such PN-pair close to the decision boundary in the image space, we compute its corresponding PN-pair in each of the feature space $\mathbb{R}^{n_i}$ for $f_i \in F$. In this experiment, we do not use the inverse feature transform to determine the feature labels in the feature space, although inverse transform for HOG-based features has been proposed in [11].

An important experimental result is that linear decision boundary is observed only for the correct parameter setting, while for incorrect parameter setting, the

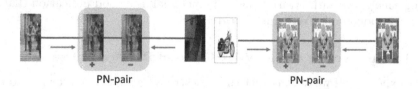

PN-pair   PN-pair

Fig. 3. Example showing PN pair recovered as the process of the bracketing. Notice that even when they appear to be very similar, one is labeled as positive sample by OpenCV person classifier and other as negative. A similar behavior is visible in the right figure where we trained HOG based SVM classifier for Motorcycle class in Caltech101 dataset [15].

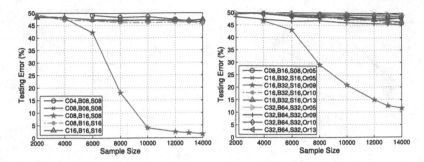

Fig. 4. LEFT: Deconstruction of OpenCV Pedestrian Detector: Classification errors for the FLD trained in five different feature spaces. The feature parameters are given in the legend (cell size, block size) and the visible decrease in classification rates is observed only in the correct feature space. **RIGHT: Deconstruction of airplane Detector.** Number of Orientations (number of bins) is also varied in this experiment, as indicated by the plots correct number of bins quite strongly impact the results

decision boundary is generally nonlinear. To efficiently and accurate detect the linear boundary in these high-dimensional feature spaces, we use Fisher linear discriminant (FLD). Specifically, for the labeled PN-pairs in each candidate feature space, we train a Fisher linear discriminant. If the labeled features are indeed linearly separable, the Fisher linear discriminant would detect it by correctly classifying large portion of the label features. Furthermore, in the right feature space, as we generate more PN-pairs that are close to true decision boundary, the linear classifier provided by FLD will move closer to the true linear classifier. This latter statement is easily visualized and its rigorous justification seems straightforward. In particular, the linear classifier determined by FLD provides good approximations to the weight (normal) vector and the bias of the true linear classifier. On the other hand, in the wrong feature space, the decision boundary would be nonlinear and the trained FLD is not expected to correctly classify large portion of the labeled features, regardless the number of PN-pairs generated. Experimental confirmations of these observations are shown in Figs. 4 and 5. In Fig. 4, the classification error of the trained FLD decreases only in the correct feature space. And in Fig. 5, 2D projections of the labeled PN-pairs in three different feature spaces are displayed and linear separability is clearly shown only for features from the correct feature space. The weight (normal) vector recovered using FLD with 10,000 PN-pairs has the normalization correlation of 0.99 with the ground truth, i.e., with an angular difference of roughly $2°$.

4   The Case and Outlook for Deconstructive Learning

Image-based classifications such as face, pedestrian and various object detections and scene recognition are important computer vision applications that have begun to have visible and noticeable impact in our daily life. Indeed, with

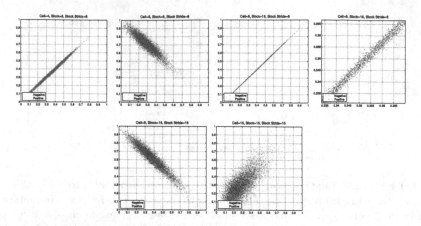

Fig. 5. 2D projections of the labeled PN-pairs in three different feature spaces. The 2-D projected subspace is spanned by the normal vector determined by FLD and the first singular vector for the collection of features. The results from the correct feature space is shown as the second pair, the two plots display the projections in two different scales.

the current trend in technology development, it is not difficult to envision a not-so-distant future in which the world is partially powered by such applications. In the backdrop of such futuristic vision, deconstructive learning points to an interesting and uncharted territory, perhaps a promising new direction with potential for generating important impacts. Several potential consequences of this new capability are interesting to ponder. A case in point is the OpenCV's HOG-based pedestrian detector. To develop such an application, the designers must have spent weeks if not months of effort in, among other things, gathering useful training images, managing other often time-consuming logistic matters and tuning both the feature parameters (cell/block/bin sizes) and the learning algorithm in order to obtain the best (linear) classifier. However, as demonstrated in this paper, the detector can be completely deconstructed in a few hours and the user of the deconstruction algorithm only requires to collect a few positive images to start the deconstruction process, since the negative images can be obtained randomly (with labels provided by the classifier **C**). The result is certainly not surprising since it basically mirrors the well-known fact that finding a solution is always more time-consuming than checking the solution. However, its implications are multiple and perhaps profound. For example, the result of months or even years of hard work can be deconstructed in a matter of a few hours, even when it is hidden under the seemingly impenetrable binary codes. On a more practical side, we believe that deconstructive learning could provide greater flexibility to the users of AI/machine learning products in the future because it allows the users to determine the full extent of an AI/ML program/system, and therefore, create his/her own adaptation or modification of the given system for specific and specialized tasks. For example, how would an ACCV reviewer know that a submitted binary code of a paper really does implement the algorithm proposed in the paper, not some clever implementation of some known algorithm? Deconstructive learning proposed in this paper offers a possible solution by explicitly deconstructing the submitted code. Finally, perhaps the most compelling reason for studying deconstructive learning is inscribed by the famous motto uttered by David Hilbert more than eighty years ago: we must know and we will know! Indeed, when presented with a black-box classifier (especially the one with great repute), we have found the problem of determining the secret of its inner working by simply querying it with images both fascinating and challenging, a problem with its peculiar elegance and charm.

In this paper, we have demonstrated the viability of deconstructive learning. Although the classifier list C consists of only two families, both SVM and linear cascades are widely-used classifiers in computer vision applications. Work is currently ongoing to expand the feature and classifier lists $\mathcal{F}, C$ to include structured SVM [17], dictionary-learning-based classifier [18], bag of words features [19] and others. Recently, neural network-based classifiers such as those emerged from the deep learning community [20,21] has gained considerable interest and popularity. At the first glance, the direct approach proposed in this paper seems insufficient and inadequate for deconstructing this type of classifiers. However, we believe that more indirect approaches and formulations are possible, with the aim of identifying crucial information that are necessary for the deconstruction process.

5   Conclusions

We have proposed a novel framework for deconstructing binary classifiers that follow the common two-component design: a feature-transform component followed by a feature-classification component. Experimental results have confirmed both the viability and practicality of the proposed deconstruction algorithm. While much work remains for the future, the results in our paper perhaps serve as a small but substantial step towards a better understanding of deconstructive learning, hitherto an uncharted territory that seems ripe for further exploration.

Acknowledgement. We in particular would like to thank one of the reviewers for his/her helpful comment and enthusiasm for our paper.

References

1. Ali, M., Rushdi, M., Ho, J.: Deconstructing kernel machines. In: Calders, T., Esposito, F., Hüllermeier, E., Meo, R. (eds.) ECML PKDD 2014, Part I. LNCS, vol. 8724, pp. 34–49. Springer, Heidelberg (2014)
2. LeCun, Y., Bottou, L., Bengio, Y., Haffner, P.: Gradient-based learning applied to document recognition. Proc. IEEE **86**, 2278–2324 (1998)
3. Benenson, R., Mathias, M., Timofte, R., Van Gool, L.: Pedestrian detection at 100 frames per second. In: CVPR (2012)

4. Viola, P., Jones, M.: Rapid object detection using a boosted cascade of simple features. In: Proceedings of the 2001 IEEE Computer Society Conference on Computer Vision and Pattern Recognition, CVPR 2001, vol. 1, p. I-511. IEEE (2001)

5. Fei-Fei, L., Perona, P.: A bayesian hierarchical model for learning natural scene categories. In: IEEE Computer Society Conference on Computer Vision and Pattern Recognition, CVPR 2005, vol. 2, pp. 524–531. IEEE (2005)

6. Bosch, A., Zisserman, A., Muñoz, X.: Scene classification via pLSA. In: Leonardis, A., Bischof, H., Pinz, A. (eds.) ECCV 2006. LNCS, vol. 3954, pp. 517–530. Springer, Heidelberg (2006)

7. Lowd, D., Meek, C.: Adversarial learning. In: Proceedings of the Eleventh ACM SIGKDD International Conference on Knowledge Discovery in Data Mining, pp. 641–647. ACM (2005)

8. Dasgupta, S.: Analysis of a greedy active learning strategy. In: Advances in Neural Information Processing Systems (2004)

9. Balcan, M., Beygelzimer, A., Langford, J.: Agnostic active learning. In: Proceedings of the International Conference Machine Learning (ICML) (2006)

10. Balcan, M.-F., Broder, A., Zhang, T.: Margin based active learning. In: Bshouty, N.H., Gentile, C. (eds.) COLT. LNCS (LNAI), vol. 4539, pp. 35–50. Springer, Heidelberg (2007)

11. Vondrick, C., Khosla, A., Malisiewicz, T., Torralba, A.: Hoggles: Visualizing object detection features. In: Proceedings of the International Conference on Computer Vision (2013)

12. Heath, M.: Scientific Computing. The McGraw-Hill Companies Inc., New York (2002)

13. Dalal, N., Triggs, B.: Histograms of oriented gradients for human detection. In: IEEE Computer Society Conference on Computer Vision and Pattern Recognition, CVPR 2005, vol. 1, pp. 886–893. IEEE (2005)

14. Lowe, D.G.: Object recognition from local scale-invariant features. In: The Proceedings of the Seventh IEEE International Conference on Computer vision, vol. 2, pp. 1150–1157. IEEE (1999)

15. Fei-Fei, L., Fergus, R., Perona, P.: One-shot learning of object categories. IEEE Trans. Pattern Anal. Mach. Intell. **28**, 594–611 (2006)

16. Bradski, G.: The OpenCV library. Dr. Dobb's J. Softw. Tools **25**, 120–126 (2000)

17. Tsochantaridis, I., Hofmann, T., Joachims, T., Altun, Y.: Support vector machine learning for interdependent and structured output spaces. In: Proceedings of the Twenty-First International Conference on Machine Learning, p. 104. ACM (2004)

18. Mairal, J., Bach, F., Ponce, J., Sapiro, G., Zisserman, A.: Discriminative learned dictionaries for local image analysis. In: IEEE Conference on Computer Vision and Pattern Recognition, CVPR 2008, pp. 1–8. IEEE (2008)

19. Csurka, G., Dance, C., Fan, L., Willamowski, J., Bray, C.: Visual categorization with bags of keypoints. In: Workshop on Statistical Learning in Computer Vision, ECCV, vol. 1, pp. 1–2 (2004)

20. Bengio, Y.: Learning deep architectures for ai. Found. Trends® Mach. Learn. **2**, 1–127 (2009)

21. Hinton, G.E., Osindero, S., Teh, Y.W.: A fast learning algorithm for deep belief nets. Neural Comput. **18**, 1527–1554 (2006)

Effective Drusen Segmentation from Fundus Images for Age-Related Macular Degeneration Screening

Huiying Liu[✉], Yanwu Xu, Damon Wing Kee Wong, and Jiang Liu

Institute for Infocomm Research, A*STAR, Singapore, Singapore
liuhy@i2r.a-star.edu.sg

Abstract. Automatic screening of Age-related Macular Degeneration (AMD) is important for both patients and ophthalmologists. The major sign of contracting AMD at the early stage is the appearance of drusen, which are the accumulation of extracellular material and appear as yellow-white spots on the retina. In this paper, we propose an effective approach for drusen segmentation towards AMD screening. The major novelty of the proposed approach is that it employs an effective way to train a drusen classifier from a weakly labeled dataset, meaning only the existence of drusen is known but not the exact locations or boundaries. We achieve this by employing Multiple Instance Learning (MIL). Moreover, our proposed approach also tracks the drusen boundaries by using Growcut, with the output of MIL as initial seeds. Experiments on 350 fundus images with 96 of them with AMD demonstrates that our approach outperforms the state-of-the-art methods on the task of early AMD detection and achieves satisfying performance on the task of drusen segmentation.

1 Introduction

Age-related Macular Degeneration (AMD), after cataract and glaucoma, is the third leading cause of blindness worldwide and the first leading cause in the elderly [1,2]. It is a kind of maculopothy that usually affects older adults and results in a loss of vision in the center of the visual field. Approximately 10 % of patients 66 to 74 years of age will have findings of macular degeneration. The prevalence increases to 30 % in patients 75 to 85 years of age. According to the statistical data of World Health Organization, till 2010, there were nearly 2 million occurrences of AMD in the United States. The number is projected to be over 5 million in 2050 (http://www.who.int/research/en/).

Population based AMD screening is in necessity for its increasing prevalence. However, symptoms (e.g., vision scotoma and distortion) at the early stage of AMD are generally not obvious to be observed. So it is usually late when patients are found out to have contracted AMD. As a result of that, the vision of those patients may be permanently lost. Therefore, it is of great importance to detect AMD at the early stage, and patients can thus take treatment to prevent it from

© Springer International Publishing Switzerland 2015
D. Cremers et al. (Eds.): ACCV 2014, Part III, LNCS 9005, pp. 483–498, 2015.
DOI: 10.1007/978-3-319-16811-1_32

getting worse. For the patients already diagnosed with AMD, accurate grading is important to customize a suitable treating strategy. Regular screening is a potential way to detect early AMD and grade AMD. However, manual detection and grading of AMD are time consuming and labor intensive. More importantly, because the grading is usually subjective (graded by human clinicians), a certain degree of inaccuracy may be introduced.

Automatic AMD screening brings profits for both patients and ophthalmologists, hence it has attracted much research effort in these years. The major sign of early AMD is the appearance of drusen [3,4]. Drusen appear as yellow-white spot on digital fundus image, which is the mainstream and most popular imaging modality for AMD diagnosis. Examples of drusen are shown in Fig. 1(b) and (c). Drusen detection has significant importance for early AMD detection, while drusen segmentation is important for AMD grading. Here we refer to drusen detection as identifying the existence of drusen in a fundus image, while drusen segmentation as finding the location and boundary of drusen.

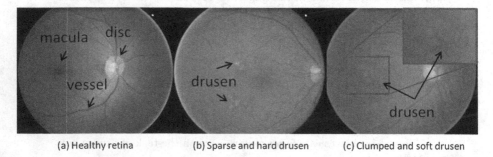

(a) Healthy retina   (b) Sparse and hard drusen   (c) Clumped and soft drusen

Fig. 1. Examples of fundus images with and without drusen. (a) A healthy fundus image. (b) A fundus image with sparse drusen. (c) A fundus image with clumped drusen, of poor image quality (Color figure online).

In this paper, we propose a novel method which is not only able to detect early AMD but also segment drusen at the same time. The flowchart of the proposed method is shown in Fig. 2. Our method first extracts local extreme points, i.e., maximum points and minimum points, in scale space. The maximum points are considered as potential drusen candidates. Edge Direction Histogram (EDH), SPIN feature, Gabor coefficients, intensity, position, and contrast are extracted at these maximum points. Then Multiple Instance Learning (MIL) is used to train a classifier from the weakly labeled data to classify each maximum points as drusen or non-drusen [5]. For a fundus image, if drusen are detected, it will be classified as early AMD. Finally, if drusen are detected, Growcut is employed to segment drusen [6]. The maximum points classified as drusen are used as foreground seeds. The ones classified as non-drusen, together with the minimum points, are used as background seeds. These seeds are fed into Growcut to get boundaries of drusen.

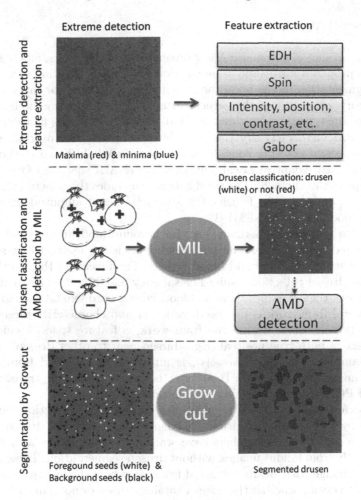

Fig. 2. The flowchart of the proposed method.

The contribution of this paper is that we propose an effective approach of drusen segmentation for AMD screening. The major contributions of this approach are as follows. (1) It is not only able to detect AMD but also to track the locations and boundaries of drusen for further AMD grading. (2) It employs Multiple Instance Learning (MIL) to train the detectors from a weakly labeled dataset thus significantly reduces the need for manual labeling. (3) It employs Growcut to track the boundaries of drusen, by using the output of MIL as initial seeds.

In the rest of this paper, we will review the state-of-the-art methods in Sect. 2. Then we will detail in Sect. 3 the proposed drusen segmentation approach, including extreme points detection, feature descriptors, classification using MIL, and segmentation using Growcut. In Sect. 4, we will show the experimental results on both AMD detection and drusen segmentation. Finally, we will conclude this paper with future work in Sect. 5.

2   Related Work

For the importance of automatic AMD screening, in recent years, lots of methods have been proposed for drusen segmentation and AMD detection. The existing drusen segmentation methods can be classified into three major categories. The first category, consisting of the earliest drusen segmentation methods, is based on local maxima, e.g., the geodesic method [7]. These methods first detect local maxima, then further classify the candidates according to contrast, size and shape. The second category consists of the local threshold based methods, e.g., Histogram based Adaptive Local Thresholding (HALT) [8], and Otsu method based adaptive threshold [9]. The third category includes the ones from frequency domain, e.g., wavelet [10], Fourier transform [11], and amplitude-modulation frequency modulation (AM-FM) [12].

There are some other methods, e.g., background modeling method [13] and saliency based method [11]. The background modeling method first segments the healthy structure of eye and blood vessels. The inverse of the healthy parts provide the drusen detection result. The saliency based method first detects the salient regions then classifies them as blood vessel, hard exudates or drusen. In [14], a general framework is proposed to detect and characterize target lesions almost instantaneously. Within the framework, a feature space, including the confounders of both true positive (e.g., dursen near to other drusen) and false positive samples (e.g., blood vessels), is automatically derived from a set of reference image samples. Then Haar filter is used to build the transformation space and PCA is used to generate the optimal filter.

The performance of drusen segmentation based AMD detection methods is restricted by the accuracy of drusen segmentation. To bypass drusen segmentation, in recent years, researchers have started to seek for methods detecting AMD directly from fundus images, without drusen segmentation. These methods describe an image with locally extracted features, where the features are fed into a classifier to decide whether the image contains drusen or not. An early attempt in this direction was a histogram based representation followed by Case-Based Reasoning [15]. Good results were produced, however observations indicated that relying on the retinal image colour distribution alone was not sufficient. Thus, the authors further proposed a method by using a spatial histogram technique to include colour and spatial information [16]. The latest work from the same team comprises a hierarchical image decomposition mechanism, founded on either a circular and angular partitioning or a pyramid partitioning. The resulting decomposition is then stored in a tree structure to which a weighted frequent sub-tree mining algorithm is applied. The identified sub-graphs are then incorporated into a feature vector representation (one vector per image) to which classification techniques can be applied [17,18]. The latest methods in this category include Biologically Inspired Feature (BIF) based method [19] and Hierarchical Word Image representation and SPIN features based method named Thalia [20].

Although the methods detecting AMD without drusen segmentation show some progress, drusen segmentation has its importance in AMD grading. The severity of AMD is usually measured according to position, size, type (hard or soft), together with geographic atrophy and other symptoms. The overlap of drusen with macula is used to measure the severity of AMD [21,22].

3   The Proposed Method

As shown in Fig. 1, drusen appear as yellow-white spots on fundus images. The visual properties that discriminate drusen from the other structures of retina are summarized as follows, together with the corresponding strategy adopted to describe the property.

1. Drusen appear brighter than the healthy part, except the optical disk, of the retina (Fig. 1). However, the light on the fundus image is not uniform thus drusen are not globally brighter. We detect local maximum points as drusen candidates and use contrast as a feature for classification.
2. Drusen don't have exact size thus we extract local maxima at multiple scales to detect drusen of different sizes.
3. Drusen are near round spots. Shape distinguishes drusen from the regions near vessels which are likely to be detected as drusen but drusen don't have rigid shape (Fig. 1(b) and (c)). We adopt edge direction histogram to describe shape and adopt SPIN feature to describe the color-spatial structure of drusen.
4. Drusen may appear differently due to different imaging conditions (Fig. 1(c)). Thus we adopt local texture, which is more robust to lighting condition than color. Gabor coefficients are used for this purpose.

The above detected and described maximum points are fed into multiple instance learning to train a classifier, which is used for drusen classification.

Tracking drusen boundaries is facing two difficulties. First, drusen have two types, hard drusen and soft drusen. Soft drusen usually don't have sharp boundary thus result in the difficulty to obtain the boundary. Second, in severe condition, drusen may clump together thus increase the difficulty of drusen segmentation. Figure 1(c) shows an example of soft and clumped drusen. To address these difficulties, we employ Growcut, with the detected drusen position as seeds, to track drusen boundaries.

The flowchart of the proposed approach is shown in Fig. 2. The details of the methods are stated in the rest of this section.

3.1   Extremum Points Detection

Like SIFT [23], we detect local extrema in the scale space. We first construct the Gaussian space of the image. At each level, the image is convolved with a Gaussian function,

$$L(i, j, \sigma_k) = G(i, j, \sigma_k) * I(i, j), \qquad (1)$$

where I is the input image, (i, j) is the position in the image, $G(i, j, \sigma_k)$ is a Gaussian function with standard variance of σ_k, and $*$ is the convolution operator. Then from the Gaussian space,we construct the Laplacian space as follow,

$$D(i,j,\sigma_k) = (G(i,j,\sigma_k) - G(i,j,\sigma_{k+1})) * I(i,j)$$
$$= L(i,j,\sigma_k) - L(i,j,\sigma_{k+1}), \tag{2}$$

The Laplacian space has one less level than the Gaussian Space. We adopt $\sigma = \sqrt{2}^{\{-1,0,1,\ldots,12\}}$. A pixel is determined to be a maximum if it is a local maximum in the Laplacian space. The local window used to determine the maximum is $3 \times 3 \times 3$. Thus, we detect maximum points at scales $\sigma = \sqrt{2}^{\{0,1,\ldots,10\}}$.

In Eq. (2), $D(i,j,\sigma) = 0$ when $i^2 + j^2 = \frac{2a^2\sigma^2 \log(a^2)}{a^2-1}$. Here $a = \frac{\sigma_{k+1}}{\sigma_k}$. When $a = \sqrt{2}$, the radius of detected drusen at scale σ is $r = 1.67\sigma$. Thus the minimal and maximal diameters of detected drusen are 3 and 108 pixels respectively. Figure 2 (the top left block) illustrates an example of detected extreme points.

3.2   Feature Description

The characteristics distinguishing drusen from the background are intensity, shape, size, contrast and texture. Further, drusen usually distribute around macula. The following features are adopted to describe these characteristics.

Edge Direction Histogram is used to describe the shape of the local maxima at the corresponding scale. The histogram is weighted by the gradient magnitude and the Gaussian function. The edge direction histogram of a maximum point is

$$H(i,j,o,\sigma) = \sum_{(i',j')\in I, O(i',j',\sigma)=o} M(i',j',\sigma) \times G(i',j',\sigma) \tag{3}$$

where $O(i,j,\sigma)$ and $M(i,j,\sigma)$ are respectively the orientation and magnitude of gradient at position (i,j) and scale σ. In our experiment, the number of bins of the histogram is set as 8.

Intensity. Drusen are bright spots on the fundus thus intensity is an useful visual descriptor of drusen. We adopt intensity at the Gaussian space at corresponding scale instead of the original image for better robustness.

Contrast. Drusen are locally brighter than neighbors thus contrast is an important indicator of drusen. The value of each maximum at the Laplacian space is used as contrast.

Size. The size of drusen is in general different compared to the optic disc and vessels. In our method, the scales of the maxima are used to indicate size.

Hessian. In SIFT, the ratio of the maximum and minimum eigen values of the Hessian matrix is used to discriminate edge and spot. We adopt this value to distinguish blood vessels and drusen.

Distance to macula. Drusen usually appear near the macula. Furthermore, the drusen nearer to the macula are more clinically important than the ones farther away. Therefore, spatial distance to macula is used as a feature for drusen classification.

Gabor coefficients. Gabor coefficients at 5 scales and 8 orientations are used as features to describe the local texture.

SPIN feature. Drusen typically appear as circular, roundish spots in the retina. To make use of this characteristic, SPIN features is used to embed local neighborhood context [24]. The SPIN feature encodes the distribution of image brightness values in the neighborhood of a particular reference (center) point. This is achieved by a soft-assigned histogram of the intensity values of pixels located at a distance d from the pixel (i,j). That is,

$$f_{(i,j)}(d,v) = \sum_{(i',j')\in\Gamma(i,j)} \exp\left(-\frac{(\|(i',j')-(i,j)\|-d)^2}{2\alpha^2} - \frac{\|I(i',j')-v\|^2}{2\beta^2}\right) \quad (4)$$

here $\|.\|$ means Euclid distance. $\Gamma(i,j)$ is the neighborhood of (i,j). v is the gray value of the pixels. α and β are the parameters representing the soft width of the bins. In our implementation, the number of color bins is 8. The number of location bins and the scales are consistent with he ones used for extrema detection.

3.3   Classification by MIL

After detecting the local maxima, we adopt multiple instance learning to train a drusen detector [5]. MIL is a good choice for weakly labeled data. For MIL, each bag of samples share a label. A bag is labelled as positive if at least one sample in it is positive, conversely it is labelled as negative if all the samples in it are negative. It has been used in object detection and image categorization with good performance [25]. For drusen detection, labelling the presence of drusen is much easier than marking the boundary of drusen. Therefore, we employ multiple instance learning to train a drusen classifier from the weakly labeled data. The mi-SVM algorithm [26] is used in our work. This algorithm formulates multiple instance learning as a maximum margin problem which can be solved by an extension of the generalized Support Vector Machines (SVM).

In mi-SVM, each instance label is subjected to constraints defined by the (positive) bag labels. This is to ensure label consistency with the bag label. The goal is then to maximize the soft-margin jointly over hidden label variables and a kernelized discriminant function. The mixed integer objective function formulation of mi-SVM as a generalized soft-margin SVM in its primal form is defined as:

$$\min_{\{y_i\}} \min_{\mathbf{w},b,\xi} \frac{1}{2}\|\mathbf{w}\|^2 + C\sum_i \xi_i,$$

$$s.t. \begin{cases} \forall i: & y_i(\langle\mathbf{w},x_i\rangle+b) \geq 1-\xi_i, \\ & \xi_i \geq 0, \\ & y_i \in \{-1,1\}, \\ \forall I: & \sum_{i\in I}\frac{y_i+1}{2} \geq 1, \; if \; Y^I = 1 \\ & y_i = -1|_{i\in I}, \; if \; Y^I = -1. \end{cases} \quad (5)$$

where $\mathbf{w} \in \mathbb{R}^d, b \in \mathbb{R}, \xi$ are the weight vector, offset and slack variables of SVM.

As y_i is a discrete variable, solving the mi-SVM problem to find the optimal labels and hyperplane, is a combinatorial mixed integer programming problem. The heuristic quadratic programming (QP) scheme proposed by [26] to optimize this objective function begins by initializing all instance labels from the positive labeled bags to be 1 and alternates between optimizing the parameters w and b for the SVM solution with the current imputed labels, and assigning y based on the resulting classification boundary. After each step, the constraints in Eq. 5 are checked and re-enforced.

3.4 Segmentation by Growcut

After classification, we obtain the locations of drusen, without boundary. We employ Growcut to track the drusen boundary. While local threshold and region grow methods are employed in other works, we found that local threshold method fails in the situation of clumped drusen and region grow has the problem of leaking. Growcut is able to track the boundary with small number of seeds [6]. It was verified to be effective in medical image segmentation.

Growcut is a celluar automata based image segmentation method. A cellular automaton is a triplet $A = (S, N, \delta)$, where S is an non-empty state set, N is the neighbor hood system, and $\delta : S^N \rightarrow S$ is the local transition function (rule). This function defines the rule of calculating the cell's state at $t + 1$ time step, given the states of the neighborhood cells at previous time step t. The cell state S_p in our case is actually a triplet $(l_p, \theta_p, \overrightarrow{C}_p)$ - the label l_p of the current cell, 'strength' of the current cell $\theta_p \in [0, 1]$, and cell feature vector $\overrightarrow{C}_p$, defined by the image (the RGB color vector). Growcut is an iterative method. At each step, the seeds attack their neighbors until all the pixels are labeled.

Growcut was designed as an interactive foreground segmentation algorithm, with users manually mark several foreground seeds and background seeds. In [27], unsupervised Growcut, with random seeds and labels, is used for medical image segmentation. We apply it in a supervised mode, with the seeds and labels determined in the classification process.

While detecting the extremum points, the minimum points are almost all non-drusen. Among the maximum points, some (most) of them are non-drusen and classified correctly as non-drusen. These points are then used as background seeds. and the points classified as drusen are used as foreground seeds. These seeds are fed into Growcut to track the boundary of drusen [6]. An example of Growcut seeds and segmentation result can be found in Fig. 2.

While labeling, we found that if the whole image is labelled at one time, Growcut is not able to give satisfying result. Therefore, for each drusen seed, we perform Growcut on the local rectangle patch, which is the minimum bounding box covering the drusen seeds and at least 5 non-drusen seeds.

4 Experiments

The experiments are performed on ACHIKO-D350 [28], which is, as far as we know, the only dataset with drusen boundaries marked. It consists of 350 population-based images from the Singapore Eye Malay Study, consisting of 96 clinically verified drusen images and 254 non-drusen images. Each image has a resolution of 3072 × 2048 and had been acquired using a 45 FOV Canon CR-DGi retinal fundus camera with a 10D SLR backing. Among the 96 images, 45 ones of left eyes and 51 ones of right eyes. The boundary of drusen are semi-manually marked out. Besides drusen boundaries, the position of the macula is also manually marked. In experiments, the images are resized to 1024*683.

The measurements adopted in experiments include sensitivity, specificity, average precision (the average of sensitivity and specificity), and the Area Under Curve (AUC) of the Receiver Operating Characteristic (ROC). Sensitivity (true positive rate) and specificity (true negative rate) are defined in Eq. 6.

$$Sensitivity = \frac{True\, positives}{Positives},$$
$$specificity = \frac{True\, negatives}{Negatives}. \tag{6}$$

Receiver operating characteristic is the true positive rate (sensitivity) vs. false positive rate (1-specificity) curve.

4.1 Computing Time

In our method, the drusen classifier using MIL is trained off-line. After training the classifier, our workflow consists of four main steps: (i) extreme point detection; (ii) feature description; (iii) multiple instance learning; and (iv) drusen segmentation using growcut. We recorded the computational time of each step for processing one image of 1024*768 as follows: 14 s, 7 s, 1.5 s, and 10 s for (i), (ii), (iii) and (iv), respectively. So, the total time for one image is 32.5 s. Note that our method is implemented with unoptimized MATLAB code on a workstation with 2.4 GHz dual CPU and 64 GB memory. The time cost can be largely reduced by optimizing the code and using an upgraded server, which easily make our method acceptable for clinical application.

4.2 Feature Selection

The features used in our work are of four types, Edge Direction Histogram (EDH), Macula Related Feature (MRF, consists of distance to macula, scale, intensity, contrast, and Hessian value), Gabor, and SPIN. The performances of the single features are shown in Table 1. From the result, we can see that (1) EDH and macula related feature are able to provide higher sensitivity with lower specificity and (2) in means of average precision, macula related feature gives the best performance.

The combination of all four types of features is used in our paper, because it gives better performance than any other forms of combinations, as shown in Table 2. We can see that the result is consistent with the one in Table 1.

Summing up the results in Tables 1 and 2, we can draw the conclusion that the macula related feature performs the best. It is able to provide high sensitivity

Table 1. Performance of single features

Feature	Sensitivity	Specificity	Average precision
EDH	80.44	55.61	68.03
MRF	90.06	75.79	82.93
Gabor	76.75	82.7	79.72
SPIN	82.67	78.86	80.76

Table 2. Performance of feature combinations

Feature combination	Sensitivity	Specificity	Average precision
MRF+EDH+Gabor+SPIN	90.62	86.86	88.74
- MRF	84.84	85.17	85
- EDH	90.59	86.87	88.73
- Gabor	90.92	83.24	87.08
- SPIN	88.43	86.03	87.23

but relatively lower specificity. Other features combined are able to keep the high sensitivity while increase the specificity.

4.3   Results on AMD Detection

To test the performance of AMD detection, we compare our method with the BIF [19] based method and the Thalia system [20]. The results of these two methods, on the same dataset, are reported in their papers. To make the comparison fair and objectively, in experiment, we adopt the same setting with the two methods, meaning randomly choose 50 positive sample and negative samples as training data and the left ones as test data. The experiments are run 10 times. The means and standard deviations of sensitivity, specificity, the average precision, and AUC are shown in Table 3. From the table, we can see that our method outperforms the two methods on the task of AMD detection. It is worth to point out that our approach achieves the high sensitivity of 100 %, with the high specificity of 96.76. The standard deviation of our method is also the lowest.

Table 3. Performance comparison on early AMD detection

	Sensitivity	Specificity	Average precision	AUC
BIF [19]	86.3 ± 3.2	91.9 ± 3.1	89.11 ± 1.35	NA
Thalia [20]	NA*	NA	95.46 ± 0.94	NA
Proposed	100 ± 0	96.76 ± 1.16	98.38 ± 0.58	97.26 ± 0.98

*NA means Not Available.

Figure 3 shows the top 10 images that are most likely to have AMD and the 10 images that are least likely to have AMD. All the 20 images are correctly classified. From the result, we can see that the approach is robust to image condition.

4.4 Results of Drusen Segmentation

Then we further evaluate the performance of drusen segmentation, by means of sensitivity, specificity, and average precision. Since drusen classification, meaning

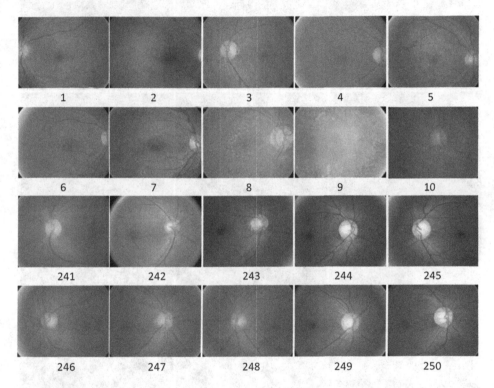

Fig. 3. Examples of AMD detection. The top two rows: the 10 images that are most likely to have AMD. The bottom two rows: the 10 images that are least likely to have AMD. The number below each image is the ranking number in the classification result.

Table 4. The performance of the proposed method

	Classification			Segmentation		
	Sensitivity	Specificity	Average precision	Sensitivity	Specificity	Average precision
SVM	90.23 ± 0.60	87.08 ± 0.28	88.66 ± 0.32	67.77 ± 0.51	94.36 ± 0.12	81.07 ± 0.24
MIL	50.59 ± 6.93	90.89 ± 3.37	70.74 ± 2.11	40.54 ± 6.26	96.17 ± 1.44	67.85 ± 2.48

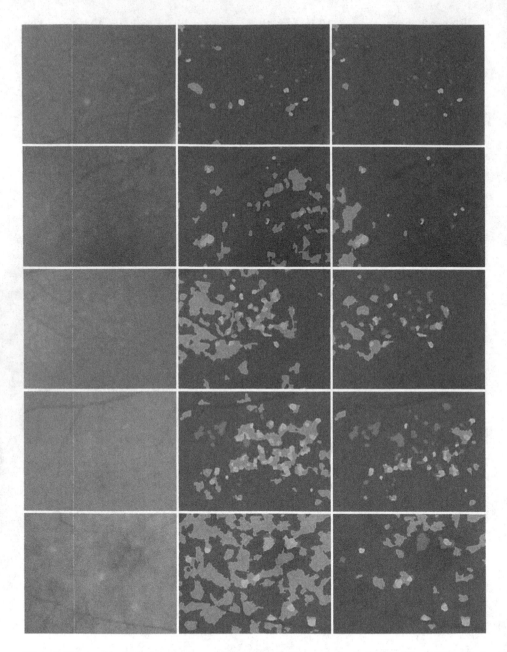

Fig. 4. Examples of drusen segmentation. The image are the 1–5th in Fig. 3. The first column shows the drusen regions of the fundus images. The second and third columns show the drusen segmentation results of the SVM based method and the MIL based method. The green background is the green channel of the fundus image, the regions in blue are the false negative. The regions in purple are the true positive and the ones in orange are false positive (Color figure online).

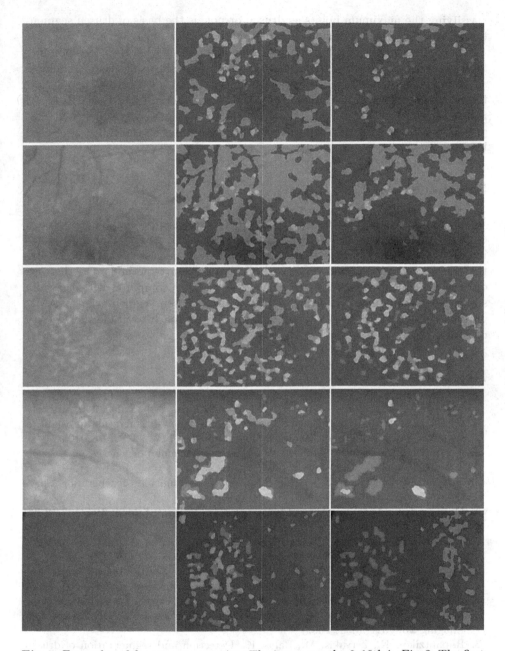

Fig. 5. Examples of drusen segmentation. The image are the 6–10th in Fig. 3. The first column shows the drusen regions of the fundus images. The second and third columns show the drusen segmentation results of the SVM based method and the MIL based method. The green background is the green channel of the fundus image, the regions in blue are the false negative. The regions in purple are the true positive and the ones in orange are false positive (Color figure online).

classifying the maximum points as drusen or not, is the basis of drusen segmentation, we also show the results of drusen classification.

As our method is weakly supervised, we compare it with the corresponding fully supervised method, meaning support vector machine using the manual label as training data. The comparison result is shown in Table 4. Figures 4 and 5 show the drusen segmentation result of the SVM based method and the MIL based method. Refer to Table 4, Figs. 4 and 5, we find that the weakly supervised MIL gives lower sensitivity but higher specificity compared to the fully supervised learning SVM.

5   Conclusion

In this paper, we propose an effective AMD screening approach. This approach employs multiple instance learning to reduce the need for manual labelling training data. As shown by the experimental results, on the task of AMD detection, the proposed approach outperforms the state-of-the-art methods. On the task of drusen segmentation, its performance is satisfying compared with the fully supervised result. One important application of drusen segmentation is AMD grading. In our future work, we will extend our approach to grade the severity of AMD.

References

1. Kawasaki, R., Yasuda, M., Song, S.J., Chen, S.J., Jonas, J.B., Wang, J.J., Mitchell, P., Wong, T.Y.: The prevalence of age-related macular degeneration in asians: a systematic review and meta-analysis. Ophthalmology **117**, 921–927 (2010)
2. Jager, R.D., Mieler, W.F., Miller, J.W.: Age-related macular degeneration. N. Engl. J. Med. **358**, 2606–2617 (2008)
3. Bressler, N.M., Bressler, S.B., Fine, S.L.: Age-related macular degeneration. Surv. Ophthalmol. **32**, 375–413 (1988)
4. De Jong, P.T.: Age-related macular degeneration. N. Engl. J. Med. **355**, 1474–1485 (2006)
5. Dietterich, T.G., Lathrop, R.H., Lozano-Pérez, T.: Solving the multiple instance problem with axis-parallel rectangles. Artif. Intell. **89**, 31–71 (1997)
6. Vezhnevets, V., Konouchine, V.: Growcut: interactive multi-label nd image segmentation by cellular automata. In: Proceedings of Graphicon, pp. 150–156 (2005)
7. Ben Sbeh, Z., Cohen, L.D., Mimoun, G., Coscas, G.: A new approach of geodesic reconstruction for drusen segmentation in eye fundus images. IEEE Trans. Med. Imaging **20**, 1321–1333 (2001)
8. Rapantzikos, K., Zervakis, M., Balas, K.: Detection and segmentation of drusen deposits on human retina: potential in the diagnosis of age-related macular degeneration. Med. Image Anal. **7**, 95–108 (2003)
9. Smith, R.T., Chan, J.K., Nagasaki, T., Ahmad, U.F., Barbazetto, I., Sparrow, J., Figueroa, M., Merriam, J.: Automated detection of macular drusen using geometric background leveling and threshold selection. Arch. Ophthalmol. **123**, 200 (2005)

10. Brandon, L., Hoover, A.: Drusen detection in a retinal image using multi-level analysis. In: Ellis, R.E., Peters, T.M. (eds.) MICCAI 2003. LNCS, vol. 2878, pp. 618–625. Springer, Heidelberg (2003)
11. Ujjwal, K., Chakravarty, A., Sivaswamy, J.: Visual saliency based bright lesion detection and discrimination in retinal images. In: IEEE 10th International Symposium on Biomedical Imaging: From Nano to Macro, pp. 1428–1431 (2013)
12. Barriga, E., Murray, V., Agurto, C., Pattichis, M., Russell, S., Abramoff, M., Davis, H., Soliz, P.: Multi-scale am-fm for lesion phenotyping on age-related macular degeneration. In: IEEE International Symposium on Computer-Based Medical Systems, pp. 1–5 (2009)
13. Köse, C., Sevik, U., Gencalioglu, O., Ikibas, C., Kayikicioglu, T.: A statistical segmentation method for measuring age-related macular degeneration in retinal fundus images. J. Med. Syst. **34**, 1–13 (2010)
14. Quellec, G., Russell, S.R., Abràmoff, M.D.: Optimal filter framework for automated, instantaneous detection of lesions in retinal images. IEEE Trans. Med. Imaging **30**, 523–533 (2011)
15. Hijazi, M.H.A., Coenen, F., Zheng, Y.: Retinal image classification using a histogram based approach. In: IEEE International Joint Conference on Neural Networks, pp. 3501–3507
16. Hijazi, M.H.A., Coenen, F., Zheng, Y.: Retinal image classification for the screening of age-related macular degeneration. In: Research and Development in Intelligent Systems XXVII, pp. 325–338 (2011)
17. Hijazi, M.H.A., Jiang, C., Coenen, F., Zheng, Y.: Image classification for age-related macular degeneration screening using hierarchical image decompositions and graph mining. In: Gunopulos, D., Hofmann, T., Malerba, D., Vazirgiannis, M. (eds.) ECML PKDD 2011, Part II. LNCS, vol. 6912, pp. 65–80. Springer, Heidelberg (2011)
18. Zheng, Y., Hijazi, M.H.A., Coenen, F.: Automated "disease/no disease" grading of age-related macular degeneration by an image mining approach. Invest. Ophthalmol. Vis. Sci. **53**, 8310–8318 (2012)
19. Cheng, J., Wong, D.W.K., Cheng, X., Liu, J., Tan, N.M., Bhargava, M., Cheung, C.M.G., Wong, T.Y.: Early age-related macular degeneration detection by focal biologically inspired feature. In: IEEE International Conference on Image Processing, pp. 2805–2808 (2012)
20. Wong, D.W., Liu, J., Cheng, X., Zhang, J., Yin, F., Bhargava, M., Cheung, G.C., Wong, T.Y.: Thalia-an automatic hierarchical analysis system to detect drusen lesion images for amd assessment. In: IEEE International Symposium on Biomedical Imaging, pp. 884–887 (2013)
21. Medhi, J.P., Nath, M.K., Dandapat, S.: Automatic grading of macular degeneration from color fundus images. In: World Congress on Information and Communication Technologies, pp. 511–514 (2012)
22. Liang, Z., Wong, D.W., Liu, J., Chan, K.L., Wong, T.Y.: Towards automatic detection of age-related macular degeneration in retinal fundus images. In: IEEE International Conference on Engineering in Medicine and Biology Society (2010)
23. Lowe, D.: Distinctive image features from scale-invariant keypoints. Int. J. Comput. Vis. **60**, 91–110 (2004)
24. Johnson, A.E., Hebert, M.: Using spin images for efficient object recognition in cluttered 3d scenes. IEEE Trans. Pattern Anal. Mach. Intell. **21**, 433–449 (1999)
25. Qi, G.J., Hua, X.S., Rui, Y., Mei, T., Tang, J., Zhang, H.J.: Concurrent multiple instance learning for image categorization. In: IEEE Conference on Computer Vision and Pattern Recognition, pp. 1–8 (2007)

26. Andrews, S., Tsochantaridis, I., Hofmann, T.: Support vector machines for multiple instance learning. In: Advances in Neural Information Processing Systems (NIPS) (2003)
27. Ghosh, P., Antani, S.K., Long, L.R., Thoma, G.R.: Unsupervised grow-cut: cellular automata-based medical image segmentation. In: IEEE International Conference on Healthcare Informatics, Imaging and Systems Biology (HISB), pp. 40–47 (2011)
28. Liu, H., Xu, Y., Wong, D.W.K., Laude, A., Lim, T.H., Liu, J.: Achiko-d350: a dataset for early amd detection and drusen segmentation. In: Ophthalmic Medical Image Analysis (MICCAI Workshop) (2014)

Recognizing People by Their Personal Aesthetics: A Statistical Multi-level Approach

Cristina Segalin[1](✉), Alessandro Perina[2], and Marco Cristani[1]

[1] University of Verona, Verona, Italy
cristina.segalin@univr.it
[2] Istituto Italiano di Tecnologia (IIT), Genova, Italy

Abstract. This paper presents a study on personal aesthetics, a recent soft biometrics application where the goal is to recognize people by considering the images they like. Here we propose a multi-level approach, where each level is intended as a low-dimensional space where the images preferred by a user can be projected, and similar images are mapped nearby, namely a Counting Grid. Multiple levels are generated by adopting Counting Grids at different resolutions, corresponding to analyze images at different grains. Each level is then associated to an exemplar Support Vector Machine, which separates the images of an individual from the rest of the users. Putting together multiple levels gives a battery of classifiers whose performances are very good: on a dataset of 200 users, and 40 K images, using 5 preferred images as biometric template gives 97 % of probability of guessing the correct user; as for the verification capability, the equal error rate is 0.11. The approach has also been tested with diverse comparative methods and different features, showing that color image properties are crucial to encode the personal aesthetics, and that high-level information (as the objects within the images) could be very effective, but current methods are not robust enough to catch it.

1 Introduction

Understanding the aesthetical preferences of a person, and specifically the images that he/she likes, is a noteworthy ability of the human beings; usually linked to high-level concepts such as the objects being portrayed in an image ("Jeff prefers photos of cars instead of landscapes"), it can be also based to apparent low-level visual properties such as having black/white colors, or full colors.

Having this capability transferred into a machine is without doubts of great benefit for many applications: from recommender systems that suggest images of interest to a particular user, to social aggregators which foster connections among individuals sharing similar aesthetical preferences. Among these applications, a novel one is emerging in these last years in the field of soft biometrics, aimed at identifying or verifying a person given a set of preferred images, dubbed *personal aesthetics* [1]. In general, soft biometric patterns differ from standard biometrics since they do not require a voluntary cooperation of the user in providing identification cues such as the face, the fingerprints etc.; even more notably, the

© Springer International Publishing Switzerland 2015
D. Cremers et al. (Eds.): ACCV 2014, Part III, LNCS 9005, pp. 499–513, 2015.
DOI: 10.1007/978-3-319-16811-1_33

identification or verification operation can be conducted without letting the user know about what is going on [2].

Soft biometrics can be partitioned into *physical/physyiological* (age, gender, ethnicity, height etc.) and *behavioral* biometrics, that is, encoding a characteristic linked to how a person does diverse mental/physical tasks [3]. This last class can be further exploded into *authorship-based* (linked to style peculiarities of the individual - how he/she writes a text), *motor skill-based* (how a person performs a particular physical task), *purely behavioral* (how a person solves a mental task) and *HCI-based* biometrics. HCI-based biometrics assumes that every person has a unique way to interact with an hardware device (a laptop, a smartphone or a simple touchscreen). For example, some approaches use the mouse or keystrokes dynamics to identify an individual [4,5]; some other more recent methods focused on how Internet applications are utilized, like chatting [6] or browsing histories [7].

Personal aesthetics assumes that, given a set of preferred images of a user, it is possible to extract a set of features which are discriminative for him/her; these patterns can be used as biometric template, and employed for identification and verification. Personal aesthetics fits surely into the behavioral soft biometrics, while at a lower level of specification do not match with any of the previous categories. For these reasons, it could be good to have a "preference-based" category, whose approaches assume that a user may be identified by means of his/her preferences on multimedia data.

The motivations of why focusing on personal aesthetics, and in particular on images, are at least three; first of all, the huge presence of images in Internet: at the moment this article is being written, 55M of new images are daily uploaded on Instagram, with 1.2 B of "*likes*" distributed over 16 B of globally shared images (See http://instagram.com/press/); on Flickr, each of the 87M users has, on average, around 2 K views per day (http://statsr.net/flickr-stats/); in the past year, 128 B of images have been uploaded on Facebook (http://goo.gl/0tWf.), accessible to an audience of 1.26 B users (http://expandedramblings.com/.). The second motivation is the enormous diffusion of the "liking" activities, since liking multimedia material is one of the most common social activities [8].

The third motivation is that, psychology and neuroscience have investigated the interrelation of individual characteristics on aesthetic preferences [9], finding that there are consistent ties between aesthetic appreciation and personality [10]; this last, being a stable characteristic of humans, ensures that personal aesthetics are somewhat *permanent*, a desirable property for soft biometric traits [2].

In this paper, a novel approach for personal aesthetics is proposed, which is based on the projection of the images into different latent spaces, each one of them representing a particular level with which to consider the preferred images. These spaces are 2D Counting Grids (CGs) [11], that is, smooth manifolds where visually similar pictures are mapped nearby. In the details, each CG is characterized by a particular resolution, that in rough words models how much visually similar should be the images in order to be close on the grid: the higher the resolution, the stronger the visual similarity of close images. The presence of multiple resolutions brings to evaluate differently grained similarity relations among images.

The approach assumes to have a set of users and some images preferred by them, which compose a gallery and a probe image set; it consists in a serial pipeline of initialization, enrollment and identification/verification stages.

In the initialization stage, multiple levels correspond to CGs of different resolutions, which are learned with the gallery images of all the users, without using ID labels. In the enrollment, the training data of a single user is projected on the CGs at different resolutions, resulting in different *embedding maps*. These maps are then fed into Support Vector Machines (SVMs), one for each CG. In particular the SVMs are trained as exemplar SVM, that is, using a single map as positive sample, and as negative samples all the maps of the other users at that CG resolution. In the identification/verification stage, probe images are projected into the CGs, forming another set of maps which are then classified by each of the SVMs, and producing a joint prediction; this last is used to provide or verify the identity of the user. It is worth noting that our method works with a varying number of images, both for the enrollment and the identification/verification stage, providing a versatile approach.

Through some explicative experiments, it is easy to capture the advantages of our methods. The use of the 2D CGs allows to see the kind of images liked by some users and disliked by the others; projecting on low-dimensional spaces permits to use any kind and number of counting features for encoding images (see more on this topic later on), contrarily to our previous approaches [1,12,13] which are based on an explicit cues weighting; having CGs at multiple resolutions avoids to deal with model selection issues (deciding a "correct" resolution for a CG is a problem [11]). The approach is also effective; in particular, the tests have been performed on the only real dataset currently available in the literature [1], composed by 40000 images which belong to 200 users chosen at random from the Flickr community. For each user, 200 preferred images (his "favorites") have been retained. As identification performance, using 5 preferred test images as biometric signature gives 97 % of probability of guessing the correct user (state of the art was 83 %); as for the verification capability, an equal error rate of 0.11 (best results was 0.25) is reached. Other than [12], we compared with several other baselines and alternative strategies, including a simple PCA baseline and multidimensional counting grids. Finally, we performed an extensive on the kind of features which can be used to describe an images: overall, the features are grouped into four families (see Table 1), i.e. *color, composition, content* and *textural properties*, according to the taxonomy proposed in [14]. Our experiments showed that using color and composition cues gives the best results, together with some interesting observations about high level features.

The rest of the paper is organized as follows: in Sect. 2 a summarization of the Counting Grid generative model is reported; in Sect. 3 the proposed approach is detailed, explaining how it can be customized for the identification and verification tasks. The approach is thoroughly tested in Sect. 4, and, finally, conclusions future perspectives are given in Sect. 5.

2   Mathematical Background: The Counting Grid Model

The Counting Grid (CG) is a generative model originally aimed at analyzing image collections [11]. It assumes that images are i.i.d. random variables represented as histograms (or bags-of-features) $\{c_z\}_{z=1,\dots,Z}$, where each c_z is a counting variable which enumerates the occurrences of the z-th feature.

In its 2D version, a CG π is a 2D finite discrete grid (a flattened torus with wrap-around at its extrema), spatially indexed by $\mathbf{i} = (x, y) \in [1\dots E]\times[1\dots E]$, and containing normalized feature counts $\{\pi_{\mathbf{i},z}\}$, indexed by $z = 1,\dots,Z$. Therefore, $\sum_z \pi_{\mathbf{i},z} = 1$ for every location $\mathbf{i}$ on the grid. The generative process underling the CG is as follows: an image (i.e. its BoF $\{c_z\}$) is generated by selecting a certain location $\mathbf{k}$ over the grid, calculating the distribution $h_{\mathbf{k},z} = \frac{1}{S^2}\sum_{\mathbf{i}\in W_{\mathbf{k}}}\pi_{\mathbf{i},z}$ by averaging all the words counts within the window $W_{\mathbf{k}}$ (of dimensions $S \times S$ and such that $\mathbf{k}$ is its upper left corner) and then drawing features counts from this distribution. In practice, a small window is located in the grid, averaging the feature counts within it to obtain a local probability mass function over the features, and then generating from it an appropriate number of features in the bag $\{c_z\}$. In simpler terms, a CG could be think as a mixture model, where the components are overlapping windows indexed by $\mathbf{k}$.

This said, it appears clear that the position of the window $\mathbf{k}$ in the grid is a latent variable; given $\mathbf{k}$, the likelihood of $\{c_z\}$ is

$$p(\{c_z\}|\mathbf{k}) = \prod_z (h_{\mathbf{k},z})^{c_z} = \frac{1}{S^2}\prod_z \Big(\sum_{\mathbf{i}\in W_{\mathbf{k}}} \pi_{\mathbf{i},z}\Big)^{c_z}. \tag{1}$$

Given that the ratio between the grid size $E \times E$ of a Counting Grid and the window size $W \times W$, is smaller than number of images, this forces windows linked to different images to overlap, and to co-exist by finding a shared compromise in the feature counts located in their intersection. The overall effect of these constraints is to produce locally smooth transitions between strongly different feature counts by gradually phasing features in/out in the intermediate locations. In practice, local neighborhoods in the grid represent similar concepts and images mapped in close locations are somehow similar.

To learn a Counting Grid, the likelihood over all training images T needs to be maximized, and this can be written as

$$p(\{\{c_z^t\}, \mathbf{k}^t\}_{t=1}^T) \propto \prod_{t=1}^T \prod_{z=1}^Z \Big(\sum_{\mathbf{i}\in W_{\mathbf{k}}} \pi_{\mathbf{i},z}^t\Big)^{c_z^t}. \tag{2}$$

The sum over $\mathbf{k}$ makes it difficult to perform assignment to the latent variables (i.e., the components of the mixture) and so to estimate the model parameters and it is necessary to employ an EM algorithm. The procedure is a bit complicated and involves different variational distributions; for this study it is only necessary to quote the posterior distribution, calculated in the E step,

$$p(\mathbf{k}^t|\{c_z^t\}) = q_{\mathbf{k}}^t \propto \exp \sum_z c_z^t \cdot \log h_{\mathbf{k},z} \tag{3}$$

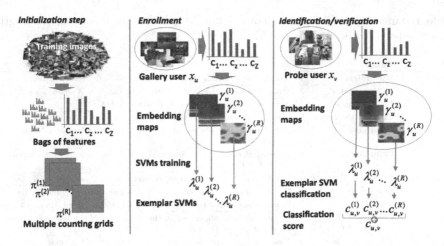

Fig. 1. The proposed approach, composed by three stages: *initialization*, where the multi-resolution Counting Grid is learnt; *enrollment*, where the classifiers for each user are trained, and *identification/verification* stages, where unknown personal aesthetics are matched with the gallery.

which is a probabilistic mapping of the t-th bag to the grid windows $\mathbf{k}$. This mapping is usually peaky, i.e. each image tends to map to a few nearby locations in the grid. For details on the learning algorithm and on its efficiency, the reader can refer to the original paper [11].

3   The Proposed Approach

The proposed three-step approach is sketched in Fig. 1. The initialization step is applied on the training image set: it consists on creating a bag of features for each image, and learning a set of Counting Grids, each at a different window size (i.e., the resolution of the CG). In the enrollment stage, the preferred images of each user x_u, $u = 1, \ldots, U$ of the gallery set are mapped on the CG latent spaces, and the resulting maps (one for each CG space) are fed into a discriminative classifier. In the identification/verification stage, the test images of a probe subject are transformed into bags of features, and projected into the CGs; in particular, in the identification scenario, the resulting maps are given as input to all the U gallery classifiers, producing U identification scores. These scores are used to decide the best gallery user. In the case of the verification task, the maps are given to a single gallery classifier (the one which is supposed to match the identity of the probe), which accepts or rejects the signature considering a given threshold.

3.1   Initialization Stage: Creating the Bags of Features

For the sake of comparison, we adopted the dataset used in [12], composed by 40000 images belonging to 200 users, chosen randomly from the Flickr social

Table 1. Summary of all features. The column 'L' indicates the feature vector length for each type of feature.

Category	Name	L	Short Description
Color	Use of light	1	Average pixel intensity of V channel [16]
	HSV statistics	3	Mean of S channel and standard deviation of S, V channels [14]
	Emotion-based	3	Amount of *Pleasure, Arousal, Dominance* [14,17]
	Circular Variance	1	*Circular variance* of the H channel in the IHLS color space [18]
	Colorfulness	1	Colorfulness measure based on Earth Mover's Distance (EMD) [14,16]
	Color Name	11	Amount of *Black, Blue, Brown, Green, Gray, Orange, Pink, Purple, Red, White, Yellow* [14]
Composition	Edges	1	Total number of edge points, extracted with Canny [1]
	Level of detail	1	Number of regions (after mean shift segmentation) [19,20]
	Regions	1	Average *size* of the regions (after mean shift segmentation) [19,20]
	Low depth of field (DOF)	3	Amount of focus sharpness in the inner part of the image w.r.t. the overall focus [14,16]
	Rule of thirds	2	Mean of S, V channels in the inner rectangle of the image [14,16]
	Image parameters	1	Size of the image [1,16]
Texture	Entropy	1	Image entropy [1]
	Wavelet textures	12	Level of spatial graininess measured with a three-level (L1, L2, L3) Daubechies wavelet transform on the HSV channels [16]
	Tamura	3	Amount of *Coarseness, Contrast, Directionality* [21]
	GLCM-features	12	Amount of *Contrast, Correlation, Energy, Homogeneity* for each HSV channel [14]
Content	Objects	28	Objects detectors [15]: in particular, here are the objects for which detectors are available: *people, plane, bike, bird, boat, bottle, bus, car, cat, dog, table, horse, motorbike, chair*. In all the cases we kept the number of instances and their average bounding box *size*
	Faces	2	Number and *size* of faces after Viola-Jones face detection algorithm [22]

network. For each user, the 200 last "favored" pictures have been retained, that is, pictures of other photographers that have meet his/her preferences. Repeated favored images across users are less than the 0.05 %.

As for the features, we consider those of [12] for comparability, here reorganized as in the computational aesthetics taxonomy of [14] (see Table 1); 4 categories are present: *color* (distribution, diversity, purity, emotional content, etc.), *composition* (size and number of homogeneous regions, amount of edges, depth of field, rule of thirds, etc.), *textures* (spatial distribution of visual properties) and *content*, which individuate semantic entities (cars, chairs and the like); in this last case, robust probabilistic object detectors have been employed [15] (for a complete list of all the detectable objects, see Table 1); other than the number of instances of objects in an image, the average area of their bounding boxes is considered.

It is worth noting that each feature extracted in the proposed approach indicates the level of presence of a particular cue, i.e. an enumeration value or an intensity count. This is needed for the modeling with the Counting Grid.

3.2 Initialization Stage: Multi-view Counting Grid Training

Given the bags of features of the training images, the extent E of the Counting Grid and its window size S, a multi-resolution CG is learned. This amounts to learn $R = E - S$ Counting Grids, starting at resolution $r = 1$ (the lowest resolution level) with the window of size $E - 1$, decreasing the window size of one pixel at each time, until the minimum size S (the highest resolution level $r = R$) is reached. At each resolution level r (except the first one), we used the CG learnt at the previous step, i.e., $\pi^{(r-1)}$ as initialization for $\pi^{(r)}$. At the first resolution level, the initialization is random.

Using different windows sizes corresponds to vary the topology of the CG latent spaces: a large window size leads to an embedding map where loosely similar images are near-uniformly distributed over a large area and only the very different images are strongly separated. Conversely, a small window size will create a peaked map, where only highly similar images are projected nearby, and weakly similar pictures are separated. Initializing a model training using the CG of the previous level allows to mitigate local minima problems (as in the case of a too sparse CG, with many images mapped very close) ensuring to use all the CG extent for the mapping. In addition, this initialization strategy permits to show how the mapping evolves at the different resolutions, refining spread and unfocused projections into defined and intuitive thematic regions.

Obviously, the Counting Grids can not be directly visualized (each location contains a distribution of features), but it is possible to create an image mosaic using those images $\{c_z^t\}$ which give the highest posterior at each location $\mathbf{k}$, i.e., $p(\mathbf{k}^t | \{c_z^t\})$, at a given resolution level r. Adopting this visualization strategy, Fig. 2(left) shows CGs with $E = 45$ at resolutions r $= 5$ (S $= 40$) and 35 (S $= 10$): while going from coarse (top) to finer (bottom) resolutions, the semantics of the CG emerge as peaked regions, where each region carries out a different type of images. In this case a set of images where the orange is predominant are highlighted. As visible, at the coarser resolution the orange images lie in two regions, where other tonalities are also present. Going to the highest resolution has the effect of packing nearby those images into a compact area. On Fig. 2(center) the CG at the highest resolution is reported.

Such a representation is shown in Fig. 2(center) for a Counting Grid with $E = 45$ at resolution $r = R$ (S $= 10$, maximum resolution). As visible, close images are visually similar, and semantic topics do emerge.

3.3 Enrollment Stage

Once the different Counting Grids are learnt, the images of each gallery user can be projected within it, obtaining R maps per user, one map for each resolution. The projection corresponds to a generative embedding, calculating a posterior probability at each location $\mathbf{k}$; once we have fixed a user u and a resolution r the posterior is

$$\gamma_u^{(r)} = \sum_{t \in T_u} p(\mathbf{k}^t | \{c_z^t\}, \pi^{(r)}) \tag{4}$$

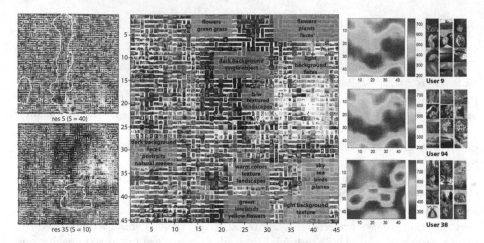

Fig. 2. Visualization of Counting Grids: on the left, CGs with E = 45 at resolutions r = 5 (S = 40, top) and 35 (S = 10, bottom). On the center, the $S = 10$ grid is visualized as a collage of images (see the text for the details on how the collage is created). On the right, the embedding maps of a single resolution level (r=R) are reported for three subjects, together with some random images preferred by them (better viewed in colors) (Color figure online).

where T_u identifies the set of images of the user u: T_u can be different, depending on how many gallery images are available for user u. Roughly speaking, the main idea is to sum all the mappings of the images belonging to a given user, thus highlighting the zones of the latent space where the images have been located. The presence of Counting Grids at multiple resolutions allows to map the preferences of the user from a very rough resolution (on the Counting Grids obtained with large windows) until the finest resolution (the Counting Grid being learned with a small sized window), where the map is usually peaked.

A graphical explanation of the mapping process is shown in Figs. 2 and 3; in Fig. 2, together with the collage of the CG, on the right are reported the

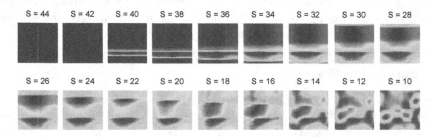

Fig. 3. Embedding maps for user 38 of Fig. 2. Starting from the lowest resolution (r = 1, S = 44) and going towards higher resolutions, the maps show refined blobs and areas, identifying more precisely semantic areas, easily interpretable, on the grid.

embedding maps of a single resolution level (the maximum, i.e., r=R) for three subjects, together with some random images preferred by them. One can notice two facts: (1) given a user, looking at his map and at the CG collage as reference, does allow to easily understand which kind of images are his preferred; (2) comparing the maps of different users, one can understand possible similarities: first two users from the top appear to share much the same preferences, while the third one has radically diverse preferences. This fact is confirmed by checking the random pictures of the users, on the right.

In Fig. 3 are reported the R mappings for the user 38 of Fig. 2. Starting from very blurred and unstructured maps corresponding to the lower resolutions, going toward higher resolution maps, blobs and distinct areas start to emerge, refining the "semantic" knowledge of the preferences a user exhibits.

After the mapping step, the maps $\{\gamma_u^{(r)}\}_{r=1,...,R}$ can be used as ID template for user u; to this sake, a battery of exemplar SVMs $\{\lambda_u^{(r)}\}_{r=1,...,R}$ are learnt (one for each resolution), using as positive samples the maps $\gamma_u^{(r)}$ at the different resolutions r (one map for each SVM) and as negative samples the maps of the other users. In this study, Support Vector Machines with radial basis functions have been employed. This step concludes the enrollment stage.

3.4 Identification and Verification Stage

In the identification/verification stage, all the probe images of a user v are first encoded as bags of features. Subsequently, they are mapped on the multiresolution CG, and the resulting maps $\{\gamma_v^{(r)}\}_{r=1,...,R}$ are used as input of the SVMs related to the gallery user u; they classify the maps producing R scores $\{c_{u,v}^{(r)}\}_{r=1,...,R}$ that, once mediated, provide a single classification score $c_{u,v}$. In other words, each user produces R probe maps; each of them is given as test input to the correspondent SVM of the gallery user, providing a confidence score (the distance from the separating hyperplane). Averaging these scores over all the resolutions gives the final confidence score. In the identification case, a confidence score is associated to each gallery user; this allows to rank the scores, keeping the highest ranked user as the best match with the probe. In the verification of the probe user, assumed to be the v−th, the confidence score given by the v−th classifier is simply evaluated, accepting o rejecting the signature depending on a threshold opportunely decided.

4   Experimental Evaluation

Several experiments are carried out to understand the potentialities of our approach. First of all, we investigate the ability of the features in capturing what is liked by an user, ensuring the highest identification and verification performance. Then, we compare our approach against a set of competitors, including our previous work [12]: to this sake, the same experiments carried out in [12] have been taken into account. Finally, we analyze how beneficial is to exploit CGs at different resolutions, capturing also how informative is each single resolution.

Identification and verification applications are considered: in the identification task the goal is to select the identity of an individual among a set of gallery users, given a pool of images liked by him/her; the verification task amounts to verify the identity of a particular user by means of his/her preferred images, considering his/her gallery images. In both the cases, the parametrization of the Counting Grids is the same: the size is fixed at $E = 45$ pixels for all of them, while the (smallest) window size is set to $S = 10$; this generates a set of 35 maps per user. The extraction of the image features takes 60 min per user (100 images), on a not optimized MATLAB code run on a 3.4 GHz processor with 16 Giga of RAM. The learning of the Counting Grid at a single resolution takes in total 2 min, while the mapping + SVM training operation requires 3 s for $N = 100$ images of the same user, on the same computer. Regarding the variability of the results in relation to the E and S values, the proposed approach maintains similar performance when the ratio between E and S (also dubbed "capacity" in [11]) is bounded in the interval [3, 5]. Even if E and S respect the capacity ratio, performances seem to decrease when $E < 10$ and $E > 70$.

4.1   Feature Analysis

Following the Table 1, we divide the features in four categories: *color, composition, texture* and *content*. For each category, we instantiate a identification task: given a probe signature built from an image or a set of images, the goal is to guess the gallery user who tagged them; to do that, fixing a gallery user, the average of the confidence scores produced by the exemplar SVMs (one score for each resolution) is calculated. Hopefully, the gallery user with highest averaged score corresponds to the probe user. As identification figure of merits, we use the Cumulative Matching Characteristic (CMC) curve [23]; given a probe signature of a user and the matching confidence score, the curves tells the rate at which the correct user is found within the first k matches, with all possible k spanned on the x-axis (they are also called *ranks*). In all the following experiments CMC plots are obtained averaging the CMC curves of 5 different experiments with different gallery/probe splits. In this experiment, we use 100 images as forming the gallery signatures, and 5 images for the probe signatures.

Table 2. CMC scores for the identification task, 100 images fo reach gallery user and 5 images for the probe user

Category	rank 1	rank 5	rank 20	rank 50	nAUC
Color	0.38 ± 0.21	0.65 ± 0.01	0.86 ± 0.01	0.97 ± 0.01	0.96 ± <0.01
Composition	0.11 ± 0.01	0.25 ± 0.02	0.45 ± 0.02	0.69 ± 0.12	0.81 ± 0.01
Texture	0.10 ± 0.01	0.21 ± 0.01	0.39 ± 0.03	0.64 ± 0.02	0.79 ± 0.01
Content	0.10 ± 0.01	0.20 ± 0.01	0.38 ± 0.03	0.61 ± 0.03	0.78 ± 0.01
All	0.36 ± 0.02	0.64 ± 0.02	0.86 ± 0.01	0.97 ± <0.01	0.96 ± <0.01
Color + Composition + Textures	0.37 ± 0.02	0.64 ± 0.02	0.86 ± 0.01	0.98 ± 0.01	0.96 ± <0.01
Color + Composition	**0.42 ± 0.02**	**0.71 ± 0.02**	**0.91 ± 0.01**	**0.99 ± 0.01**	**0.97 ± <0.01**

In Table 2 are reported the CMC values at different ranks, together with the normalized Area Under the Curve (nAUC). As visible, the color category is the most significant, followed by composition, texture and content. The poor performance of the content features, that is, object detectors, is due to the fact that object detectors produce many errors, both in precision and recall: this is due to the nature of the Flickr photos, which are artistic and not reminiscent those of the object recognition benchmark (PASCAL, CALTECH and the like). We evaluate all the possible combinations of group of features (some of them are reported in the table), with the best one formed by color and composition, which will be sued in the following. Interesting, the textures seem to slightly degrade the performances.

4.2 Identification Results

The results of the identification task are carried out following the protocol of [12]. We cross-validate the parameters of the SVM classifier with Gaussian kernel obtaining the best configuration with $C = 1000$ and $g = 0.001$. As competitors, we report the performance of [12] (with the acronym $LASSO$) and [13] (PaD). In addition, we set up some baselines, which may help in motivating some technical choices we have made with our framework. The $Ensemble$ method is the same as our proposal, with the only difference that the CGs are learned independently, without sharing their parameters; the PCA approach, which actually uses Principal Component Analysis to create a low dimensional space projection space where all the images can be projected. Once the projection of a probe signature is performed, the resulting map containing the projected images (opportunely quantized in order to be of the same dimension irrespective of the nature and cardinalities of the signatures) is fed into the exemplar SVMs. In Fig. 4(left) the various CMC curves are reported by fixing the number of gallery images to 100, and the number of probe images to 5. As visible, our approach overcomes all the competitors.

In Table 3 we report (in the upper part) the performance of our approach while varying the number of test images used to compose the probe signature of a user, while keeping the number of images used to build the gallery signature fixed to 100; in the lower part we report the analogue figure while varying the cardinality of the gallery signatures and keeping fixed to 100 the cardinality of the probe signature. Intuitively, augmenting the cardinality of the gallery/probe signature does ameliorate the identification performance.

To test the importance of having different CG resolutions, we perform a set of identification trials while using 100 images of gallery and 100 of probe, with 1, 2, 5, 10, 20 and 35 different resolutions (35 is the total number of resolutions employed). In the case of a single resolution, all the S windows size between 10 and $E - 1 = 44$ have been independently evaluated, averaging their recognition performance. For evaluating higher numbers of resolutions, different windows size have been sampled without replacement (depending on the cardinality being evaluated) and ranked in descending order. After that, the window with the largest size has been learned with random initialization; the obtained CG has

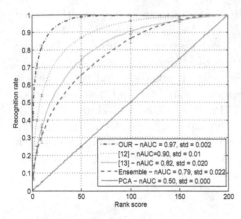

Table 3. Identification results, varying the number T_{te}/T_{tr} of images of gallery/probe signatures (and fixing the other cardinality to 100 for each user). All the results are with a variance of less than the 1 %.

Fig. 4. Comparative results for the identification task, with 5 images for the probe signatures and 100 images for the gallery signatures.

T_{te}	rank 1	rank 5	rank 20	rank 50	nAUC
1	0.19	0.42	0.66	0.86	0.90
5	0.42	0.71	0.71	0.99	0.97
20	0.63	0.87	0.7	1.00	0.99
100	0.73	0.92	0.98	1.00	0.99
T_{tr}	rank 1	rank 5	rank 20	rank 50	nAUC
5	0.29	0.59	0.83	0.94	0.95
10	0.46	0.80	0.95	0.99	0.98
20	0.63	0.89	0.98	1.00	0.99
50	0.71	0.93	0.99	1.00	0.99
100	0.71	0.92	0.98	1.00	0.99

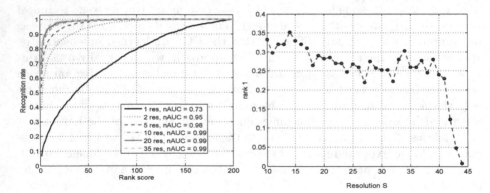

Fig. 5. Identification scores while varying the number of resolution employed, and analysis at rank 1.

been used as prior for the second ranked one and so on. Results (averaged over 35 gallery/probe splits) are portrayed in Fig. 5.

As expected, increasing the number of resolution levels does augment the identification capabilities. To better understand the role of each resolution, each one of them has been evaluated independently (under the same experimental protocol, $T_{tr} = T_{te} = 100$, 35 repetitions), reporting in Fig. 5 the rank-1 identification score (standard deviation <1 % in all the cases). It emerges that performance is better while going toward higher resolutions, even if no one of them can reach the same score one can get when using the joint framework (that is, 0.71, see Table 3). This means that every resolution level carries out a different complementary analysis of the images.

4.3 Verification Results

In the verification scenario, the capability of the system to verify if a signature matches a given identity is evaluated. For this purpose, a ROC curve is computed for every user u, where client images are taken from the probe set of the user u and impostor images are taken from all the other probe sets. Depending on the number of images taken into account, different kind of client/impostor maps may be built. Given an "authentication threshold", i.e., a value over which the subject is authenticated, sensitivity (true positive rate) and specificity (true negative rate) can be computed. By varying this threshold the ROC curve is finally obtained. In Fig. 6 the authentication ROC curves are portrayed; other than AUC, the equal error rate (EER) is also reported, which models the error when sensitivity and 1-specificity have an equal value.

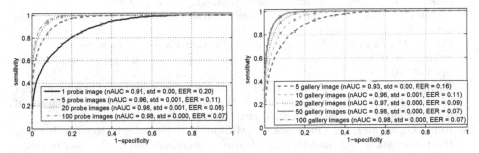

Fig. 6. Verification scores: the ROC curves (together with AUC and EER score) are reported while varying the number of probe (left) and gallery (right) images employed.

Even in this case, augmenting the number of test images per signatures increments the performance; as for varying the number of images used for the gallery signatures, and the number of resolutions for producing the multi-scale CG, analogue results than those obtained for the recognition task can be observed, so the results have been omitted.

5   Conclusions

Personal aesthetics is a recent soft biometrics trait that emerged thanks to the large diffusion of images in Internet and to the possibility of liking them. The idea of capturing the identity of people using their aesthetical preferences underlies the capability of understanding their personal tastes. This approach does both the things in a satisfying fashion: Counting Grids allow to project images in a latent space where similar pictures are mapped nearby, so that semantic areas can emerge and being observed and interpreted. In this respect, future work should focus on the kind of features to use, and in particular on how medium-high level features can be crafted, since object detection have shown to be unreliable; we think that deep learning could be well suited for this aim. On the other side, our method shows that CGs induce latent representations (the embedding maps) very informative for discriminating users by means of kernel machines, especially when multiple images preferred by a single individual are available. In this regard, future work should be spent in testing a real application where personal aesthetics are exploited, encouraging their use in genuine soft/biometric scenarios.

References

1. Lovato, P., Perina, A., Sebe, N., Zandonà, O., Montagnini, A., Bicego, M., Cristani, M.: Tell me what you like and i'll tell you what you are: Discriminating visual preferences on flickr data. In: Lee, K.M., Matsushita, Y., Rehg, J.M., Hu, Z. (eds.) ACCV 2012, Part I. LNCS, vol. 7724, pp. 45–56. Springer, Heidelberg (2013)
2. Dantcheva, A., Velardo, C., D'angelo, A., Dugelay, J.L.: Bag of soft biometrics for person identification. Multimed. Tools Appl. **51**, 739–777 (2011)
3. Yampolskiy, R.V., Govindaraju, V.: Behavioural biometrics: a survey and classification. Int. J. Biometrics **1**, 81–113 (2008)
4. Pusara, M., Brodley, C.E.: User re-authentication via mouse movements. In: Proceedings of ACM workshop on Visualization and data mining for computer security, pp. 1–8 (2004)
5. Rybnik, M., Tabedzki, M., Saeed, K.: A keystroke dynamics based system for user identification. In: 7th Computer Information Systems and Industrial Management Applications, CISIM 2008, pp. 225–230. IEEE (2008)
6. Roffo, G., Segalin, C., Vinciarelli, A., Murino, V., Cristani, M.: Reading between the turns: Statistical modeling for identity recognition and verification in chats. In: 10th IEEE International Conference on Advanced Video and Signal Based Surveillance, AVSS, pp. 99–104 (2013)
7. Olejnik, L., Castelluccia, C., Janc, A., et al.: Why johnny can't browse in peace: On the uniqueness of web browsing history patterns. In: 5th Workshop on Hot Topics in Privacy Enhancing Technologies (HotPETs) (2012)
8. Jin, X., Wang, C., Luo, J., Yu, X., Han, J.: Likeminer: a system for mining the power of 'like' in social media networks. In: Proceedings of the 17th ACM SIGKDD International Conference on Knowledge Discovery and Data Mining, pp. 753–756 (2011)
9. Joshi, D., Datta, R., Fedorovskaya, E., Luong, Q.T., Wang, J., Li, J., Luo, J.: Aesthetics and emotions in images. IEEE Sig. Process. Mag. **28**, 94–115 (2011)
10. Furnham, A., Walker, J.: The influence of personality traits, previous experience of art, and demographic variables on artistic preference. Personality Individ. Differ. **31**, 997–1017 (2001)
11. Perina, A., Jojic, N.: Image analysis by counting on a grid. In: IEEE Conference on Computer Vision and Pattern Recognition (CVPR), pp. 1985–1992 (2011)
12. Lovato, P., Bicego, M., Segalin, C., Perina, A., Sebe, N., Cristani, M.: Faved! biometrics: Tell me which image you like and i'll tell you who you are. IEEE Trans. Inf. Forensics Secur. **9**, 364–374 (2014)
13. Segalin, C., Perina, A., Cristani, M.: Biometrics on visual preferences: A "Pump and Distill" regression approach. In: IEEE International Conference on Image Processing (ICIP) (2014)
14. Machajdik, J., Hanbury, A.: Affective image classification using features inspired by psychology and art theory. In: International Conference on Multimedia, pp. 83–92. ACM (2010)

15. Felzenszwalb, P., Girshick, R., McAllester, D., Ramanan, D.: Object detection with discriminatively trained part-based models. IEEE Trans. Pattern Anal. Mach. Intell. **32**, 1627–1645 (2010)
16. Datta, R., Joshi, D., Li, J., Wang, J.Z.: Studying aesthetics in photographic images using a computational approach. In: Leonardis, A., Bischof, H., Pinz, A. (eds.) ECCV 2006. LNCS, vol. 3953, pp. 288–301. Springer, Heidelberg (2006)
17. Valdez, P., Mehrabian, A.: Effects of color on emotions. J. Exp. Psychol. Gen. **123**, 394 (1994)
18. Mardia, K., Jupp, P.: Directional Statistics. Wiley, Chichester (2009)
19. Comaniciu, D., Meer, P.: Mean shift: A robust approach toward feature space analysis. IEEE TPAMI **24**, 603–619 (2002)
20. Georgescu, C.: Synergism in low level vision. In: International Conference on Pattern Recognition, pp. 150–155 (2002)
21. Tamura, H., Mori, S., Yamawaki, T.: Texture features corresponding to visual perception. IEEE Trans. Syst. Man Cybern. **8**, 460–473 (1978)
22. Viola, P., Jones, M.: Rapid object detection using a boosted cascade of simple features. In: IEEE Conference on CVPR, pp. 511–518 (2001)
23. Moon, H., Phillips, P.J.: Computational and performance aspects of PCA-based face-recognition algorithms. Perception-London **30**, 303–322 (2001)

FASA: Fast, Accurate, and Size-Aware Salient Object Detection

Gökhan Yildirim[✉] and Sabine Süsstrunk

School of Computer and Communication Sciences,
École Polytechnique Fédérale de Lausanne, Lausanne, Switzerland
{gokhan.yildirim,sabine.susstrunk}@epfl.ch

Abstract. Fast and accurate salient-object detectors are important for various image processing and computer vision applications, such as adaptive compression and object segmentation. It is also desirable to have a detector that is aware of the position and the size of the salient objects. In this paper, we propose a salient-object detection method that is fast, accurate, and size-aware. For efficient computation, we quantize the image colors and estimate the spatial positions and sizes of the quantized colors. We then feed these values into a statistical model to obtain a probability of saliency. In order to estimate the final saliency, this probability is combined with a global color contrast measure. We test our method on two public datasets and show that our method significantly outperforms the fast state-of-the-art methods. In addition, it has comparable performance and is an order of magnitude faster than the accurate state-of-the-art methods. We exhibit the potential of our algorithm by processing a high-definition video in real time.

1 Introduction

When we examine an image without specifying a task, our visual system attends mostly to the low-level distinctive or *salient* regions. Visual saliency can thus be defined as how much a certain image region visually stands out, compared to its surrounding area.

Low-level visual saliency deals with color and texture contrast, and their spatial constraints. The studies on these types of saliency-extraction techniques are, in general, inspired by the human visual system (HVS). A leading investigation in this field was done by Itti et al. [1], where, to generate a saliency map, center-to-surround differences in color, intensity, and orientations are combined at different scales with a non-maximum suppression.

One of the branches of visual saliency is salient-object detection. It is a popular and extensively studied topic in the computer vision community. It has the ability to mimic the human visual attention by *rapidly* finding important regions in an image. Therefore, similar to how the human brain operates [2], various applications, such as video compression [3], image retargeting [4], video retargeting [5,6] and object detection [7], can allocate the processing resources according to saliency maps given by the detectors. As saliency detection is a

© Springer International Publishing Switzerland 2015
D. Cremers et al. (Eds.): ACCV 2014, Part III, LNCS 9005, pp. 514–528, 2015.
DOI: 10.1007/978-3-319-16811-1_34

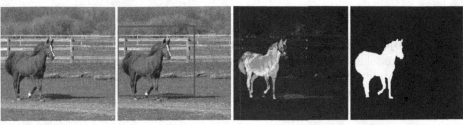

(a) Original image   (b) Position & size   (c) Saliency map   (d) Ground truth

Fig. 1. FASA processes (a) the 400 × 400 pixel image in 6 ms and outputs (b) the parameters of rectangles that enclose the salient objects and (c) a saliency map, which is comparable to (d) the ground truth.

pre-processing step, it should process the image in an efficient and accurate manner and provide as much information as possible for the successive step.

In this paper, we satisfy the efficiency, accuracy, and information criteria by introducing a **F**ast, **A**ccurate, and **S**ize-**A**ware (FASA) salient object detector. To achieve these goals, our method first performs a color quantization and forms a histogram in perceptually uniform CIEL*a*b* color space. It then uses the histogram to compute the spatial center and variance of the quantized colors via an efficient bilateral filtering approach. We show that the said variables are related to the position and the size of the salient object. Our method builds a probabilistic model of salient-object sizes and positions in an image. In order to compute the probability of saliency, the spatial center and variance of the colors are used in this model. The saliency probabilities are then multiplied with a global contrast value that is efficiently calculated using the quantized color differences. Finally, to obtain a full-resolution saliency map, the saliency values are linearly interpolated and are assigned to individual pixels using their quantization (histogram) bins.

On average, our method computes the saliency maps in 4.3 milliseconds (ms), when it uses the SED-100 [8] dataset and in 5.5 ms, when it uses the MSRA-1000 dataset [9]. On the same datasets, we show that our method is one order of magnitude faster than the accurate state-of-the-art methods and has a comparable performance in salient-object detection. Furthermore, it performs significantly better than other fast saliency-detection methods. In addition to fast computation and accurate saliency maps, our method also supplies the position and the size of the salient regions. We demonstrate the potential of our algorithm on a public high-definition (HD) video by detecting the saliency maps in *real time* (over 30 frames per second), as well as the position and the size of the salient object. In Fig. 1, the outputs of our algorithm are illustrated with an example.

The outline of our paper is as follows: In Sect. 2, we summarize the recent research that is related to our method. In Sect. 3, we explain and discuss our efficient saliency detection method and its outputs. In Sect. 4, we present numerical and visual results of our method and compare it with other techniques on the MSRA-1000 [9] and SED-100 [8] datasets. In Sect. 5, we recapitulate the main points of our paper and explain possible future research directions.

2   Related Work

The main objective of a salient-object detector is to *rapidly* and *accurately* generate a pixel-precision map of visually distinctive objects and to provide additional information about them. We thus divide the previous studies on salient-object detection into two groups.

2.1   Fast Methods

One approach to accelerate saliency detection without introducing undesirable loss of accuracy is to quantize the intensity levels and/or compute the histogram of an image. In Zhai et al. [10], global color contrast is calculated using separate histograms for each channel. Whereas, in Cheng et al. [11], the color contrast is computed using a joint histogram. Both of the methods rely on global color contrast as the primary measure of visual saliency and they perform color quantization in sRGB color space. As sRGB is not perceptually uniform, histograms require a large number of quantization bins, otherwise they can suffer from large quantization errors. In order to avoid this, in our method, we perform the color quantization in CIEL*a*b* color space and, consequently, need fewer quantization bins. This provides faster, more accurate, and perceptually uniform color-contrast estimations.

Another approach for fast saliency estimation is to analyze the frequency content of the images with salient objects. Achanta et al. [9] show that visual distinctiveness is related to almost all frequency bands. Thus, saliency can be detected by simply computing the color contrast between image pixels and the average color of the scene. This corresponds to a band-pass filter. This method is limited to the images, where average scene color is sufficiently different from the color of the salient object. It does not suppress multi-colored backgrounds very well. Our modeling of the spatial center and variances of colors overcomes this limitation.

2.2   Accurate Methods

Other studies have focused on the accuracy of the saliency map and ignored the computational efficiency. In order to estimate the visual saliency, Perazzi et al. [12] fuse the spatial variance of a color of a superpixel and its contrast with its local surroundings. The study in [11] is extended in Cheng et al. [13], where a Gaussian mixture model with a spatial constraint is introduced for a spatially-aware (non-global) color quantization. This step is followed by a further color clustering for calculating the spatial variance and contrast of the colors in a scene. To achieve an initial foreground and background segregation, Yang et al. [14] form a superpixel graph and combine the saliency maps with different image boundary queries. They find the final saliency map by querying the initial foreground estimation.

Similar to ours, some of the techniques use the spatial variance of a color [12,13]. They assume that the spatial variance of a salient object is smaller than the background. Therefore, they inversely correlate the variance and saliency, and introduce a bias towards detecting smaller objects as more salient. In Sects. 3.2 and 3.5, we discuss this relationship and introduce a statistical model based on salient-object position and size to correctly address the problem.

Salient-object detection is a pre-processing step. In order to properly allocate the processing resources for higher-level tasks, such as object detection and recognition, the detectors should rapidly detect the salient regions. Therefore, we propose that the efficiency of salient object detectors is as important as their accuracy.

3   Our Method

Our saliency-detection method, FASA, combines a probability of saliency with a global contrast map. Figure 2 provides a scheme illustrating our method. For computational efficiency, our algorithm first quantizes an image to reduce the number of colors. Then, in order to estimate the position and the size of the salient object, the spatial center and variances of the quantized colors are calculated. These values are put in an object model to compute the probability of saliency. The same quantized colors are used to generate global contrast values as well. Finally, the saliency probabilities of the colors and the contrast values are fused into a single saliency map.

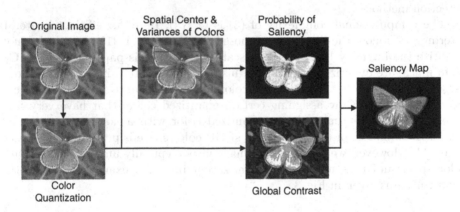

Fig. 2. Scheme of our method.

3.1   Spatial Center and Variances of a Color

One of the prominent components of visual saliency is the spatial variance of a color in a scene [12,13]. In order to compute it, we first define a position and a color vector notation.

$$\mathbf{p}_i = \begin{bmatrix} x_i \\ y_i \end{bmatrix}, \mathbf{C}_i = \begin{bmatrix} L^*(\mathbf{p}_i) \\ a^*(\mathbf{p}_i) \\ b^*(\mathbf{p}_i) \end{bmatrix} \tag{1}$$

Here, $\mathbf{p}_i$ is the position vector, which represents the coordinates (x_i, y_i) of the ith pixel. $\mathbf{C}_i$ is the color vector of the pixel at position $\mathbf{p}_i$ in CIEL*a*b* color space. The spatial center $\{m_x(\mathbf{p}_i), m_y(\mathbf{p}_i)\}$ and the horizontal and vertical variances $\{V_x(\mathbf{p}_i), V_y(\mathbf{p}_i)\}$ of a color can be calculated using the following equation:

$$m_x(\mathbf{p}_i) = \frac{\sum_{j=1}^{N} w^c(\mathbf{C}_i, \mathbf{C}_j) \cdot x_j}{\sum_{j=1}^{N} w^c(\mathbf{C}_i, \mathbf{C}_j)}$$

$$V_x(\mathbf{p}_i) = \frac{\sum_{j=1}^{N} w^c(\mathbf{C}_i, \mathbf{C}_j) \cdot \left(x_j - m_x(\mathbf{p}_i)\right)^2}{\sum_{j=1}^{N} w^c(\mathbf{C}_i, \mathbf{C}_j)} \qquad (2)$$

Similar calculations can be done for y dimension. Here, N is the total number of pixels in an image, and $w^c(\mathbf{C}_i, \mathbf{C}_j)$ are the color weights and are calculated using a Gaussian function.

$$w^c(\mathbf{C}_i, \mathbf{C}_j) = e^{-\frac{||\mathbf{C}_i - \mathbf{C}_j||^2}{2\sigma_c^2}} \qquad (3)$$

Here, σ_c is a parameter to adjust the effect of the color difference. If we look at (2), we can notice that w^c in both of the equations depends on the spatial coordinates. These calculations correspond to a bilateral filter with a color kernel, namely $w^c(\mathbf{C}_i, \mathbf{C}_j)$. For computational efficiency, the spatial kernel (or support) is chosen to be the whole image, which turns our algorithm into a global saliency-detection method.

The computational complexity of (2) is $O(N^2)$. Here, for efficient bilateral filtering, we follow the approach proposed by Yang et al. [15], in which they quantize the intensity levels of a grayscale image. In this paper, the colors $\mathbf{C}_i$ of an image are quantized (i.e., a color histogram is created) into a set of colors $\{\mathbf{Q}_k\}_{k=1}^{K}$, where K is the number of colors after the quantization. In practice, we can minimize K by assigning certain quantized colors that have very few pixels to the perceptually closest quantized color with a non-zero number of pixels. A similar color quantization in sRGB color space is performed in Cheng et al. [11]. However, we quantize the image in perceptually uniform CIEL*a*b* color space and thus need fewer quantization bins. An example of the color quantization is given in Fig. 3.

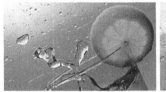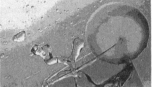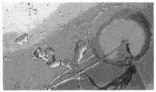

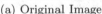
    (a) Original Image   (b) 175 quantized colors   (c) 50 quantized colors

Fig. 3. The L*a*b* histogram (8 bins in each channel, $8^3 = 512$ bins in total) of (a) the original image contains (b) 175 quantized colors with non-zero histogram bins and (c) 50 quantized colors that can cover 95 % of the image pixels.

In our paper, $\mathbf{C}_i \rightarrow \mathbf{Q}_k$ indicates that the color of the pixel at $\mathbf{p}_i$ falls to the kth color histogram bin after the quantization. If we quickly calculate the color histogram of the image and precompute $w^c(\mathbf{Q}_k, \mathbf{Q}_j)$, we can efficiently estimate the spatial center and variances of the quantized colors as follows:

$$m'_{xk} = \frac{\sum_{j=1}^{K} w^c(\mathbf{Q}_k, \mathbf{Q}_j) \cdot \sum_{\forall x_i | \mathbf{C}_i \rightarrow \mathbf{Q}_j} x_i}{\sum_{j=1}^{K} h_j \cdot w^c(\mathbf{Q}_k, \mathbf{Q}_j)}$$

$$V'_{xk} = \frac{\sum_{j=1}^{K} w^c(\mathbf{Q}_k, \mathbf{Q}_j) \cdot \sum_{\forall x_i | \mathbf{C}_i \rightarrow \mathbf{Q}_j} (x_i - m'_{xk})^2}{\sum_{j=1}^{K} h_j \cdot w^c(\mathbf{Q}_k, \mathbf{Q}_j)} \tag{4}$$

Similar calculations can be performed for y dimension. Here, $\{m'_{xk}, m'_{yk}\}$ is the spatial center and $\{V'_{xk}, V'_{yk}\}$ are the spatial variances of the kth quantized color. $h_k = |\forall x_i | \mathbf{C}_i \rightarrow \mathbf{Q}_k|$ is the number of pixels in the kth color histogram bin. The spatial center and variances at each pixel in (2) can be estimated as follows:

$$m_x(\mathbf{p}_i) \approx m'_{xk} \quad \forall \mathbf{p}_i | \mathbf{C}_i \rightarrow \mathbf{Q}_k$$
$$V_x(\mathbf{p}_i) \approx V'_{xk} \quad \forall \mathbf{p}_i | \mathbf{C}_i \rightarrow \mathbf{Q}_k \tag{5}$$

Similar calculations can be performed for y dimension. We reduce the complexity of the bilateral filtering in (2) to $O(K^2)$ via the color quantization in (4). In addition, as explained in Sect. 3.2, $\{m'_{xk}, m'_{yk}\}$ and $\{V'_{xk}, V'_{yk}\}$ provide valuable position and size cues about the salient object.

3.2 The Center and the Size of a Salient Object

The spatial center $\{m'_{xk}, m'_{yk}\}$ shows the color-weighted center of mass of kth quantized color of the image. The spatial variances $\{V'_{xk}, V'_{yk}\}$ depict how spatially distributed the same quantized color is within the image. In addition, it also gives us an idea about the "size" of that color. In order to show this relationship, in Fig. 4(a), we illustrate a test image of size 256×256 pixels that includes a red and a blue rectangle.

In this image, we have three dominant colors, i.e. $k \in \{red, green, blue\}$. As there is sufficient global color contrast between these colors, we can assume $w^c(\mathbf{Q}_k, \mathbf{Q}_j) \approx 0$ for $k \neq j$ and we know that $w^c(\mathbf{Q}_k, \mathbf{Q}_k) = 1$. By using this, we can rewrite (4) and estimate the center of the objects as follows:

$$m'_{x,rect} \approx \frac{1}{h_{rect}} \sum_{\forall x_i | \mathbf{C}_i \rightarrow \mathbf{Q}_{rect}} x_i = r_{xc} \tag{6}$$

Here r_{xc} is the x coordinate of the center of the red rectangle. As rectangles are symmetrical in both horizontal and vertical dimensions, we can easily compute the center of the red rectangle (r_{xc}, r_{yc}) using (6). The size of an object can be calculated as follows:

$$V'_{x,rect} \approx \frac{1}{h_{rect}} \sum_{\forall x_i | \mathbf{C}_i \rightarrow \mathbf{Q}_{rect}} (x_i - r_{xc})^2 \approx \frac{r_{yl} \cdot \int_{-r_{xl}/2}^{r_{xl}/2} x^2 \cdot dx}{r_{yl} \cdot r_{xl}} = \frac{r_{xl}^2}{12} \tag{7}$$

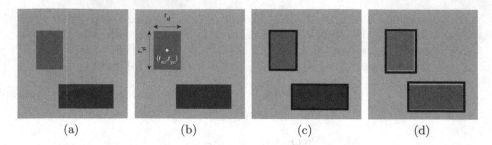

Fig. 4. (a) A test image with two salient rectangles with (b) the center and size parameters of the red rectangle. (c) The estimated position and sizes are shown with black bounding rectangle. (d) The accuracy of the center and the size estimation degrades, when the color of the objects are similar (Color figure online).

Here, r_{xl} and r_{yl} are the width and the height of the red rectangle, respectively. Similar equations can be derived for the y dimension. As we can see from (6) and (7), given sufficient color contrast, we are able to estimate the center and the size of both rectangles and ellipses, which is illustrated with black boundaries in Fig. 4(c).

Conventionally, a bounding rectangle is used to represent a detected object. However, in some cases, it could be useful to represent the objects using a bounding ellipse instead. The central position of a bounding ellipse can be computed using (6). To estimate the dimensions of an ellipse, we slightly modify (7):

$$V'_{x,ellipse} \approx \frac{\pi/4 \cdot e_{yl} \cdot \int_{-e_{xl}/2}^{e_{xl}/2} x^2 \sqrt{1 - \frac{x^2}{(e_{xl}/2)^2}} \cdot dx}{\pi^2/16 \cdot e_{yl} \cdot e_{xl}} = \frac{e_{xl}^2}{16} \tag{8}$$

Here, e_{xl} and e_{yl} are the width and the height of an ellipse, respectively. The equation for estimating the height is similar to (8).

Natural images often contain non-rectangular objects and the color of the objects might interfere with each other as shown in Fig. 4(d). However, the spatial center and variances still give us an idea about the position and the size of an object (or background), so that we can better calculate the saliency value. Moreover, this additional information is beneficial for object detection applications, as demonstrated in Sect. 4.4.

3.3   Computing Probability of Saliency

The salient objects tend to be smaller then their surrounding background. As they do not calculate the position and the size of an object, Perazzi et al. [12] and Cheng et al. [13] favor small spatial variations by using an inverting function to map the spatial variance to visual saliency. This creates a bias towards smaller objects.

In our method, we estimate the position and the size of the salient object, thus we can statistically model a mapping from these variables to a saliency probability. To generate our model, we use the MSRA-A dataset [16] that includes over

20,000 images with salient objects and their enclosing rectangles marked by three persons. The MSRA-1000 dataset is derived from the MSRA-A dataset. Therefore, to generate unbiased statistics, we exclude the images of the MSRA-1000 from the MSRA-A dataset. In Fig. 5, we illustrate the probability distributions in terms of the width and the height of the salient objects, as well as their distance to the image center.

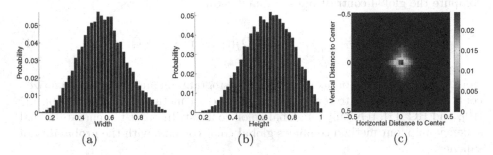

(a)   (b)   (c)

Fig. 5. Distributions of object (a) width (b) height, and (c) distance to image center in the MSRA-A dataset [16] based on the ground truth rectangles. All values are normalized by using the image dimensions.

We can see in Fig. 5 that all probability distributions resemble a Gaussian distribution. Therefore, we model their joint distribution with a multivariate Gaussian function given as follows:

$$P(\mathbf{p}_i) = \frac{1}{(2\pi)^2\sqrt{|\mathbf{\Sigma}|}} \exp\left(-\frac{(\mathbf{g}_i - \boldsymbol{\mu})^T \mathbf{\Sigma}^{-1}(\mathbf{g}_i - \boldsymbol{\mu})}{2}\right)$$

$$\mathbf{g}_i = \left[\frac{\sqrt{12 \cdot V_x(\mathbf{p}_i)}}{n_w} \quad \frac{\sqrt{12 \cdot V_y(\mathbf{p}_i)}}{n_h} \quad \frac{m_x(\mathbf{p}_i) - n_w/2}{n_w} \quad \frac{m_y(\mathbf{p}_i) - n_h/2}{n_h}\right]^T \tag{9}$$

Here, $P(\mathbf{p}_i)$ is the probability of saliency of an input image with dimensions n_w and n_h. Note that the factor 12 in $\mathbf{g}_i$ comes from (7).

The mean vector and the covariance matrix of the joint Gaussian model that is illustrated in Fig. 5 are given as follows:

$$\boldsymbol{\mu} = \begin{bmatrix} 0.5555 \\ 0.6449 \\ 0.0002 \\ 0.0063 \end{bmatrix}, \quad \mathbf{\Sigma} = \begin{bmatrix} 0.0231 & -0.0010 & 0.0001 & -0.0002 \\ -0.0010 & 0.0246 & -0.0000 & 0.0000 \\ 0.0001 & -0.0000 & 0.0115 & 0.0003 \\ -0.0002 & 0.0000 & 0.0003 & 0.0080 \end{bmatrix} \tag{10}$$

If we analyze $\boldsymbol{\mu}$ in (10), we can see that the average height is larger than the average width. This could be due to a tendency of the photographers to take landscape photographs over portraits, in order to emphasize salient objects.

In addition, the average position is very close to the image center, thus validating the well-known center-bias phenomenon [17].

3.4 Global Contrast

High color-contrast is widely used as a measure of saliency [1,9–14]. Once we have the quantized colors and the color differences $w^c(\mathbf{Q}_k, \mathbf{Q}_j)$, we can easily compute the global contrast of each quantized color as follows:

$$R(\mathbf{p}_i) = \sum_{j=1}^{K} h_j \cdot ||\mathbf{Q}_k - \mathbf{Q}_j||_2, \quad \forall \mathbf{p}_i | \mathbf{C}_i \rightarrow \mathbf{Q}_k \qquad (11)$$

Here, h_j is the number of pixels in the jth histogram bin and $\mathbf{Q}_j$ is the quantized color that corresponds to that bin. State-of-the-art methods, such as FT [9], LC [10], and HC [11], rely only on global color contrast. In order to generate a final saliency map, our method combines global color contrast with the probability of saliency.

3.5 Computing the Final Saliency Map

In order to combine the probability of saliency and the global contrast into a single saliency map, we use the following approach:

$$S(\mathbf{p}_i) = \frac{\sum_{j=1}^{K} w^c(\mathbf{Q}_k, \mathbf{Q}_j) \cdot P(\mathbf{p}_i) \cdot R(\mathbf{p}_i)}{\sum_{j=1}^{K} w^c(\mathbf{Q}_k, \mathbf{Q}_j)}, \quad \forall \mathbf{p}_i | \mathbf{C}_i \rightarrow \mathbf{Q}_k \qquad (12)$$

Here, $S(\mathbf{p}_i)$ is the saliency value of the pixel at $\mathbf{p}_i$. All of the computations for $P(\mathbf{p}_i)$, $R(\mathbf{p}_i)$, and $S(\mathbf{p}_i)$ can be done using quantized colors. Therefore, our implementation performs the calculations by using K colors and assigns the corresponding saliency values to individual pixels based on their color quantization bins. The final computational complexity of our method is $O(N)+O(K^2)$, where $O(N)$ comes from the histogram computation and $O(K^2)$ comes from the bilateral filtering and other quantization related computations. A color weighting is used in (12) for smoother saliency values. After computing the final saliency map, we normalize the map between 0 and 1.

4 Experiments

In this section, to show the most recent state-of-the-art performance on the MSRA-1000 [9] and the SED-100 [8] datasets, we compare our **FASA** method to fast saliency detection methods, such as FT [9], LC [10], HC [11], as well as accurate methods, such as GC [13], SF [12], RC [11], and GMR [14]. FASA performs efficient and image-dependent quantization in CIEL*a*b* color space and benefits from a statistical object model. Therefore, it is one order of magnitude faster than accurate methods while significantly outperforming other fast techniques.

4.1 Experimental Setup

Given an input image, we quantize its colors in CIEL*a*b* color space. We use 8 bins in each channel. In order to minimize the quantization errors, instead of using the full range of CIEL*a*b* (for example $L^* \in [0, 100]$), we divide the range, defined by the minimum and the maximum value of each channel, into 8 bins. This gives us a histogram of size $8^3 = 512$. We further reduce the number of colors to a set of colors that represents 95 % of the image pixels. We reassign the excluded non-zero color histogram bins to the perceptually closest bins. There are, on average, 55 and 60 colors per image in the MSRA-1000 and the SED-100 datasets, respectively. We use $\sigma_c = 16$ to calculate the color weights $w^c(\mathbf{Q}_k, \mathbf{Q}_j)$. For all methods, we run the corresponding author's implementations using an Intel Core i7 2.3 GHz with 16 GB RAM.

4.2 Performance Comparisons

The color quantization step, prior to the bilateral filtering, greatly reduces the computational complexity of our method while still retaining the saliency accuracy. Our algorithm estimates the visual saliency of an image in the MSRA-1000 and the SED-100 datasets in, on average, 5.5 and 4.3 ms, respectively. The comparison of execution times is given in Table 1. Note that the most time consuming step (superpixel segmentation) in GMR is implemented in C++ and it processes the MSRA-1000 images in approximately 200 ms, on average.

Table 1. Average computation time (in miliseconds) for the MSRA-1000 (12×10^4 pixels per image) and the SED-100 (8.7×10^4 pixels per image) datasets.

	Accurate				Fast			
	GMR [14]	SF [12]	RC [11]	GC [13]	FT [9]	HC [11]	LC [10]	**FASA**
MSRA-1000	262	241	180	68	16	12	3	**5.5**
SED-100	214	198	121	50	13	10	3	**4.3**
Code	Matlab/C++	C++	C++	C++	C++	C++	C++	C++

To reduce the computation time, the methods LC, HC, RC, and GC execute a color quantization step that is similar to ours. They quantize the colors in sRGB space by using either 255 bins (LC, independent histograms for each channel) or 12 bins (HC, RC, GC) per channel. Instead, we perform the quantization in the perceptually more uniform CIEL*a*b* color space and adjust the histogram using the minimum and the maximum values of L*a*b* channels of the processed image. Consequently, we need only 8 bins per channel and obtain a better and faster representation of the image.

In Fig. 6, we compare the precision and recall curves of our method with the other methods on the MSRA-1000 and SED-100 datasets. As it can be seen from Fig. 6(a) and (b), our algorithm significantly outperforms the fast methods, such as FT, LC, and HC, because they only take the color contrast (global

and/or local) into account. The local saliency-detection methods, such as SF
and GC, also use the spatial variance as a part of their saliency computation.
However, as stated before, they directly favor smaller objects by assuming an
inverse correlation between the spatial variance and the object saliency. We use,
instead, the position and the size information in a statistical model and, even
though our method is global, we achieve an accuracy comparable to SF, GC,
and RC and we are one order of magnitude faster.

As we state in Sect. 2.2, saliency detection is a pre-processing step for successive applications. Therefore, the speed of a salient-object detector can be as
essential as its accuracy. In this paper, we focus on the efficiency and present
a method that is 50 times faster than GMR, which is one of the most accurate
state-of-the-art salient-object detectors.

Our method outputs additional position and size information about salient
objects, which can be considered as an "objectness" measure. Therefore, we compare the object-detection capabilities of FASA to well-known objectness measuring methods, such as Alexe et al. [18] and BING [19]. The object-detection rate

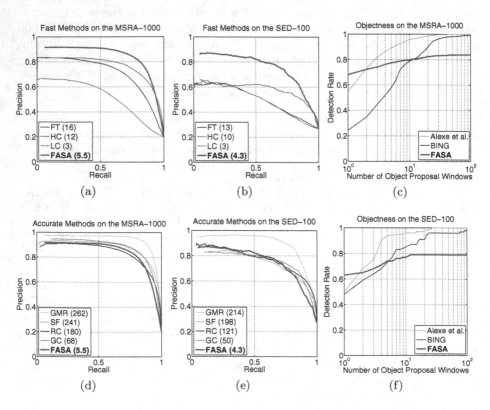

Fig. 6. Salient object detection performance of our method are compared to fast and
accurate methods in (a, b, d, e). The numbers in parentheses indicate the execution
times of the corresponding methods. The objectness detection rate of our method is
compared to other methods in (c) and (e).

(probability of detecting an object) versus the number of object proposal windows for the MSRA-1000 and the SED-100 datasets are illustrated in Fig. 6(c) and Fig. 6(f), respectively. Our method is more accurate if we just consider the first proposal window. This is logical as our method focuses on (and is optimized for) estimating the salient objects and provides object center and size as additional information. This property can be helpful to provide single and accurate proposals for object detection and tracking.

4.3 Visual Comparisons

We visually compare the saliency maps generated by different methods in Fig. 7. Due to the accurate quantization in CIEL*a*b* color space, our saliency maps are more uniform than the maps of LC and HC. Moreover, the background suppression of the probability of saliency is better than FT. Compared to the other fast methods, FASA generates visually better results.

Our maps are visually comparable to the maps of the accurate methods, such as RC, GC, SF, and even GMR. Considering that FASA is one order of magnitude faster than these methods, our method may be preferable for time-critical applications.

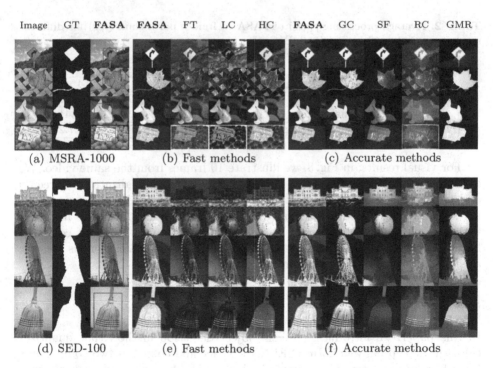

Fig. 7. Four example images from the MSRA-1000 and the SED-100 datasets. (a, d) FASA estimates the position and the size of the objects (red rectangles). (b, e) Our saliency maps are better than the maps of the fast methods and (c, f) they are visually comparable to the maps of the accurate state-of-the-art methods (GT: GroundTruth) (Color figure online).

4.4 Application to Videos

Our method is fast enough to use it as a real-time salient-object detector in videos. Furthermore, it provides the position and size information for the salient and non-salient parts of the image. This property can be used in applications such as object tracking in videos [20,21].

In order to demonstrate the potential of FASA, we estimate, using different resolutions, the saliency of the publicly available video "Big Buck Bunny"[1]. We are able to process the HD version (1280 × 720) of the video with a speed of 30 frames per second (fps). Given that the frame-rate of the video is 24 fps, our method estimates the saliency map and the center and the size of the objects in real time. The fps values under different resolutions are given in Table 2. The fps value linearly changes with the number of pixels in a single video frame. In other words, the number of pixels our method can process in a second ($N\times$ fps) is largely independent from the resolution of the image. This shows that our method has a computational complexity of $O(N) + O(K^2) \approx O(N)$, where K is the number of colors after quantization and $K^2 \ll N$. Note that our method is optimized to perform saliency detection in images and individually processes each video frame.

Table 2. Average processing speed of FASA in frames per second (fps) for different resolutions of the video "Big Buck Bunny".

		Resolution		
		1920 × 1080	1280 × 720	854 × 480
fps	Frames per second	13.7	**30.7**	66.5
N	Number of megapixels	2.07	0.92	0.41
$N\times$ fps	Number of megapixels per second	28.4	28.3	27.2

For visual results, in Fig. 8, we illustrate 10 frames from the same video. We encircle the most salient regions (saliency > 0.75 after normalization between 0 and 1) using their estimated positions and sizes, and we display the corresponding saliency maps. Due to its global nature, our method is accurate in scenes with a single salient object or multiple salient objects with different colors. It has a limited performance when color interference or a complex scene is present, as shown in the last two frames in Fig. 8.

5 Conclusion

In this paper, we introduce a salient-object detection method that quantizes colors in perceptually uniform CIEL*a*b* space and combines two components for a fast and accurate estimation of saliency. The first component deals with the spatial center and variances of the quantized colors via an efficient bilateral filtering. This component also produces a probability of saliency based on a

---

[1] http://www.bigbuckbunny.org/index.php/download/.

statistical object model that is extracted from the MSRA-A dataset [16]. The center and variance values are shown to be related to the position and the size of the salient objects. The second component computes the global color contrast. The final saliency map is calculated by linearly interpolating the product of the two components. Our method performs significantly better than other fast state-of-the-art methods and it is an order of magnitude faster than the methods with similar precision-recall performances on the MSRA-1000 [9] and SED-100 [8] datasets. We also present the potential of our method by generating saliency maps and by computing the position and the size of salient objects in 30 fps on an HD video.

For computational efficiency, our algorithm globally detects the visual saliency. This can create limitations in scenes with multiple salient objects and multi-colored salient objects, because colors interfere with each other during the estimation of saliency. In order to generate more accurate saliency maps, we can enforce spatial constraints to our color histogram through bilateral filtering or to our contrast computation, without significantly sacrificing the execution time. Another future research direction is to calculate temporally-aware color histograms for video processing.

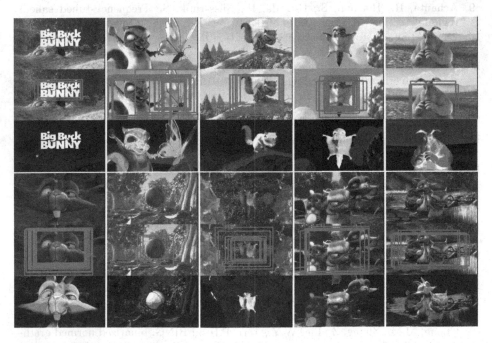

Fig. 8. 10 frames from the video "Big Buck Bunny". The first row shows the original frame, the second row position and the size of the most salient objects, and the third row the saliency map of the frame.

Acknowledgement. This work was supported by the Swiss National Science Foundation under grant number 200021-143406/1.

References

1. Itti, L., Koch, C., Niebur, E.: A model of saliency-based visual attention for rapid scene analysis. IEEE Trans. PAMI **20**, 1254–1259 (1998)
2. Anderson, J.R.: Cognitive Psychology and Its Implications, 5th edn. Worth, New York (2000)
3. Itti, L.: Automatic foveation for video compression using a neurobiological model of visual attention. IEEE Trans. Image Process. **13**, 1304–1318 (2004)
4. Achanta, R., Süsstrunk, S.: Saliency detection for content-aware image resizing. In: Proceedings of IEEE ICIP, pp. 1001–1004 (2009)
5. Xiang, Y., Kankanhalli, M.S.: Video retargeting for aesthetic enhancement. In: Proceedings of ACM Multimedia, pp. 919–922 (2010)
6. Wolf, L., Guttmann, M., Cohen-Or, D.: Non-homogeneous content-driven video-retargeting. In: Proceedings of IEEE ICCV, pp.1–6 (2007)
7. Oliva, A., Torralba, A., Castelhano, M., Henderson, J.: Top-down control of visual attention in object detection. In: Proceedings of IEEE ICIP, vol. 1, pp. 253–256 (2003)
8. Alpert, S., Galun, M., Basri, R., Brandt, A.: Image segmentation by probabilistic bottom-up aggregation and cue integration. In: Proceedings of IEEE CVPR, pp. 1–8 (2007)
9. Achanta, R., Hemami, S., Estrada, F., Süsstrunk, S.: Frequency-tuned salient region detection. In: Proceedings of IEEE CVPR, pp. 1597–1604 (2009)
10. Zhai, Y., Shah, M.: Visual attention detection in video sequences using spatiotemporal cues. In: Proceedings of ACM Multimedia, pp. 815–824 (2006)
11. Cheng, M., Zhang, G., Mitra, N.J., Huang, X., Hu, S.: Global contrast based salient region detection. In: Proceedings of IEEE CVPR, pp. 409–416 (2011)
12. Perazzi, F., Krahenbuhl, P., Pritch, Y., Hornung, A.: Saliency filters: contrast based filtering for salient region detection. In: Proceedings of IEEE CVPR, pp. 733–740 (2012)
13. Cheng, M.M., Warrell, J., Lin, W.Y., Zheng, S., Vineet, V., Crook, N.: Efficient salient region detection with soft image abstraction. In: IEEE ICCV (2013)
14. Yang, C., Zhang, L., Lu, H., Ruan, X., Yang, M.: Saliency detection via graph-based manifold ranking. In: Proceedings of IEEE CVPR, pp. 3166–3173 (2013)
15. Yang, Q., Tan, K., Ahuja, N.: Real-time O(1) bilateral filtering. In: Proceedings of IEEE CVPR, pp. 557–564 (2009)
16. Liu, T., Yuan, Z., Sun, J., Wang, J., Zheng, N., Tang, X., Shum, H.: Learning to detect a salient object. IEEE Trans. PAMI **33**, 353–367 (2011)
17. Borji, A., Sihite, D.N., Itti, L.: Salient object detection: a benchmark. In: Fitzgibbon, A., Lazebnik, S., Perona, P., Sato, Y., Schmid, C. (eds.) ECCV 2012, Part II. LNCS, vol. 7573, pp. 414–429. Springer, Heidelberg (2012)
18. Alexe, B., Deselaers, T., Ferrari, V.: Measuring the objectness of image windows. IEEE Trans. PAMI **34**, 2189–2202 (2012)
19. Cheng, M.M., Zhang, Z., Lin, W.Y., Torr, P.H.S.: BING: binarized normed gradients for objectness estimation at 300fps. In: Proceedings of IEEE CVPR (2014)
20. Zia, K., Balch, T., Dellaert, F.: MCMC-based particle filtering for tracking a variable number of interacting targets. IEEE Trans. PAMI **27**, 1805–1819 (2005)
21. Stalder, S., Grabner, H., Van Gool, L.: Cascaded confidence filtering for improved tracking-by-detection. In: Daniilidis, K., Maragos, P., Paragios, N. (eds.) ECCV 2010, Part I. LNCS, vol. 6311, pp. 369–382. Springer, Heidelberg (2010)

Gesture Modeling by Hanklet-Based
Hidden Markov Model

Liliana Lo Presti[1]([✉]), Marco La Cascia[1], Stan Sclaroff[2], and Octavia Camps[3]

[1] DICGIM, Universitá degli Studi di Palermo, Palermo, Italy
liliana.lopresti@unipa.it
[2] Computer Science Department, Boston University, Boston, USA
[3] Department of Electrical and Computer Engineering, Northeastern University,
Boston, USA

Abstract. In this paper we propose a novel approach for gesture modeling. We aim at decomposing a gesture into sub-trajectories that are the output of a sequence of atomic linear time invariant (LTI) systems, and we use a Hidden Markov Model to model the transitions from the LTI system to another. For this purpose, we represent the human body motion in a temporal window as a set of body joint trajectories that we assume are the output of an LTI system. We describe the set of trajectories in a temporal window by the corresponding Hankel matrix (Hanklet), which embeds the observability matrix of the LTI system that produced it. We train a set of HMMs (one for each gesture class) with a discriminative approach. To account for the sharing of body motion templates we allow the HMMs to share the same state space. We demonstrate by means of experiments on two publicly available datasets that, even with just considering the trajectories of the 3D joints, our method achieves state-of-the-art accuracy while competing well with methods that employ more complex models and feature representations.

1 Introduction

The detection, recognition and analysis of gestures is of great interest for the computer vision community in well studied fields like surveillance [1–4] and human-computer interaction [5] and in emerging fields like assistive technologies [6], computational behavioral science [7,8] and consumer behavior analysis [9].

In this paper, we propose to represent a gesture as a temporal series of body motion templates. A body motion template may be either an ordered set of trajectories (i.e. trajectories of body parts such as hands, arms, legs, head, torso) or motion descriptors (bag-of-words, histogram of flow, histogram of dense trajectories, etc.) within a temporal window.

As for the gesture temporal structure, there are dynamics regulating the sequence of motion templates; for example, handshaking may require the following ordered sequence of movements: moving the whole body for approaching the other person, raising the arm, and shaking the hand.

Many previous works have extracted global features for action recognition and trained models for each gesture-class [10–13]. Some works have focused on

© Springer International Publishing Switzerland 2015
D. Cremers et al. (Eds.): ACCV 2014, Part III, LNCS 9005, pp. 529–546, 2015.
DOI: 10.1007/978-3-319-16811-1_35

discriminative learning of models such as HMM [11,14,15] and CRF [16–18]. Most of them assume the gestures "live" in different state spaces. However, gestures may share body motion templates while having different temporal structures. In this paper, each body motion template is assumed to be the output of a linear time invariant (LTI) system and described by means of a Hankel matrix, which embeds the parameters of the LTI system [19].

A gesture is modeled by an HMM where the observations are Hankel matrices computed in a sliding window across time. In the following, we refer to such Hankel matrices as Hanklets. Each hidden state of the HMM represents an LTI system for which only a Hanklet is known. To account for the sharing of body motion templates, we train a set of gesture models that have the same state space but different dynamics, priors and conditional distributions over the observed Hanklets. The parameters of the gesture models are jointly learnt via a discriminative approach.

To summarize, the main contributions of this paper are:

– a novel gesture representation as sequence of Hanklets and
– a novel discriminative learning approach that allows different HMMs to share the same state space.

We show how a gesture can be modeled as a sequence of outputs from atomic LTI systems that are regulated by a Markov process. We describe each LTI system in terms of a Hankel matrix. This is different from other approaches such as [20], which represent body pose frame-by-frame. Instead the observations for our model are body motion templates with an intrinsic temporal duration.

To evaluate our method, we implemented a version of the formulation that takes 3D skeleton tracking data as input. Therefore, our body motion template is a set of trajectories of the 3D joints within a temporal window. Figure 1 shows examples of body motion templates and gestures. As the figure highlights, gestures may share body motion templates. In experiments with two publicly-available gesture datasets, our approach attains state-of-the-art classification accuracies.

The rest of the paper is organized as follows. In Sect. 2 we report previous works in gesture recognition. In Sect. 3 we present our novel feature representation for body motion. In Sect. 4 we discuss our gesture model and present inference and learning approaches. In Sect. 5 we present experimental results. Finally, in Sect. 6 we present conclusions and future work.

2   Related Work

With the introduction of the Kinect sensor and the seminal work by Shotton, et al. [21] for estimating the joint locations of a human body, there has been a proliferation of works on gesture recognition. Most of these works introduce novel body pose representations. Some works [20,22] use only the joint locations, while others [23,24], mix descriptors from depth, motion and skeleton data. These

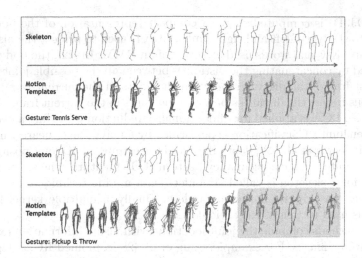

Fig. 1. Samples for two gestures from the MSRA3D-Action dataset. In each box, the first row shows the sequence of skeletons, the second row gives an idea of motion templates. Each image represents the super-imposition of skeletons detected in a temporal window. The last motion templates in the two gestures are generated by the same LTI-system during test; hence the corresponding action models share the same state.

works in general use state-of-the-art machinery to learn the temporal structure of gestures and/or to classify them.

Li et al. [24] proposed an action graph for depth action recognition. The depth map is projected onto three orthogonal Cartesian planes. A sub-sampled set of points uniformly distributed are extracted and used as a bag of 3D points to encode the body pose. Each of these bags is a node in the action graph, which is used to model the dynamics of the actions. In Wang et al. [25], a 3D action sequence is treated as a 4D shape and a Random Occupancy Patterns (ROP) feature is extracted. Sparse coding and an Elastic-Net regularized classification model are used to classify the sequences. In Vieira et al. [26], space-time occupancy patterns are adopted to represent depth sequences. The features are computed by binarizing the space and time axes and computing what cells are occupied. Then a nearest neighbor classifier is applied for action recognition. In a similar way, Oreifej et al. [13] described the depth sequence as histograms of oriented surface normals (HON4D) captured in the 4D volume, based on depth and spatial coordinates. The quantization of the normals is non-uniform. Classification is performed by SVM classifier. In [27], each action is represented by spatio-temporal motion trajectories of the joints. Trajectories are represented as curves in the Riemannian manifold of open curve shape space; trajectories are compaired by an elastic distance between their corresponding points in shape space. Classification is performed by KNN on the Riemannian manifold. Other works focus on body pose representation of the given the 3D joint skeleton. In Xia et al. [20] a histogram of the locations of 12 manually selected 3D skeleton joints (HOJ3D) is computed to get a compact representation of the body pose invariant to the use of left and right limbs. LDA is used to project the histogram and compute K visual words used as states of an HMM. In [22], the body pose is represented by concatenating the distances between all the possible joint pairs in the current frame, the distances between the joints in the current frame and in the previous frame, the distances between the joints in the current frame and in a neutral pose. PCA is applied for dimensionality reduction providing a descriptor called EigenJoints. Classification is performed by a naive-Bayes nearest neighbor classifier. In Wang et al. [23], depth data and the estimated 3D joint positions are used to compute the local occupancy pattern (LOP) feature. The set of features computed for a skeleton is called actionlet. Data mining techniques are used to discover the most discriminative actionlets. Finally, a multiple kernel learning approach is used to weight the actionlets.

Other methods combine the joint locations with visual information extracted from the RGB images. For example, Sung et al. [28] combined RGB, depth and hand positions, body pose and motion features extracted from skeleton joints. HOG [29] is used as the descriptor for both RGB and depth images. Then, a two-layer maximum-entropy Markov model is adopted for classification.

In contrast with previous works, we do not present a body pose representation. Instead we adopt the Hanklet representation [19] to describe body motion. Our method only uses body part trajectories (such as locations of joints in a skeleton) to represent a gesture as the output of a sequence of Linear Time Invariant (LTI) systems. We use an HMM to model the transition from one LTI system to another across time. HMM have been widely used for action modeling, for example in [11,20,30–33]. Another model often used for action recognition is Conditional Random Fields (CRF)[16–18], which is a discriminative approach and has proven to be successful for recognition task. It has been shown that discriminative approaches tend to achieve better performance with respect to the standard HMM. Therefore, previous works [34,35] have tried to learn the parameters of the HMM with a discriminative approach. In this paper, we adopt an HMM to model a gesture and learn its parameters in a discriminative way. The main difference between our approach and the standard HMM is that we allow classes' models to share the same state space.

Our approach is related to both linear parameter varying model identification [36] and switched system identification [37]. In linear parameter varying models, the parameters of each autoregressive model may change over time based on a scheduling variable. Our method may be considered as a discretization of linear parameter varying models; we model the switching of the LTI systems as a Markov process and, instead of estimating the scheduling variable, we infer the atomic LTI system that may have generated the given observation. In this sense, our method is more similar to piecewise models and Markovian jump linear models [37–39] where there is a stochastic process that regulates the switching from one LTI system to another. Unlike previous methods [38,39], our goal is not that of segmenting the sequence in outputs of different LTI systems; instead, we parse the sequence with a sliding window of fixed duration, and model probabilistically the switching among atomic LTI systems to capture the temporal structure of the whole gesture. Finally, there is an interesting connection with [40]. In [40], each video sequence is associated with a dynamical model. Then a metric is learned in order to optimally classify these dynamical models. Instead, we represent a video as a sequence of dynamical models and learn the parameters of an HMM that may regulate this sequence of atomic models.

3   Gesture Representation

We propose to represent a gesture as a sequence of body motion templates each one produced by an LTI system with unknown parameters. In our framework, each LTI system is represented by a Hanklet corresponding to an exemplar output. Associations between observed body motion templates and LTI systems is performed by comparing Hanklets.

Differently than methods like [13,24,25], we do not propose a body pose representation, but a new discriminative HMM model for gesture recognition. The novelty of our work stands in the decomposition of a gesture into atomic LTI systems by means of the decoding procedure used at inference time. In this sense, our method implicitly models the gesture as a switched dynamic system where each state is an LTI system. Furthermore, we formulate a discriminative HMM that can model the transition from one LTI system to another.

In the following we summarize the approach proposed in [41] to represent a trajectory and how we employ this descriptor for gesture representation.

3.1   Trajectory Representation by Hanklets

A trajectory may be represented as the output of a linear time invariant (LTI) system. LTIs are dynamic systems where the state and the measurement equations are linear, the matrices A and C are constant over time, and $w_k \sim N(0, Q)$ is uncorrelated zero mean Gaussian measurement noise:

$$x_{k+1} = A \cdot x_k + w_k;$$
$$y_k = C \cdot x_k. \tag{1}$$

In these equations, $x_k \in R^u$ is the u-dimensional hidden state, while $y_k \in R^v$ is the v-dimensional measurement. To associate output measurements with the generating LTI system, we should apply system identification techniques to estimate the parameters of the LTI system, as in [42]. Instead, in our approach, we describe the trajectories produced by the dynamic system through a Hankel matrix. Given a sequence of output measurements $[y_o, \ldots, y_T]$ from (1), its associated (block) Hankel matrix is

$$H = \begin{bmatrix} y_0, & y_1, & y_2, & \ldots, & y_m \\ y_1, & y_2, & y_3, & \ldots, & y_{m+1} \\ \ldots & \ldots & \ldots & \ldots & \ldots \\ y_n, & y_{n+1}, & y_{n+2}, & \ldots, & y_T \end{bmatrix}, \tag{2}$$

where n is the maximal order of the system, T is the temporal length of the sequence, and it holds that $T = n + m - 1$.

As explained in [41], the Hankel matrix embeds the observability matrix Γ of the system, that is $H = \Gamma \cdot X$, where X is the sequence of hidden states of the system. Therefore H provides information about the dynamics of the temporal sequence. As H is also invariant to affine-transformations of the trajectory points [41], it is particularly appealing to adopt such a descriptor for gesture recognition.

In contrast with [41], which proposes a standard bag-of-words and SVM approach on Hanklet histograms, we propose to model the dynamics that regulates sequences of Hanklets. We adopt a trajectory representation that is similar to the one used in [41]; while [41] computes a histogram of Hanklets for each action based on the set of detected dense trajectories, we compute a single Hanklet based on all the body joints together in a sliding window approach.

For the sake of demonstrating our idea, we use the 3D joints of the detected skeletons as input to our algorithm; the Hankel matrices are computed using the joint locations in a sliding window, where the temporal window is composed of T frames and the shift of the window happens frame by frame. We believe that the approach may be extended to the case when the skeleton is unknown, for example by detecting and tracking the body parts or correlated features (i.e. optical flow) from the RGB data. The same framework may also be used with frame-based body pose representations. These extensions remain a topic of future investigation.

3.2   Hanklet Computation and Comparison

A Hankel matrix is a powerful mathematical tool that embeds salient information about the dynamics of trajectories generated by LTI systems with unknown parameters. Hankel matrices have been successfully used in previous works on action recognition [41], tracking [43] and dynamic textures [42]. Our approach differs from these previous works in that we use the Hankel matrix space as an intermediary space where it is possible to compare body motion templates and LTI systems. In contrast to [41], which considers the velocities as measurements, we directly consider the joint locations as input measurements. We have empirically found that this representation is more informative than the one suggested in [41] for our gesture recognition task. We have also noticed that a better local representation (i.e. within the temporal window) is achieved by considering Hankel matrices with order lower than 5.

Given a temporal sequence $[y_0, \ldots, y_T]$, where y_t is a vector of the concatenated 3D joint locations in the skeleton at time t, and T is the number of frames in the temporal window, we center the sequence by taking off its average as in [41]. We compute the Hankel matrix and normalize it by its Frobenius norm. Our Hanklet representation for the given temporal sequence is the following:

$$H_p = \frac{H_p}{||H_p||_F}. \tag{3}$$

In contrast to [41], which considers the covariance matrix $H_p \cdot H_p'$ to represent a trajectory, we directly use the Hankel matrix H_p. The matrix $H_p \cdot H_p'$ is invariant to the direction in which the state changes and may not be suitable for gesture recognition. The Frobenius norm may be computed as:

$$||H_p||_F = \sqrt{\sum_{i,j}(H_p(i,j)^2)}. \tag{4}$$

Once we represent the trajectories by means of their corresponding Hankel matrices, we need a way to establish if two trajectories have been generated by the same LTI system or not. We do this by comparing their Hankel matrices. To convey the degree to which two Hanklets may be considered similar, we use an approximate score similar to that proposed in [41], defined as follows:

$$d(H_p, H_q) = 2 - ||H_p + H_q||_F. \tag{5}$$

4 Hanklet-Based Hidden Markov Model

We assume that a gesture is a sequence of body motion templates produced by a set of LTI systems. Each LTI system is represented by a Hanklet S of an exemplar output sequence that the system has produced. The probability that a given sequence of measurements is produced by an LTI system is modeled by the following exponential distribution:

$$p(H|S) = \lambda \cdot e^{-\lambda \cdot d(H,S)} \tag{6}$$

where H is the Hanklet corresponding to the given sequence of measurements, S is the Hanklet used for representing the LTI system, $d(H, S)$ is the dissimilarity score in Eq. (5), λ is a parameter to learn.

We assume that the measurements in a gesture come from a sequence of LTI systems. The switching process that generates a gesture is assumed to be a Markovian process and therefore we employ an HMM to model the transitions from one LTI system to another. The transition matrix T is a stochastic matrix where $T(i, j) = p(S_t^j|S_{t-1}^i)$, and is a parameter of the model. The prior probability π, such that $\pi(i) = p(S_0^i)$, is the probability that the measurement in the first temporal window ($t = 0$) has been generated by the i-th LTI model.

Given these definitions, the joint probability of the sequence of N observed Hankel matrices $H = \{H_t\}_{t=0}^N$ (computed from the observations) and the sequence of LTI systems, represented by means of the corresponding Hanklets $S = \{S_t\}_{t=0}^N$ is:

$$p(H, S|T, \pi, \Lambda) = \prod_{t=0}^N p(H_t|S_t) \cdot \prod_{t=1}^N P(S_t|S_{t-1}) \cdot \pi(S_0) \tag{7}$$

where $\Lambda = \{\lambda_S\}$ is the set of parameters λ associated with each state.

Algorithm 1. Inference of Gesture-Class

Input : $\{H_t\}_{t=0}^{T}$ test sequence;
$\{\Lambda^c\}_{c=1}^{N}$, $\{T^c\}_{c=1}^{N}$, $\{\pi^c\}_{c=1}^{N}$ parameters of the HMMs;
$\{S_i\}_{i=1}^{M}$ state space
Output: C_P predicted label

for $i \leftarrow 1$ **to** M **do**
    for $j \leftarrow 1$ **to** T **do**
      | $D(i,j) \leftarrow d(S_i, H_j)$ (Eq. 5);
    end
end
for $c \leftarrow 1$ **to** N **do**
    | $LL(c) \leftarrow$applyViterbi$(D, \Lambda^c, T^c, \pi^c)$
end

$C_P \leftarrow \text{argmin}(LL)$

4.1 Inference and Classification

Given a gesture model with parameters $\{\Lambda^c, T^c, \pi^c\}$, where c is the label of the gesture to which the model refers, the inference of the sequence of LTI-systems is performed via the Viterbi algorithm [44]. This well-known algorithm is based on Dynamic Programming and attempts to maximize the log-likelihood of the joint probability of the states and the observations sequentially.

The inference of the label to assign to a sequence of measurements is performed by maximum likelihood. The predicted label C_P is computed solving:

$$C_P = \min_c \{- \log p(H, S^c | T^c, \pi^c, \Lambda^c)\}. \tag{8}$$

The label corresponding to the model providing the highest likelihood is assigned to the sequence of observations.

Algorithm 1 shows how the classification of an input Hanklet sequence is performed. As all the models share the state space, it is necessary to compute the matrix of dissimilarity scores between the Hanklets and the shared states only once. Then the Viterbi algorithm is applied N times, once for each gesture class. The negative log-likelihood score is normalized to account for different lengths of the sequences.

4.2 Discriminative Learning

The traditional learning approach for the HMM parameters uses the Baum-Welch algorithm [44]. In many applications, e.g. [34,35], it has been demonstrated that discriminative learning of the HMM parameters results in better performance. We therefore apply this approach to the parameter learning of our models. The learning procedure learns the parameters of all the HMMs simultaneously while encouraging correct predictions and penalizing the wrong ones.

Discriminative learning tries to minimize the mis-classification measure for an input training sample H defined as follows:

$$loss(H) = \max\{0, g^k(H, \Lambda^k, T^k, \pi^k) - \min_{j \neq k}\{g^j(H, \Lambda^j, T^j, \pi^j)\} + 1\} \quad (9)$$

where g^k represents the negative log-likelihood returned by the correct model k, and $\min_j\{g^j\}$ is the negative log-likelihood of the most competitive but incorrect model. The difference of these two terms represents the margin of the classifier and the loss function in Eq. 9 is the hinge loss. Minimizing this mis-classification error corresponds to increasing the inter-class distances on a training set. Whenever the loss is greater than 0, then the prediction is incorrect and it is necessary to update the parameters. The negative log-likelihood g is defined as:

$$g(H, \Lambda, T, \pi) = -\log(p(H, S|T, \pi, \Lambda)) = \quad (10)$$

$$-\sum_{t=0}^{N} log(p(H_t|S_t)) - \sum_{t=1}^{N} \log(P(S_t|S_{t-1})) - \log(\pi(S_0)), \quad (11)$$

which may be written as:

$$g(H, \Lambda, T, \pi) = \sum_{t=0}^{N}(\lambda_{S_t} \cdot d(H_t|S_t) - \log(\lambda_{S_t})) - \sum_{t=1}^{N} \alpha_{S_t|S_{t-1}} - \beta_{S_0}, \quad (12)$$

where the variables α and β represent the logarithms of the transition probabilities and priors respectively, and we use Eq. (6) for the observation probabilities. As the priors and the transition probabilities must be positive and must sum to one, the original optimization problem should be constrained. As in previous works, such as [45], we consider that α and β do not have any constraints and perform the optimization directly on these variables. Before doing inference, these variables are transformed back to obtain the parameters of the model π and T. In particular, for π we get:

$$\pi(S) = \frac{e^{\beta_S}}{\sum_s e^{\beta_s}}. \quad (13)$$

A similar transformation holds for T.

We minimize the loss over all the samples in the training set via a quasi-Newton strategy with limited-memory BFGS updates where a block-coordinate descent approach is used in turn for updates to the parameters Λ, T and the prior π. In practice we have observed that the block-coordinate descent results in faster convergence of the training procedure.

Algorithm 2 shows the pseudo-code for our training procedure. After initializing all the models with the same parameters (uniform distributions for T and π and 1 for λ), the method iteratively minimizes the objective function $f(\cdot)$ by block-coordinate descent. The function check_convergence() checks if some convergence criteria is met. The variable p_set is used to identify the active parameter subset, that is the subset of parameters considered when minimizing the

---

Algorithm 2. Discriminative learning of the Parameters

Input : $\{Y_i\}_{i=1}^{W}$: training set of Hanklet sequences;
    labels: gesture-classes for each training sequence;
    $\{S_i\}_{i=1}^{M}$ state space
Output: $\{\Lambda^c\}_{c=1}^{N}$, $\{T^c\}_{c=1}^{N}$, $\{\pi^c\}_{c=1}^{N}$ parameters of the HMMs;

%% Parameter initialization;
for $c \leftarrow 1$ **to** N **do**
    $\lambda^c \leftarrow$ all-ones vector of dimension M;
    $T^c \leftarrow M \times M$ stochastic matrix with uniform distribution on each row;
    $\pi^c \leftarrow$ uniform distribution over the M states;
end

iter $\leftarrow 1$;
converged $\leftarrow false$;

%% Apply Block-Coordinate Gradient Descent to each active parameter subset
(p_set);
while $iter < Max\_Iter$ & $!converged$ **do**
    %% Optimize with respect to $\{\Lambda^c\}_{c=1}^{N}$;
    p_set $\leftarrow$ lambdas;
    $\{\Lambda^c\}_{c=1}^{N} \leftarrow \operatorname{argmin} f(\{Y_i\}_{i=1}^{W}, \text{labels}, \{\Lambda^c\}_{c=1}^{N}, \{T^c\}_{c=1}^{N}, \{\pi^c\}_{c=1}^{N}, \{S_i\}_{i=1}^{M},$
    p_set);

    %% Optimize with respect to $\{T^c\}_{c=1}^{N}$;
    p_set $\leftarrow$ transition matrices;
    $\{T^c\}_{c=1}^{N} \leftarrow \operatorname{argmin} f(\{Y_i\}_{i=1}^{W}, \text{labels}, \{\Lambda^c\}_{c=1}^{N}, \{T^c\}_{c=1}^{N}, \{\pi^c\}_{c=1}^{N}, \{S_i\}_{i=1}^{M},$
    p_set);

    %% Optimize with respect to $\{\pi^c\}_{c=1}^{N}$;
    p_set $\leftarrow$ priors;
    $\{\pi^c\}_{c=1}^{N} \leftarrow \operatorname{argmin} f(\{Y_i\}_{i=1}^{W}, \text{labels}, \{\Lambda^c\}_{c=1}^{N}, \{T^c\}_{c=1}^{N}, \{\pi^c\}_{c=1}^{N}, \{S_i\}_{i=1}^{M},$
    p_set);

    converged $\leftarrow$ check_convergence($\{\Lambda^c\}_{c=1}^{N}, \{T^c\}_{c=1}^{N}, \{\pi^c\}_{c=1}^{N}$);
    iter $\leftarrow$ iter $+ 1$;
end

---

objective function within the block-coordinate schema. Algorithm 3 summarizes the main steps to evaluate the cumulative loss function over the training set. For each sample, it computes the negative log-likelihood of the correct model and the negative log-likelihood returned by the most likely incorrect model. If the loss is positive, then the models have produced a wrong prediction; therefore the gradients are accumulated and returned to the L-BFGS algorithm to update the parameters. The variable p_set allows us to accumulate the gradients only for the current active parameter subset.

Algorithm 3. f() : Objective Function to Minimize

Input   : $\{Y_i\}_{i=1}^{W}$: training set of Hanklet sequences;
labels: gesture-classes for each training sequence;
$\{S_i\}_{i=1}^{M}$ state space;
$\{\Lambda^c\}_{c=1}^{N}$, $\{T^c\}_{c=1}^{N}$, $\{\pi^c\}_{c=1}^{N}$ parameters of the HMMs;
p_set: active parameter subset
Output: Cum_loss: loss over all the samples in the dataset; Grad: gradients

%% Accumulate loss for all the sequences in the training set;
Cum_loss ← 0;
for i ← 1 **to** W **do**

> %% Compute loss for the i-th sequence;
> D ← compute dissimilarity score matrix between Y_i and $\{S_i\}_{i=1}^{M}$;
> k ← labels(i);
> $[g^k, z^k]$ ← applyViterbi$(D, \Lambda^k, T^k, \pi^k)$;
> $[g^c, z^c]$ ← $\min_{c \neq k}$ applyViterbi$(D, \Lambda^c, T^c, \pi^c)$;
> loss ← $\max(0, g^k - g^c + 1)$;
> Cum_loss ← Cum_loss + loss;
>
> %% If the sequence is misclassified, accumulate gradients. The optimization
> %% algorithm will use the gradients to update the active parameter subset;
> **if** *loss*> 0 **then**
>> Accumulate gradients Grad for the active parameter subset p_set along
>> the inferred paths z^k and z^c for classes k and c respectively
> **end**

end

4.3   Initialization of the State Space

The state space initialization is performed by considering, for each class, a subset of video sequences in the training set. Then the corresponding Hanklets are clustered via K-medoids and the K medoids are used to compose the state space. Therefore, given N classes, the state space has a dimensionality equal to $K \cdot N$.

We have tested two strategies: online learning the state representation while learning the parameters of the model versus not learning the state representation. Learning of the state is done by re-clustering the Hankel matrices, that is, for each state we consider all the observed Hankel matrices that have been generated by that state and we compute the medoid of this set of matrices. Our experiments have shown a small change in the performance when learning vs non-learning the state representation. As learning the state representation increases the time complexity, in this paper we do not update the state space online.

In our implementation the number of states is defined a priori. Computing the state space by allowing the introduction of new states, merging/removing of existing states could be certainly done, e.g. using a reversible jump Markov chain Monte Carlo [46] to decide when to add/merge/remove a state. However, this is beyond the scope of this paper and remains a topic for future investigation.

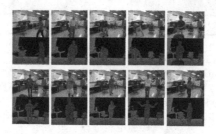

Fig. 2. Samples from the UTKinect-Action dataset (source:UTKinect-Action website)

Table 1. Accuracy on the MSRA-3D action dataset.

Methods	[47][a]	[10][a]	[11][a]	[12]	[24]	[48][b]	[13][b]	[25]	[23]	[13][b]	Ours
Accuracy:	42.5 %	54 %	63 %	65.7 %	74.7 %	85.5 %	85.8 %	86.5 %	87.2 %	88.9 %	**89 %**

[a] Results reported in [12].
[b] Different splitting of training and test set. We note that [10] uses dynamic time warping, while [11] uses a standard HMM.

5 Experiments

We evaluated our method on two datasets: MSRAction3D [23] and UTKinect-Action [20]. The first dataset provides skeleton and depth data; examples of the detected skeletons are shown in Fig. 1. The second dataset also provides RGB data and sample images are shown in Fig. 2. We used only the skeleton data; such data are corrupted by various levels of noise, which affects the recognition accuracy. The code of our implementation has been written in Matlab[1].

5.1 Setting of Parameters and Initialization

The maximal order of the LTI systems (that is the number of rows of the Hankel matrix) determines the minimal length of the temporal window needed to build a square Hankel matrix (8 if the order is 3; 15 if the order is 4). In the datasets we used, some sequences contain fewer than 15 frames. To guarantee a fair comparison with previous methods we have chosen to set the order to 3 instead of removing the shorter training/test sequences.

The state space has been computed by applying the K-medoid algorithm to subsets of Hanklets. For each class we have selected randomly 20 videos and we have clustered the oberved Hankel matrices. The number of centroids K has been set to 5. Thus, we used a state space composed of 100 Hankel matrices for the MSRA-3D dataset and 50 Hankel matrices for the UTKinect-Action dataset.

5.2 Experiments on the MSRA3D Dataset

The MSRAction3D dataset[2] provides the skeleton (20 joints) for 20 gestures performed 2 or 3 times by 10 subjects. The dataset contains 3D coordinates

---

[1] Code available at http://www.dicgim.unipa.it/cvip/people/lopresti/.

[2] http://research.microsoft.com/en-us/um/people/zliu/actionrecorsrc/.

Table 2. Confusion matrix for the MSRA-3D dataset.

T vs P	HW	HoW	Ham	HC	FP	HT	DX	DT	DC	HC	2HW	SB	Bend	FK	SK	Jog	TSw	TSe	GSw	P-T
HW	58.3	33.3	0	0	0	0	0	0	0	0	0	0	0	0	0	0	8.3	0	0	0
HoW	0	100	0	0	0	0	0	0	0	0	0	0	0	0	0	0	0	0	0	0
Ham	0	0	100	0	0	0	0	0	0	0	0	0	0	0	0	0	0	0	0	0
HC	0	8.3	8.3	58.3	16.7	0	0	0	0	0	0	0	0	0	0	0	8.3	0	0	0
FP	0	0	0	0	63.6	0	0	9.1	0	0	0	0	0	0	0	0	0	27.3	0	0
HT	9.1	0	0	0	0	63.6	0	0	0	0	0	0	0	0	0	0	0	0	27.3	0
DX	0	0	0	0	0	0	100	0	0	0	0	0	0	0	0	0	0	0	0	0
DT	6.7	0	0	0	0	0	0	93.3	0	0	0	0	0	0	0	0	0	0	0	0
DC	0	0	0	0	0	0	0	0	100	0	0	0	0	0	0	0	0	0	0	0
HC	0	0	0	0	0	0	0	0	0	93.3	6.7	0	0	0	0	0	0	0	0	0
2HW	0	0	0	0	0	0	0	0	0	0	100	0	0	0	0	0	0	0	0	0
SB	6.7	0	0	0	0	0	0	0	0	0	0	73.8	0	6.7	0	0	13.3	0	0	0
Bend	0	0	0	0	0	0	0	0	0	0	0	0	100	0	0	0	0	0	0	0
FK	0	0	0	0	0	0	0	0	0	0	0	0	0	100	0	0	0	0	0	0
SK	0	0	0	0	0	0	0	0	0	0	0	0	0	9.1	90.9	0	0	0	0	0
Jog	0	0	0	0	0	0	0	0	0	0	0	0	0	0	0	100	0	0	0	0
TSw	0	0	0	0	0	0	0	0	0	0	0	0	0	0	0	0	100	0	0	0
TSe	0	0	0	0	0	0	0	0	0	0	0	0	0	0	0	0	0	100	0	0
GSw	0	0	0	0	0	0	0	0	0	0	0	0	0	0	0	0	0	0	100	0
P-T	0	0	0	0	0	0	0	0	0	0	0	0	35.7	0	0	0	0	0	0	64.3

from 557 sequences of the following gestures: high arm wave, horizontal arm wave, hammer, hand catch, forward punch, high throw, draw x, draw tick, draw circle, hand clap, two hand wave, side-boxing, bend, forward kick, side kick, jogging, tennis swing, tennis serve, golf swing, pickup and throw.

We use the same setting reported on the authors' website: 10 sequences have been filtered out because of the excessive noise on the skeletons; the splitting of the data in training and test set is as follows: subjects 1, 3, 5, 7, and 9 for training, the others for test.

Table 1 shows the comparison between our proposed approach and previous works in terms of classification accuracy (number of correctly classified sequences over number of sequences). On this dataset our method performs the best. Tables 2 and 3 show the confusion matrix and the classification accuracies per class respectively. For half of the actions, our method attains 100 % of accuracy. Only for some classes, namely High Arm Waving and Hand Clap, the performance decreases. As for the action High Arm Waving, most of the confusion is with Horizontal Arm Waving. The decrease of performance in this case may be ascribable to the fact we are not considering the relative position of the 3D joints when training our models. Most of the previous works we compare

Table 3. Accuracy on the MSRA-3D dataset per class.

Acc.	HW	HoW	Ham	HC	FP	HT	DX	DT	DC	HC	2HW	SB	Bend	FK	SK	Jog	TSw	TSe	GSw	P-T
[12]	NA	NA	0	0	NA	14.3	35.7	NA	20	100	100	NA	NA	100	NA	NA	NA	100	100	NA
[23]	91.7	100	83.9	25	72.7	72.7	53.8	100	100	100	100	86.7	93.3	100	100	100	100	100	100	64.3
Ours	58.3	100	100	58.3	63.6	63.6	100	93.3	100	93.3	100	73.3	100	100	90.9	100	100	100	100	64.3

Table 4. Accuracy on the UTKinect-Action dataset.

Accuracy	Walk	SitDown	StandUp	PickUp	Carry	Throw	Push	Pull	WHands	CHands	Avr
[27]	90 %	100 %	100 %	100 %	68.4 %	**95 %**	90 %	100 %	100 %	80 %	**91.5 %**
[20]	**96.5 %**	91.5 %	93.5 %	97.5 %	**97.5 %**	59 %	81.5 %	92.5 %	100 %	100 %	90.9 %
Ours	63.16 %	100 %	100 %	100 %	83.33 %	61.11 %	90 %	100 %	85 %	85 %	86.76 %

to, i.e. [23] or [13], use more complicated feature representation or machinery. In contrast, we only use information about the dynamics of the 3D skeleton joints.

5.3　Experiments on the UTKinect-Action Dataset

The UTKinect-Action dataset[3] provides the skeleton (20 joints) for 10 actions performed twice by 10 subjects. The dataset contains 200 sequences of the following gestures: walk, sit down, stand up, pick up, carry, throw, push, pull, wave and clap hands. Six sequences were too short to compute the Hankel matrices and have been filtered out. As done in [20], we performed the experiments in leave-one-out cross-validation (LOOCV). In this dataset, one of the subject is left-handed and there is a very high variance in the length of the sequences (the length ranges from 5 to 120 frames). Moreover, there is a significant variation among different realizations of the same action: some actors pick up objects with one hand, while others pick up the objects with both hands. The individuals can toss an object with either their right or left arm, producing different trajectories. Finally, actions have been taken from different views and, therefore, the body orientation varies.

Table 5. Confusion matrix for the UTKinect-Action dataset.

True vs Predicted	Walk	SitDown	StandUp	PickUp	Carry	Throw	Push	Pull	WaveHands	ClapHands
Walk	**63.16 %**	0	0	0	31.58 %	0	5.26 %	0	0	0
SitDown	0	**100 %**	0	0	0	0	0	0	0	0
StandUp	0	0	**100 %**	0	0	0	0	0	0	0
PickUp	0	0	0	**100 %**	0	0	0	0	0	0
Carry	16.67 %	0	0	0	**83.33 %**	0	0	0	0	0
Throw	0	0	5.56 %	5.56 %	0	**61.11 %**	16.67 %	0	5.56 %	5.56 %
Push	5 %	0	0	0	0	5 %	**90 %**	0	0	0
Pull	0	0	0	0	0	0	0	**100 %**	0	0
WaveHands	0	0	0	0	0	0	0	0	**85 %**	15 %
ClapHands	0	5 %	0	0	0	0	0	0	10 %	**85 %**

As shown in Table 4, our method attains performance that approaches that reported by [20,27]. Considering the challenges in this dataset, and the limited number of sequences available for training, the accuracy we get is quite high. Accuracy is somewhat limited in this experiment because the Hanklets are sensitive to the order the joints are considered, therefore it cannot discriminate

---

[3] http://cvrc.ece.utexas.edu/KinectDatasets/HOJ3D.html.

between two samples of the same action in which one involves a left limb and the other one a right limb (i.e. in the class Throw).

In this experiment, we use the same joints as in [20]. We center the points on the hip center at each frame and use the remaining 11 joints to compute the descriptors. Table 5 reports the confusion matrix for the 10 classes. Most of the confusion is between the actions walk and carry. This is probably due to the fact that these actions, in terms of the dynamics of many of the joints involved in the actions, are pretty indistinguishable. In such cases, features capturing the 3D joint spatial configuration may help to disambiguate.

6   Conclusions and Future Work

We have proposed a novel representation of a gesture in terms of temporal sequence of body motion templates. We have assumed that each motion template represents the output of an atomic LTI system and can be represented by a Hankel matrix. We have adopted a discriminative HMM to model the transition from one LTI system to the next. We have allowed the discriminative HMMs to share the same state space. This enables the gesture models to share LTI systems and, therefore, body motion templates.

In experiments on two challenging gesture recognition benchmarks, our method achieves state-of-the-art accuracy by considering only 3D joint trajectories. The experiments suggest that dynamics of a suitable body pose/shape descriptor may help to disambiguate in cases where 3D joints dynamics are too similar.

In future work, we will extend the Hanklet-based representation in order to account for the temporal warping in the observed data. A limitation of the Hanklet is that it is sensitive to the order the joints are used when computing the Hankel matrix. This is problematic in cases where the same gesture can be performed either with left or right limbs. We will investigate new techniques to formulate the Hankel matrix that may overcome these limitations.

As for our discriminative HMM, we will investigate techniques that enable the state space to adapt online by adding, removing or merging existing states. We will also investigate the use of more complex dynamic Bayesian networks to account for the temporal warping and switching of the LTI systems, thereby removing the need for a sliding window approach.

Acknowledgement. This work was partially supported by Italian MIUR grant PON01 01687, SINTESYS - Security and INTElligence SYStem and by US NSF grant 1029430.

References

1. Kwak, S., Han, B., Han, J.: Scenario-based video event recognition by constraint flow. In: 2011 IEEE Conference on Computer Vision and Pattern Recognition (CVPR), pp. 3345–3352. IEEE (2011)

2. Gaur, U., Zhu, Y., Song, B., Roy-Chowdhury, A.: A string of feature graphs model for recognition of complex activities in natural videos. In: 2011 IEEE International Conference on Computer Vision (ICCV), pp. 2595–2602. IEEE (2011)

3. Park, S., Aggarwal, J.: Recognition of two-person interactions using a hierarchical Bayesian network. In: First ACM SIGMM International Workshop on Video Surveillance, pp. 65–76. ACM (2003)

4. Junejo, I., Dexter, E., Laptev, I., Pérez, P.: View-independent action recognition from temporal self-similarities. IEEE Trans. Pattern Anal. Mach. Intell. **33**, 172–185 (2011)

5. Duric, Z., Gray, W., Heishman, R., Li, F., Rosenfeld, A., Schoelles, M., Schunn, C., Wechsler, H.: Integrating perceptual and cognitive modeling for adaptive and intelligent human-computer interaction. Proceeding of the IEEE **90**(7), 1272–1289 (2002)

6. Chang, Y.J., Chen, S.F., Huang, J.D.: A kinect-based system for physical rehabilitation: a pilot study for young adults with motor disabilities. Res. Dev. Disabil. **32**, 2566–2570 (2011)

7. Rehg, J.M., Abowd, G.D., Rozga, A., Romero, M., Clements, M.A., Sclaroff, S., Essa, I., Ousley, O.Y., Li, Y., Kim, C., et al.: Decoding children's social behavior. In: 2013 IEEE Conference on Computer Vision and Pattern Recognition (CVPR), pp. 3414–3421. IEEE (2013)

8. Lo Presti, L., Sclaroff, S., Rozga, A.: Joint alignment and modeling of correlated behavior streams. In: The IEEE International Conference on Computer Vision Workshops (ICCVW), pp. 730 - 737 (2013)

9. Jung, N., Moon, H., Sharma, R.: Method and system for measuring shopper response to products based on behavior and facial expression. US Patent 8,219,438 (2012)

10. Müller, M., Röder, T.: Motion templates for automatic classification and retrieval of motion capture data. In: Proceedings of the 2006 ACM SIGGRAPH/Eurographics symposium on Computer animation, pp. 137–146. Eurographics Association (2006)

11. Lv, F., Nevatia, R.: Recognition and segmentation of 3-D human action using HMM and multi-class AdaBoost. In: Leonardis, A., Bischof, H., Pinz, A. (eds.) ECCV 2006. LNCS, vol. 3954, pp. 359–372. Springer, Heidelberg (2006)

12. Masood, S.Z., Ellis, C., Tappen, M.F., LaViola, J.J., Sukthankar, R.: Exploring the trade-off between accuracy and observational latency in action recognition. Int. J. Comput. Vis. **101**, 420–436 (2013)

13. Oreifej, O., Liu, Z., Redmond, W.: HON4D: histogram of oriented 4D normals for activity recognition from depth sequences. In: Computer Vision and Pattern Recognition (CVPR), pp. 716–723 (2013)

14. Yamato, J., Ohya, J., Ishii, K.: Recognizing human action in time-sequential images using hidden Markov Model. In: 1992 IEEE Computer Society Conference on Computer Vision and Pattern Recognition. Proceedings CVPR 1992, pp. 379–385. IEEE (1992)

15. Starner, T., Pentland, A.: Real-time American sign language recognition from video using hidden Markov models. In: Shah, M., Jain, R. (eds.) Motion-Based Recognition. CIV, vol. 9, pp. 227–243. Springer, Heidelberg (1997)

16. Wang, Y., Mori, G.: Max-margin hidden conditional random fields for human action recognition. In: IEEE Conference on Computer Vision and Pattern Recognition. CVPR 2009, pp. 872–879. IEEE (2009)

17. Vail, D.L., Veloso, M.M., Lafferty, J.D.: Conditional random fields for activity recognition. In: Proceedings of the 6th International Joint Conference on Autonomous Agents and Multiagent Systems, pp. 1331–1338, ACM (2007)
18. Wang, S.B., Quattoni, A., Morency, L., Demirdjian, D., Darrell, T.: Hidden conditional random fields for gesture recognition. In: 2006 IEEE Computer Society Conference on Computer Vision and Pattern Recognition, vol. 2, pp. 1521–1527. IEEE (2006)
19. Li, B., Ayazoglu, M., Mao, T., Camps, O.I., Sznaier, M.: Activity recognition using dynamic subspace angles. In: 2011 IEEE Conference on Computer Vision and Pattern Recognition (CVPR), pp. 3193–3200. IEEE (2011)
20. Xia, L., Chen, C.C., Aggarwal, J.: View invariant human action recognition using histograms of 3D joints. In: 2012 IEEE Computer Society Conference on Computer Vision and Pattern Recognition Workshops (CVPRW), pp. 20–27. IEEE (2012)
21. Shotton, J., Sharp, T., Kipman, A., Fitzgibbon, A., Finocchio, M., Blake, A., Cook, M., Moore, R.: Real-time human pose recognition in parts from single depth images. Commun. ACM 56, 116–124 (2013)
22. Yang, X., Tian, Y.: Eigenjoints-based action recognition using Naive-Bayes-Nearest-Neighbor. In: 2012 IEEE Computer Society Conference on Computer Vision and Pattern Recognition Workshops (CVPRW), pp. 14–19. IEEE (2012)
23. Wang, J., Liu, Z., Wu, Y., Yuan, J.: Mining actionlet ensemble for action recognition with depth cameras. In: 2012 IEEE Conference on Computer Vision and Pattern Recognition (CVPR), pp. 1290–1297. IEEE (2012)
24. Li, W., Zhang, Z., Liu, Z.: Action recognition based on a bag of 3D points. In: 2010 IEEE Computer Society Conference on Computer Vision and Pattern Recognition Workshops (CVPRW), pp. 9–14. IEEE (2010)
25. Wang, J., Liu, Z., Chorowski, J., Chen, Z., Wu, Y.: Robust 3D action recognition with random occupancy patterns. In: Fitzgibbon, A., Lazebnik, S., Perona, P., Sato, Y., Schmid, C. (eds.) ECCV 2012, Part II. LNCS, vol. 7573, pp. 872–885. Springer, Heidelberg (2012)
26. Vieira, A.W., Nascimento, E.R., Oliveira, G.L., Liu, Z., Campos, M.F.: Stop: space-time occupancy patterns for 3D action recognition from depth map sequences. In: Alvarez, L., Mejail, M., Gomez, L., Jacobo, J. (eds.) Progress in Pattern Recognition, Image Analysis, Computer Vision, and Applications. LNCS, vol. 7441, pp. 252–259. Springer, Heidelberg (2012)
27. Devanne, M., Wannous, H., Berretti, S., Pala, P., Daoudi, M., Del Bimbo, A.: Space-time pose representation for 3D human action recognition. In: Petrosino, A., Maddalena, L., Pala, P. (eds.) ICIAP 2013. LNCS, vol. 8158, pp. 456–464. Springer, Heidelberg (2013)
28. Sung, J., Ponce, C., Selman, B., Saxena, A.: Unstructured human activity detection from RGBD images. In: 2012 IEEE International Conference on Robotics and Automation (ICRA), pp. 842–849. IEEE (2012)
29. Dalal, N., Triggs, B.: Histograms of oriented gradients for human detection. In: IEEE Computer Society Conference on Computer Vision and Pattern Recognition. CVPR 2005, vol. 1, pp. 886–893. IEEE (2005)
30. Weinland, D., Boyer, E., Ronfard, R.: Action recognition from arbitrary views using 3D exemplars. In: IEEE 11th International Conference on Computer Vision. ICCV 2007, pp. 1–7. IEEE (2007)
31. Martinez-Contreras, F., Orrite-Urunuela, C., Herrero-Jaraba, E., Ragheb, H., Velastin, S.A.: Recognizing human actions using silhouette-based HMM. In: Sixth IEEE International Conference on Advanced Video and Signal Based Surveillance. AVSS 2009, pp. 43–48. IEEE (2009)

32. Lan, T., Wang, Y., Yang, W., Mori, G.: Beyond actions: discriminative models for contextual group activities. NIPS **4321**, 4322–4325 (2010)
33. Wilson, A.D., Bobick, A.F.: Parametric hidden Markov models for gesture recognition. IEEE Trans. Pattern Anal. Mach. Intell. **21**, 884–900 (1999)
34. Sha, F., Saul, L.K.: Large margin hidden Markov models for automatic speech recognition. Adv. Neural Inf. Process. Syst. **19**, 1249 (2007)
35. Collins, M.: Discriminative training methods for hidden Markov models: theory and experiments with perceptron algorithms. In: Proceedings of the ACL-02 Conference on Empirical Methods in Natural Language Processing, vol. 10, pp. 1–8. Association for Computational Linguistics (2002)
36. Bamieh, B., Giarre, L.: Identification of linear parameter varying models. Int. J. Robust Nonlinear Control **12**, 841–853 (2002)
37. Paoletti, S., Juloski, A.L., Ferrari-Trecate, G., Vidal, R.: Identification of hybrid systems a tutorial. Eur. J. Control **13**, 242–260 (2007)
38. Sontag, E.D.: Nonlinear regulation: the piecewise linear approach. IEEE Trans. Autom. Control **26**, 346–358 (1981)
39. Gupta, V., Murray, R.M., Shi, L., Sinopoli, B.: Networked sensing, estimation and control systems. California Institute of Technology Report (2009)
40. Cuzzolin, F., Sapienza, M.: Learning pullback HMM distances. IEEE Trans. Pattern Anal. Mach. Intell. **36**, 1483–1489 (2013)
41. Li, B., Camps, O.I., Sznaier, M.: Cross-view activity recognition using Hankelets. In: 2012 IEEE Conference on Computer Vision and Pattern Recognition (CVPR), pp. 1362–1369. IEEE (2012)
42. Doretto, G., Chiuso, A., Wu, Y.N., Soatto, S.: Dynamic textures. Int. J. Comput. Vis. **51**, 91–109 (2003)
43. Dicle, C., Camps, O.I., Sznaier, M.: The way they move: tracking multiple targets with similar appearance, pp. 2304–2311 (2013)
44. Rabiner, L.: A tutorial on hidden Markov models and selected applications in speech recognition. Proc. IEEE **77**, 257–286 (1989)
45. Chang, P.C., Juang, B.H.: Discriminative training of dynamic programming based speech recognizers. IEEE Trans. Speech Audio Process. **1**, 135–143 (1993)
46. Green, P.J.: Reversible jump Markov Chain Monte Carlo computation and Bayesian model determination. Biometrika **82**, 711–732 (1995)
47. Martens, J., Sutskever, I.: Learning recurrent neural networks with Hessian-free optimization. In: Proceedings of the 28th International Conference on Machine Learning (ICML-11), pp. 1033–1040 (2011)
48. Yang, X., Zhang, C., Tian, Y.: Recognizing actions using depth motion maps-based histograms of oriented gradients. In: Proceedings of the 20th ACM International Conference on Multimedia, pp. 1057–1060. ACM (2012)

A Novel Face Spoofing Detection Method Based on Gaze Estimation

Lijun Cai[✉], Chunshui Xiong, Lei Huang, and Changping Liu

Institute of Automation, Chinese Academy of Sciences, Beijing, China
cailijun2013@ia.ac.cn

Abstract. Since gaze is a kind of behavioral biometrics which is difficult to be detected by the surveillance due to the ambiguity of visual attention process, it can be used as a clue for anti-spoofing. This work provides the first investigation in research literature on the use of gaze estimation for face spoofing detection. Firstly, a gaze estimation model mapping the gaze feature to gaze position is established for tracking user's gaze trajectory. Secondly, gaze histogram is obtained by quantifying and encoding the gaze trajectory. Finally, information entropy on gaze histogram suggests the uncertainty level of user's gaze movement and estimates the liveness of the user. Our basic assumption is that the gaze trajectory of genuine access has higher uncertainty level than that of attack. Therefore, the greater the entropy, the more probable the user is genuine. Experimental results show that the proposed method obtains competitive performance in distinguishing attacks from genuine access.

1 Introduction

Due to the requirement of information security, face spoofing detection is attracting more and more attention and research nowadays. Generally speaking, there are three common manners to spoof face recognition system: photograph, video and 3D model of a valid user. Among them, photograph and video faces are the most popular because invaders can easily obtain the faces of valid users through mobile phones or surveillance cameras. With the aid of modern technology, 3D face composition is no more difficult. For example, the service of ThatMyFace.com can realizes 3D face reconstruction and model order by uploading a front and side photos. Compared with real faces, photograph faces are planar, as well as having quality degradation and blurring problems. Video faces are reflective and 3D face models are rigid. Based on these clues, face anti-spoofing techniques can be roughly classified into three categories: motion based methods, texture based methods and fusion methods.

Motion based anti-spoofing methods hypothesize that planar objects move significantly different with real faces, which are 3D objects. K. Kollreider et al. [1] present a lightweight novel optical flow to analyze the trajectories of certain parts of a real face against a fake one. Bao et al. [2] estimate four basic types of optical

© Springer International Publishing Switzerland 2015
D. Cremers et al. (Eds.): ACCV 2014, Part III, LNCS 9005, pp. 547–561, 2015.
DOI: 10.1007/978-3-319-16811-1_36

flow field and heuristically detect attacks by calculating the difference degree. Anjos et al. [3] compute the correlations between personal's head movements and scene context based on the pixel difference of adjacent two frames. Later, the same authors present a similar method [4] based on motion direction correlation instead of pixel intensity. In addition to involuntary head movement, other liveness traits, such as eye-blinks or mouth-movements, are also used for spoofing detection. Pan et al. [5] formulate blink detection as an undirected conditional graphical framework and propose to use scene context information to avoid video replay.

Another commonly used facial clue is texture analysis. The key idea is that the local micro textures are changed during image recapture. Jukka et al. [6] adapt multi-scale local binary pattern and nonlinear support vector machine to classify real and fake faces. Later, the same authors [7] propose to fuse texture and shape features for spoofing detection. Tan et al. [8] propose two strategies to extract the essential information of a live human face or a photograph by Lambertian model and train a complex classifier. Komulainen et al. [9] introduces the first investigation on the use of dynamic texture for face spoofing detection.

Motion based methods can effectively distinguish photographs from genuine access, while invalid to warped photograph and video attacks. Texture based methods can effectively obtain the discriminative models for differentiating real and fake faces, while can't take full advantage of adjacent frames information. Nowadays, more and more researchers are focusing their attention on the fusion methods which can defense multiple kinds of attacks by complementary advantages. Yan et al. [10] propose three clues including non-rigid motion, face-background consistency and imaging banding effect to conduct an effective face spoofing detection. Komulainen et al. [11] present the complementary countermeasures by studying fusion of motion and texture.

Besides above methods, multi-mode information [12–14] and multi-spectra [15–17] also offer useful clues for spoofing detection. However, they require extra devices or user cooperation.

Therefore, non-intrusive methods without extra devices and human cooperation are preferable in practice, since they can be embedded into a face recognition system, which is usually only equipped with a generic webcam. Gaze is a kind of biometric metrical information which can avoid spoofing with following characteristics [18]. Firstly, it does not require physical contact between user and device. Secondly, gaze is difficult to be obtained by surveillance camera and other equipment. Ali et al. [19–21] present the first time to use gaze clue for anti-spoofing, in which user is required to follow a moving point showed on the computer screen. Features based on the collinearity of gaze are used to discriminate between genuine access and attack. Experiments show that these methods are effective on small scale collected database by screening samples. However, they are invalid for still photographs and uncooperative users. What's more, the process of collecting samples lasts 130s, which is far beyond the users' patience. To my knowledge, except for the methods proposed by Ali et al. [19–21], there is no other work to introduce gaze into face spoofing detection.

In this paper, we propose a novel and appealing approach for face spoofing detection based on gaze estimation, which is non-intrusive and doesn't require extra device and user cooperation. Because of the ambiguity of the visual attention process, real faces has higher uncertainty level of gaze trajectory in a period of time compared with the fake faces. Our key idea is to make a statistical analysis on gaze trajectory for liveness estimation by gaze tracking. This work provides the first investigation in research literature on the use of gaze estimation for face spoofing detection. Extensive experimental analysis on databases show that gaze estimation offers a new and effective tool for anti-spoofing.

2   General Framework

The general framework of the proposed method is illustrated in Fig. 1, which consists of two sections: establishment of gaze estimation model and spoofing detection.

In the first section, gaze estimation model mapping gaze feature to gaze position, a 2D coordinate, on the computer screen is established. This paper formulates the model as a nonlinear regression problem. In the second section, spoofing detection based on gaze estimation is conducted. It includes three stages: (I) gaze tracking, (II) gaze quantification and encoding, and (III) liveness estimation. Firstly, a video clip lasting 3–5 s of a test user is obtained and gaze trajectory (the gaze locations of each frame in the video clip) can be estimated according to the gaze estimation model. Secondly, quantification and encoding of gaze trajectory is performed to form the gaze histogram, which is convenient for statistics and robust to attacks of warped photograph. Finally, information entropy of the gaze histogram is used to analyze the uncertainty level of gaze trajectory and estimate the liveness of test user. Our hypothesis is that compared with attacks, the gaze uncertainty level of genuine accesses are higher. Therefore, the greater the information entropy value is, the more probable the user is judged to be a genuine access.

3   Gaze Estimation Model

The existing gaze estimation methods can be roughly classified into two categories: feature-based methods and appearance-based methods. Feature-based methods [22,23] map the gaze feature (for example iris outline, pupil, cornea) to gaze position. However, this kind of methods generally require high quality camera, even multiple light sources. Appearance-based [24,25] methods firstly locate eye region, then directly map the whole eye region to gaze position, which takes full advantage of gaze information. Considering our proposed method is conducted under the condition of the nature light and a generic camera, in this paper we choose appearance-based method to establish the gaze estimation model.

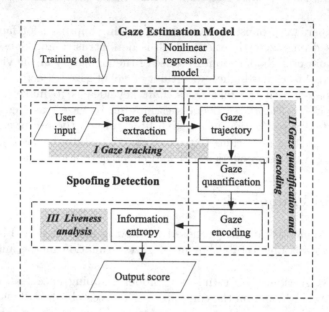

Fig. 1. System architecture.

3.1 Data Collection

To obtain training data for gaze estimation model, we develop a system on a desktop composed of a 19-inch computer screen with 1440 × 900 resolution and a generic webcam with 640 × 480 resolution. The user is asked to sit in front of the computer screen (about 50 cm–60 cm) and keep his head stable with the help of a chinrest. There are nine fixed makers on the computer screen. The setup of our system is shown in Fig. 2(a) and the positions of markers are illustrated in Fig. 2(b).

In the process of data collection, the system captures the user's frontal appearance while his gaze is focusing on the each marker shown on the screen. In this paper there are 50 users and 30 images are captured at each marker for each user, totally 13500 frontal images. By artificially removing eye-closed images, there are 12698 frontal images left. Considering the negative effect of optical reflection, users are required to remove glasses during the data collection.

3.2 Gaze Feature Extraction

We want to find a function that map the gaze feature to the corresponding marker on the computer screen. In this paper gaze feature is obtained based on micro-texture analysis of eye image.

Firstly we introduce an eye image extraction method consisting of two steps: eye corners detection and eye region alignment. In the first step, the face region and inner and outer eye corners are detected by adaptive boosting algorithm [26] (Fig. 3(a), left eye is used in this paper). In the second step, to deal with

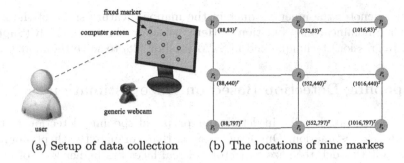

(a) Setup of data collection   (b) The locations of nine markes

Fig. 2. Data collection system for gaze estimation.

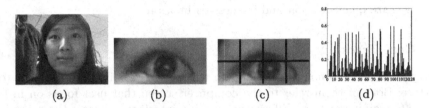

(a)   (b)   (c)   (d)

Fig. 3. Gaze feature extraction. (a) Face and eye corners detection. (b) Eye image (64×32). (c) Uniform partition of eye image. (d) Gaze feature (128D)

small head motion, an additional alignment procedure is performed. Firstly we define an eye image template with 64×32 size, and the location of inner eye corner is (54, 20) and outer corner (9, 20). The aligned eye image is obtained by rotating and scaling the face region based on the locations of eye corners in template (Fig. 3(b)).

In the procedure of feature extraction, to fully use the micro-texture difference between fake faces and real faces, the eye image is divided into $r \times c$ subregions (4×2 in this paper, Fig. 3(c)) and for each subregion dual histogram local binary pattern (DH-LBP) [27] is extracted as feature. The feature of eye image is formed by concatenating features of subregions (Fig. 3(d)). DH-LBP is the improved version of LBP and its local texture descriptor reduces the dimensions of LBP as well as maintains the discriminate ability.

3.3   Model Building and Solving

Given data set $\{x_i, y_i\}_{i=1}^N$, $x_i \in R^n$ ($n = 128$) is gaze feature and $y_i = (p_{x,i}, p_{y,i})^T$ $\in R^2$ is the corresponding gaze position (one of the fixed markers in Fig. 2(b)), $N = 12698$ is the data number. Considering gaze estimation under non-high quality camera is a complex nonlinear problem, we use regression model in the following to establish the function f mapping gaze feature to gaze position.

$$y = f(x) = (w \cdot \phi(x)) + b \tag{1}$$

where $(\cdot)$ denotes the inner product in the mapped feature space of the input space via a nonlinear map function ϕ. Here, we adapt the robust SVR (Support Vector Regression) technique and libSVM toolbox [28] to solve the model.

4   Spoofing Detection Based on Gaze Estimation

In this section, we describe in details our proposed spoofing detection method based on gaze estimation. Our hypothesis is that compared with photograph, video and 3D model, the gaze trajectory of real faces has higher level of uncertainty. Information entropy is used to evaluate the the uncertainty level and estimate the liveness of user. The proposed method has three main steps: gaze tracking, gaze quantification and liveness estimation.

4.1   Gaze Tracking

Firstly we define two nouns used later in this paper: training interface and test interface. Both of them refer to the computer screen that user focus on in the process of training or test. Differently, training interface indicates the computer screen adapted in Fig. 2(a) for gaze estimation model, and test interface indicates the one adapted in test phrase. Since the establishment of gaze estimation model is offline, training interface and test interface may have different resolutions. Considering the mapping of two different resolutions, for the same user, the predict gaze trajectories are different, but the relative gaze positions are invariable.

(1) Test interface has the same resolution with the training interface. Assuming there are M frontal images captured for the user in front of camera, by extracting gaze feature, we can directly get the gaze trajectory $\{\hat{y}_i = (\hat{p}_{x,i}, \hat{p}_{y,i})^{\mathrm{T}}\}_{i=1}^{M}$ according to function f obtained by solving Eq. (1).

(2) Test interface has the different resolution with the training interface. In this case, we should perform affine transformation on $\{\hat{y}_i = (\hat{p}_{x,i}, \hat{p}_{y,i})^{\mathrm{T}}\}_{i=1}^{M}$ to get the final gaze trajectory. Assuming the final gaze trajectory is $\{\hat{z}_i = (\hat{q}_{x,i}, \hat{q}_{y,i})^{\mathrm{T}}\}_{i=1}^{M}$ and the affine transformation matrix is $T = \begin{pmatrix} a_{00} & a_{01} & b_{00} \\ a_{10} & a_{11} & b_{10} \end{pmatrix}$, we have

$$(\hat{z}_1 \cdots \hat{z}_M) = T(\hat{y}_1 \cdots \hat{y}_M)$$

$$= \begin{pmatrix} a_{00} & a_{01} & b_{00} \\ a_{10} & a_{11} & b_{10} \end{pmatrix} \begin{pmatrix} \hat{p}_{x,1} & \cdots & \hat{p}_{x,M} \\ \hat{p}_{y,1} & \cdots & \hat{p}_{y,M} \\ 1 & \cdots & 1 \end{pmatrix} \tag{2}$$

T can be obtained by three pairs of corresponding points between training interface and test interface.

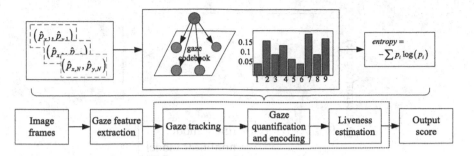

Fig. 4. The flowchart of the proposed spoofing detection algorithm.

4.2 Gaze Quantification and Encoding

The quantization step is important because it not only simplify the statistics for gaze trajectory of real faces but also may robust to that of warped photograph attack. Gaze codebook is firstly constructed as base points for further quantification. In this paper gaze codebook is obtained by performing affine transformation on the nine fixed makers belonging to the training interface of Fig. 2(a). Given $\{P_1, \cdots, P_9\}$ presented in Sect. 3.1 and transformation matrix T obtained in Sect. 4.1, we have

$$(Q_1 \cdots Q_9) = T \begin{pmatrix} P_1 & \cdots & P_9 \\ 1 & \cdots & 1 \end{pmatrix} \tag{3}$$

$\{Q_1, \cdots, Q_9\}$ forms the gaze codebook. Then, gaze quantification is performed by classifying each gaze position of gaze trajectory to its nearest Q_i and gaze encoding is conducted by voting and normalization to form gaze histogram.

4.3 Liveness Estimation

In information theory, entropy is the indicator of information quantity. The greater the entropy is, the larger quantity the information contains. In this paper, we use information entropy to estimate the liveness of user. The greater the information entropy is, the higher the uncertainty level of gaze trajectory is, and the more probable the user is judged as a live person.

For gaze histogram $H = \{p_1, p_2, \cdots, p_9\}$ satisfying $\sum_{i=1}^{9} p_i = 1, 0 \leq p_i \leq 1$, according to the definition of information entropy

$$entropy = - \sum_{i=1}^{9} p_i log(p_i) \tag{4}$$

if $\exists\ p_{i_0} = 1$, then $entropy = -\sum_{i=1}^{9} p_i log(p_i) = -p_{i_0} log(p_{i_0}) = 0$. if $\exists\ \{0 < p_{i_k} < 1\}_{k=1}^{l}, 1 < l \leq 9,\ entropy = -\sum_{i=1}^{9} p_i log(p_i) = -\sum_{k=1}^{l} p_{i_k} log(p_{i_k}) > 0$. $entropy = log(9) \approx 2.1972$ obtains the maximum if and only if $p_1 = p_2 = \cdots = p_9 = \frac{1}{9}$.

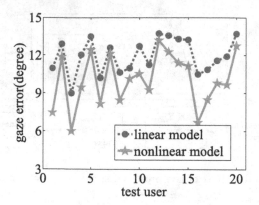

Fig. 5. Average gaze error of 20 test users by linear and nonlinear regression model.

By above analysis, if the user keeps gaze still in a period of time, then *entropy* = 0. If he moves his attention and changes the gaze, then *entropy* > 0, and if the user casts his gaze on the neighborhood of each Q_i uniformly, then *entropy* gets the maximum.

To sum up, for a test user, our proposed spoofing detection method based on gaze estimation includes the following procedures: (1) Capture video frames of user from generic webcam. (2) Gaze feature extraction. (3) Spoofing detection based on gaze trajectory analysis: gaze tracking, gaze quantification and encoding, and liveness estimation. (4) Output entropy as liveness score. Figure 4 shows the flowchart of the proposed method.

5   Experiments

5.1   Evaluation of Gaze Estimation Model

Gaze error [25] is commonly used to evaluate the gaze estimation model.

$$error = arctan\left(\frac{\|y - \hat{y}\|_2}{d_{user}}\right) \tag{5}$$

where $\|y - \hat{y}\|_2$ represents the Euclidean distance between real and predict value, and d_{user} refers to the distance between user's eye with computer screen.

In this experiment, we compare adapted nonlinear model solved by SVR with linear model solved by least square method. Experiment is performed by separating the collected data in Sect. 3.1 into two parts: 30 persons for training gaze estimation model and 20 persons for test. Figure 5 illustrates the average gaze error on nine makers of 20 test users. Experimental results show that nonlinear model has lower average gaze error. Compared with SVR, (1) Least square method is sensitive to outer points of fitting curve. (2) Least square method only minimizes the empirical risk and doesn't generalize well. It should be noted that all the existing gaze estimation model presented under the condition of

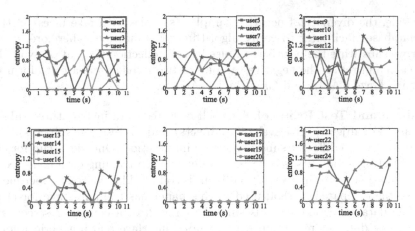

Fig. 6. The variation of gaze directions under user's involuntary state.

nature light and a generic webcam can be embedded into our spoofing detection method.

5.2 Gaze Analysis of Real Faces Under Involuntary State

This section studies the gaze change of real faces under involuntary state. Involuntary state means that there is no interference from outside. We collect 24 video clips with 15 fps (Frames Per Second) from 24 users, and each clip lasts about 10 s (Second). Different from the setup showed in Fig. 2(a), the video collection setup has no fixed markers on the computer screen. Considering the detection efficiency, we choose time window with 15 frames for evaluation. Figure 6 gives the entropy values for each time window of 24 users.

Experimental results show that different users have different uncertainly level of gaze trajectory. For example, user 1–4, 5, 8, 10, 12, 16 and 21 change their gaze in the first 1 s. However, user 18–20 and 24 keeps gaze still during all the 10 s. Therefore, to ensure the efficiency of applicant system, extra stimulus showed on the test interface is needed to attract the attention of genuine access for gaze change, which avoids mistakenly judging the real faces as attacks.

5.3 Effectiveness of Proposed Spoofing Detection Method

To my knowledge, there is no suitable database which is public available to evaluate our proposed method. In this section, we construct two databases by combing self-collected data with parts of two public databases. CASIA [29] and Replay-Attack [30] are commonly used databases for evaluating spoofing detection methods. They contain samples with multiple qualities (low quality, low quality and high quality) and multiple forms (photograph, iPhone and iPad play). However, the positive samples (sample with real faces) of the two databases keep gaze direction unchanged, which is unfit for proposed method. On the other side, the diversity of negative samples (samples with fake faces) in these two databases facilitates to verify algorithm generalization. Therefore, in this paper we substitute the positive samples by self-collection for that of two public databases and retain the negative samples of two public databases to form two new ones: Gaze-CASIA and Gaze-Replay-Attack.

Database and Test Protocol. The self-collected data include three subsets: G-Train (50 subjects), G-Devel (30 subjects) and G-Test (30 subjects). Subjects belonging to different subsets have no intersection. One video clip for each subject lasting about 10 s is collected. Different with training data collected for gaze estimation model in Sect. 3.1, G-Train is collected for contrast experiments, because the compared method used in this paper has training stage for classifier. The data collection setup is similar to Fig. 2(a): a computer screen with the same or different resolution with training interface and a generic webcam with 640 × 480 resolution. The difference is that in Fig. 2(a), there are nine fixed markers on the computer screen, while in this section, random points is set to appear on computer screen for attacking user's attention and changing live user's gaze direction as soon as possible. It is noted that we don't force users to follow the trajectory of random points, which means that our proposed method doesn't require user's cooperation. Gaze-CASIA and Gaze-Gaze-Replay-Attack databases are constructed as follows.

(1) Gaze-CASIA is composed of two subsets: training set and test set. Their positive samples are G-Train and G-Test respectively, and the negative samples are the same with that in CASIA database (L2, L3, L4, N2, N3, N4, H2, H3 and H4, each with 20 and 30 subjects for training and test sets). L, N and H refer to low-quality camera, normal-quality camera and high-quality camera respectively. 2, 3 and 4 refer to warped photograph, photograph removing eye region and video. Thus, L2 means photograph attack in front of a low-quality camera, and so on.

(2) Gaze-Replay-Attack database is composed of three subsets: training, validation and test. Positive samples are G-Train, G-Devel and G-Test respectively, and negative samples are the same with that in Replay-Attack database. Validation is used for selecting parameters. Details are shown in Table 1.

Table 1. The decomposition of Gaze-Replay-Attack database. The numbers indicate how many videos are included in each subset (the sums indicate the amount of hand-based and fixed-support attacks).

Type	Train	Devel	Test	Total
Real-access	50	30	50	130
Print-attack	30 + 30	30 + 30	40 + 40	100 + 100
Phone-attack	60 + 60	60 + 60	80 + 80	200 + 200
Tablet-attack	60 + 60	60 + 60	80 + 80	200 + 200
Total	350	330	450	1130

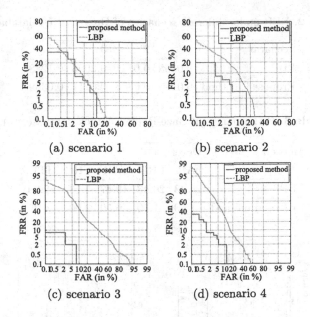

(a) scenario 1   (b) scenario 2

(c) scenario 3   (d) scenario 4

Fig. 7. DET curves under the different scenarios of the Gaze-CASIA database.

For Gaze-Replay database, to verify the effectiveness of proposed method on samples with diverse qualities, we present four scenarios similar to [29].

scenario 1: {G-Train+G-Test, L2, L3, L4};

scenario 2: {G-Train+G-Test, N2, N3, N4};

scenario 3: {G-Train+G-Test, H2, H3, H4};

scenario 4: {G-Train+G-Test, L2, L3, L4, N2, N3, N4, H2, H3, H4}. DET (Detection-Error Trade-off) curve and EER (Equal Error Rate) [29] are adapted for evaluation on each scenario. EER is the value when FRR (False Rejection Rate) equals to FAR (False Acceptance Rate).

For Gaze-Replay-Attack database, FAR, FRR and HTER (Half Total Error Rate) [30] on test set should be given under the threshold selected by minimizing EER on validation set.

Contrast Experiments. Because there is no similar methods proposed before, we can't compare our proposed method with the state of the arts on the public available databases. To verify the effective of our method, on the constructed databases Gaze-CASIA and Gaze-Replay-Attack, classical LBP-based spoofing detection method [6] is used for comparison. Figure 7 and Table 2 are the DET curves and EER of two compared methods under four scenarios of Gaze-CASIA database.

Experimental results show that compared with LBP-based method, proposed method gets lower FAR and FRR under scenario 2, 3, and 4. By contrast, the difference of two methods under scenario 1 are not apparent. It expresses that compared with low-quality photo and video, proposed method works better with

Table 2. EER under different scenarios of Gaze-CASIA database.

Scenario	1	2	3	4
LBP	0.0558	0.0821	0.2096	0.1288
Proposed method	0.0489	0.0378	0.0211	0.0359

Table 3. Performance on Gaze-Replay-Attack database (%).

Method	Devel		Test		
	FAR	FRR	FAR	FRR	HTER
LBP	26.43	26.43	19.47	5.13	12.30
Proposed method	1.50	1.50	6.50	2.00	4.25

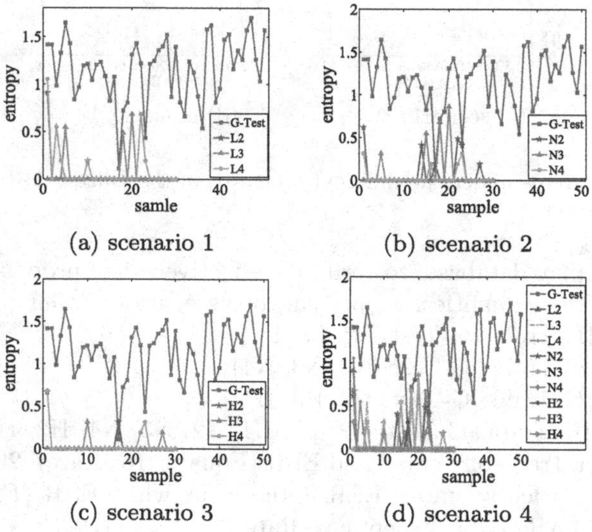

(a) scenario 1   (b) scenario 2

(c) scenario 3   (d) scenario 4

Fig. 8. The entropy values of Gaze-CASIA database.

high-quality camera. Because high-quality camera offers clear image, thus face region and eye corners can be detect accurately.

Table 3 gives the compared performance on Gaze-Replay-Attack database. Experimental results show that proposed method works better. The FAR doesn't reach 0 % may because the glasses reflectivity brings mistaken judgement.

5.4   Is Entropy a Good Indicator?

This section verifies the effectiveness of bringing into information entropy into our proposed method. Figures 8 and 9 illustrate the entropy values of samples in two databases and show that entropy values of real faces (G-Test in Fig. 8(a)–(c) and Fig. 9(a), (e)) are averagely higher than that of fake faces (L2-L4, N2-N4,

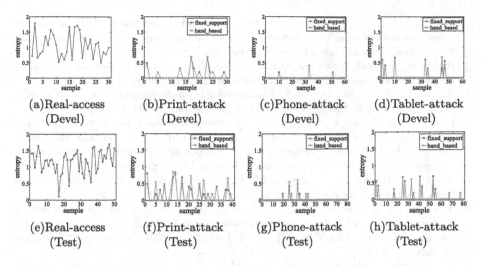

Fig. 9. The entropy values of Gaze-Replay-Attack database.

H2-H4 in Fig. 8(a)–(c) and Fig. 9 (b)–(d), (f)–(h)). Considering the fact that compared with attacks, genuine accesses have higher uncertainty level of gaze trajectory. Experimental results show that the hypothesis of proposed method matches the real case, therefore, entropy is a good indicator.

6 Conclusion and Future Work

In this paper we propose a novel spoofing detection method based on gaze estimation. To the best of my knowledge, it is the first time to present this kind of method for preventing the fake faces based on gaze tracking and analysis. Due to the ambiguity of visual attention process, real faces have no fixed gaze trajectory within a period of time. Our key idea is that compared with photograph, video and 3D model, gaze trajectory of real face has higher level of uncertainty. The proposed spoofing detection method contains three key stages: gaze tracking, gaze quantification and decoding, and liveness estimation. Gaze tracking is performed based on gaze estimation model to form gaze trajectory. Gaze quantification and decoding of gaze trajectory offers convenient way for statistics and is robust to attack of warped photograph. Information entropy is a good indicator to estimate the liveness of user. Experimental results on constructed databases show that the proposed method can effectively distinguish the attacks from genuine accesses. How to prevent video attacks with gaze changing is the future issue we will research on.

References

1. Kollreider, K., Fronthaler, H., Bigun, J.: Non-intrusive liveness detection by face images. Image Vis. Comput. **27**, 223–244 (2009)

2. Bao, W., Li, H., Li, N., Jiang, W.: A liveness detection method for face recognition based on optical flow field. In: Proceedings of the International Conference on Image Analysis and Signal Processing, pp. 233–236 (2009)
3. Anjos, A., Marcel, S.: Counter-measures to photo attacks in face recognition: a public database and a baseline. In: Proceedings of IJCB, pp. 1–7 (2011)
4. Anjos, A., Mohan, M., Marcel, S.: Motion-based counter-measures to photo attacks in face recognition. Inst. Eng. Technol. J. Biometrics **3**, 147–158 (2014)
5. Pan, G., Sun, L., Wu, Z., Wang, Y.: Monocular camera-based face liveness detection by combining eyeblink and scene context. J. Telecommun. Syst. **47**, 215–225 (2011)
6. Jukka, M.P., Hadid, A., Pietikinen, M.: Face spoofing detection from single images using micro-texture analysis. In: Proceedings of IJCB, pp. 1–7 (2011)
7. Maatta, J., Hadid, A., Pietikainen, M.: Face spoofing detection from single images using texture and local shape analysis. IET Biometrics **1**, 3–10 (2012)
8. Tan, X., Li, Y., Liu, J., Jiang, L.: Face liveness detection from a single image with sparse low rank bilinear discriminative model. In: Daniilidis, K., Maragos, P., Paragios, N. (eds.) ECCV 2010, Part VI. LNCS, vol. 6316, pp. 504–517. Springer, Heidelberg (2010)
9. Komulainen, J., Hadid, A., Pietikäinen, M.: Face spoofing detection using dynamic texture. In: Park, J.-I., Kim, J. (eds.) ACCV Workshops 2012, Part I. LNCS, vol. 7728, pp. 146–157. Springer, Heidelberg (2013)
10. Yan, J.J., Zhang, Z.W., Lei, Z., Yi, D., Li, S.Z.: Face liveness detection by exploring multiple scenic clues. In: Proceedings of the International Conference on Control Automation Robotics and Vision, pp. 188–193 (2012)
11. Komulainen, J., Hadid, A., Pietikainen, M., Anjos, A., Marcel, S.: Complementary countermeasures for detecting scenic face spoofing attacks. In: Proceedings of ICB, pp. 1–7 (2013)
12. Frischholz, R.W., Dieckmann, U.: Bioid: a multimodal biometric identification system. Computer **33**, 64–68 (2000)
13. Eveno, N., Besacier, L.: Co-inertia analysis for "liveness" test in audio-visual biometrics. In: Proceedings of the International Symposium on Image and Signal Processing and Analysis, pp. 257–261 (2005)
14. Chetty, G., Wagner, M.: Liveness verification in audio–video speaker authentication. In: Proceedings of the Australian International Conference on Speech Science and Technology, pp. 363–385 (2004)
15. Pavlidis, I., Symosek, P.: The imaging issue in an automatic face/disguise detection system. In: Proceedings of the IEEE Workshop on Computer Vision Beyond the Visible Spectrum: Methods and Applications, pp. 15–24 (2000)
16. Zhang, Z.W., Yi, D., Lei, Z., Li, S.Z.: Face liveness detection by learning multispectral reflectance distributions. In: Proceedings of the IEEE International Conference on Automatic Face and Gesture Recognition and Workshops, pp. 436–441 (2011)
17. Kim, Y., Na, J., Yoon, S., Yi, J.: Masked fake face detection using radiance measurements. J. Opt. Soc. Am. A **24**, 760–766 (2009)
18. Sireesha, M.V., Vijaya, P.A., Chellamma, K.: A survey on gaze estimation techniques. In: Proceedings of the International Conference on VLSI, Communication, Advanced Devices, Signals and Systems and Networking, pp. 353–361 (2013)
19. Ali, A., Deravi, F., Hoque, S.: Liveness detection using gaze collinearity. In: Proceedings of the International Conference on Emerging Security Technologies, pp. 62–65 (2012)
20. Ali, A., Deravi, F., Hoque, S.: Directional sensitivity of gaze-collinearity features in liveness detections. In: Proceedings of the International Conference on Emerging Security Technologies, pp. 8–11 (2013)

21. Ali, A., Deravi, F., Hoque, S.: Spoofing attempt detection using gaze colocation. In: Proceedings of the International Conference on Biometrics Special Interest Group, pp. 1–12 (2013)
22. Sigut, J.F., Sidha, S.A.: Iris center corneal reflection method for gaze tracking using visible light. IEEE Trans. Biomed. Eng. **58**, 411–419 (2011)
23. Villanueva, A., Cabeza, R.: Evaluation of corneal refraction in a model of a gaze tracking system. IEEE Trans. Biomed. Eng. **55**, 2812–2822 (2008)
24. Williams, O., Blake, A., Cipolla, R.: Sparse and semi-supervised visual mapping with the S3GP. In: Proceedings of the IEEE Computer Society Conference on Computer Vision and Pattern Recognition, pp. 230–237 (2006)
25. Feng, L., Sugano, Y., Takahiro, O., Sato, Y.: Inferring human gaze from appearance via adaptive linear regression. In: Proceedings of ICCV, pp. 153–160 (2011)
26. Viola, P., Jones, M.: Robust real-time face detection. Int. J. Comput. Vis. **57**, 137–154 (2004)
27. Ma, W.H., Huang, L., Liu, C.P.: Advanced local binary pattern descriptors for crowd estimation. In: Proceedings of the Pacific-Asia Workshop on Computational Intelligence and Industrial Application, pp. 958–962 (2008)
28. Chang, C.C., Lin, J.C.: LIBSVM: a library for support vector machines. ACM Trans. Intell. Syst. Technol. **2**, 1–27 (2011). http://www.csie.ntu.edu.tw/cjlin/libsvm
29. Zhang, Z.W., Yan, J.J., Liu, S.F., Lei, Z., Yi, D., Li, S.Z.: A face antispoofing database with diverse attacks. In: Proceedings of the IAPR International Conference on Biometrics, pp. 26–31 (2012)
30. Chingovska, I., Anjos, A., Marcel, S.: On the effectiveness of local binary patterns in face anti-spoofing. In: Proceedings of the International Conference on Biometrics Special Interest Group, pp. 1–7 (2012)

Hybrid Euclidean-and-Riemannian Metric Learning for Image Set Classification

Zhiwu Huang[1,2], Ruiping Wang[1(✉)], Shiguang Shan[1], and Xilin Chen[1]

[1] Key Laboratory of Intelligent Information Processing of Chinese Academy of Sciences (CAS), Institute of Computing Technology, CAS, Beijing 100190, China
zhiwu.huang@vipl.ict.ac.cn,
{wangruiping,sgshan,xlchen}@ict.ac.cn
[2] University of Chinese Academy of Sciences, Beijing 100049, China

Abstract. We propose a novel hybrid metric learning approach to combine multiple heterogenous statistics for robust image set classification. Specifically, we represent each set with multiple statistics – mean, covariance matrix and Gaussian distribution, which generally complement each other for set modeling. However, it is not trivial to fuse them since the mean vector with d-dimension often lies in Euclidean space $\mathbb{R}^d$, whereas the covariance matrix typically resides on Riemannian manifold Sym_d^+. Besides, according to information geometry, the space of Gaussian distribution can be embedded into another Riemannian manifold Sym_{d+1}^+. To fuse these statistics from heterogeneous spaces, we propose a Hybrid Euclidean-and-Riemannian Metric Learning (HERML) method to exploit both Euclidean and Riemannian metrics for embedding their original spaces into high dimensional Hilbert spaces and then jointly learn hybrid metrics with discriminant constraint. The proposed method is evaluated on two tasks: set-based object categorization and video-based face recognition. Extensive experimental results demonstrate that our method has a clear superiority over the state-of-the-art methods.

1 Introduction

Learning problems of classifying image sets is commonly encountered in many branches of computer vision community. In video-based face recognition, for example, each face video can be considered as an image set, which may cover large variations in a subject's appearance due to camera pose changes, non-rigid deformations, or different illumination conditions. The objective of image set classification task is to classify an unknown image set to one of the gallery image sets. Generally speaking, existing image set classification methods mainly focus on the key issues of how to quantify the degree of match between two sets and how to learn discriminant function from training image sets [1].

In the aspect of how to quantify the degree of match, image set classification methods can be broadly partitioned into sample-based methods [2–7], subspace-based methods [1,8–13] and distribution-based methods [14,15]. Sample-based methods compare sets based on matching their sample-based statistics (SAS)

D. Cremers et al. (Eds.): ACCV 2014, Part III, LNCS 9005, pp. 562–577, 2015.
DOI: 10.1007/978-3-319-16811-1_37

Table 1. Three major challenges for set modeling: arbitrary data distribution, large data variation and small set size. Here, the tick (/cross) indicates the corresponding set statistics, i.e., sample-based (SAS), subspace-based (SUS) or distribution-based (DIS) statistics, is (/not) qualified to handle the challenge in that column. The last row represents the combination of ALL above three statistics in our proposed method.

Statistics	Arbitrary distribution	Large variation	Small size
SAS	✓	✗	✓
SUS	✓	✗	✓
DIS	✗	✓	✓
ALL	✓	✓	✓

such as sample mean and affine (convex) combination of samples. This kind of methods include Maximum Mean Discrepancy (MMD)[2], Affine (Convex) Hull based Image Set Distance (AHISD, CHISD)[3] and Sparse Approximated Nearest Point (SANP) [4] etc. Subspace-based methods typically apply subspace-based statistics (SUS) to model sets and classify them with given similarity function. For example, Mutual Subspace Method (MSM) [8] represent sets as linear subspaces and match them using canonical correlations [16]. The distribution-based methods, e.g., Single Gaussian Model (SGM) [14] and Gaussian Mixture Models (GMM) [15], model each set with distribution-based statistics (DIS) (i.e., Gaussian distribution), and then measure the similarity between two distributions in terms of the Kullback-Leibler Divergence (KLD) [17].

In the real-world scenario, image sets are often of arbitrary data distribution or large data variation or small set size. As shown in Table 1, however, SAS performs poorly when sets are of large variation while SUS is not good at dealing with the challenge of small set size, though both have no assumption of data distribution. Different from them, DIS requires the set data to follow Gaussian distribution. Fortunately, the three kinds of statistics are complementary for each other: when sets contain small variation, SAS is qualified to model sets with any size and in arbitrary distribution. As a complement, SUS is able to tackle the problem of large variation but requires the set size to be large enough. In addition to the above situations, the last challenge of large variation meanwhile small set size can be overcame by DIS to some extent. This is because DIS is usually obtained by jointly estimating the mean and the covariance, which are capable of adapting to the scenario of small set size and characterizing large data variation respectively.

The other important problem in set classification is how to learn discriminant function from training image sets, which generally are sets of single vectors. The first kind of methods [1,7,11,13] is to learn the discriminant function in Euclidean space. For instance, Discriminative Canonical Correlations (DCC) [1] seeks a discriminant projection of single vectors in Euclidean space to maximizes (minimizes) the canonical correlations of within-class (between-class) sets. Set-to-Set Distance Metric Learning (SSDML) [7] learns a proper metric between pairs of single vectors in Euclidean space to get more accurate set-to-set affine hull based distance for classification. Localized Multi-Kernel Metric Learning (LMKML) [13] treats three order statistics of each set as single vectors again in Euclidean spaces and attempts to learn one metric for them by embedding Euclidean spaces into Reproducing Kernel Hilbert Spaces (RKHS). However, the higher order statistics they used such as the tensors typically lie in non-Euclidean space, which does not adhere to Euclidean geometry. Therefore, in this method, applying the kernel function induced by Euclidean metric to the higher order statistics does not always preserve the original set data structure. In contrast, the second kind of learning methods [10,12,18] treat each subspace-based statistics as a point in a specific non-Euclidean space, and perform metric learning in the same space. For example, Grassmann Discriminant Analysis (GDA) [10] and Covariance Discriminative Learning (CDL) [12] represent each linear subspace or covariance matrix as a point on a Riemannian manifold and learn discriminant Riemannian metrics on that manifold.

In this paper, we propose a new approach to combine multiple statistics for more robust image set classification. From a view of probability statistics, we model each set as sample mean, covariance matrix and Gaussian distribution, which are the corresponding instances of SAS, SUS and DIS. As discussed above, the three kinds of statistics complement each other especially in the real-world settings. Therefore, we attempt to fuse them to simultaneously deal with the challenges of arbitrary distribution, large variation and small set size, which is shown in Table 1. However, combining these multiple statistics is not an easy job because they lie in multiple heterogeneous spaces: the mean is a d-dimension vector lying in Euclidean space $\mathbb{R}^d$. As studied in [19–21], the covariance matrix is regarded as a Symmetric Positive Definite (SPD) matrix residing on a Sym_d^+ manifold. In comparison, the space of Gaussian distribution can be embedded into another Riemannian manifold Sym_{d+1}^+ by employing information geometry [22]. To fuse these multiple statistics from heterogeneous spaces, inspired by our previous work [23], we propose a Hybrid Euclidean-and-Riemannian Metric Learning (HERML) method to exploit the Euclidean and Riemannian metrics for embedding these spaces into high dimension Hilbert spaces, and jointly learn corresponding metrics of multiple statistics for discriminant objective.

2   Background

In this section, we first review the Riemannian metric of SPD matrices. This metric derives the Riemannian kernel function, which can be used to embed the Riemannian manifold into RKHS. Then, we introduce the Information-Theoretic Metric Learning method and its kernelized version.

2.1   Riemannian Metric of Symmetric Positive Definite Matrices

As mostly studied in [19–21], the space of SPD matrices is a specific Riemannian manifold Sym^+ when equipping Riemannian metric. The two most widely used Riemannain metric are the Affine-Invariant Distance (AID) [19] and the Log-Euclidean Distance (LED) [21]. In this work, we focus on the LED, which is a true geodesic distance on Sym^+ and yields a positive definite kernel as studied in [12,24].

By exploiting the Lie group structure of Sym^+, the LED for Sym^+ manifold is derived under the operation $\boldsymbol{X}_i \odot \boldsymbol{X}_j := exp(log(\boldsymbol{X}_i) + log(\boldsymbol{X}_j))$ for $\boldsymbol{X}_i, \boldsymbol{X}_j \in Sym^+$, where $exp(\cdot)$ and $log(\cdot)$ denote the common matrix exponential and logarithm operators. Under the log-Euclidean framework, a geodesic between $\boldsymbol{X}_i, \boldsymbol{X}_j \in Sym^+$ is defined as $\varsigma(t) = exp((1-t)log(\boldsymbol{X}_i) + tlog(\boldsymbol{X}_j))$. The geodesic distance between $\boldsymbol{X}_i$ and $\boldsymbol{X}_j$ is then expressed by classical Euclidean computations in the domain of matrix logarithms:

$$d(\boldsymbol{X}_i, \boldsymbol{X}_j) = \|log(\boldsymbol{X}_i) - log(\boldsymbol{X}_j)\|_F. \tag{1}$$

where $\|\cdot\|_F$ denotes the matrix Frobenius form. As studied in [12], a Riemannian kernel function on the Sym^+ manifold can be derived by computing the corresponding inner product in the space:

$$\kappa_x(\boldsymbol{X}_i, \boldsymbol{X}_j) = tr(log(\boldsymbol{X}_i) \cdot log(\boldsymbol{X}_j)) \tag{2}$$

2.2 Information-Theoretic Metric Learning

Information-Theoretic Metric Learning (ITML) [25] method formulates the problem of metric learning as a particular Bregman optimization, which aims to minimize the LogDet divergence subject to linear constraints:

$$\min_{\boldsymbol{A} \succeq 0, \boldsymbol{\xi}} \quad D_{\ell d}(\boldsymbol{A}, \boldsymbol{A}_0) + \gamma D_{\ell d}(diag(\boldsymbol{\xi}), diag(\boldsymbol{\xi}_0))$$
$$s.t. \quad tr(\boldsymbol{A}(\boldsymbol{x}_i - \boldsymbol{x}_j)(\boldsymbol{x}_i - \boldsymbol{x}_j)^T) \leq \boldsymbol{\xi}_{ij}, \quad (i,j) \in S \tag{3}$$
$$tr(\boldsymbol{A}(\boldsymbol{x}_i - \boldsymbol{x}_j)(\boldsymbol{x}_i - \boldsymbol{x}_j)^T) \geq \boldsymbol{\xi}_{ij}, \quad (i,j) \in D$$

where $\boldsymbol{A}, \boldsymbol{A}_0 \in \mathbb{R}^{d \times d}$, $D_{\ell d}(\boldsymbol{A}, \boldsymbol{A}_0) = tr(\boldsymbol{A}\boldsymbol{A}_0^{-1}) - logdet(\boldsymbol{A}\boldsymbol{A}_0^{-1}) - d$, d is the dimensionality of the data. $(i,j) \in S(D)$ indicates the pair of samples $\boldsymbol{x}_i, \boldsymbol{x}_j$ is in similar (dissimilar) class. $\boldsymbol{\xi}$ is a vector of slack variables and is initialized to $\boldsymbol{\xi}_0$, whose components equal to a upper bound of distances for similarity constraints and a lower bound of distances for dissimilarity constraints.

Meanwhile, ITML method can be extended to a kernel learning one. Let $\boldsymbol{K}_0$ denote the initial kernel matrix, that is, $\boldsymbol{K}_0(i,j) = \phi(\boldsymbol{x}_i)^T \boldsymbol{A}_0 \phi(\boldsymbol{x}_j)$, where ϕ is an implicit mapping from original space to high dimensional kernel space. Note that the Euclidean distance in kernel space may be written as $\boldsymbol{K}(i,i) + \boldsymbol{K}(j,j) - 2\boldsymbol{K}(i,j) = tr(\boldsymbol{K}(\boldsymbol{e}_i - \boldsymbol{e}_j)(\boldsymbol{e}_i - \boldsymbol{e}_j)^T)$, where $\boldsymbol{K}(i,j) = \phi(\boldsymbol{x}_i)^T \boldsymbol{A} \phi(\boldsymbol{x}_j)$ is the learned kernel matrix, $\boldsymbol{A}$ represents an operator in the RKHS, whose size can be potentially infinite, and $\boldsymbol{e}_i$ is the i-th canonical basis vector. Then the kernelized version of ITML can be formulated as:

$$\min_{\boldsymbol{K} \succeq 0, \boldsymbol{\xi}} \quad D_{\ell d}(\boldsymbol{K}, \boldsymbol{K}_0) + \gamma D_{\ell d}(diag(\boldsymbol{\xi}), diag(\boldsymbol{\xi}_0))$$
$$s.t. \quad tr(\boldsymbol{K}(\boldsymbol{e}_i - \boldsymbol{e}_j)(\boldsymbol{e}_i - \boldsymbol{e}_j)^T) \leq \boldsymbol{\xi}_{ij}, \quad (i,j) \in S \tag{4}$$
$$tr(\boldsymbol{K}(\boldsymbol{e}_i - \boldsymbol{e}_j)(\boldsymbol{e}_i - \boldsymbol{e}_j)^T) \geq \boldsymbol{\xi}_{ij}, \quad (i,j) \in D$$

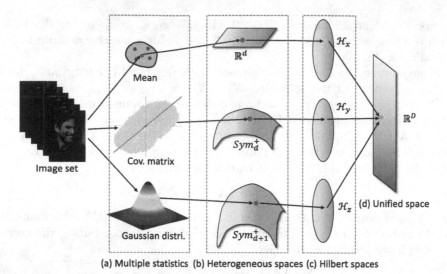

(a) Multiple statistics (b) Heterogeneous spaces (c) Hilbert spaces

Fig. 1. Conceptual illustration of the proposed Hybrid Euclidean-and-Riemannian Metric Learning framework for image set classification. (a) We first model each image set by its sample mean, covariance matrix and Gaussian distribution. (b) Then we embed the space of them into one Euclidean space $\mathbb{R}^d$ and two Riemannian manifolds Sym_d^+, Sym_{d+1}^+ respectively. Finally, by further embedding such heterogeneous spaces into Hilbert spaces (c), the hybrid points are unified in a common subspace (d) by our proposed hybrid metric learning framework.

3 Proposed Method

In this section, we first describe an overview of our proposed approach for image set classification. Then, we introduce multiple statistics for set modeling from a view of probability statistics, followed by embedding them into multiple heterogeneous spaces, i.e., one Euclidean space and two different Riemannian manifolds. Subsequently, we present the Hybrid Euclidean-and-Riemannian Metric Learning (HERML) for fusing such statistics lying in heterogeneous spaces. Finally, we give a discussion about other related work.

3.1 Overview

This paper proposes a novel Hybrid Euclidean-and-Riemannian Metric Learning (HERML) approach for more robust image set classification. As discussed in the prior sections, simultaneously exploiting the multiple statistics may improve the performance of image set classification. With this in mind, we represent each image set with multiple statistics– mean, covariance matrix and Gaussian distribution. For such different statistics, we study their spanned heterogeneous spaces: one Euclidean space $\mathbb{R}^d$ and two Riemannian manifolds Sym_d^+, Sym_{d+1}^+ respectively. Therefore, we then formulate the problem as fusing points in such three heterogeneous spaces spanned by our employed multiple statistics. Since classical multiple kernel learning algorithms cannot take hybrid Euclidean-and-Riemannian points as their direct inputs, we explore an efficient hybrid metric learning framework to fuse the multiple Euclidean-and-Riemannian points by employing the classical Euclidean and Riemannian kernel. A conceptual illustration of our approach is shown in Fig. 1.

3.2 Multiple Statistics Modeling

Let $[x_1, x_2, \ldots, x_n]$ be the data matrix of an image set with n samples, where $x_i \in \mathbb{R}^d$ denotes the i-th image sample with d-dimensional feature representation. From a naive probability statistics perspective, we model each set as the following three statistics with different properties: sample-based, subspace-based and distribution-based statistics.

Sample-based statistics (SAS): Given a set of samples characterized by certain probability distribution, mean value is often used as the sample-based statistics to measure the central tendency of the set of samples. Specifically, the mean vector m of one set containing n samples shows the averaged position of the set in the high dimensional space and is computed as:

$$m = \frac{1}{n} \sum_{i=1}^{n} x_i \tag{5}$$

Subspace-based statistics (SUS): Since the covariance matrix can be eigen-decomposed into the subspace spanned by the set of samples, it can be considered as the subspace-based statistics, which models the variations of the set data and makes no assumption about the data distribution. Given one set with n samples, the covariance matrix is calculated as:

$$C = \frac{1}{n-1} \sum_{i=1}^{n} (x_i - m)(x_i - m)^T \tag{6}$$

Distribution-based statistics (DIS): In probability theory, the Gaussian (or normal) distribution is a very commonly occurring probability distribution, which is a continuous distribution with the maximum entropy for a given mean and variance. Therefore, we can model the data distribution of set as a Single Gaussian Model (SGM) with estimated mean $\tilde{m}$ and covariance matrix $\tilde{C}$:

$$x \sim \mathcal{N}(\tilde{m}, \tilde{C}) \tag{7}$$

3.3 Heterogeneous Space Embedding

As well known, the mean vector lies in Euclidean space $\mathbb{R}^d$, where d is the dimension of the samples. Nevertheless, as studied in [19,21], the covariance matrix resides on Riemannian manifold Sym_d^+. Based on the information geometry [22,26] theory, we can embed the space of Gaussian distribution into a

Riemannian manifold Sym_{d+1}^+. In this case, our defined multiple statistics are in one Euclidean space and two different dimensional Riemannian manifolds respectively.

In the information geometry, if the random vector s follows $\mathcal{N}(0, I)$, then its affine transformation $Qx + \tilde{m}$ follows $\mathcal{N}(\tilde{m}, \tilde{C})$, where $\tilde{C}$ has a decomposition $\tilde{C} = QQ^T, |Q| > 0$, and vice versa. As such the $\mathcal{N}(\tilde{m}, \tilde{C})$ can be characterized by the affine transformation $(\tilde{m}, Q)$. Let τ_1 be the mapping from the affine group $Aff_d^+ = \{(\tilde{m}, Q)|\tilde{m} \in \mathbb{R}^d, Q \in \mathbb{R}^{d \times d}, |Q| > 0\}$ to the simple Lie group $Sl_{d+1} = \{V|V \in \mathbb{R}^{(d+1) \times (d+1)}, |V| > 0\}$ as:

$$\tau_1 : Aff_d^+ \mapsto Sl_{d+1}, \quad (\tilde{m}, Q) \mapsto |Q|^{-\frac{1}{d+1}} \begin{bmatrix} Q & \tilde{m} \\ \tilde{m}^T & 1 \end{bmatrix} \tag{8}$$

Then we denote τ_2 as the mapping from Sl_{d+1} to the space of SPD matrices $Sym_{d+1}^+ = \{P|P \in \mathbb{R}^{(d+1) \times (d+1)}, |P| > 0\}$, i.e.,

$$\tau_2 : Sl_{d+1} \mapsto Sym_{d+1}^+, \quad V \mapsto VV^T \tag{9}$$

Through the two mappings, a d-dimensional Gaussian $\mathcal{N}(\tilde{m}, \tilde{C})$ can be embedded into Sym_{d+1}^+ and thus is uniquely represented by a $(d + 1) \times (d + 1)$ SPD matrix P as:

$$\mathcal{N}(\tilde{m}, \tilde{C}) \sim P = |Q|^{-\frac{2}{d+1}} \begin{bmatrix} QQ^T + \tilde{m}\tilde{m}^T & \tilde{m} \\ \tilde{m}^T & 1 \end{bmatrix} \tag{10}$$

For detailed theory on the embedding process, please kindly refer to [26].

3.4   Hybrid Euclidean-and-Riemannian Metric Learning

Denote $X = [X_1, X_2, \ldots, X_N]$ as the training set formed by N image sets, where $X_i = [x_1, x_2, \ldots, x_{n_i}] \in \mathbb{R}^{n_i \times d}$ indicates the i-th image set, $1 \leq i \leq N$, and n_i is the number of samples in this image set. It is known that the kernel function is always defined by first mapping the original features to a high dimension Hilbert space, that is $\phi : \mathbb{R}^d \rightarrow \mathcal{F}$ (or $Sym^+ \rightarrow \mathcal{F}$), and then calculating the dot product of high dimensional features Φ_i and Φ_j in the new space. Though the mapping ϕ is usually implicit, we first consider it as an explicit mapping for simplicity. Hence, we first use Φ_i^r as the high dimensional feature of r-th statistic feature extracted from the image set X_i. Here, $1 \leq r \leq R$ and R is the number of statistics being used, which is 3 in the setting of our multiple statistics modeling. Now, given a pair of training sets X_i and X_j with the r-th statistic features Φ_i^r, Φ_j^r, we define the distance metric as:

$$d_{A_r}(\Phi_i^r, \Phi_j^r) = tr(A_r(\Phi_i^r - \Phi_j^r)(\Phi_i^r - \Phi_j^r)^T) \tag{11}$$

where A_r is the learned Mahalanobis matrix for the r-th statistic in the high dimensional Hilbert space.

By assuming the high dimensional features of multiple statistics can be mapped to a common space, we can jointly optimize the unknown A_r $(r = 1, \ldots, R)$ for the multiple statistics lying in multiple Hilbert spaces. To learn these distance metrics, we attempt to maximize inter-class variations and minimize the intra-class variations with the regularizer of the LogDet divergence, which usually prevents overfitting due to the small training set and high model complexity. In addition, as stated in [25], the LogDet divergence forces the learned Mahalanobis matrices to be close to an initial Mahalanobis matrix and keep symmetric positive definite during the optimization. The objective function for our multiple metric learning problem is formulated as:

$$\min_{A_1 \succeq 0,\ldots,A_R \succeq 0, \boldsymbol{\xi}} \quad \frac{1}{R} \sum_{r=1}^{R} D_{\ell d}(A_r, A_0) + \gamma D_{\ell d}(diag(\boldsymbol{\xi}), diag(\boldsymbol{\xi}_0)),$$

$$s.t. \quad \frac{\delta_{ij}}{R} \sum_{r=1}^{R} d_{A_r}(\boldsymbol{\Phi}_i^r, \boldsymbol{\Phi}_j^r) \leq \boldsymbol{\xi}_{ij}, \forall (i,j). \tag{12}$$

where $d_{A_r}(\boldsymbol{\Phi}_i^r, \boldsymbol{\Phi}_j^r)$ is obtained in Eq. 11 and $\boldsymbol{\xi}$ is initialized as $\boldsymbol{\xi}_0$, which is a vector with each elements equal to $\delta_{ij}\rho - \zeta\tau$, ρ is the threshold for distance comparison, τ is the margin, ζ is the tuning scale of the margin. Another variable $\delta_{ij} = 1$ if the pair of samples come from the same class, otherwise $\delta_{ij} = -1$. Since each Mahalanobis matrix A_r is symmetric and positive semi-definite, we can seek a non-square matrix $W_r = [w_1^r, \ldots, w_{d_r}^r]$ by calculating the matrix square root $A_r = W_r W_r^T$.

In general, because the form of ϕ^r is usually implicit, it is hard or even impossible to compute the distance $d_{A_r}(\boldsymbol{\Phi}_i^r, \boldsymbol{\Phi}_j^r)$ in Eq. 11 directly in the Hilbert space. Hence, we use the kernel trick method [27] by expressing the basis w_k^r as a linear combination of all the training samples in the mapped space as:

$$w_k^r = \sum_{j=1}^{N} u_j^k \boldsymbol{\Phi}_j^r \tag{13}$$

where u_j^k are the expansion coefficients. Hence,

$$\sum_{r=1}^{R} (w_k^r)^T \boldsymbol{\Phi}_i^r = \sum_{r=1}^{R} \sum_{j=1}^{N} u_j^k (\boldsymbol{\Phi}_j^r)^T \boldsymbol{\Phi}_i^r = \sum_{r=1}^{R} (u^k)^T K_{.i}^r \tag{14}$$

where u^k is an $N \times 1$ column vector and its j-th entry is u_j^k, and $K_{.i}^r$ is the i-th column of the r-th kernel matrix K^r. Here K^r is an $N \times N$ kernel matrix, calculated from the r-th statistic feature using the Euclidean kernel functions $\kappa_m(m_i, m_j) = m_i^T m_j$ or Riemannian kernel functions in Eq. 2 for different set statistic features. If we denote Mahalanobis matrices as $B_r = U_r U_r^T$ for $1 \leq r \leq R$, then Eq. 12 can be rewritten as:

$$\min_{B_1 \succeq 0,\ldots,B_R \succeq 0, \boldsymbol{\xi}} \quad \frac{1}{R} \sum_{r=1}^{R} D_{\ell d}(B_r, B_0) + \gamma D_{\ell d}(diag(\boldsymbol{\xi}), diag(\boldsymbol{\xi}_0)),$$

$$s.t. \quad \frac{\delta_{ij}}{R} \sum_{r=1}^{R} d_{B_r}(K_{.i}^r, K_{.j}^r) \leq \boldsymbol{\xi}_{ij}, \forall (i,j). \tag{15}$$

where $d_{B_r}(\boldsymbol{K}^r_{.i}, \boldsymbol{K}^r_{.j})$ indicates the distance between the i-th and j-th samples under the learned metric $\boldsymbol{B_r}$ for the r-th statistic mapping in the Hilbert space:

$$d_{B_r}(\boldsymbol{K}^r_{.i}, \boldsymbol{K}^r_{.j}) = tr(\boldsymbol{B_r}(\boldsymbol{K}^r_{.i} - \boldsymbol{K}^r_{.j})(\boldsymbol{K}^r_{.i} - \boldsymbol{K}^r_{.j})^T) \qquad (16)$$

3.5 Optimization

To solve the problem in Eq. 15, we adopt the cyclic Bregman projection method [28,29], which is to choose one constraint per iteration, and perform a projection so that the current solution satisfies the chosen constraint. In the case of inequality constraints, appropriate corrections of $\boldsymbol{B_r}$ and $\boldsymbol{\xi}_{ij}$ are also enforced. This process is then repeated by cycling through the constraints. The method of cyclic Bregman projections is able to converge to the globally optimal solution. Please kindly refer to [28,29] for more details. The updating rules for our proposed method are shown in the following proposition:

Proposition 1. *Given the solution $\boldsymbol{B}^t_r$ for $r = 1, \ldots, R$ at the t-th iteration, we update $\boldsymbol{B_r}$ and the corresponding $\boldsymbol{\xi}_{ij}$ as follows:*

$$\begin{cases} \boldsymbol{B}^{t+1}_r = \boldsymbol{B}^t_r + \beta_r \boldsymbol{B_r}(\boldsymbol{K}^r_{.i} - \boldsymbol{K}^r_{.j})(\boldsymbol{K}^r_{.i} - \boldsymbol{K}^r_{.j})^T \boldsymbol{B_r}, & (17) \\[2mm] \xi^{t+1}_{ij} = \dfrac{\gamma \xi^t_{ij}}{\gamma + \delta_{ij}\alpha \xi^t_{ij}}, & (18) \end{cases}$$

where $\beta_r = \delta_{ij}\alpha/(1 - \delta_{ij}\alpha d_{B^t_r}(\boldsymbol{K}^r_{.i}, \boldsymbol{K}^r_{.j}))$ and α can be solved by:

$$\frac{\delta_{ij}}{R} \sum_{r=1}^{R} \frac{d_{B^t_r}(\boldsymbol{K}^r_{.i}, \boldsymbol{K}^r_{.j})}{1 - \delta_{ij}\alpha d_{B^t_r}(\boldsymbol{K}^r_{.i}, \boldsymbol{K}^r_{.j})} - \frac{\gamma \xi^t_{ij}}{\gamma + \delta_{ij}\alpha \xi^t_{ij}} = 0. \qquad (19)$$

Proof. Based on the cyclic projection method [28, 29], we formulate the Lagrangian form of Eq. 15 and set the gradients to zero w.r.t $\boldsymbol{B}^{t+1}_r$, ξ^{t+1}_{ij} and α to get the following update equations:

$$\begin{cases} \nabla D(\boldsymbol{B}^{t+1}_r) = \nabla D(\boldsymbol{B}^t_r) + \delta_{ij}\alpha(\boldsymbol{K}^r_{.i} - \boldsymbol{K}^r_{.j})(\boldsymbol{K}^r_{.i} - \boldsymbol{K}^r_{.j})^T, & (20) \\[2mm] \nabla D(\xi^{t+1}_{ij}) = \nabla D(\xi^t_{ij}) - \dfrac{\delta_{ij}\alpha}{\gamma}, & (21) \\[2mm] \dfrac{\delta_{ij}}{R} \sum_{r=1}^{R} tr(\boldsymbol{B}^{t+1}_r(\boldsymbol{K}^r_{.i} - \boldsymbol{K}^r_{.j})(\boldsymbol{K}^r_{.i} - \boldsymbol{K}^r_{.j})^T) = \xi^{t+1}_{ij}. & (22) \end{cases}$$

Then, we can derive Eq. 17 and Eq. 18 from Eq. 20 and Eq. 21, respectively. Substituting Eqs. 17 and 18 into Eq. 22, we obtain the Eq. 19 related to α.

The resulting algorithm is given as Algorithm 1. The inputs to the algorithm are the starting Mahalanobis matrices $\boldsymbol{B}_1, \ldots, \boldsymbol{B}_R$, the constraint data, the slack parameter γ, distance threshold ρ, margin parameter τ and tuning scale ζ. If necessary, the projections can be computed efficiently over a factorization $\boldsymbol{U}$ of each Mahalanobis matrix, such that $\boldsymbol{B_r} = \boldsymbol{U}^T_r \boldsymbol{U}_r$. The main time cost is to update $\boldsymbol{B}^{t+1}_r$ in Step 5, which is $O(RN^2)$ (N is the number of samples) for each constraint projection. Therefore, the total time cost is $O(LRN^2)$ where L is the total number of the updating in Step 5 executed by the algorithm.

Algorithm 1. Hybrid Euclidean-and-Riemannian Metric Learning

Input: Training pairs $\{(\boldsymbol{K}^r_{\cdot i}, \boldsymbol{K}^r_{\cdot j}), \delta_{ij}\}$, and slack parameter γ, input Mahalanobis matrix $\boldsymbol{B}_0$, distance thresholds ρ, margin parameter τ and tuning scale ζ

1. $t \leftarrow 1$, $\boldsymbol{B}^1_r \leftarrow \boldsymbol{B}_0$ for $r = 1, \ldots, R$, $\lambda_{ij} \leftarrow 0$, $\xi_{ij} \leftarrow \delta_{ij}\rho - \zeta\tau, \forall(i,j)$
2. **Repeat**
3. Pick a constraint (i, j) and compute the distances $d_{\boldsymbol{B}^t_r}(\boldsymbol{K}^r_{\cdot i}, \boldsymbol{K}^r_{\cdot j}))$ for $r = 1, \ldots, R$.
4. Solve α in Eq.19 and set $\alpha \leftarrow min(\alpha, \boldsymbol{\eta}_{ij})$ and $\boldsymbol{\eta}_{ij} \leftarrow \boldsymbol{\eta}_{ij} - \alpha$
5. Update $\boldsymbol{B}^{t+1}_r$ by using Eq. 17 for $r = 1, \ldots, R$.
6. Update ξ^{t+1}_{ij} by using Eq. 18.
7. **Until** convergence

Output: Mahalanobis matrices $\boldsymbol{B}_1, \ldots, \boldsymbol{B}_R$.

3.6 Discussion About Related Work

The original kernelized version of ITML [25] method implicitly solves the metric learning problem in a single high dimensional Hilbert space by learning the optimal kernel matrix $\boldsymbol{K}^*$. In contrast, our proposed method explicitly learns multiple metrics $\{\boldsymbol{B}^*_1, \ldots, \boldsymbol{B}^*_R\}$ on multiple Hilbert spaces for fusing hybrid Euclidean-and-Riemannian features. To some extent, our proposed metric learning framework is a generalized version of ITML. When the type of kernel function is linear and meanwhile the data lie in a single space, the proposed framework can be reduced to the original ITML.

In addition, there are a couple of previous works [13,30–35] for multiple kernel/metric learning in the literature. Nevertheless, most of these works mainly focus on fusing multiple homogeneous Euclidean (or Riemannian) features, while our method attempts to study the new problem of learning hybrid metrics for fusing heterogeneous Euclidean and Riemannian features. Thus, their problem domains are different from ours.

4 Experiments

In this section, we evaluate our proposed approach on two image set classification applications: set-based object categorization and video-based face recognition. The following describes the experiments and results.

4.1 Databases and Settings

For the set-based object categorization task, we use the database ETH-80 [36]. It consists of 8 categories of objects with each category including 10 object instances. Each object instance has 41 images of different views from one set. The task is to classify an image set of an object into a known category. The images were resized to 20×20 as [12,13] and the intensities were used for features.

For the video-based face recognition task, we consider two public datasets: YouTube Celebrities [37] and COX [38]. The YouTube is a quite challenging and widely used video face dataset. It has 1,910 video clips of 47 subjects collected from YouTube. Most clips contains hundreds of frames, which are often low resolution and highly compressed with noise and low quality. The COX is a large scale video dataset involving 1,000 different subjects, each of which has 3 videos captured by different camcorders. In each video, there is around $25 \sim 175$ frames of low resolution and low quality, with blur, and captured under poor lighting. Each face in YouTube was resized to a 20×20 image as [12,13] while the faces in COX were resized to 32×40. For all faces in the two datasets, histogram equalization was implemented to eliminate lighting effects.

On the three datasets, we followed the same protocol as the prior work [3,12,13], which conducted ten-fold cross validation experiments, i.e., 10 randomly selected gallery/probe combinations. Finally, the average recognition rates of different methods were reported. Specifically, for ETH-80, each category had 5 objects for gallery and the other 5 objects for probes. For YouTube, in each fold, one person had 3 randomly chosen image sets for the gallery and 6 for probes. Different from ETH and YouTube, COX dataset does also contain an additional independent training set [38], where each subject has 3 videos. Since there are 3 independent testing sets of videos in COX, each person had one video as the gallery and the remaining two videos for two different probes, thus in total 6 groups of testing need to be conducted.

4.2   Comparative Methods and Settings

We compared our approach with three categories of the state-of-the-art image set classification methods as following. Note that, we add ITML to sample-based methods as it performs metric learning on single samples/images, which can be considered as a kind of sample-based statistics here. Since ITML also has a kernel version, we feed our proposed kernel function of distribution-based statistics (DIS) to it for additional comparison.

1. Sample-based method:
   Maximum Mean Discrepancy (MMD)[2], Affine (Convex) Hull based Image Set Distance (AHISD, CHISD)[3], Set-to-Set Distance Metric Learning (SS-DML) [7] and Information Theoretic Metric Learning (ITML)[25].
2. Subspace-based method:
   Mutual Subspace Method (MSM) [8], Discriminant Canonical Correlations (DCC)[1], Manifold Discriminant Analysis (MDA)[11], Grassmann Discriminant Analysis (GDA) [10], Covariance Discriminative Learning (CDL)[12] and Localized Multi-Kernel Metric Learning (LMKML)[13].
3. Distribution-based method:
   Single Gaussian Models (SGM) [14], Gaussian Mixture Models (GMM) [15] and kernel version of ITML [25] with our DIS-based set model (DIS-ITML).

Except SGM and GMM, the source codes of above methods are provided by the original authors. Since the codes of SGM and GMM are not publicly available, we carefully implemented them using the code[1] to generate Gaussian

---

[1] https://engineering.purdue.edu/~bouman/software/cluster/.

model(s). For fair comparison, the important parameters of each method were empirically tuned according to the recommendations in the original references: For MMD, we used the edition of Bootstrap and set the parameters $\alpha = 0.1, \sigma = -1$, the number of iteration to 5. For ITML, we used the default parameters as the standard implementation. For AHISD, CHISD and DCC, PCA was performed by preserving 95 % energy to learn the linear subspace and corresponding 10 maximum canonical correlations were used. For MDA, the parameters were configured according to [11]. For GDA, the dimension of Grassmannian manifold is set to 10. For CDL, since KPLS works only when the gallery data is used for training, the setting of COX prevent it from working. So, we use KDA for discriminative learning and adopt the same setting as [12]. For SSDML, we set $\lambda_1 = 0.001, \lambda_2 = 0.5$, numbers of positive and negative pairs per set is set to 10 and 20. For LMKML, we used median distance heuristic to tune the widths of Gaussian kernels. For our method HERML[2], we set the parameters $\gamma = 1$, ρ as the mean distances, τ as the standard variations and the tuning range of ζ is $[0.1, 1]$.

4.3   Results and Analysis

We present the rank-1 recognition results of comparative methods on the three datasets in Table 2. Each reported rate is an average over the ten-fold trials. Note that, since the LMKML method is too time-consuming to run in the setting of COX dataset, which has a large scale dataset, we alternately use 100 of 300 subject's data for training and 100 of 700 remaining subject's sets for testing.

Firstly, we are interested in the classification results of methods with different degree of match. Here, we focus on the comparison between those unsupervised methods MMD, AHISD, CHISD, MSM, SGM, GMM. On the ETH-80, the subspace-based method MSM and the distribution-based methods SGM, GMM outperform the sample-based methods MMD, AHISD, CHISD. This is mainly because the ETH-80 contains many sets of large variations. In this setting, MSM, SGM and GMM can capture the pattern variations, which are more robust to outlier and noise than MMD, AHISD and CHISD. In other two datasets, YouTube and COX, it is also reasonable that the three kinds of methods achieve comparable results for their used statistics are all effective for set modeling.

Secondly, we also care about which way to learn a discriminant function is more effective. So, we compare the results of the supervised methods SSDML, ITML, DCC, MDA, GDA, CDL. On the three datasets, GDA and CDL methods have clear advantage over SSDML, ITML, DCC and MDA. This is because ITML performs the metric learning and classification on single samples, which neglects the specific data structure of sets. SSDML, DCC and MDA methods learn the discriminant metrics in Euclidean space, whereas most of them classify the sets in non-Euclidean spaces. In contrast, GDA and CDL extract the subspace-based statistics in Riemannian space and match them in the same space, which is more favorable for the set classification task [10].

---

[2] The source code is released on the website: http://vipl.ict.ac.cn/resources/codes.

Table 2. Average recognition rate (%) of different image set classification methods on ETH-80, YouTube and COX-S2V datasets. Here, COX-ij represent the test using the i-th set of videos as gallery and the j-th set of videos as probe.

Method	ETH-80	YouTube	COX-12	COX-13	COX-23	COX-21	COX-31	COX-32
MMD [2]	77.5	52.6	36.4	19.6	8.90	27.6	19.1	9.60
AHISD [3]	77.3	63.7	53.0	36.1	17.5	43.5	35.0	18.8
CHISD [3]	73.5	66.3	56.9	30.1	15.0	44.4	26.4	13.7
SSDML [7]	80.0	68.8	60.1	53.1	28.7	47.9	44.4	27.3
ITML [25]	77.2	65.3	50.9	46.0	35.6	39.6	37.1	34.8
MSM [8]	87.8	61.1	45.5	21.5	11.0	39.8	19.4	9.50
DCC [1]	90.5	64.8	62.5	66.1	50.6	56.1	64.8	45.2
MDA [11]	89.0	65.3	65.8	63.0	36.2	55.5	43.2	30.0
GDA [10]	92.3	65.9	68.6	77.7	71.6	66.0	76.1	74.8
CDL [12]	**94.5**	69.7	**78.4**	**85.3**	**79.7**	**75.6**	**85.8**	**81.9**
LMKML [13]	90.0	**70.3**	66.0	71.0	56.0	74.0	68.0	60.0
SGM [14]	81.3	52.0	26.7	14.3	12.4	26.0	19.0	10.3
GMM [15]	89.8	61.0	30.1	24.6	13.0	28.9	31.7	18.9
DIS-ITML [25]	87.8	68.4	47.9	48.9	36.1	43.1	35.6	33.6
HERML	**94.5**	**74.6**	**94.9**	**96.9**	**94.0**	**92.0**	**96.4**	**95.3**

Thirdly, we compare the state-of-the-art methods with our approach and find they are impressively outperformed by ours on the three datasets. Several reasons are figured out as following: In terms of set modeling, as stated in Sect. 1, our combining of multiple complementary statistics can more robustly model those sets of arbitrary distribution, large variation and small size in the three datasets. In terms of discriminant function learning, by encoding the heterogeneous structure of the space of such statistics, our method jointly learns hybrid metrics to fuse them for more discriminant classification. In comparison, LMKML neglects the non-Euclidean data structure of two higher order statistics, i.e., the covariance matrix and the tensor. Thus, our proposed method is more desirable to learn metrics for non-Euclidean data and has a clear advantage over LMKML. In addition, the results also shows that our novel hybrid metric learning method has an impressive superiority over the original ITML.

In addition, we also compare the discriminative power of our proposed sample-based, subspace-based and distribute-based statistics (SAS, SUS, DIS) for image set classification. For each statistic, we performed our proposed method to train and classify sets with NN classifier. Table 3 tabulates the classification rates of multiple statistics. We can observe that the DIS achieves the best recognition performance than other two statistics because it jointly model the mean and the covariance matrix in a Gaussian distribution. Additionally, the results of combining of SAS and SUS sometimes are better than those of DIS on COX-S2V. This is because the dataset may contain some sets not in Gaussian distribution. Since the multiple statistics complement each other, the performance can be improved by our proposed metric learning with all of statistic models.

Table 3. Average recognition rate (%) of different statistics (SAS, SUS, DIS), combining SAS and SUS (SAS+SUS), fusing all multiple statistics (ALL) with our metric learning method on ETH-80, YouTube and COX-S2V. Here, COX-ij indicates the test using the i-th set of videos as gallery and the j-th set of videos as probe.

Statistics	ETH-80	YouTube	COX-12	COX-13	COX-23	COX-21	COX-31	COX-32
SAS	83.5	64.1	86.2	92.0	82.8	83.2	86.9	84.9
SUS	93.5	70.2	88.8	93.6	90.3	86.4	94.0	93.1
DIS	**94.3**	**73.5**	92.8	94.7	92.2	89.0	94.7	94.4
SAS+SUS	92.0	71.6	**93.1**	**95.2**	**93.1**	**91.2**	**95.2**	**95.0**
ALL	**94.5**	**74.6**	**94.9**	**96.9**	**94.0**	**92.0**	**96.4**	**95.3**

Table 4. Computation time (seconds) of different methods on the YouTube dataset for training and testing (classification of one video).

Method	MMD	SSDML	ITML	DCC	CDL	LMKML	SGM	GMM	**HERML**
Train	N/A	433.3	2459.7	11.9	4.3	17511.2	N/A	N/A	27.3
Test	0.1	2.6	0.5	0.1	0.1	247.1	0.4	1.9	0.1

Lastly, on the YouTube dataset, we compared the computational complexity of different methods on an Intel(R) Core(TM) i7-3770 (3.40 GHz) PC. Table 4 lists the time cost for each method. The presentation of training time is only required by discriminant methods. For testing, we report the classification time of one video. Since ITML has to train and test on large number of samples from sets and classify pairs of samples, it has high time complexities. Except DCC and CDL, our method is much faster than other methods especially the LMKML method. This is because it transformed the covariance matrices and third-order tensors to vectors, which lies in very high dimension Euclidean spaces. As a result, it is very time-consuming to perform metric learning and classification.

5   Conclusions

In this paper, we proposed a novel hybrid Euclidean-and-Riemannian metrics method to fuse multiple complementary statistics for robust image set classification. The extensive experiments have shown that our proposed method outperforms the state-of-the-art methods in both terms of accuracy and efficiency. To our best knowledge, the problem of hybrid metric learning across Euclidean and Riemannian spaces has not been investigated before and we made the first attempt to address this issue in this paper. In the future, it would be interesting to explore other possible metric learning methods to fuse multiple complement statistics or pursue more robust statistics to model image sets with different structures in real-world scenario.

Acknowledgement. The work is partially supported by Natural Science Foundation of China under contracts nos.61390511, 61379083, and 61222211.

References

1. Kim, T., Kittler, J., Cipolla, R.: Discriminative learning and recognition of image set classes using canonical correlations. IEEE Trans. PAMI **29**, 1005–1018 (2007)
2. Gretton, A., Borgwardt, K.M., Rasch, M.J., Schölkopf, B., Smola, A.: A kernel two-sample test. JMLR **13**, 723–773 (2012)
3. Cevikalp, H., Triggs, B.: Face recognition based on image sets. In: CVPR (2010)
4. Hu, Y., Mian, A., Owens, R.: Sparse approximated nearest points for image set classification. In: CVPR (2011)
5. Yang, M., Zhu, P., Gool, L., Zhang, L.: Face recognition based on regularized nearest points between image sets. In: FG (2013)
6. Huang, Z., Zhao, X., Shan, S., Wang, R., Chen, X.: Coupling alignments with recognition for still-to-video face recognition. In: ICCV (2013)
7. Zhu, P., Zhang, L., Zuo, W., Zhang, D.: From point to set: extend the learning of distance metrics. In: ICCV (2013)
8. Yamaguchi, O., Fukui, K., Maeda., K.: Face recognition using temporal image sequence. In: FG (1998)
9. Wang, R., Shan, S., Chen, X., Dai, Q., Gao, W.: Manifold-Manifold distance and its application to face recognition with image sets. IEEE Trans. Image Proces. **21**, 4466–4479 (2012)
10. Hamm, J., Lee, D.D.: Grassmann discriminant analysis: a unifying view on subspace-based learning. In: ICML, pp. 376–383 (2008)
11. Wang, R., Chen, X.: Manifold discriminant analysis. In: CVPR (2009)
12. Wang, R., Guo, H., Davis, L., Dai, Q.: Covariance discriminative learning: a natural and efficient approach to image set classification. In: CVPR (2012)
13. Lu, J., Wang, G., Moulin, P.: Image set classification using holistic multiple order statistics features and localized multi-kernel metric learning. In: ICCV (2013)
14. Shakhnarovich, G., Fisher III, J.W., Darrell, T.: Face recognition from long-term observations. In: Heyden, A., Sparr, G., Nielsen, M., Johansen, P. (eds.) ECCV 2002. LNCS, vol. 2352, pp. 851–865. Springer, Heidelberg (2002)
15. Arandjelovic, O., Shakhnarovich, G., Fisher, J., Cipolla, R., Darrell, T.: Face recognition with image sets using manifold density divergence. In: CVPR (2005)
16. Hotelling, H.: Relations between two sets of variates. Biometrika **28**, 312–377 (1936)
17. Cover, T.M., Thomas, J.A.: Elements of Information Theory. Wiley, New York (1991)
18. Harandi, M.T., Sanderson, C., Shirazi, S., Lovell, B.C.: Graph embedding discriminant analysis on Grassmannian manifolds for improved image set matching. In: CVPR (2011)
19. Pennec, X., Fillard, P., Ayache, N.: A Riemannian framework for tensor computing. IJCV **66**, 41–66 (2006)
20. Tuzel, O., Porikli, F., Meer, P.: Region covariance: a fast descriptor for detection and classification. In: Leonardis, A., Bischof, H., Pinz, A. (eds.) ECCV 2006, Part II. LNCS, vol. 3952, pp. 589–600. Springer, Heidelberg (2006)
21. Arsigny, V., Fillard, P., Pennec, X., Ayache, N.: Geometric means in a novel vector space structure on symmetric positive-definite matrices. SIAM J. Matrix Anal. Appl. **29**, 328–347 (2007)

22. Amari, S.I., Nagaoka, H.: Methods of Information Geometry. Oxford University Press, Oxford (2000)
23. Huang, Z., Wang, R., Shan, S., Chen, X.: Learning Euclidean-to-Riemannian metric for point-to-set classification. In: CVPR (2014)
24. Jayasumana, S., Hartley, R., Salzmann, M., Li, H., Harandi, M.: Kernel methods on the Riemannian manifold of symmetric positive definite matrices. In: CVPR (2013)
25. Davis, J.V., Kulis, B., Jain, P., Sra, S., Dhillon, I.S.: Information-theoretic metric learning. In: ICML (2007)
26. Lovrić, M., Min-Oo, M., Ruh, E.A.: Multivariate normal distributions parametrized as a Riemannian symmetric space. J. Multivar. Anal. **74**, 36–48 (2000)
27. Baudat, G., Anouar, F.: Generalized discriminant analysis using a kernel approach. Neural Comput. **12**, 2385–2404 (2000)
28. Bregman, L.M.: The relaxation method of finding the common point of convex sets and its application to the solution of problems in convex programming. USSR Comput. Math. Math. Phys. **7**, 200–217 (1967)
29. Censor, Y., Zenios, S.: Parallel Optimization: Theory, Algorithms, and Applications. Oxford University Press, Oxford (1997)
30. Rakotomamonjy, A., Bach, F.R., Canu, S., Grandvalet, Y.: SimpleMKL. J. Mach. Learn. Res. (JMLR) **9**, 2491–2521 (2008)
31. McFee, B., Lanckriet, G.: Learning multi-modal similarity. JMLR **12**, 491–523 (2011)
32. Xie, P., Xing, E.P.: Multi-modal distance metric learning. In: IJCAI (2013)
33. Vemulapalli, R., Pillai, J.K., Chellappa, R.: Kernel learning for extrinsic classification of manifold features. In: CVPR (2013)
34. Cui, Z., Li, W., Xu, D., Shan, S., Chen, X.: Fusing robust face region descriptors via multiple metric learning for face recognition in the wild. In: CVPR (2013)
35. Jayasumana, S., Hartley, R., Salzmann, M., Li, H., Harandi, M.: Combining multiple manifold-valued descriptors for improved object recognition. In: DICTA (2013)
36. Leibe, B., Schiele, B.: Analyzing appearance and contour based methods for object categorization. In: CVPR (2003)
37. Kim, M., Kumar, S., Pavlovic, V., Rowley, H.: Face tracking and recognition with visual constraints in real-world videos. In: CVPR (2008)
38. Huang, Z., Shan, S., Zhang, H., Lao, S., Kuerban, A., Chen, X.: Benchmarking still-to-video face recognition via partial and local linear discriminant analysis on COX-S2V dataset. In: Lee, K.M., Matsushita, Y., Rehg, J.M., Hu, Z. (eds.) ACCV 2012, Part II. LNCS, vol. 7725, pp. 589–600. Springer, Heidelberg (2013)

Size and Location Matter: A New Baseline for Salient Object Detection

Long Zhao[1], Shuang Liang[1]([✉]), Yichen Wei[2], and Jinyuan Jia[1]

[1] Tongji University, Shanghai, China
shuangliang@tongji.edu.cn
[2] Microsoft Research, Beijing, China

Abstract. Recent years have seen many complex models proposed for salient object detection and progressing results. However, less has been done to justify the need for such complex models as there lacks sufficient comparison to simple baselines on more challenging datasets. In this work, we propose a new baseline method for saliency detection. It simply considers a large region close to the image center as salient, and defines the saliency of a region as the product of its size and centerness. As accurate image segmentation problem is difficult by itself, we propose novel techniques that can estimate these attributes using superpixels in a soft manner, without the need to perform hard image segmentation. Our approach is based on very simple concepts and implementation, but already achieves very competitive results, especially on challenging datasets. It is further shown highly complementary with the state-of-the-art. Therefore we believe our method serves as a strong baseline and would enhance the problem understanding for future work.

1 Introduction

Salient object detection has attracted a lot of research interests in recent years [1]. The problem is inherently ambiguous since there lacks common definitions and criteria of "what a salient object is". Consequently, the research in this area presents a great amount of diversity, from low level features to high level methodologies. While many new methods have been proposed and steady improvements in evaluation have been shown, it is still unclear to tell how well and to what extent this problem has been solved.

We observed two issues in the current field: complex methodologies and insufficient evaluation. First, recent works adopt more complex models. The saliency models have evolved from the earlier simple contrast based methods [2–5] and frequency analysis based methods [6,7], to more complex ones such as gaussian mixture appearance models [8], low rank matrix recovery [9], multi-scale segmentation and optimization [10], graph based manifold ranking [11], formulation as a submodular optimization [12], hypergraph modelling [13], Markov Chain [14], learning based [15], and fusion of multiple models [16]. All of these models are well motivated and explained from their own viewpoints, and have been shown working well. However, due to their high complexities and large differences, it is

© Springer International Publishing Switzerland 2015
D. Cremers et al. (Eds.): ACCV 2014, Part III, LNCS 9005, pp. 578–592, 2015.
DOI: 10.1007/978-3-319-16811-1_38

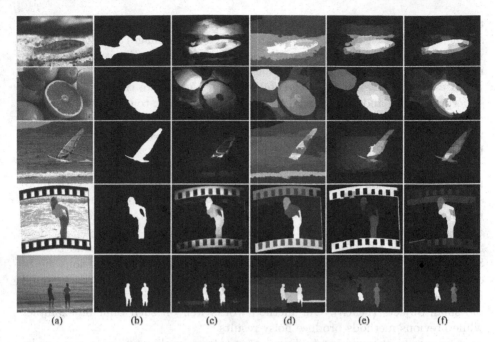

Fig. 1. Saliency detection results on challenging examples. (a) input images; (b) ground truth; (c)–(e) results from the state-of-the-art methods [10,11,19]; (f) our results.

very hard to find how different methods are related and identify what is really working for saliency detection. In other words, it is unclear whether such high complexities are essential or not.

The second issue is that evaluation is mostly performed on the simple ASD [7] or MSRA [2] datasets. It has been well recognized that these datasets are biased to contain a large object near the image center with strong contrast to the background, thus too simple. Although several other more challenging datasets have been proposed, such as SED1 [17], SED2 [17], SOD [18], and ECSSD [10], they are less used in evaluation. While the performance on the simple ASD dataset nowadays is close to saturate, it is relatively unclear whether the good models on ASD can be generalized to more challenging datasets.

This work is a try to address the above two issues by proposing a simple baseline method and showing strong results. Our method just uses two basic concepts: the size and location of a region for determining its saliency. Observing that *larger image regions closer to the image center are more salient*, we define the saliency of a region as the product of its size and centerness. Our definition is intuitive and consistent with human visual perception. The problem is how to compute such concepts reliably.

Region size is clearly informative but has been rarely used before. This is probably because accurate image segmentation problem itself is difficult and there is no good enough segmentation algorithm. While region center has been well known to be useful for saliency estimation, its usage in previous work is usually overly simple, non-adaptive (such as a gaussian centered on the image) and does not work well for images with different spatial object/background compositions. Our approach is based on a key observation that *geodesic distances between image superpixels essentially encode the segmentation information*. We therefore propose a superpixel based and unified geodesic filtering framework to compute these concepts in a simple and robust manner: (1) it computes approximate region sizes without actually performing image segmentation; (2) it estimates relative region locations with respect to the image center adaptively.

We treat our approach as a baseline because both its concept and implementation is simple, and it can be easily extended or combined with more sophisticated models. Nevertheless, our results are quite strong and encouraging. Extensive experimental comparisons on all above datasets show that our method compares favorably with many recent state-of-the-art complex models. Specifically, it is the best on SED2 [17] and SOD [18], and the second best on SED1 [17]. The examples in Fig. 1 show different challenges for previous methods: low-contrast object (fish, boat), high-contrast but off-center background region (green leaf), complex object/background composition (film), and multiple small objects (beach). Our method works well on such difficult examples while previous methods produce noisy results.

The second encouraging finding is that, after simply combining our results with others, all previous methods are significantly improved and new state-of-the-art results are achieved. Furthermore, the gaps between them before combination are also reduced. This illustrates that these concepts underlying our approach are highly effective and complementary to previous works.

To summarize, this work tackles the saliency detection problem using a basic principle: a large and central region is salient. Our baseline compares favorably and is highly complementary with much more sophisticated models across various datasets. The simplicity, when equipped with strong results, convinces us that the proposed concepts reveal more the essence of saliency detection problem and challenge the necessity of adopting more complex models. Besides the technical contribution, we also expect this work to inspire the field and encourage beneficial changes in mindset.

2   Geodesic Connectivity and Filtering

The geometric attributes such as size and location of an image region are important for determining its saliency. However, extracting good image regions is a challenging problem by itself. All off-the-shelf image segmentation algorithms have the similar problems of how to choose appropriate parameters automatically. Usually, the same parameters could produce different results over different images and this in turn leads to unstable region attributes.

We present simple methods to estimate the size and location of an image region, without actually performing an image segmentation, thus alleviating the above problems. It performs on a regular superpixel image representation. The parameters are easy-to-set and the results are stable. It is based on a continuous measure of how well any two superpixels are spatially connected, called *geodesic connectivity* in this work. Based on the connectivity measure, we further define a basic operation, called *geodesic filtering*.

An image is first decomposed into a few hundreds of superpixels (200 in our implementation) of similar sizes and regular boundaries, using the recent SLIC algorithm [20]. An undirected weighted graph is created by connecting adjacent superpixels. The edge weight $w_{i,j}$ between superpixels i and j is the Euclidean distance between the average colors of the superpixels in CIELab color space. The geodesic distance, or the length of the shortest path, between any two superpixels $geo\_dist(i,j)$ is defined as

$$geo\_dist(i,j) = \min_{i=v_1,v_2,...,v_n=j} \sum_{k=1}^{n-1} w_{v_k,v_{k+1}} \tag{1}$$

where $v_1, v_2, ..., v_n$ is a path in the graph linking nodes i and j. Without loss of generality, $geo\_dist(i,i)$ is defined as 0. We then define the *geodesic connectivity* measure as

$$geo\_con(i,j) = exp(-\frac{geo\_dist^2(i,j)}{2\sigma^2}) \tag{2}$$

The geodesic distance measures the accumulated differences in appearance between two superpixels and the geodesic connectivity characterizes how well they are spatially connected. For the superpixels in the same homogeneous region, the geodesic distance is close to 0 and the connectivity is close to 1. Otherwise, the geodesic distance is large and the connectivity is close to 0. Thus, a superpixel only has large connectivity values for superpixels in the same homogeneous region, and has near zero connectivity values for the other superpixels. Noting this, *the geodesic connectivity measure actually encodes the information of image segmentation in an implicit and soft manner*. It is intuitive, easy-to-implement, and stable. The only important parameter is σ. We found that the performance is stable when $\sigma \in [10, 20]$. It is set to 15 empirically.

We then define a *geodesic filtering* process to measure the properties of image regions from superpixels. Suppose we have a primitive region property map M in superpixel representation, that is, $M(i)$ is the property value of superpixel i, the geodesic filtering computes the property of the region that superpixel i belongs to as

$$\mathcal{GF}(M,i) = \frac{\sum_{j=1}^{N} geo\_con(i,j) \times M(j)}{\sum_{j=1}^{N} geo\_con(i,j)} \tag{3}$$

where N is the number of superpixels.

Equation (3) is a global filtering of the property map M using geodesic connectivity as weights. It aggregates and smoothes the property values within the same homogeneous region. After filtering, all superpixels in the same region have similar property values of that region. By removing the normalization part (the denominator) in Eq. (3), we obtain an un-normalized version of the filtering,

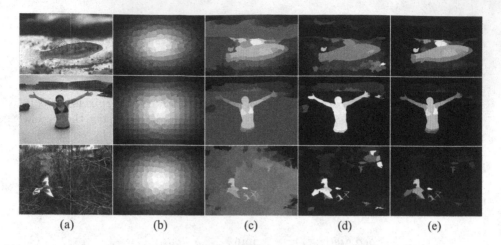

(a)   (b)   (c)   (d)   (e)

Fig. 2. Illustration of centerness computation. (a) input images; (b) superpixel based gaussian map C_{gau}; (c) geodesic filtered gaussian map SC_{gau} in Eq. (4); (d) image boundary based centerness map C_{bnd} in Eq. (5); (e) our final centerness map C in Eq. (6).

denote as $\tilde{\mathcal{GF}}$. It performs summation instead of averaging. Compared to using a hard image segmentation, our method usually produces smoother and more stable results. The example results before and after geodesic filtering are shown in Figs. 2(b) and (c).

We note that the geodesic saliency propagation approach in [21] shares certain similarity with our work because it essentially applies geodesic filtering to refine an input coarse saliency map. It therefore can be considered as a post-processing and a special case of ours. By contrast, our approach is motivated and derived from a more general viewpoint: we analyze the relation of geodesic distance and segmentation, and generalize the geodesic filtering as a framework to compute more useful region properties (size and centerness) for saliency estimation, which are novel and effective.

3   Our Approach

3.1   Adaptive Computation of Region Centerness

Many saliency methods are biased to assign image center regions with higher saliency. However, previous methods simply use a gaussian fall-off map with mean at the image center and a fixed radius. Such a map does not consider the image content and is problematic for off-center objects or multiple objects. Some methods re-estimate the mean and radius of the gaussian map from an initial saliency map and then refine the saliency map accordingly. This strategy is still not suitable for multiple objects and highly depends on the quality of the initial saliency map.

We propose a simple adaptive method to compute the *centerness* of image regions that alleviates the above problems. We start with a gaussian fall-off map with mean at image center and standard deviation equals to 10 % of the image dimension (the shorter of image width and height). This gaussian map is then turned into a superpixel based version: all the pixels in the same superpixel have their values averaged. We denote the superpixel based gaussian map as C_{gau}. It is exemplified in Fig. 2(b). This map is blocky and uneven in homogeneous image regions. It is then smoothed using geodesic filtering as

$$SC_{gau} = \mathcal{GF}(C_{gau}) \tag{4}$$

The smoothed maps are shown in Fig. 2(c). It is much better but still unsatisfactory because the large background regions usually cover the central parts of the gaussian map and still have large 'centerness' values.

To reduce such errors, we notice that the large background regions also touch the image boundaries. However, special care should be taken because the objects often also do. We further notice that background regions are more widely distributed and more heavily connected to image boundaries than objects: an object seldom touches different sides of the image boundary, while background usually does. We then define a new centerness map C_{bnd} with respect to the four sides of the image boundary, where the value of a superpixel i is computed by considering its geodesic distances to the four sides,

$$C_{bnd}(i) = \sqrt[4]{\mathcal{L}(i) \times \mathcal{T}(i) \times \mathcal{R}(i) \times \mathcal{B}(i)} \tag{5}$$

where $\mathcal{L}(i), \mathcal{T}(i), \mathcal{R}(i)$, and $\mathcal{B}(i)$ are the geodesic distances of superpixel i to the left, top, right, and bottom boundaries, respectively. We add a small constant value to the four distances to avoid the degenerate case when they are equal to 0. Example results of C_{bnd} are shown in Fig. 2(d). The large background regions in Fig. 2(c) are suppressed accordingly.

Our measure in Eq. (5) differs from the work in [11, 22] in tricky but important ways. This is illustrated in Fig. 3. The method in [22] simply uses the geodesic distance of a superpixel to the entire image boundary. This is very sensitive for touching-boundary objects, as shown in Fig. 3(b). The method in [11] uses the four boundaries separately in its first stage. However, it does not exploit the concept of geodesic connectivity but uses a complex optimization based on manifold ranking. This usually produces results that are hard to understand, as shown in Fig. 3(c). By contrast, our measure better retains the boundary-touching objects and removes most large backgrounds, as shown in Fig. 3(d).

The two centerness maps in Eqs. (4) and (5) are complementary. Our final centerness map is obtained as the product of the two,

$$C = SC_{gau} \times C_{bnd} \tag{6}$$

Example centerness maps are shown in Fig. 2(e). It is more reasonable than the maps in Figs. 2(c) and (d): the objects in the image center are of higher values and large backgrounds are removed.

Our centerness measure in Eq. (6) is highly adaptive to the image content. It can naturally capture off-center objects and multiple objects, as exemplified in Figs. 1, 2 and 3. This is mainly why our approach outperforms previous methods on images with multiple objects.

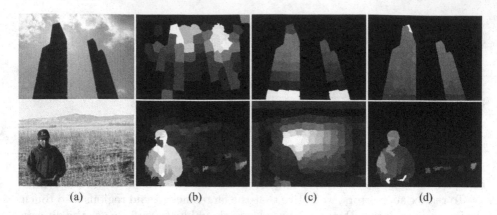

(a)   (b)   (c)   (d)

Fig. 3. Illustration of the advantage of our centerness map C_{bnd}. (a) input images; (b) results in [22]; (c) first stage results in [11]; (d) our results of C_{bnd} in Eq. (5).

3.2   Approximate Computation of Region Size

Although the concept of region size is intuitive, it is seldom used in previous work. One possible reason is that it is almost impossible to compute the region size accurately, as image segmentation could be unstable and generate inaccurate regions.

We point out that an accurate segmentation may be unnecessary. Since the superpixels are of similar sizes and shapes, our basic idea is to count the number of superpixels in a homogeneous region and use it as an approximate size of the region. This is done in a soft manner using the geodesic filtering approach in Sect. 2. Let N be the number of superpixels, we denote U as a uniform map that has the same normalized area $\frac{1}{N}$ for all the superpixels. We compute the region size map as

$$A = \tilde{\mathcal{GF}}(U) \qquad (7)$$

Note that we use the un-normalized version of geodesic filtering so for each superpixel it "sums" all superpixels in the same homogeneous region of it, which is the region size. Compared to hard image segmentation methods, our "soft" approach produces more stable and smoother results. This is exemplified in Fig. 4. We tested one of the most widely used image segmentation method in [23]. It has a few parameters. We tried different values and found it is hard to find common parameters that produce reasonable results for different images. We also tried normalized cut and mean shift segmentation algorithms, and found the similar problem. By contrast, our method computes stable and smooth region size maps and does not have the difficult parameter selection problem.

Our final saliency map is simply defined as the product of region size and centerness, as

$$S(i) = C(i) \times \sqrt{A(i)} \qquad (8)$$

Note that we use the square root of region size to make the product less sensitive to the region size, which is found useful heuristically.

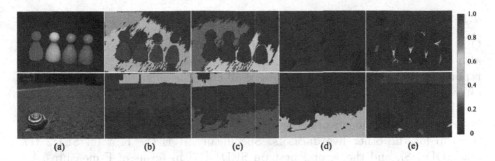

Fig. 4. (Better viewed in color) Example results of computing regions' size using a segmentation method and our method. (a) input images; (b) – (d) region size maps using the segmentation method in [23] with different parameters; (e) region size map of our method. The region size values are normalized to [0, 1] and visualized in color (Color figure online).

4   Experiments

In the experiments, we use six standard benchmark datasets, ASD [7], MSRA [2], SED1 [17], SED2 [17], SOD [18] and ECSSD [10]. ASD [7] and MSRA [2] are relatively simple as there is only one large object near the image center. Note that we obtain the pixel-wise labeling of the MSRA dataset from [15]. The remaining four datasets are more challenging. SED1 [17] and SED2 [17] each contain 100 images with great diversity in object sizes and locations. SOD [18] includes 300 images of complex scenes and multiple objects. It is considered as the most difficult dataset in [1]. ECSSD [10] is a recent dataset extended from CSSD [10]. It includes 1000 images of complex scenes.

We use the standard precision-recall curves (PR curves) and F-measures as evaluation metrics. Given a saliency map, a PR curve is obtained by generating binary masks with a threshold varying from 0 to 255 and comparing these masks against the ground truth. The PR curves are then averaged on each dataset. We follow [7] to compute F measure. For each saliency map, an adaptive threshold (1.5 times of the average saliency) is used to generate a binary mask and precision/recall value. F-measure is then computed as

$$F_\beta = \frac{\left(1 + \beta^2\right) \times Precision \times Recall}{\beta^2 \times Precision + Recall} \tag{9}$$

We set $\beta^2 = 0.3$ as in [7] to highlight precision.

We compare with eight recent state-of-the-art methods: saliency filter (SF) [5], geodesic saliency (GS_SP, short for GS) [22], soft image abstraction (SIA) [8], low rank saliency (LRS) [9], hierarchical saliency (HS) [10], dense and sparse reconstruction (DSR) [19], salient region detection by UFO (UFO) [16] and manifold ranking (MR) [11]. There are many other methods in the literature. They are worse than the above methods and not compared for conciseness.

4.1   Comparison with State-of-the-art

Our baseline method is compared with the eight methods. Those methods are also combined with ours, by simply multiplying the two saliency maps. Figure 5 reports the PR curves and F-measures of all methods on all datasets, before and after combining our method.

We can make several interesting observations. Firstly, our method compares favorably with previous works. Besides ASD dataset, our method is always at the top for the other five datasets. Specifically, it is the best on SED2 [17] and SOD [18], and the second best on SED1 [17] in terms of F-measures. We conjecture that this is because other complex methods are more or less over fitted to the simple ASD dataset and do not generalize as well to others. Secondly, after combination all previous methods are significantly improved. The improved results are new state-of-the-art on all datasets. This indicates that our method is highly complementary to previous methods. Especially, SF, GS, SIA and LRS are all improved to a large extent. Lastly, the performance gaps between previous methods are much smaller after combination. For example, while GS and LRS are much worse before combination, they are mostly comparable to the best methods after being improved. Example results of previous methods before and after combining our approach are shown in Fig. 6.

Table 1. The F-measure improvements on different datasets and overall, caused by combining one method to all the other methods, averaged on all other methods. The top two most complementary methods on each dataset are highlighted in bold and underlined bold, respectively.

	ASD [7]	MSRA [2]	SED1 [17]	SED2 [17]	SOD [18]	ECSSD [10]	All
SF [5]	0.0295	−0.0184	−0.1026	0.0537	−0.0582	−0.0686	−0.0274
GS [22]	0.0510	0.0450	0.0237	0.0505	0.0415	0.0356	0.0412
MR [11]	**0.0783**	**0.0693**	**0.0618**	0.0378	0.0528	0.0675	0.0613
DSR [19]	0.0632	0.0659	0.0538	**0.0594**	**0.0653**	**0.0753**	**0.0638**
LRS [9]	0.0377	0.0361	0.0059	0.0307	0.0237	0.0298	0.0273
UFO [16]	0.0675	0.0594	0.0298	0.0347	0.0301	0.0465	0.0447
SIA [8]	0.0422	0.0314	0.0342	0.0153	−0.0054	0.0135	0.0219
HS [10]	0.0654	0.0586	0.0505	0.0508	0.0430	0.0565	0.0541
Ours	<u>**0.0682**</u>	0.0699	0.0697	0.0882	<u>**0.0647**</u>	<u>**0.0742**</u>	0.0725

Table 2. Average running time (seconds per image) of different methods, tested on an Intel 3.39 GHz Quad-core CPU. For previous methods, we obtained the implementation from the original authors. SIA and HS are in C++ and others are in Matlab.

Ours	SF [5]	GS [22]	MR [11]	DSR [19]	LRS [9]	UFO [16]	SIA [8]	HS [10]
0.260	0.248	0.323	0.825	4.686	12.147	19.209	0.022	0.217

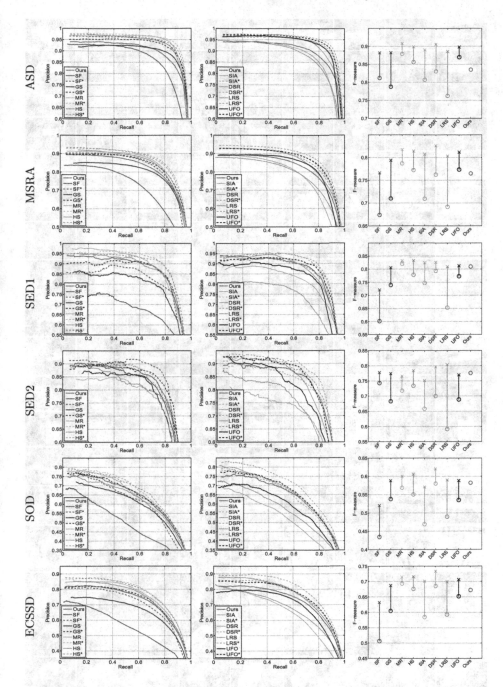

Fig. 5. (Better viewed in color) Precision-recall curves (left, middle) and F-measures (right) of various methods. In the PR curves, results of dotted lines and (*) are obtained by combining our results. In the F-measure, the circle and cross markers are the results before and after combining ours, respectively (Color figure online).

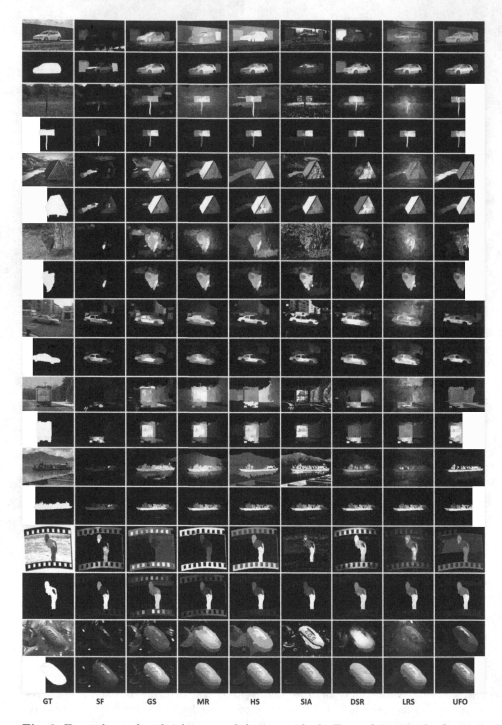

GT   SF   GS   MR   HS   SIA   DSR   LRS   UFO

Fig. 6. Example results of eight state-of-the-art methods. For each image, the first row shows the input image and their original results. The second row shows the ground truth and their improved results after combining our approach.

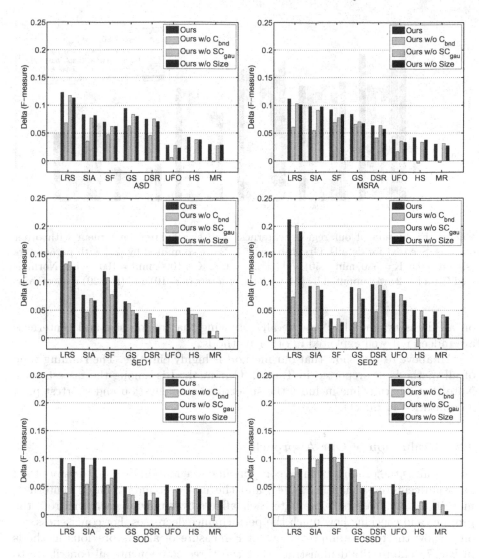

Fig. 7. The relative improvement of F-measure of eight methods caused by our method, our method without using boundary based centerness C_{bnd}, our method without using smoothed gaussian centerness SC_{gau}, and our method without using region size.

We note that it is possible that combining any two good models could produce improvement, as pointed out in [1]. To truly and fairly evaluate how complementary one method is, we report the F-measure improvements by combining it to other methods on the six datasets, averaged on all other methods. Results are shown in Table 1. Indeed, these state-of-the-art methods can improve each other (besides SF), and our method is the most complementary (among the top two

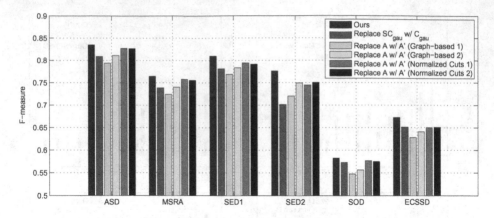

Fig. 8. Evaluation of our region centerness and size by replacing them with other options. See text for details. Graph-based 1 & 2 are computed by [23] with parameters (sigma = 0.5, K = 500, min = 50) and (sigma = 0.5, K = 1000, min = 100), while Normalized Cuts 1 & 2 are computed by [24] with parameters (n = 10) and (n = 20) respectively.

on all datasets, and the best overall), showing that region size and centerness are indeed not well exploited in other methods.

All above results show that our method is highly effective. The running time of all methods are reported in Table 2. Our method is among the fastest ones. Note that our run time includes the superpixel segmentation and shortest path computation in Eq. (1).

4.2   Evaluation of Our Approach

Our result is the product of three components: size map in Eq. (7), the smoothed gaussian centerness map in Eq. (4), and the image boundary based centerness map in Eq. (5). We firstly evaluate their effects by removing each one from the product and checking how much the performance decreases. For conciseness, we only show the relative improvement of F-measure of all the previous methods in Fig. 7. The results demonstrate that the three components all contribute to the improvement and removing any of them would cause performance drop. The results on PR curves are similar.

Evaluation of Geodesic Filtering for Gaussian Centerness Map. To evaluate the effectiveness of applying geodesic filtering in Eq. (4), we remove the filtering and use C_{gau} instead of SC_{gau}, while fixing the other components the same. The results in Fig. 8 show that not using the geodesic filtering clearly decreases the performance.

Evaluation of Region Size. To compare with our 'soft' computation of region size A in Eq. (7), we also compute another region size map A' using hard image segmentation. We segment an image using [23,24], compute the exact size of each region (number of pixels in it), assign each pixel the size of the region enclosing it, and normalize A' so that its summed value is equal to ours to remove any affection due to magnitude. We then replace A with A' while fixing the other components the same. We test four versions of A': two methods [23, 24] and each with two sets of parameters. Results in Fig. 8 show that our soft region size is better and more stable than hard computation of region size, because it is difficult to find good image segmentation parameters for different images.

5 Conclusions

We present a new baseline saliency method. It uses basic principle and concepts of region size and location. We demonstrated how to estimate these attributes with simple techniques, without requiring performing image segmentation. Our method works well across different datasets, including the most challenging ones. It compares favorably with the state-of-the-art and can be easily combined for further improvement. We hope this work can enhance the understanding of salient object detection problem and encourage more works of using simple models that generalize well.

Acknowledgement. This research work was supported by the National Science Foundation of China (No.61272276, No.61305091), the National Twelfth Five-Year Plan Major Science and Technology Project of China (No.2012BAC11B01-04-03), Special Research Fund of Higher Colleges Doctorate (No.20130072110035), the Fundamental Research Funds for the Central Universities (No.2100219038), and Shanghai Pujiang Program (No.13PJ1408200).

References

1. Borji, A., Sihite, D.N., Itti, L.: Salient object detection: a benchmark. In: Fitzgibbon, A., Lazebnik, S., Perona, P., Sato, Y., Schmid, C. (eds.) ECCV 2012, Part II. LNCS, vol. 7573, pp. 414–429. Springer, Heidelberg (2012)
2. Liu, T., Sun, J., Tang, X., Shum, H.Y.: Learning to detect a salient object. In: CVPR (2007)
3. Goferman, S., Manor, L., Tal, A.: Context-aware saliency detection. In: CVPR (2010)
4. Cheng, M., Zhang, G., Mitra, N., Huang, X., Hu, S.: Global contrast based salient region detection. In: CVPR (2011)
5. Perazzi, F., Krahenbuhl, P., Pritch, Y., Hornung, A.: Saliency filters: contrast based filtering for salient region detection. In: CVPR (2012)
6. Hou, X., Zhang, L.: Saliency detection: a spectral residual approach. In: CVPR (2007)
7. Achanta, R., Hemami, S., Estrada, F., Susstrunk, S.: Frequency-tuned salient region detection. In: CVPR (2009)
8. Cheng, M.M., Warrell, J., Lin, W.Y., Zheng, S., Vineet, V., Crook, N.: Efficient salient region detection with soft image abstraction. In: ICCV (2013)
9. Shen, X., Wu, Y.: A unified approach to salient object detection via low rank matrix recovery. In: CVPR (2012)

10. Yan, Q., Xu, L., Shi, J., Jia, J.: Hierarchical saliency detection. In: CVPR (2013)
11. Yang, C., Zhang, L., Lu, H., Ruan, X., Yang, M.H.: Saliency detection via graph-based manifold ranking. In: CVPR (2013)
12. Jiang, Z., Davis, L.S.: Submodular salient region detection. In: CVPR (2013)
13. Li, X., Li, Y., Shen, C., Dick, A., van den Hengel, A.: Contextual hypergraph modelling for salient object detection. In: ICCV (2013)
14. Jiang, B., Zhang, L., Lu, H., Yang, C., Yang, M.H.: Saliency detection via absorbing markov chain. In: ICCV (2013)
15. Jiang, H., Wang, J., Yuan, Z., Wu, Y., Zheng, N., Li, S.: Salient object detection: a discriminative regional feature integration approach. In: CVPR (2013)
16. Jiang, P., Ling, H., Yu, J., Peng, J.: Salient region detection by UFO: uniqueness, focusness and objectness. In: ICCV (2013)
17. Alpert, S., Galun, M., Basri, R., Brandt, A.: Image segmentation by probabilistic bottom-up aggregation and cue integration. In: CVPR (2007)
18. Movahedi, V., Elder, J.H.: Design and perceptual validation of performance measures for salient object segmentation. In: 2010 IEEE Computer Society Conference on Computer Vision and Pattern Recognition Workshops (CVPRW), pp. 49–56. IEEE (2010)
19. Li, X., Lu, H., Zhang, L., Ruan, X., Yang, M.H.: Saliency detection via dense and sparse reconstruction. In: ICCV (2013)
20. Achanta, R., Shaji, A., Smith, K., Lucchi, A., Fua, P., Susstrunk, S.: Slic superpixels compared to state-of-the-art superpixel methods. PAMI **34**, 2274–2281 (2012)
21. Fu, K., Gong, C., Gu, I., Yang, J.: Geodesic saliency propagation for image salient region detection. In: ICIP (2013)
22. Wei, Y., Wen, F., Zhu, W., Sun, J.: Geodesic saliency using background priors. In: Fitzgibbon, A., Lazebnik, S., Perona, P., Sato, Y., Schmid, C. (eds.) ECCV 2012, Part III. LNCS, vol. 7574, pp. 29–42. Springer, Heidelberg (2012)
23. Felzenszwalb, P.F., Huttenlocher, D.P.: Efficient graph-based image segmentation. IJCV **59**, 167–181 (2004)
24. Shi, J., Malik, J.: Normalized cuts and image segmentation. PAMI **22**, 888–905 (2000)

Learning Hierarchical Feature Representation in Depth Image

Yazhou Liu[1]([✉]), Pongsak Lasang[2], Quansen Sun[1], and Mel Siegel[3]

[1] Nanjing University of Science and Technology, Nanjing, China
{yazhouliu,sunquansen}@njust.edu.cn
[2] Panasonic R&D Center Singapore, Singapore, Singapore
Pongsak.Lasang@sg.panasonic.com
[3] Carnegie Mellon University, Pittsburgh, USA
mws@cmu.edu

Abstract. This paper presents a novel descriptor, geodesic invariant feature (GIF), for representing objects in depth images. Especially in the context of parts classification of articulated objects, it is capable of encoding the invariance of local structures effectively and efficiently. The contributions of this paper lie in our multi-level feature extraction hierarchy. (1) Low-level feature encodes the invariance to articulation. Geodesic gradient is introduced, which is covariant with the non-rigid deformation of objects and is utilized to rectify the feature extraction process. (2) Mid-level feature reduces the noise and improves the efficiency. With unsupervised clustering, the primitives of objects are changed from pixels to superpixels. The benefit is two-fold: firstly, superpixel reduces the effect of the noise introduced by depth sensors; secondly, the processing speed can be improved by a big margin. (3) High-level feature captures nonlinear dependencies between the dimensions. Deep network is utilized to discover the high-level feature representation. As the feature propagates towards the deeper layers of the network, the ability of the feature capturing the data's underlying regularities is improved. Comparisons with the state-of-the-art methods reveal the superiority of the proposed method.

1 Introduction

Photometric local descriptor [1] is one of the most powerful tools for image and video analysis. It has attracted extensive research efforts in recent years, and remarkable progress has been achieved [2–7]. Local descriptor encodes the microstructure or statistical information of a region and generates a new description of it. Ideally, this description should be at least partially invariant to photometric (changes in brightness, contrast, saturation or color balance) and geometric (mainly affine transformations, like translations, rotations and scale changes) transforms [8]. Therefore, it has a wide variety of applications in the fields of object detection and classification [9], texture analysis [10], image retrieval [11,12], object tracking [13,14], and face recognition [15,16].

© Springer International Publishing Switzerland 2015
D. Cremers et al. (Eds.): ACCV 2014, Part III, LNCS 9005, pp. 593–608, 2015.
DOI: 10.1007/978-3-319-16811-1_39

Recently, with the rapid development of range sensors, such as Kinect and SwissRanger, 3D depth information can be readily obtained with low cost. These devices use either the structured light or time-of-flight (ToF) to measure the distance between objects and cameras. The images that captured by these devices are known as range/depth images. Since depth image resolves the distance ambiguities which exist in the photometric image, a large number of recent applications have emerged based on it. For instance, 3D scanning and reconstruction [17,18], pose and action recognition [19–22].

Comparing depth images with photometric images, the differences exist in the following aspects.

(1) *Geometrical structure.* Pixels in a depth image indicate calibrated depth in the scene, rather than a measure of intensity or color [23]. Therefore, depth images capture the geometrical structure information and resolve the depth ambiguities, which can greatly simplify some processing step such as background subtraction.

(2) *Weak texture.* In the depth image, the color and texture variations induced by clothing, hair, and skin are not observable.

(3) *High noise.* Comparing with the advanced photometric image sensors, the noise rates of depth sensors are relatively higher, especially in the environments of strong ambient light.

(4) *Low resolution.* The lateral resolution of time-of-flight cameras is generally low compared to the standard 2D video cameras, with most commercially available devices at 320×240 pixels or less. Kinect claims its lateral resolution as 640×480.

With these essential differences, the well-developed local descriptors for the photometric images cannot be readily applied for the depth images. For example, scale invariant feature transform (SIFT) [7] descriptor and its variants [2] encode the gradient distribution with respect to the orientations within a local region. However, without photometric texture, the interest points with distinct local structure and statistics cannot be identified in depth images. Local binary pattern (LBP) descriptor [24] and its variants represent the statistics of micro structures of a region. For depth images, the meaningful structures only exist at the boundary regions of objects. Therefore, different parts within the objects cannot be differentiated successfully.

Finding a descriptor that can encode the local information of depth images effectively is the motivation and target of this paper. In order to achieve this target, the properties of depth images and their special targeting applications must be considered during the feature design process. The desirable properties of the depth descriptors are summarized as follows: Firstly, the descriptors in the depth should have some invariant properties which are preferable for the specific applications. Secondly, because the depth images are noisy and texture-less, the units that being processed should be changed from pixels to some middle level representations, which might reduce the processing time and improve the robustness of the descriptor. Thirdly, in order to capture the nonlinear nature of the feature, some high level representations should be discovered to improve the discriminant of the feature.

The contribution of this paper lies in the multi-level feature extraction hierarchy for depth images. The above targeting properties have been addressed in the different levels of the hierarchy.

Low-level representation encodes the invariance to the articulate motion. An active research topic based on depth image is pose and action recognition [20–22]. In this context, most of the interested objects are non-rigid and consist of multiple parts, for instance, human/animal body contains torso and limbs, and human hands contain fingers. Parts of the objects are connected by joints and have multiple degree of freedoms (DOFs). The overall motion patterns of objects are articulate motion. It is desirable that the descriptors can provide consistent representations of the parts in different poses and gestures. The object is model as a map whose nodes correspond to the pixels on the object and whose edges represent the neighborhood relationship between the pixels. Based on this map model, the geodetic gradient is introduced to rectify the feature extraction which is supposed to be invariant to the articulate motion as long as the local connection relationship does not change during the motion.

Mid-level representation reduces the computation cost. By unsupervised clustering, the pixels of the depth image are grouped into clusters according to their 3D positions in the scene. And the clustering result is referred to as superpixel representation, which is used to replace the rigid structure of the pixel grid. On the one hand, this representation provides a convenient primitive from which to compute image features and greatly reduce the complexity of subsequent image processing tasks [25]. Especially for the texture-less depth image, in which only the pixels on the boundaries of objects have the distinct structural information, the superpixel based representation reduces the image redundancy dramatically. On the other hand, since the noise level of depth sensors is higher than photometric sensors, superpixels can suppress the noise effect of the individual pixels and yield a more robust representation.

High-level representation captures the nonlinear information. Because of the complexity of data distribution, nonlinear mapping which maps the data from their original space to some latent feature space is used to achieve better discriminant. Deep learning [26–29] is utilized to find high order dependency between the dimensions of the feature, which has been successfully applied in many fields including computer vision [30–32], natural language processing and speech recognition [33–35]. In this work, the employed deep network is based on stacked denoising autoencoders (SdA), as the feature evolved towards the deeper layers of SdA, two desirable properties for classification have been observed: sparsity and better discrimination.

The overall processing flow of the method is shown in Fig. 1. The rest of the paper is structured as follows. Section 2 introduces the proposed geodesic invariance feature (GIF) in detail and Sect. 3 extends GIF to the superpixel based mid-level representation. Section 4 presents a deep learning based method for feature mining. Experimental results and comparisons are provided in Sect. 5. Finally, we conclude this work in Sect. 6.

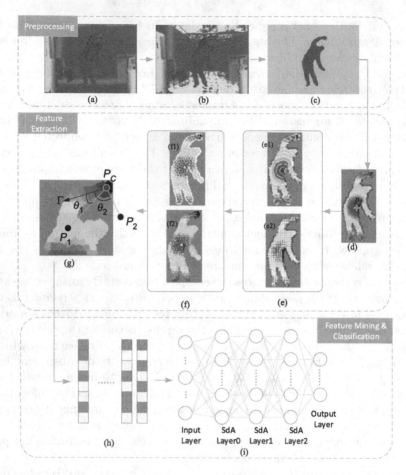

Fig. 1. The processing flow of the proposed method (Best viewed in color). (a) The input depth image. (b) Floor and ceiling detection (c) The foreground segmentation result. (d) Geodesic distance map of the foreground object. (e) Low-level feature: geodesic invariant feature extraction: (e1) is the isoline map and (e2) is the geodesic gradient map. (f) Mid-level feature: superpixel constrained geodesic invariant feature extraction: (f1) is the superpixel segmentation result and (f2) is the geodesic gradient map of the superpixels. (g) Orientation regularized binary feature calculation. (h) Binary feature strings. (i) High-level feature: depth network for feature mining (Color figure online).

2   Geodesic Invariant Feature (GIF)

The proposed method is inspired by the early works [3, 21, 23] which use the binary strings generated by pairwise comparisons to represent a local patch. In [3], the comparisons are based on the intensity of pixels and in [21, 23] the comparisons are based on the depth values of pixels. The difference of the proposed method is that the geodesic gradient is used to rectify the pairwise comparisons process, which endows the feature with the robustness to the articulate motion.

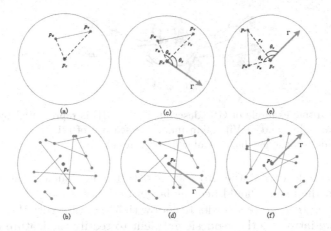

Fig. 2. Using the geodesic gradient to rectify the feature extraction. (a) Comparison between the two points generates one bit binary feature value. (b) A region is represented by the binary string produced by the multiple random comparisons which have been used in [21,23]. (c) Random points generated with respect to the canonical direction Γ. (d) Descriptor contains multiple pair comparisons. (e)~(f) the random point-pairs are covariant with the canonical direction Γ.

Given a depth image I, $I(p)$ represents the pixels depth value at position $p = (x, y)^T$. $D_{C_{p_c,r},F}$ denotes a local descriptor which determined by two parameters: coverage $C_{p_c,r}$ and feature list F. $C_{p_c,r}$ represents the coverage region of a local descriptor within the image, where p_c is the center and r is the radius of the coverage region. $F = \{P_i, \ldots, P_n\}$ denotes the list of random feature pairs where $P_i = (p_u^i, p_v^i)$ is a pair of random positions and n is the number of position pairs. The simple comparison function is defined as follows:

$$\tau(p_u, p_v) = \begin{cases} 1, & \text{if } |I(p_u) - I(p_v)| > t \\ 0, & \text{otherwise} \end{cases} \tag{1}$$

where (p_u, p_v) is a random pair from the list F and t is the comparison threshold.

By applying the comparison function $\tau(\cdot)$ to the feature list F, a binary string $f \in \{0,1\}^n$ is obtained and serves as the feature vector of the descriptor $D_{C_{p_c,r},F}$ as shown in Fig. 2(a)~(b). In [21,23], f is used to train the randomized decision forests and regression forests.

Distance Invariance. In order to make a descriptor be invariant to distance variation, the coverage of the descriptor should be constant in the *real world* space. Based on the knowledge of projection geometry, the radius r of feature coverage $C_{p_c,r}$ on the image should be defined as:

$$r = \frac{\alpha}{I(p_c)} \tag{2}$$

where $I(p_c)$ is the depth value of center pixel p_c, and α is a constant determined by the size of the coverage in the *real world* space and imaging focus. Intuitively,

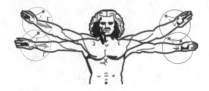

Fig. 3. An intuitive example of GIF descriptor: the GIF is represented by the circles (green) on the right hand of Vitruvian man; the feature of [21,23] is represented by the circles (blue) on the left hand (Color figure online).

this equation tells that if the object is closer to the camera, the size of the descriptor on the image should become larger and vice versa.

Articulation Invariance. In order to endow the descriptor with the articulation invariance, we introduce the geodesic gradient to rectify the feature extraction, which is referred to as canonical direction Γ. Now we are going to introduce how to calculate the feature with the geodesic gradient. The properties of geodesic gradient will be presented in the following parts.

By assigning a consistent orientation to each descriptor based on local properties, the descriptor can be represented relative to this orientation and therefore achieve invariance to the rotation [7]. For a geodesic invariance descriptor, its coverage is denoted by $C_{p_c,r,\Gamma}$, where Γ is used to represents the canonical direction of the descriptor. The random point-pairs are generated in the polar coordinates where p_c is the origin and Γ is the polar axis, as shown in Fig. 2(c)~(d). Take random point p_u for instance, it determined by two parameters, the angle $\theta_u \in [0, 2\pi)$ and the distance $r_u \in [0, r)$. Since θ_u represents the relative angle between the point p_u and Γ, all the point-pairs are covariant with the canonical direction Γ, as shown in Fig. 2(e)~(f).

Figure 3 gives an intuitive example which shows the contribution of the canonical direction Γ. The feature which covers the right hand of the Vitruvian man is the GIF descriptor and the one covers the left hand represents the feature of [21,23]. This example shows that the variation introduced by the articulation is canceled out by the canonical direction Γ, therefore the positions of the given point pair are relatively stable with respect to the local body parts. But for the feature of [21,23], this invariance cannot be readily maintained.

Calculation of canonical direction Γ is inspired by the insight that geodesic distances on a surface mesh are largely invariant to mesh deformations and rigid transformations [36]. More intuitively, the distance from the left hand of a person to the right hand along the body surface is relatively unaffected by her/his posture. For the given object, f_g represents the foreground object segmentation results as shown in Fig. 1(c). p_0 represents the centroid pixel of f_g which marked as the red cross in Fig. 1(d). Calculation of canonical direction Γ contains following steps:

1. The geodesic distance map I_d is generated by calculating geodesic distances between the pixels on the f_g and p_0 using Dijkstra's algorithm, as shown in the first column (from left) of Fig. 4.

Geodesic distance map   Isoline map   Geodesic gradient map   Covariance feature extraction

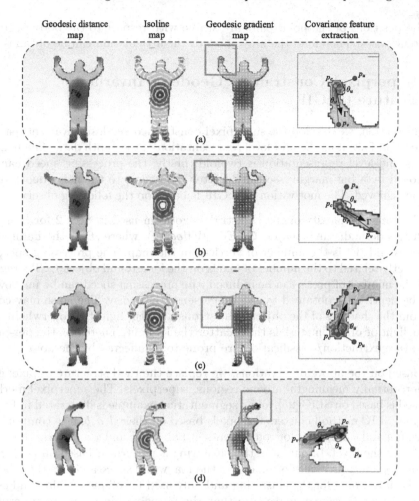

Fig. 4. Geodesic invariance feature. (a)~(d) show the invariance of a GIF descriptor under four different poses. The geodesic distance map, isoline map, geodesic gradient map and feature extraction are shown from left to right.

2. The pixels with equal geodesic distances to p_0 are marked in the isoline map as shown in the second column (from left) of Fig. 4.
3. For each pixel, canonical direction can be either calculated as

$$\Gamma = \arctan\left(\frac{\partial I_d}{\partial x}, \frac{\partial I_d}{\partial y}\right) \tag{3}$$

or as the direction that pointing along the shortest path obtained from step 1. In this paper, we adopt the second approach and the examples of canonical direction are shown in the third column (from left) of Fig. 4.

The nature of canonical direction Γ is presented in the right most column of Fig. 4, in which the hand patches of four different poses are shown. Rectified by

Γ, the positions of the point-pairs are stable with respect to the body parts in different poses. Therefore, the invariance to the articulation can be obtained.

3 Superpixel Constrained Geodesic Invariant Feature (ScGIF)

In this section, we develop the superpixel constrained geodesic invariant feature (ScGIF) and use it as the mid-level representation of the depth data. The benefit of this mid-level representation is twofold: firstly, the processing speed can be improved by a big margin; secondly, better robustness to the noisy depth data can be achieved. The motivation of ScGIF is based on the following observations:

1. The time complexity of the Dijkstra's algorithm used in Sect. 2 for building the geodesic distance map is $O(|E| + |V|log|V|)$, where $|E|$ is the number of edges and $|V|$ is the number of vertices in the map. The processing speed is directly related to the number of pixels on the foreground object f_g. Therefore, if the number of pixels can be reduced, the processing speed can be improved.
2. The depth data obtained by the range sensor are noisy. The noise may come from the shadows of the objects, the strong ambient light that overwhelm the IR light or object materials that scatter the IR light. Therefore, the per-pixel feature extraction/classification are prone to be affected by the noise.

Based on the above observations, we replace the rigid structure of pixel grid by perceptually meaningful atomic regions, superpixels. The superpixel method we used is based on SLIC [25], and a segmentation example is illustrated in Fig. 5. Original SLIC method clusters the pixels based on their $[l, a, b, x, y]$ components where l, a and b are the color components in Lab space and x and y are the coordinates of the pixel. In our case, the clustering is performed based on $[x, y, z, L]$ where x, y and z are the coordinates in the real world space and L is the label of pixel. L is optional for the clustering and only used for offline training and evaluation. Using L, we can make sure that the pixels within the same superpixel have consistent labels, as shown in Fig. 5(a)~(b). During online classification, only real world coordinate $[x, y, z]$ is used for superpixel segmentation.

For each superpixel, we record the mean depth value of all the pixels that belongs to it. The random point pair comparison is replaced by the superpixel

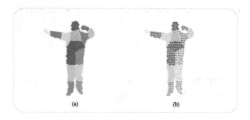

(a)   (b)

Fig. 5. Superpixel segmentation results. (a) Ground truth label of the depth data. (b) SLIC superpixel segmentation of the data.

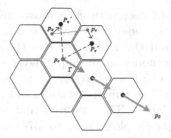

Fig. 6. Feature calculation for the superpixels.

pair comparison. As illustrated in Fig. 6, the point pair (p_u, p_v) is mapped to their corresponding superpixel (p'_u, p'_v), and comparison is carried out between their mean depth values. The canonical direction Γ pointing along to the shortest path towards the object centroid p_0.

By SLIC clustering, the unit being processed is changed from pixel to superpixel. For depth frame with VGA size, the foreground objects may contains tens of thousands pixels, but this lead to only a few hundreds of superpixels. Therefore, the processing load is reduced dramatically. In additional, using the mean value to replace the individual pixel depth can further improve the robustness to the noise. These improvements are going to be verified in the experimental section.

4 Feature Mining Through Deep Network

Generally, high dimensional data have complex distribution in their feature space. If the nonlinearity of the data is handled properly, the performance can be improved dramatically. There are two possible approaches to exploit nonlinearity of the data. The first approach is to leave this task to the classifiers, such as support vector machines (SVM) which use kernel functions to build nonlinear classifiers to model the complex data distribution. The second approach is to use an intermediate stage, between the original feature and the classifier, to map the feature from its original space to some latent feature space where the data may have more compact distribution. The second approach also called representation learning or feature learning which is the essence of deep learning. The sequential training manner makes it especially suitable for learning task under the big data environment.

In this section, we attempt to exploit the high order nonlinearity of the data by deep networks. Specifically, the employed deep network is based on stacked denoising autoencoders (SdA) [37–39]. Through SdA, the data are projected nonlinearly from its original feature space to some latent representations. We refer to these representations as SdA-layer$x$ feature spaces. SdA can eliminate the irrelevant variation of the input data while preserving the discriminant information that can be used for classification and recognition. Meanwhile, the propagation process of the data from the top layers to the deep layers of the SdA generates a series of latent representations with different abstraction ability. The deeper the layer, the higher level of abstraction.

The structure of our SdA deep network is illustrated in Fig. 7(a). It contains five layers: 1 input layer, 3 hidden/SdA layers and 1 output layer. Each layer contains a set of nodes and the nodes between the adjacent layers are fully connected. The number of nodes in the input layer equals to n, which is the number of random pairs. The binary strings of ScGIF are feed directly to the network as the input layer. The number of nodes in the output layer is d which equals to the number of labels. The rationale and training details of SdA is beyond the scope of this paper, please refer to [37–39] for more details.

Since we have claimed that the representations learnt by SdA can eliminate the irrelevant variation of the input data while preserving the information that is useful for the final classification task, it is important to investigate what actually have been learnt through this deep feature hierarchies. We plot the features of different layers of SdA in Fig. 7(b)∼(e), which provide us with some insight of SdA learning. Figure 7(b) is the binary string of ScGIF descriptor which feed directly to the input layer. Figure 7(c)∼(e) are the features that have been learnt by SdA layer 0 ∼ 2. A very interesting observation is that as the data propagate towards the deeper layers of the network, a trend of sparsity can be clearly observed. Until final layer of SdA, the number of no-zero entries reduced to 331, which accounts for only 16.6 % of the 2000-dimentional feature space.

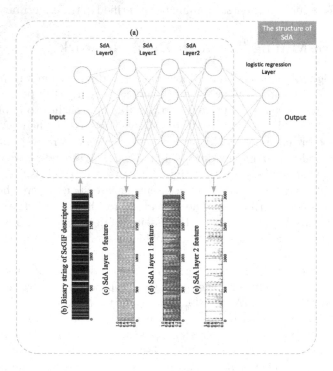

Fig. 7. The structure of SdA and its layer outputs. As the feature propagate from the SdA-layer0 feature space to the SdA-layer2, a trend of sparsity can be clearly observed.

5   Experiments

In this section, we present the details of parameter setting, dataset, and the comparison results with the state-of-the-art methods.

Dataset. We collect a depth image dataset using Kinect sensor. Four actors perform different poses and actions. There are 6930 depth frames of VGA size. For each human body, 15 body parts are labeled. An example of the ground truth label is illustrated in Fig. 5(a). The total number of labeled pixels is around 80 million. We randomly select 50 % frames for training, 10 % frames for validation, and the rest 40 % frames for testing.

Baselines. The first baseline descriptor that we used is the accumulative geodesic extrema descriptor proposed by Christian et al. [36], and it is referred as to AGEX. The second baseline descriptor is presented by Shotton et al. [21,23] which is variant of the BRIEF [3] descriptor in the depth image. Therefore, this descriptor is referred to as BRIEFd. The geodesic invariant feature presented in Sect. 2 is denoted as GIF, the superpixel constrained geodesic invariant feature in Sect. 3 is denoted as ScGIF, and the feature obtained by deep learning in Sect. 4 is denoted as ScGIF+SdA.

5.1   Contribution of Canonical Direction Rectification

To highlight performance improvement obtained by using the canonical direction, we compare the BRIEFd and GIF in more details. Both of these two methods are pixel-wise descriptors and the only difference between them is with or without canonical direction rectification. Random forests are learnt as the classifiers which contain 3 random trees and the maximum level of each tree is 20.

The confusion matrices are illustrated in Fig. 8, in which (a) is the confusion matrix of BRIEFd and (b) is the results of GIF. Average accuracy is increased

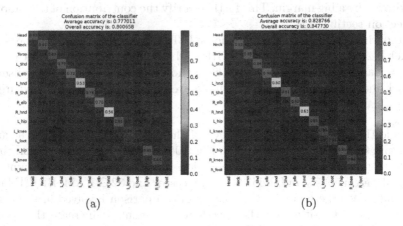

(a)   (b)

Fig. 8. Confusion matrix of the classification results (random forest): (a) Confusion matrix obtained using the BRIEFd feature. (b) Confusion matrix of the GIF feature.

from 77.7 % to 82.9 % and overall accuracy is improved from 80.0 % to 84.8 %. From these results, two observation can be obtained.

1. With the help of canonical direction, about 5 % accuracy improvement can be achieved for both overall accuracy and average accuracy.
2. The improvements for parts on the limbs are higher than the parts on the torso. A possible explanation is that the articulate variation are more prominent on the limbs, and canonical direction can counteract these variations effectively.

5.2   Comparison with the State-of-the-art Methods

The detailed comparison of the per-class classification accuracy are presented in Fig. 9. Regarding the AGEX method [36], since we are working on the classification task, we use their patch based descriptor without the geodesic EXtrema detector. The random forest is used as the classifier and the training process is very similar to BRIEFd and GIF. The only difference is that we replace the random pair comparison with the random dictionary patch filtering. Following the setting in [40], 2000 random sub-patches for each joint are randomly generated and used as the dictionary. The error bars of all the methods are obtained by 5-round of cross validation. The visualization of the classification results of ScGIF and ScGIF+SdA are illustrated in Fig. 10(a) and (b). From this result, we have following observations:

1. Among all the five methods, the performance of the dictionary patch matching based descriptor (AGEX) is lower with the others. One possible explanation is that the dictionary patches for the depth data are lack of textures and cannot provide enough discrimination information [40].
2. The proposed GIF descriptor and its two variants can outperform the other baseline methods. Especially for the hands and feet, accuracies have been improved by a big margin. This further verify the contribution of the canonical direction rectification.
3. Comparing the pixel based methods (BRIEFd and GIF) with the superpixel based methods (ScGIF, ScGIF+SdA), improvements for both of the mean classification accuracy and the standard deviation have been observed, which indicate superpixel is helpful for resenting the noise and texture less depth data.

In addition, we analyze the efficiency of the proposed methods. The accuracy versus rum time figure is illustrated in Fig. 10(c). Here, only classification time is considered and the foreground segmentation time is not took into account. The testing platform consist of Intel i7 3.7 G processor and 32 G RAM. BRIEFd is the fastest one since there are only simple pixel comparison involved in the evaluation. Superpixel is critical for the speed improvement. It increase the speed of GIF from 3.7 fps to 30 fps (ScGIF). This verifies another assumption about the superpixel: the superpixel based representation can reduce the image redundancy

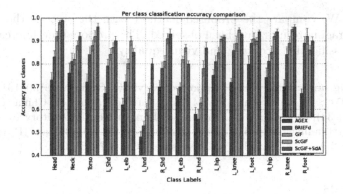

Fig. 9. Comparison results of each body parts.

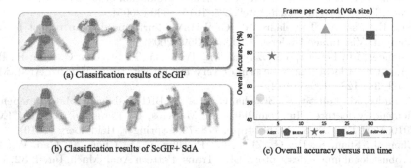

Fig. 10. Classification results of superpixel and superpixel+SdA.

and improve the processing speed dramatically. The accuracy winner ScGIF+SdA runs at 15 fps on a GTX 780i GPU using python lib theano (only the SdA part is running on GPU, superpixel is still on CPU). Since the evaluation process of the deep networks has high parallelism, the GPU time (including copy the data from host to device) for each frame is only 28.7 ms.

6 Conclusion

In this work, we presented a geodesic invariant feature and its two variants to encoding the local structure of the depth data. These new descriptors were applied in the context of human body parts recognition. Specially, the proposed descriptors form a multi-level feature extraction hierarchy: pixel based low-level representation addressed the articulation variation of human motion by introducing the canonical direction to rectify the feature extraction process; superpixel based mid-level representation replaced the rigid structure of the pixel grid by perceptually meaningful atomic regions which reduced the computation cost and improve the robustness to the noise; high-level feature exploit the nonlinearity of the data by deep networks which further improve the performance of the descriptor. We compare the proposed method with the state-of-the-art methods. Encouraging results have been observed. The proposed method can achieve superior classification accuracy and visual quality.

Acknowledgment. This work is supported by NSFC (Grant No 61300161, 61371168 and 61273251), Doctoral Fund of Ministry of Education of China (Grant No 20133219120033), Open Project Program of Jiangsu Key Laboratory of Image and Video Understanding for Social Safety (Grant No JSKL201306) and Programme of Introducing Talents of Discipline to Universities (Grant NoB13022).

References

1. Mikolajczyk, K., Schmid, C.: A performance evaluation of local descriptors. IEEE Trans. Pattern Anal. Mach. Intell. **27**, 1615–1630 (2005)
2. Bay, H., Ess, A., Tuytelaars, T., Gool, L.V.: Surf: speeded up robust features. Comput. Vis. Image Underst. **110**, 346–359 (2008)
3. Calonder, M., Lepetit, V., Ozuysal, M., Trzcinski, T., Strecha, C., Fua, P.: Brief: computing a local binary descriptor very fast. IEEE Trans. Pattern Anal. Mach. Intell. **34**, 1281–1298 (2012)
4. Calonder, M., Lepetit, V., Strecha, C., Fua, P.: BRIEF: binary robust independent elementary features. In: Daniilidis, K., Maragos, P., Paragios, N. (eds.) ECCV 2010, Part IV. LNCS, vol. 6314, pp. 778–792. Springer, Heidelberg (2010)
5. Chen, J., Shan, S., He, C., Zhao, G., Pietikinen, M., Chen, X., Gao, W.: Wld: a robust local image descriptor. IEEE Trans. Pattern Anal. Mach. Intell. **32**, 1705–1720 (2009)
6. Ke, Y., Sukthankar, R.: PCA-SIFT: a more distinctive representation for local image descriptors (2004)
7. Lowe, D.G.: Distinctive image features from scale-invariant keypoints. Int. J. Comput. Vis. **60**, 91–110 (2004)
8. Valle, E.: Local-Descriptor Matching for Image Identification Systems. Thesis (2008)
9. Felzenszwalb, P.F., Girshick, R.B., McAllester, D., Ramanan, D.: Object detection with discriminatively trained part-based models. IEEE Trans. Pattern Anal. Mach. Intell. **32**, 1627–1644 (2010)
10. Chen, J., Zhao, G., Salo, M., Rahtu, E., Pietikinen, M.: Automatic dynamic texture segmentation using local descriptors and optical flow. IEEE Trans. Image Process. **22**, 326–339 (2013)
11. Rahmani, R., Goldman, S.A., Zhang, H., Cholleti, S.R., Fritts, J.E.: Localized content based image retrieval. IEEE Trans. Pattern Anal. Mach. Intell. **30**, 1902–1912 (2008)
12. Shen, X., Lin, Z., Brandt, J., Wu, Y.: Detecting and aligning faces by image retrieval (2013)
13. Subrahmanyam, M., Maheshwari, R., Balasubramanian, R.: Local maximum edge binary patterns: a new descriptor for image retrieval and object tracking. Sig. Process. **92**, 1467–1479 (2012)
14. Ta, D.N., Chen, W.C., Gelfand, N., Pulli, K.: Surftrac: efcient tracking and continuous object recognition using local feature descriptors (2009)

15. Ahonen, T., Hadid, A., Pietikainen, M.: Face description with local binary patterns: application to face recognition. IEEE Trans. Pattern Anal. Mach. Intell. **28**, 2037–2041 (2006)
16. Zhang, W., Shan, S., Gao, W., Chen, X., Zhang, H.: Local gabor binary pattern histogram sequence (LGBPHS): a novel non-statistical model for face representation and recognition (2005)
17. Izadi, S., Kim, D., Hilliges, O., Molyneaux, D., Newcombe, R., Kohli, P., Shotton, J., Hodges, S., Freeman, D., Davison, A., Fitzgibbon, A.: Kinectfusion: real-time 3D reconstruction and interaction using a moving depth camera (2011)
18. Newcombe, R.A., Izadi, S., Hilliges, O., Molyneaux, D., Kim, D., Davison, A.J., Kohli, P., Shotton, J., Hodges, S., Fitzgibbon, A.: Kinectfusion: real-time dense surface mapping and tracking (2011)
19. Helten, T., Baak, A., Bharaj, G., Mller, M., Seidel, H.P., Theobalt, C.: Personalization and evaluation of a real-time depth-based full body tracker (2013)
20. Lallemand, J., Pauly, O., Schwarz, L.: Multi-task forest for human pose estimation in depth images (2013)
21. Shotton, J., Girshick, R., Fitzgibbon, A., Sharp, T., Cook, M., Finocchio, M., Moore, R., Kohli, P., Criminisi, A., Kipman, A., Blake, A.: Efficient human pose estimation from single depth images. IEEE Trans. Pattern Anal. Mach. Intell. **35**, 2821–2840 (2013)
22. Ye, M., Yang, R.: Real-time simultaneous pose and shape estimation for articulated objects using a single depth camera (2014)
23. Shotton, J., Fitzgibbon, A., Cook, M., Sharp, T., Finocchio, M., Moore, R., Kipman, A., Blake, A.: Real-time human pose recognition in parts from single depth images. In: Cipolla, R., Battiato, S., Farinella, G.M. (eds.) Machine Learning for Computer Vision, vol. 411, pp. 119–135. Springer, Heidelberg (2011)
24. Ojala, T., Pietikinen, M., Menp, T.: Multiresolution gray scale and rotation invariant texture analysis with local binary patterns. IEEE Trans. Pattern Anal. Mach. Intell. **24**, 971–987 (2002)
25. Achanta, R., Shaji, A., Smith, K., Lucchi, A., Fua, P., Ssstrunk, S.: Slic superpixels compared to state-of-the-art superpixel methods. IEEE Trans. Pattern Anal. Mach. Intell. **34**, 2274–2282 (2012)
26. Arel, I., Rose, D.C., Karnowski, T.P.: Deep machine learning a new frontier in artificial intelligence research. IEEE Comput. Intell. Mag. **5**, 13–18 (2010)
27. Bengio, Y.: Learning deep architectures for AI. Found. Trends Mach. Learn. **2**, 1–127 (2009)
28. Bengio, Y., Courville, A., Vincent, P.: Representation learning: a review and new perspectives. IEEE Trans. Pattern Anal. Mach. Intell. **35**, 1798–1828 (2013)
29. Bergstra, J., Breuleux, O., Bastien, F., Lamblin, P., Pascanu, R., Desjardins, G., Turian, J., Warde-Farley, D., Bengio, Y.: Theano: a CPU and GPU math expression compiler (2010)
30. Farabet, C., Couprie, C., Najman, L., LeCun, Y.: Learning hierarchical features for scene labeling. IEEE Trans. Pattern Anal. Mach. Intell. **35**, 1915–1929 (2013)
31. Kavukcuoglu, K., Sermanet, P., Boureau, Y.L., Gregor, K., Mathieu, M., LeCun, Y.: Learning convolutional feature hierarchies for visual recognition (2010)
32. Krizhevsky, A., Sutskever, I., Hinton, G.E.: Imagenet classification with deep convolutional neural networks (2012)
33. Bordes, A., Glorot, X., Weston, J., Bengio, Y.: Joint learning of words and meaning representations for open-text semantic parsing (2012)
34. Socher, R., Huang, E.H., Pennington, J., Ng, A.Y., Manning, C.D.: Dynamic pooling and unfolding recursive autoencoders for paraphrase detection (2011)

35. Socher, R., Pennington, J., Huang, E.H., Ng, A.Y., Manning, C.D.: Semi-supervised recursive autoencoders for predicting sentiment distributions (2011)
36. Plagemann, C., Ganapathi, V., Koller, D., Thrun, S.: Real-time identification and localization of body parts from depth images (2010)
37. Bengio, Y., Lamblin, P., Popovici, D., Larochelle, H.: Greedy layer-wise training of deep networks (2007)
38. Vincent, P., Larochelle, H., Bengio, Y., Manzagol, P.A.: Extracting and composing robust features with denoising autoencoders (2008)
39. Vincent, P., Larochelle, H., Lajoie, I., Bengio, Y., Manzagol, P.A.: Stacked denoising autoencoders: learning useful representations in a deep network with a local denoising criterion. J. Mach. Learn. Res. **11**, 3371–3408 (2010)
40. Torralba, A., Murphy, K.P., Freeman, W.T.: Sharing features: efficient boosting procedures for multiclass object detection (2004)

Automatic Wrinkle Detection Using Hybrid Hessian Filter

Choon-Ching Ng$^{(\boxtimes)}$, Moi Hoon Yap, Nicholas Costen, and Baihua Li

School of Computing, Mathematics & Digital Technology,
Manchester Metropolitan University, Manchester, UK
choon.c.ng@mmu.ac.uk

Abstract. Aging as a natural phenomenon affects different parts of the human body under the influence of various biological and environmental factors. The most pronounced changes that occur on the face is the appearance of wrinkles, which are the focus of this research. Accurate wrinkle detection is an important task in face analysis. Some have been proposed in the literature, but the poor localization limits the performance of wrinkle detection. It will lead to false wrinkle detection and consequently affect the processes such as age estimation and clinician score assessment. Therefore, we propose a hybrid Hessian filter (HHF) to cope with the identified problem. HHF is composed of the directional gradient and Hessian matrix. The proposed filter is conceptually simple, however, it significantly increases the true wrinkle localization when compared with the conventional methods. In the experimental setup, three coders have been instructed to annotate the wrinkle of 2D forehead image manually. The inter-reliability among three coders is 93 % of Jaccard similarity index (JSI). In comparison to the state-of-the-art Cula method (CLM) and Frangi filter, HHF yielded the best result with a mean JSI of 75.67 %. We noticed that the proposed method is capable of detecting the medium to coarse wrinkle but not the fine wrinkle. Although there is a gap between human annotation and automated detection, this work demonstrates that HHF is a remarkably strong filter for wrinkle detection. From the experimental results, we believe that our findings are notable in terms of the JSI.

1 Introduction

Quantitative assessment of skin condition has been an area of intense activity. There is a great interest in supplementing the dermatologist's diagnostic visual assessment of skin with objective measures [1]. These techniques are also valuable for the efficient development of effective pharmaceutical treatments. Many skin assessments have been developed over the past few years. For example, analysis of the skin surface around pores on the face [2], evaluation of facial wrinkle development over the lifetime [3], assessing facial wrinkles using automatic detection and quantification method [4]. Most of these assessments were based on clinician perspective (subjective assessment) instead of computer vision (objective assessment). Judgements are typically made on neutral-expression images.

© Springer International Publishing Switzerland 2015
D. Cremers et al. (Eds.): ACCV 2014, Part III, LNCS 9005, pp. 609–622, 2015.
DOI: 10.1007/978-3-319-16811-1_40

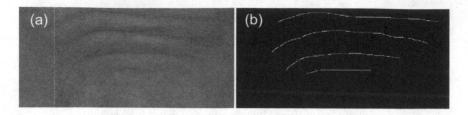

Fig. 1. Result of manual annotation. (a) and (b) present the original forehead image and the corresponding mask of manual annotation, respectively.

Clinician perspective focuses on the level of wrinkle severity which is assessed using either descriptive or photographically-calibrated scales, but in computer vision, the concern is on how a wrinkle is located correctly against the ground truth [5]. The well-known shortcomings of subjective assessment limit the scientific study of treatment and environmental effects on skin aging. Therefore, this work may result as an additional tool for them.

Assume a 2D forehead image consists of four observed wrinkles as shown in Fig. 1, but an automated method might estimate less or more than that, it will lead to false detection. This will highly influence the processes such as age estimation and clinician score assessment. Cula et al. [4] claimed that an automatic facial wrinkle detection method (hereinafter referred to as CLM) has been developed with the advantage of high correlation between clinician score and the computed wrinkle index (WI). Although CLM sounds promising, further quantification is needed to localize the wrinkle and distinguish it from image noise such as illumination, hair or scar. Therefore, in this work, a novel method is highlighted on how to detect the wrinkle accurately by assessing how closely a wrinkle is located through the Jaccard Similarity Index (JSI).

The rest of this paper is organized as follows. Section 2 reviews the state-of-the-art methods of wrinkle detection. Section 3 presents the proposed method HHF. Section 4 depicts the experimental results, and Sect. 5 concludes the paper.

2   Related Works

Automated detection of wrinkles in 2D images is an important step in age estimation [6] and synthesis [7,8]. Aznar-Casanova et al. [9] investigated the influence of wrinkles on facial age judgments. Their results indicated that the number of wrinkles and the depth of furrows are highly correlated with the perceived facial age. Choi et al. [10] explored the accurate wrinkle representation scheme for skin age estimation. The proposed scheme shows that it may be possible to estimate skin aging automatically from skin images. Huang et al. [11] presented a robust facial expression recognition method with skin wrinkles. The side-view profile plus skin wrinkles can correctly differentiate the expressions however acted facial expressions is used instead of spontaneous expression under complex illumination condition. Bando et al. [12] proposed a simple method for modelling wrinkles on human skin. They demonstrated the ability of the proposed method to model realistic wrinkle shapes by comparing them with real wrinkles. Despite the fact that it is a simple method to easily model wrinkles on human skin, but this work is lack of validation against the modelled wrinkles. Batool et al. [13] investigated the forehead wrinkles as curve patterns for their discriminative power as a soft biometric. Several metrics based on Hausdorff distance and curve-to-curve correspondences are introduced to quantify the similarity. However, the information of relative positions of the curves within the pattern was not included in the experiment.

Wrinkle detection is basically a line or ridge detection problem. Few methods have been proposed in the literature. A class of popular approaches to wrinkle detection is snake-based method which use the active contour map to initialize and localize the wrinkles [6,10,13]. Kwon and Lobo [6,14] computed wrinkles from face images to separate young adults from senior adults. The wrinkles were computed in several regions, such as on the forehead, next to the eyes, and near the cheek bones. The presence of wrinkles in a region is based on the detection of curves in that region. However, the random initialization and multiple thresholds resulted in implementation difficulty. Filtering-based method exploits the local orientation and optimizes the response to ridge-like structures. Hayashi et al. [15] utilized the edge detection method and Digital Template Hough Transform (DTHT) to extract both shorter and longer wrinkles on the face. This method is not reliable because wrinkle detection is not a boundary detection problem. Among the various wrinkle detection methods, the CLM is representative and simple. Cula et al. [4] explored the first-order derivative and Gabor filter for detecting the wrinkle length and depth, respectively. The estimation is based on the orientation and frequency of elongated spatial features. They defined the wrinkle index (WI) as the product of both wrinkle length and wrinkle depth. Wrinkle depth is derived from the Gabor filter responses. The authors claimed that the WI is highly correlated between clinical scores and outputs of CLM. However, from computer vision perspective, this work is deficient in detailed quantification of line segment localization. Therefore, this work is carried out to validate the detected lines in a 2D forehead image.

Frangi et al. [16] proposed a vessel enhancement filter as Frangi filter (FRF) for extracting the vessel and the Magnetic Resonance Angiography (MRA) dataset of cerebral vasculature. It has been widely used in retinal vessel detection [17,18], but not in wrinkle detection. Since both wrinkle detection and vessel enhancement present similar line patterns as shown in Fig. 1, it would be interesting to find out the performance of FRF on wrinkle detection. The idea of FRF is based on second-order partial derivatives for ridge detection. Eigenvalues of Hessian matrix are utilized to extract the principal directions in which the local second-order structure of the image can be decomposed. Although both vessel and wrinkle present similar curve patterns, the underlying image quality is different. The vessel image was captured by the TopCon TRV-50 fundus camera at a 35° field of view (FOV), which were digitized with 24-bit grayscale resolution and a spatial resolution of 700×605 pixels. In contrast, the original image of wrinkles were acquired with a normal light camera with the image resolution of 1600×1200. Higher resolution image contains more noise. Therefore, the proposed method has to deal with the pepper noise and illumination without damaging the region of interest. In addition, a retinal scan involves using a low-intensity light source through an optical coupler to scan the unique patterns of the retina [19]. Retinal scanning can be quite accurate but does not require the user to look into a receptacle and focus on a given point. As a result, these images present constant intensity across the dataset. In contrast to retinal vessels images, skin images present different challenges. Skin surface consists of pore, hair and pigmentation signal, among these attributes wrinkles present significant variations such as curve pattern, length, thickness and orientation with varied waviness and roughness.

CLM employs the local dominant orientation of first-order derivative for detecting the peak responses, it does not recognize a distinction between wrinkle and noise. Since FRF is capable on determining locally the likelihood that a ridge is present, this problem can be minimized by looking at the maximum image intensity in the direction of maximal curvature through directional gradient of image, and hence the wrinkle location can be correctly located. Therefore, a novel method namely hybrid Hessian filter (HHF) is proposed in this work. The following sections will describe the method in detail.

3   Hybrid Hessian Filter

Wrinkles are considered as stochastic spatial arrangements of line segment sequences, reasonably similar with those in retinal blood vessels. Wrinkle should not be confused with edge. Edge is the border between two areas while wrinkle is a line that is either darker or lighter than their neighbourhood. Therefore, edge detection methods such as Canny and Sobel are not suitable for wrinkle detection because it will produce wrinkle boundaries, not the wrinkle. In this work, we explored the multiscale second order local structure of an image. A measure of ridge-likeliness is obtained on the basis of all eigenvalues of the Hessian matrix. The eigenvalues of the Hessian matrix evaluated at each point quantify the rate of change of the gradient field in various directions. The eigenvalues are independent vector measures by the components of the second derivatives of the field at each point (x, y). A small eigenvalue indicates a low change rate of the field in the corresponding eigen-direction, and vice versa [16].

Figure 2 shows the proposed HHF for wrinkle detection. Given a 2D forehead image $I(x, y)$ as illustrated in Fig. 2(a), it is converted into grayscale as shown in Fig. 2(b). The directional gradient $\left(\frac{\partial I}{\partial x}, \frac{\partial I}{\partial y}\right)$ is computed from the grayscale image and the $\frac{\partial I}{\partial y}$ is illustrated as in Fig. 2(c). Let $\frac{\partial I}{\partial y}$ denoted as $\mathcal{I}$, due to $\mathcal{I}$ emphasizes the horizontal line, it is used as the input for calculating the Hessian matrix $\mathcal{H}$. The Hessian matrix $\mathcal{H}$ at scale σ is defined as

$$\mathcal{H}(x, y, \sigma) = \begin{bmatrix} \mathcal{H}_a & \mathcal{H}_b \\ \mathcal{H}_b & \mathcal{H}_c \end{bmatrix} \tag{1}$$

where $\mathcal{H}_a$, $\mathcal{H}_b$ and $\mathcal{H}_c$ are the outputs of second derivative [16]. Each approximates the convolution of $\mathcal{I}$ by the Gaussian kernels $\mathcal{G}_1(\sigma)$, $\mathcal{G}_2(\sigma)$ as

$$\mathcal{H}_a(x, y, \sigma) = \mathcal{I}(x, y) * \mathcal{G}_1(\sigma) \tag{2}$$

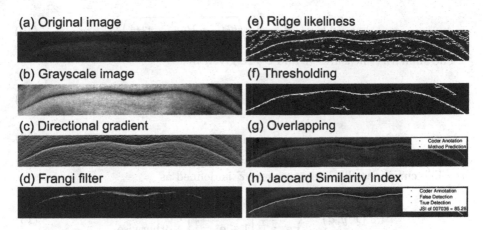

Fig. 2. Hybrid Hessian filter. (a) Original image was cropped from the Bosphorus dataset [20]. (b) Colour image was converted into grayscale image. (c) Gaussian filter was used to derive the directional gradient from grayscale image. (d) FRF was applied on directional gradient image to approximate the structure around each pixel at certain scale. (e) Image vectors less than zero was preserved as ridge-like pattern. (f) Ridge image was thresholded in a degree that only wrinkle-like patterns are extracted. (g) The overlapping between coder annotation (red line) and method estimation (blue line). (h) JSI was calculated based on the intersection area only (green line) (Color figure online).

$$\mathcal{H}_b(x, y, \sigma) = \mathcal{I}(x, y) * \mathcal{G}_2(\sigma) \tag{3}$$

$$\mathcal{H}_c = [\mathcal{H}_a]^T \tag{4}$$

The second derivative of a Gaussian kernel at scale σ generates a probe kernel that measures the contrast at the selective scale in the direction of the derivative. They are given by

$$\mathcal{G}_1(i, j, \sigma) = \frac{1}{2\pi\sigma^4} \left[\frac{\mathcal{M}_{i,j}^2}{\sigma^2} - 1 \right] e^{\frac{-\mathcal{M}_{i,j}^2 + \mathcal{N}_{i,j}^2}{2\sigma^2}} \tag{5}$$

$$\mathcal{G}_2(i, j, \sigma) = \frac{1}{2\pi\sigma^6} [\mathcal{M}_{i,j}\mathcal{N}_{i,j}] e^{\frac{-\mathcal{M}_{i,j}^2 + \mathcal{N}_{i,j}^2}{2\sigma^2}} \tag{6}$$

where $\mathcal{M}$ and $\mathcal{N}$ are the kernels with vertical and horizontal directions as

$$\mathcal{M}_{i,j} = \sum_{i=-3\sigma}^{3\sigma} \sum_{j=-3\sigma}^{3\sigma} i \tag{7}$$

$$\mathcal{N}_{i,j} = \sum_{i=-3\sigma}^{3\sigma} \sum_{j=-3\sigma}^{3\sigma} j \tag{8}$$

To categorize the texture pattern, eigenvalues λ_1 and λ_2 of the Hessian at specific scale and coordinates are given by

$$\lambda_1 = \frac{1}{2} \left[\mathcal{H}_a + \mathcal{H}_c + \left(\sqrt{(\mathcal{H}_a - \mathcal{H}_c)^2 + 4\mathcal{H}_b^2} \right) \right] \tag{9}$$

$$\lambda_2 = \frac{1}{2} \left[\mathcal{H}_a + \mathcal{H}_c - \left(\sqrt{(\mathcal{H}_a - \mathcal{H}_c)^2 + 4\mathcal{H}_b^2} \right) \right] \tag{10}$$

The similarity measures $\mathcal{R}$ and $\mathcal{S}$ are given by

$$\mathcal{R} = \left(\frac{\lambda_1}{\lambda_2} \right)^2 \tag{11}$$

$$\mathcal{S} = \lambda_1^2 + \lambda_2^2 \tag{12}$$

where λ_2 is set to $eps \approx 2^{(-52)}$ if $\lambda_2 == 0$. This is to avoid the λ_1 divided by zero. The curvilinear likeliness measure $\mathcal{E}$ is defined as

$$\mathcal{E}(x, y, \sigma) = \begin{cases} 0 & \text{if } \lambda_2 < 0 \\ e^{-\frac{\mathcal{R}}{2\beta_1^2}} \left[1 - e^{-\frac{\mathcal{S}}{2\beta_2^2}} \right] & \text{otherwise} \end{cases} \tag{13}$$

Due to the ridge is analyzed at different scales σ, the response of the filter $\mathcal{L}$ will be maximum of all scales that approximately matches the size of the ridge to detect as

$$\mathcal{L}(x, y) = \max_{\sigma_{min} \leqslant \sigma \leqslant \sigma_{max}} [\mathcal{E}(x, y, \sigma)] \tag{14}$$

where σ_{min} and σ_{max} are the minimum and maximum scales at which relevant structure are expected to be found (as shown in Fig. 2(d)). In this work, we are interested on the curvilinear pattern which represents the wrinkles. λ_1 and λ_2 highlights the data of interest and discards the noisy patterns [16]. In all scales, if λ_2 appears to be negative, then the wrinkle is detected. Moreover, if $\mathcal{E}$ appears exactly as zero, then the wrinkle is detected as well. Once the curvilinear is derived from the Eq. 14, the wrinkle-like pattern is preserved. The initial wrinkle mask $\mathcal{B}$ is generated as shown in Fig. 2(e) and it is defined as

$$\mathcal{B}(x, y) = \begin{cases} 0 & \text{if } \mathcal{L}(x, y) > 0 \\ 1 & \text{otherwise} \end{cases} \tag{15}$$

Next, each region of interest (8-connected pixels) is filtered by an area threshold where regions less than 250 pixels are removed and the output is the estimated forehead wrinkle as shown in Fig. 2(f). Note that the area threshold is based on the initial image resolution.

In this work, we set the kernel scale σ to 1, 3, 5, 7; β_1 controls the sensitivity of the filter to the measure $\mathcal{R}$ and the default value is 0.5; β_2 depends on the greyscale range of the ridge of interest and controls the sensitivity of the filter to the measure $\mathcal{S}$ and the default value is 15 (refer to [16]).

Figure 2(g) illustrated the overlapping between manual annotation and predicted wrinkle of the HHF. A polynomial fitting is implemented on the predicted wrinkle to localize the center line of the wrinkle and it is used for calculating the JSI denoted as Eq. (16). In computer vision, we are interested in how each method estimates correctly a line/segment. In this context, we used the JSI [21] to measure the reliability of wrinkle detection method. The Jaccard index $\mathcal{J}$ is

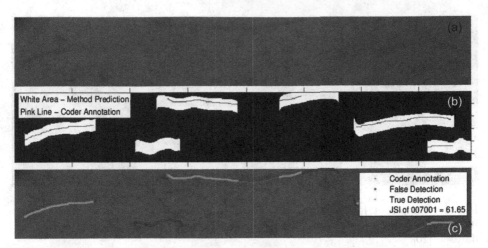

Fig. 3. Pixel overlapping between coders. (a) Original image. (b) Method annotation (or white area) has expanded nine pixels to top and bottom from its original location as shown in (c) as blue and green line. Pink line represents the coder's annotation. (c) Blue line represents the false detection and green line shows the true prediction. The image JSI is 61.65 % (Color figure online).

calculated by the intersection of $\mathbb{A}$ and $\mathbb{B}$ divided by the union of $\mathbb{A}$ and $\mathbb{B}$. $\mathbb{A}$ and $\mathbb{B}$ are annotations of two different coders, respectively.

$$\mathcal{J}(\mathbb{A}, \mathbb{B}) = \frac{|\mathbb{A} \cap \mathbb{B}|}{|\mathbb{A} \cup \mathbb{B}|} \tag{16}$$

Figure 2(h) shows how the JSI is calculated, red represents the manual annotation or ground truth, blue means the false detection and green is the true detection. In this work, we utilized the expansion threshold of nine pixels when calculating the JSI. From the experiment, we noticed that nine pixels produced the best overlapping in between the ground truth and estimated line. Small number of pixels will fail to hit the estimated line and large number of pixels will bias the result due to certain wrinkles are close to each other. Figure 3 illustrates an example of how the method annotation is expanded with nine pixels to top and bottom from its original location. The white area in Fig. 3(b) is an expansion of the method prediction and it is represented by the blue and green lines in Fig. 3(c).

4   Results and Discussion

In order to assess the performance of the wrinkle detection algorithm, images were selected from the Bosphorus dataset [20]. This dataset consists of 106 subjects and the 2D face images were acquired under good illumination conditions with a normal light camera. According to Batool and Chellappa [13], it is easier to generate the ground truth by hand labelling and wrinkles are more obvious

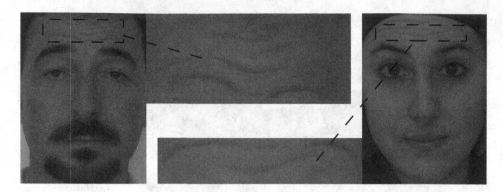

Fig. 4. Sample of forehead image. The dash lines show the portion of forehead image cropped from the original facial image. The image source was from Bosphorus dataset [20].

on the forehead in most of the images. Therefore, we repeated the same procedure by manually cropping the forehead images from the Bosphorus dataset. For each image, the forehead was manually cropped with a rectangle selector as shown in Fig. 4. Rectangle size varied from one to another. Resizing images was not included because the manual cropping was considered sufficient unless the wrinkle length and width are needed. In total we collected 100 random forehead images from the Bosphorus dataset and each forehead image is annotated with hand-labelling as the ground truth. Three coders have been instructed to do the annotation in Matlab under a controlled environment as illustrated in Fig. 5 (Microsoft Windows 7 Enterprise 64-bit SP1, Intel Core i7-3770 CPU @ 3.40 GHZ, 8.0 GB RAM, NVIDIA Quadro 200, lab with similar lighting condition). They were instructed how to use the annotation tool, annotating on the interior center line of the wrinkle according to what they see as a wrinkle. Center line of a wrinkle means the deepest wrinkle area. The reason for this is to minimize the factors such as lighting, screen size and the noise interference while annotating the wrinkles. In this work, we are interested in horizontal wrinkles as most forehead wrinkles are horizontal. Wrinkles are annotated only within those less than 45°. One pixel line was used for each manual annotation. Figure 1(b) illustrates the mask of manual annotation.

4.1   Manual Annotation

In the first experiment, we validated the reliability of manual annotation among coders. Coders were given the forehead images in the computer and they performed the wrinkle annotation by saving the wrinkle mask in the logical format of Matlab. Then, the annotated masks were used for calculating the JSI between coders as shown in Fig. 6. In this work, we used JSI threshold equals to 40 % as a benchmark of reliability [22]. Any overlapping above this threshold is considered reliable. For the coder A and B, almost 99 % of the JSI is above the threshold and the standard deviation (STD) is 14.27; for the coder A and C, 92 % of the

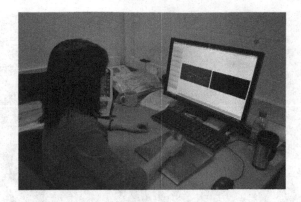

Fig. 5. Coder is doing wrinkle annotation in Matlab.

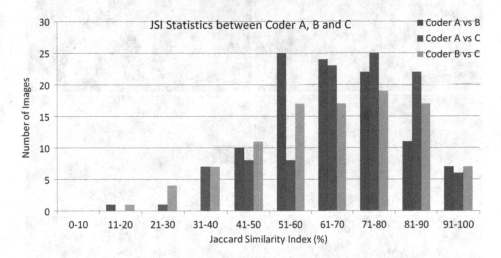

Fig. 6. JSI between coders: A and B, A and C, B and C.

JSI is above the threshold and STD is 16.77; and for the coder B and C, 88 % of the JSI is above the threshold and STD is 18.61. The average reliability of manual annotation between coder A, B and C is 93 %. We noticed that most of the coarse wrinkles were correctly annotated, but not the fine wrinkles. This experiment shows the inconsistency among coders. Figure 7 shows the samples of manual annotation between three coders. As we noticed that coder B did not annotate certain lines of all images as wrinkles but coder A did annotate it such as *img* i, ii and iv. Such contradictions resulted in the variations of annotation and hence yielded different JSI results. Moreover, this result demonstrates the difficulty of wrinkle localization and the high technical challenge for automatic wrinkle detection.

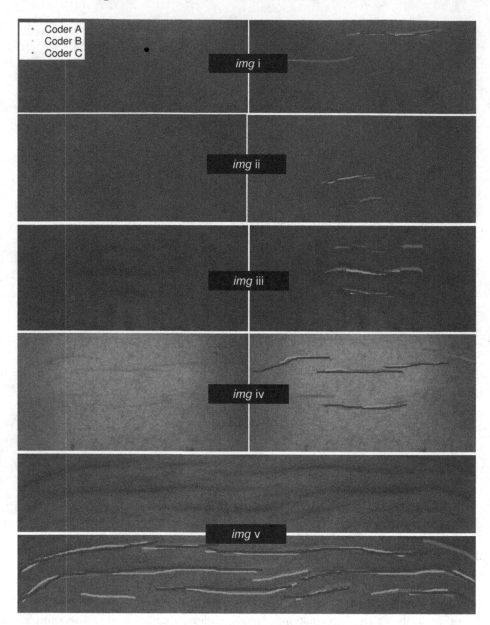

Fig. 7. Samples of Manual Annotation. Each row shows an original image (left) and annotated image of three coders (right). Red line represents coder A, green line is coder B and blue line is coder C. *img* i, ii, iii, iv, v mean different images (Color figure online).

4.2   Performance Assessment Against Benchmark Algorithm

Figure 8 shows the automatic detection output of coarse wrinkles. Top right is the CLM output with JSI 18.41 %, bottom left is the FRF output with JSI

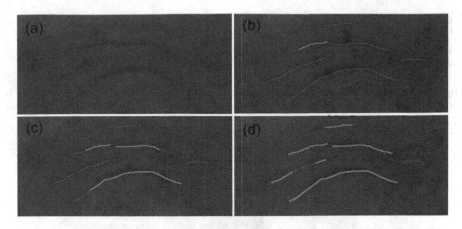

Fig. 8. Automatic detection of coarse wrinkles. (a) Original image. (b), (c) and (d) are the wrinkle detection by CLM, FRF and HHF, respectively. Red: ground truth, green: true positive, blue: false positive (Color figure online).

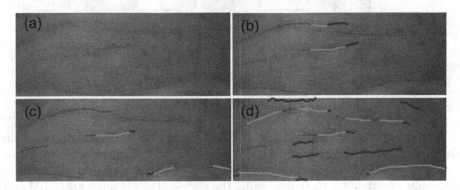

Fig. 9. Automatic detection of medium wrinkles. (a) Original image. (b), (c) and (d) are the wrinkle detection by CLM, FRF and HHF, respectively. Red: ground truth, green: true positive, blue: false positive (Color figure online).

49.23 %, and bottom right is the HHF output with JSI 64.14 %. HHF increased the true positive rate, but it also generated false wrinkle.

Figure 9 illustrates the outputs of wrinkle detection for medium wrinkles. Top left is the original image, top right is the CLM output with JSI 12.22 %, bottom left is the FRF output with JSI 19.44 %, and bottom right is the HHF output with JSI 48.68 %. In this case, the wrinkles are less visible than the image of Fig. 8.

Figure 10 presents the outputs of fine wrinkle detection. Left is the original image and right is the HHF output with JSI 10.31 %. Other methods failed to detect any wrinkles. The wrinkles in this image are very blurred compared to the previous examples. This is what we meant by low visibility where the coders might have large variations of annotations.

Fig. 10. Automatic detection of fine wrinkles. Left is the original image and right is the HHF output. Red: ground truth, green: true positive, blue: false positive (Color figure online).

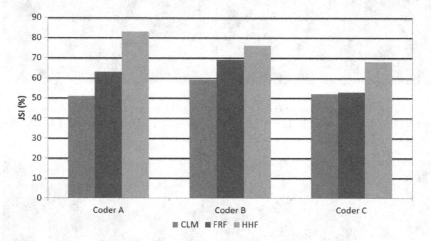

Fig. 11. JSI of automatic wrinkle detection.

In this experiment, we repeated the CLM and FRF experiments based on our understanding and certain functions were derived from the available sources in [23,24]. All derived functions used the default parameters. Figure 11 shows the results of wrinkle detection by using the state-of-the-art methods (CLM and FRF) and the proposed method HHF. As we observed HHF appears to perform better than CLM and FRF. The average of CLM, FRF and HHF are 54.00 %, 61.67 % and 75.67 %; the STD are 4.36, 8.08 and 7.51, respectively. One reason for this might be that in HHF the directional gradient has greatly smoothed the image and preserved the data of interest. Cula et al. [4] argued that red channel of image and histogram equalization will strengthen the wrinkle image, but the CLM result was poor. Histogram equalization is good when the histogram of the image is confined to a particular region, but it is not useful on certain images which have large intensity variations where the histogram covers a large region.

This experiment illustrates that the HHF is capable of detecting the wrinkles compared to the conventional edge detection methods. It is worth to mention that the proposed HHF is having the ability to preserve the horizontal wrinkles and discard the noises. Although HHF is outperformed, further investigation is needed on the issues of over-segmentation and sensitivity to the fine wrinkles. In order to reduce the false alarm, more efforts are needed to improve second order structure of Hessian matrix at each scale. In addition, the distribution of ridge likeliness is another aspect which could be explored. In future work, this experiment will be extended to detect the wrinkles on the face especially around the crows feet and mouth corner. Moreover, the relationship between the detected wrinkles and facial aging will be investigated.

5   Conclusion

In this work, we addressed some of the limitations in automatic wrinkle detection. Traditionally, the objective quantification was missing to validate the detection accuracy. Such implementation require significant user interactions where results are subjective, depending on user's expertise. This paper contributes to the groundwork of automated wrinkle detection using a new approach with objective quantification, which will bring advancements to the research in facial aging, cosmetics and soft biometrics. We described a novel method hybrid Hessian filter (HHF) for wrinkle detection in 2D facial image. It is based on the directional gradient and Hessian matrix. This matrix is computed for all the pixels on the image. The maximum eigenvalues of the Hessian matrix will indicate if a point belongs to a ridge regardless of the ridge orientation. We compared the proposed method with the Cula method (CLM) and Frangi filter (FRF). The experimental results demonstrated that HHF outperforms state-of-the-art methods with an average JSI of 75.67 %. Although there is a gap between human observation and automatic wrinkle detection, the proposed HHF significantly increases the number of true detection and wrinkles can be correctly localized at the desired location. In future, we will collaborate with skin biology expert to determine the correlation in between the clinician score and automatic detection. Then, we will apply the proposed method to the whole face and find out the interesting patterns which could be used in age estimation or synthesis.

Acknowledgement. This work was supported by Manchester Metropolitan University's PhD Studentship. The authors gratefully acknowledge the contribution of reviewers' comments. They would also like to thank the Savran et al. [20] for providing the Bosphorus dataset.

References

1. Gartstein, V., Shaya, S.A.: Image analysis of facial skin features. In: Application of Optical Instrumentation in Medicine XIV and Picture Archiving and Communication Systems (PACS IV) for Medical Applications, pp. 284–289. International Society for Optics and Photonics (1986)
2. Mizukoshi, K., Takahashi, K.: Analysis of the skin surface and inner structure around pores on the face. Skin Res. Technol. **20**, 23–29 (2014)
3. Luebberding, S., Krueger, N., Kerscher, M.: Comparison of validated assessment scales and 3D digital fringe projection method to assess lifetime development of wrinkles in men. Skin Res. Technol. **20**, 30–36 (2014)
4. Cula, G.O., Bargo, P.R., Nkengne, A., Kollias, N.: Assessing facial wrinkles: automatic detection and quantification. Skin Res. Technol. **19**, e243–e251 (2013)

5. Batool, N., Chellappa, R.: Detection and inpainting of facial wrinkles using texture orientation fields and markov random field modeling. IEEE Trans. Image Process. **23**, 3773–3788 (2014)
6. Kwon, Y., da Vitoria Lobo, N.: Age classification from facial images. Comput. Vis. Image Underst. **74**, 1–21 (1999)
7. Ramanathan, N., Chellappa, R., Biswas, S.: Computational methods for modeling facial aging: a survey. J. Vis. Lang. Comput. **20**, 131–144 (2009)
8. Fu, Y., Guo, G., Huang, T.: Age synthesis and estimation via faces: a survey. IEEE Trans. Pattern Anal. Mach. Intell. **32**, 1955–1976 (2010)
9. Aznar-Casanova, J., Torro-Alves, N., Fukusima, S.: How much older do you get when a wrinkle appears on your face? modifying age estimates by number of wrinkles. Aging Neuropsychol. Cogn. **17**, 406–421 (2010)
10. Choi, Y.H., Tak, Y.S., Rho, S., Hwang, E.: Accurate wrinkle representation scheme for skin age estimation. In: 5th FTRA International Conference on Multimedia and Ubiquitous Engineering (MUE), pp. 226–231. IEEE (2011)
11. Huang, Y., Li, Y., Fan, N.: Robust symbolic dual-view facial expression recognition with skin wrinkles: local versus global approach. IEEE Trans. Multimedia **12**, 536–543 (2010)
12. Bando, Y., Kuratate, T., Nishita, T.: A simple method for modeling wrinkles on human skin. In: Proceedings of the 10th Pacific Conference on Computer Graphics and Applications, pp. 166–175. IEEE (2002)
13. Batool, N., Chellappa, R.: Modeling and detection of wrinkles in aging human faces using marked point processes. In: Fusiello, A., Murino, V., Cucchiara, R. (eds.) ECCV 2012 Ws/Demos, Part II. LNCS, vol. 7584, pp. 178–188. Springer, Heidelberg (2012)
14. Kwon, Y., da Vitoria Lobo, N.: Age classification from facial images. In: Proceedings of the IEEE Computer Society Conference on Computer Vision and Pattern Recognition, pp. 762–767. IEEE (1994)
15. Hayashi, J.i., Yasumoto, M., Ito, H., Koshimizu, H.: Age and gender estimation based on wrinkle texture and color of facial images. In: Proceedings of the 16th International Conference on Pattern Recognition. vol. 1, pp. 405–408. IEEE (2002)
16. Frangi, A.F.: Three-dimensional model-based analysis of vascular and cardiac images. Ph.D. thesis, University Medical Center, Utrecht (2001)
17. Sofka, M., Stewart, C.V.: Retinal vessel centerline extraction using multiscale matched filters, confidence and edge measures. IEEE Trans. Med. Imaging **25**, 1531–1546 (2006)
18. Martinez-Perez, M.E., Hughes, A.D., Thom, S.A., Bharath, A.A., Parker, K.H.: Segmentation of blood vessels from red-free and fluorescein retinal images. Med. Image Anal. **11**, 47–61 (2007)
19. Liu, S., Silverman, M.: A practical guide to biometric security technology. IT Prof. **3**, 27–32 (2001)
20. Savran, A., Sankur, B., Taha Bilge, M.: Regression-based intensity estimation of facial action units. Image and Vision Computing **30**, 774–784 (2012)
21. Jaccard, P.: Distribution de la flore alpine dans le bassin des drouces et dans quelques regions voisines. Bulletin de la Socit Vaudoise des Sciences Naturelles **37**, 241–272 (1901)
22. Real, R.: Tables of significant values of Jaccard's index of similarity. Miscel. lània Zoològica **22**, 29–40 (1999)
23. Kovesi, P.: Matlab and octave functions for computer vision and image processing. http://www.csse.uwa.edu.au/~pk/, Accessed on March 2014
24. Kroon, D.J.: Hessian based frangi vesselness filter. (Matlab Central, http://www.mathworks.co.uk/), Accessed on January 2014

Transductive Transfer Machine

Nazli Farajidavar[✉], Teofilo de Campos, and Josef Kittler

CVSSP, Univeristy of Surrey, Guildford, Surrey GU2 7XH, UK
n.farajidavar@surrey.ac.uk

Abstract. We propose a pipeline for transductive transfer learning and demonstrate it in computer vision tasks. In pattern classification, methods for transductive transfer learning (also known as unsupervised domain adaptation) are designed to cope with cases in which one cannot assume that training and test sets are sampled from the same distribution, i.e., they are from different domains. However, some unlabelled samples that belong to the same domain as the test set (i.e. the target domain) are available, enabling the learner to adapt its parameters. We approach this problem by combining three methods that transform the feature space. The first finds a lower dimensional space that is shared between source and target domains. The second uses local transformations applied to each source sample to further increase the similarity between the marginal distributions of the datasets. The third applies one transformation per class label, aiming to increase the similarity between the posterior probability of samples in the source and target sets. We show that this combination leads to an improvement over the state-of-the-art in cross-domain image classification datasets, using raw images or basic features and a simple one-nearest-neighbour classifier.

1 Introduction

In many machine learning tasks, such as object classification, it is often not possible to guarantee that the data used to train a learner offers a good representation of the distribution of samples in the test set. Furthermore, it is often expensive to acquire vast amounts of labelled training samples in order to provide classifiers with a good coverage of the feature space. Transfer learning methods can offer low cost solutions to these problems, as they do not assume that training and test samples are drawn from the same distribution [1]. Such techniques are becoming more popular in Computer Vision, particularly after Torralba and Efros [2] discovered significant biases in object classification datasets. However, much of the work focuses on *inductive* transfer learning problems, which assume that labelled samples are available both in source and target domains. In this paper we focus on the case in which only unlabelled samples are available in the target domain. This is a *transductive* transfer learning (TTL) problem, i.e., the joint

---

Electronic supplementary material The online version of this chapter (doi:10. 1007/978-3-319-16811-1_41) contains supplementary material, which is available to authorized users.

© Springer International Publishing Switzerland 2015
D. Cremers et al. (Eds.): ACCV 2014, Part III, LNCS 9005, pp. 623–639, 2015.
DOI: 10.1007/978-3-319-16811-1_41

probability distribution of samples and classes in the source domain $P(\mathbf{X}^{src}, \mathbf{Y}^{src})$ is assumed to be different, but related to that of a target domain joint distribution $P(\mathbf{X}^{trg}, \mathbf{Y}^{trg})$, but labels $\mathbf{Y}^{trg}$ are not available in the target set. We follow a similar notation to that of [1] (see Table 1). Some papers in the literature refer to this problem as Unsupervised Domain Adaptation.

TTL methods can potentially improve a very wide range of classification tasks, as it is often the case that a domain change happens between training and application of algorithms, and it is also very common that unlabelled samples are available in the target domain. For example, in image classification, the training set may come from high quality images (e.g. from DSLR cameras) and the target test set may come from mobile devices. Another example is action classification where training samples are from tennis and test samples are from badminton. TTL methods can potentially generalise classification methods for a wide range of domains and make them scalable for big data problems.

In this paper, we propose Transductive Transfer Machine (TTM), a framework that combines methods that adapt the marginal and the conditional distribution of the samples, so that source and target datasets become more similar, facilitating classification. A key novelty is a sample-based adaptation method, TransGrad, which enables a fine adjustment of the probability density function of the source samples. Our method obtains state-of-the-art results in cross-domain vision datasets using a simple nearest neighbour classifier, with a significant gain in computational efficiency in comparison to related methods.

Table 1. Notation and acronyms used most frequently in this paper (also used in [3]).

$\mathbf{X} = [\mathbf{x}^1, \cdots, \mathbf{x}^i, \cdots, \mathbf{x}^n]^\top \in \mathbb{R}^{n \times f}$	Input data matrix with n samples of f features
$\mathbf{x}^i = (x_1^i, \cdots, x_j^i, \cdots, x_f^i)^\top$	Feature vectors
$\mathbf{Y} = (y^1, \cdots, y^n)^\top$	Array of class labels associated to $\mathbf{X}$
$\mathcal{Y} = \{1, \cdots, C\}$	Set of classes
$\mathbf{X}^{src} \in \mathbb{R}^{n_{src} \times f}$, $\mathbf{X}^{trg} \in \mathbb{R}^{n_{trg} \times f}$	Source and target data matrices
Λ_{src}	Classification model trained with $\mathbf{X}^{src}$
$G(\mathbf{X})$	Transformation function
θ	transfer rate parameter
T	Number of iterations
$\lambda = \{w_k, \boldsymbol{\mu}_k, \Sigma_k, k = 1, \cdots, K\}$	GMM parameters with K components
$E^{src}[x_j, y^i]$, $E^{trg}[x_j, y^i]$	Joint expectation of feature j and label y^i
$D(p, q)$	Dissimilarity between two distributions
$\nabla_{\mathbf{b}^i} \mathcal{L}(\lambda_{trg} \vert \mathbf{x}^{src})$	Gradient of the log likelihood with respect to $\mathbf{b}^i$
γ	TransGrad translation regulator
TL, ITL, TTL	Transfer Learning, Inductive TL, Transductive TL
MMD	Maximum Mean Discrepancy
TransGrad	Sample-based transformation using gradients
TST	Class-based Translation and Scaling Transform

In [3], we present a follow-up work which adds a step that automatically selects the most appropriated classifier and its kernel parameter. The present paper gives more details of the derivations of the methods in the pipeline and includes further evaluations of its main steps.

In the next section, we briefly review related works and give an outline of our contribution. Section 3 presents the core components of our method and further discusses the relation between them and previous works. This is followed by a description of our framework and an analysis of our algorithm. Experiments and conclusions follow in Sects. 4 and 5.

2   Related Work

According to Pan and Yang's taxonomy [1], Transfer Learning (TL) methods can be of the following types: *Inductive*, when labelled samples are available in both source and target domains, *Transductive*, when labels are only available in the source set and *Unsupervised*, when labelled data is not present. For the reasons highlighted in Sect. 1, we focus on Transductive TL problems (TTL). They relate to sample selection bias correction methods [4,5], where training and test distributions follow different distributions but the label distributions remain the same. It is common to apply semi-supervised learning methods for transductive transfer learning tasks, e.g. Transductive SVM [6]. In [7], a domain adapted SVM was proposed, which simultaneously learns a decision boundary and maximises the margin in the presence of unlabelled patterns, without requiring density estimation. In contrast, Gopalan et al. [8], used a method based on Grassmann manifold in order to generate intermediate data representations to model cross-domain shifts. In [9], Chu et al. proposed to search for an instance based re-weighting matrix applied to the source samples. The weights are based on the similarity between the source and target distributions using the Kernel Mean Matching algorithm. This method iteratively updates an SVM classifier using transformed source instances for training until convergence.

Transfer learning methods can be categorised based on *instance re-weighting* (e.g. [9,10]), *feature space transformation* (e.g. [11,12]) and *learning parameters transformation* (e.g. [7,13]). Different types of methods can potentially be combined. In this paper, we focus on *feature space transformation* and approach the TTL problem by finding a set of transformations that are applied to the source domain samples $G(\mathbf{X}^{src})$ such that the joint distribution of the transformed source samples becomes more similar to that of the target samples, i.e. $P(G(\mathbf{X}^{src}), \mathbf{Y}^{src}) \approx P(\mathbf{X}^{trg}, \mathbf{Y}^{trg*})$, where $\mathbf{Y}^{trg*}$ are the labels estimated for target domain samples.

Long et al. [12] proposed a related method which does Joint Distribution Adaptation (JDA) by iteratively adapting both the marginal and conditional distributions using a procedure based on a modification of the Maximum Mean Discrepancy (MMD) algorithm [11]. JDA uses the pseudo target labels to define a shared subspace between the two domains. At each iteration, this method requires the construction and eigen decomposition of an $n \times n$ matrix whose complexity can be up to $O(n^3)$.

Our pipeline which first searches for a global transformation such that the marginal distribution of the two domains becomes more similar and then with the same objective applies a set of local transformations to each transformed source domain sample. Finally in an iterative scheme, our algorithm aims to reduce the difference between the conditional distributions in source and target spaces where a class-based transformation is applied to each of the transformed source samples. The complexity of the latter step is linear on the number of features in the space, i.e., $O(f)$.

3 The Transductive Transfer Machine

We propose the following pipeline (see Table 1 for the notation):

1. **MMD** – A global linear transformation G^1 is applied to both $\mathbf{X}^{src}$ and $\mathbf{X}^{trg}$ such that the marginal $P(G^1(\mathbf{X}^{src}))$ becomes more similar to $P(G^1(\mathbf{X}^{trg}))$.
2. **TransGrad** – For a finer grained adaptation of the marginal, a local transformation is applied to each transformed source domain sample $G_i^2(G^1(\mathbf{x}_{src}^i))$.
3. **TST** – Finally, aiming to reduce the difference between the conditional distributions in source and target spaces, a class-based transformation is applied to each of the transformed source samples $G_{y^i}^3(G_i^2(G^1(\mathbf{x}_{src}^i)))$.

Figure 1 illustrates the effect of the three steps of the pipeline above on a dataset composed of subset of digits 1 and 2 from the MNIST and USPS datasets. The effect of step (MMD) is to bring the mean of the two distributions closer to each other while it projects the data into its principal components directions of the full data including the source and target.[1] We use a marginal distribution

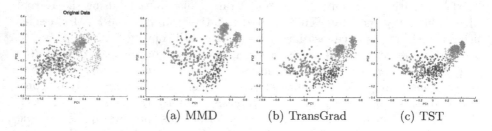

(a) MMD   (b) TransGrad   (c) TST

Fig. 1. Effect of the steps of the TTM pipeline on digits 1 and 2 of the MNIST→USPS datasets, visualised in 2D through PCA. The source dataset (MNIST) is indicated by stars, the target dataset (USPS) is indicated by circles, red indicates samples of digit 1 and blue indicates digit 2 (better viewed on the screen). This figure has been reproduced from [3] with permission.

---

[1] In Fig. 1, the feature space is visualised in 2D using PCA projection and only two classes are shown, but the MMD computation was done on a higher dimensional space on samples from 10 classes. For these reasons it may not be easy to see that the means of source and target samples became closer after MMD.

adaptation method which relates to the works of [12, 14, 15]. This uses the empirical Maximum Mean Discrepancy (MMD) to compare different distributions and compute a lower-dimensional embedding that minimises the distance between the expected values of samples in source and target domains.

For the second step of our pipeline (TransGrad), we proposed a method that distorts the source probability density function towards target clusters. We employ a sample-wise transformation that uses likelihoods of source samples given a GMM that models target data. Up to our knowledge, this is the first time a sample-based transformation is proposed for transfer learning.

In the final step (TST), the source class-conditional distributions are iteratively transformed to become more similar to their corresponding target conditionals. A related approach has been followed in [12] using pseudo-labels to iteratively update a supervised version of MMD. We adopt a method that uses insights from Arnold et al. [16], who used the ratio between the expected class-based posterior probability of target samples and the expected value of source samples per class. This effectively re-scales the source feature space. Our method is a more complex transformation, as each individual feature is both scaled and translated, with different parameters per class. We describe early experiments with TST in [17].

The next subsections detail each of the steps above.

3.1 Shared Space Detection Using MMD

In the first step of our pipeline, we look for a shared space projection that reduces dimensionality of the data whilst minimising the reconstruction error. As explained in [12], one possibility for that is to search for an orthogonal transformation matrix $A \in \mathbb{R}^{f \times k}$ such that the embedded data variance is maximised as follows:

$$\max_{A^\top A = I} tr(A^\top X H X^\top A), \tag{1}$$

where $X = [X^{src}; X^{trg}] \in \mathbb{R}^{f \times n_{src} + n_{trg}}$ is the input data matrix that combines source and target samples, $tr(\cdot)$ is the trace of a matrix and $H = I - \frac{1}{n_{src} + n_{trg}} \mathbb{1}$ is a centring matrix where $\mathbb{1}$ is a $(n_{src} + n_{trg}) \times (n_{src} + n_{trg})$ matrix of ones. The optimisation problem can be efficiently solved by eigen-decomposition. However, the above PCA-based representation may not reduce the difference between source and target domains. Following [12, 14, 15, 18] we adopt the Maximum Mean Discrepancy (MMD) as a measure to compare different distributions. This algorithm searches for a projection matrix, $A \in \mathbb{R}^{f \times k}$ which aims to minimise the distance between the samples means of the source and target domains:

$$\left\| \frac{1}{n_{src}} \sum_{i=1}^{n_{src}} A^\top x^i - \frac{1}{n_{trg}} \sum_{j=n_{src}+1}^{n_{src}+n_{trg}} A^\top x^j \right\|^2 = tr(A^T X M X^\top A) \tag{2}$$

where M is the MMD matrix and is computed as follows:

$$
M^{ij} = \begin{cases} \frac{1}{n_{src}n_{src}}, & \mathbf{x}^i, \mathbf{x}^j \in X^{src} \\ \frac{1}{n_{trg}n_{trg}}, & \mathbf{x}^i, \mathbf{x}^j \in X^{trg} \\ -\frac{1}{n_{src}n_{trg}}, & \text{otherwise.} \end{cases}
$$

The optimisation problem then is to minimise (2) such that (1) is maximised, i.e. solve the following eigen-decomposition problem: $(XMX^\top + \epsilon I)A = XHX^\top D$, obtaining the eigenvectors A and the eigenvalues on the diagonal matrix D. The effect is to obtain a lower dimensional shared space between the source and target domains. Consequently under the new representation $A^\top X$, the marginal distributions of the two domains are drawn closer to each other.

3.2   Sample-Based Adaptation with TransGrad

We propose a sample-based transformation to perform a finer PDF adaptation of the source domain. We assume that the transformation from the source to the target domain is locally linear, i.e. a sample's feature vector $\mathbf{x}$ from the source domain is mapped to the target space by

$$
G_i^2(\mathbf{x}) = \mathbf{x} + \alpha\mathbf{b}^i, \tag{3}
$$

where the f dimensional vector $\mathbf{b}^i$ represents a local offset in the target domain and α is a translation regulator. In order to impose as few assumptions as possible, we shall model the unlabelled target data, X^{trg} by a mixture of Gaussian probability density functions $p(\mathbf{x}) = \sum_{k=1}^{K} w_k p(\mathbf{x}|\lambda_k)$ whose parameters are denoted by $\lambda = \{w_k, \boldsymbol{\mu}_k, \Sigma_k, k = 1, \cdots, K\}$ where w_k, $\boldsymbol{\mu}_k$ and Σ_k denote the weight, mean and covariance matrix of Gaussian component k respectively, K denotes the number of Gaussians and $p(\mathbf{x}|\lambda_k) = \mathcal{N}(\boldsymbol{\mu}_k, \Sigma_k)$.

We formulate the problem of finding an optimal translation parameter $\mathbf{b}^i$ as one of moving the point $\mathbf{x}$ to a new location $G^2(\mathbf{x}) = \mathbf{x} + \alpha\mathbf{b}^i$ to increase its likelihood as measured using $p(\mathbf{x}|\lambda)$.

Using the Taylor expansion, in the vicinity of $\mathbf{x}$, the likelihood of the $p(\mathbf{x} + \alpha\mathbf{b}^i)$ can be expressed as:

$$
p(\mathbf{x} + \alpha\mathbf{b}^i|\lambda) = p(\mathbf{x}|\lambda) + \alpha(\nabla_\mathbf{x} p(\mathbf{x}|\lambda))^\top \mathbf{b}^i \tag{4}
$$

We wish to maximise the $p(\mathbf{x} + \alpha\mathbf{b}^i|\lambda)$ with respect to the unknown parameter $\mathbf{b}^i$. The learning problem then can be formulated as

$$
\max_{\mathbf{b}^i}\{p(\mathbf{x}|\lambda) + \alpha(\nabla_\mathbf{x} p(\mathbf{x}|\lambda))^\top \mathbf{b}^i\}
$$
$$
\text{s.t. } \mathbf{b}^{i\top}\mathbf{b}^i = 1 \tag{5}
$$

The Lagrangian of Eq. 5 is

$$
p(\mathbf{x}|\lambda) + \alpha\nabla_\mathbf{x} p(\mathbf{x}|\lambda))^\top \mathbf{b}^i - \alpha''(\mathbf{b}^{i\top}\mathbf{b}^i - 1) \tag{6}
$$

Setting the gradient of Eq. 6 with respect to $\mathbf{b}^i$ to zero

$$\nabla_{\mathbf{x}} p(\mathbf{x}|\lambda) - \gamma \mathbf{b}^i = 0, \tag{7}$$

where γ is considered as TransGrad's step size parameter and is equal to $\frac{2\alpha''}{\alpha}$.

Clearly, the source data-point $\mathbf{x}$ should be moved in the direction of maximum gradient of the function $p(\mathbf{x}|\lambda)$. Therefore, $\mathbf{b}^i$ is defined as

$$\mathbf{b}^i = \nabla_{\mathbf{x}} p(\mathbf{x}|\lambda) = \sum_{k=1}^{K} w_k p(\mathbf{x}^{src}|\lambda_k) \Sigma_k^{-1} (\mathbf{x} - \boldsymbol{\mu}_k) \tag{8}$$

In practice, equation 3 translates $\mathbf{x}^{src}$ using the combination of the translations between $\mathbf{x}^{src}$ and $\boldsymbol{\mu}_k$, weighted by the likelihood of $G^2(\mathbf{x}^{src})$ given the model parameters λ_k.

3.3   Conditional Distribution Adaptation with TST

In order to adapt the class-conditional distribution mismatch between the corresponding clusters of the two domains, we introduce a set of linear class-specific transformations. To achieve this, one can assume that a Gaussian Mixture Model fitted to the source classes can be adapted in a way that it matches to target classes. While the general GMM uses full covariance matrices, we follow Reynolds et al. [19] and use only diagonal covariance matrices. This way, the complexity of the estimation system becomes linear in f. In our experiments, we further simplify the model for this step of the pipeline by using only one Gaussian model per class.

In order to adapt the class conditional distributions one can start with an attempt to match the joint distribution of the features and labels between corresponding clusters of two domains. However, as explained in Sect. 1, labelled samples are not available in the target domain. We thus use posterior probability of the target instances to build class-based models in the target domain. We restrict our class-based adaptation method to a translation and scale transformation (abbreviated as TST). This approximation makes the computational cost very attractive.

The proposed adaptation is introduced by means of a class-based transformation $G_{y^i}(\mathbf{X})$ which aims to adjust the mean and standard deviation of the corresponding clusters from the source domain, i.e., each feature j of each sample $\mathbf{x}^i$ is adapted as follows

$$G_{y^i}(x_j^i) = \frac{x_j^i - E^{src}[x_j, y^i]}{\sigma_{j,y_i}^{src}} \sigma_{j,y_i}^{trg} + E_{\Lambda_{src}}^{trg}[x_j, y^i], \forall i = 1 : n_{src}, \tag{9}$$

where $E^{src}[x_j, y^i]$ is the joint expectation of the feature x_j and labels y^i, and σ_{j,y^i}^{src} is the standard deviation of feature x_j of the source samples labelled as y^i, defined by

$$E^{src}[x_j, y^i] = \frac{\sum_{i=1}^{n_{src}} x_j^i \mathbb{1}_{[y]}(y^i)}{\sum_{i=1}^{n_{src}} \mathbb{1}_{[y]}(y^i)}. \tag{10}$$

Here $\mathbb{1}_{[y]}(y^i)$ is an indicator function[2].

An estimation of the target join expectation is thus formulated as

$$E^{trg}[x_j, y] \approx E^{trg}_{\Lambda_{src}}[x_j, y] = \frac{\sum_{i=1}^{n_{trg}} x_j^i P_{\Lambda_{src}}(y|\mathbf{x}_i)}{\sum_{i=1}^{n_{trg}} P_{\Lambda_{src}}(y|\mathbf{x}_i)} \qquad (11)$$

and we propose to estimate the standard deviation per feature and per class using

$$\sigma^{trg}_{j,y^i} = \sqrt{\frac{\sum_{n=1}^{n_{trg}} (x_j^n - E^{trg}_{\Lambda_{src}}[x_j, y^i])^2 P_{\Lambda_{src}}(y^i|\mathbf{x}_n)}{\sum_{n=1}^{n_{trg}} P_{\Lambda_{src}}(y^i|\mathbf{x}_n)}}. \qquad (12)$$

In other words, in a common TTL problem, the joint expectation of the features and labels over source distribution, $E^{src}[x_j, y^i]$, is not necessarily equal to $E^{trg}[x_j, y^i]$. Therefore, one can argue that if the expectations in the source and target domains are similar, then the model Λ learnt on the source data will generalise well to the target data. Consequently the less these distributions differ, the better the trained model will perform.

Since the target expectation $E^{trg}_{\Lambda_{src}}[x_j, y^i]$ is only an approximation based on the target's posterior probabilities, rather than the ground-truth labels (which are not available in the target set), there is a danger that samples that would be miss-classified could lead to negative transfer. To alleviate this, we follow Arnold et al.'s [16] suggestion and smooth out the transformation by applying the following:

$$G_{y^i}^3(x_j^i) = (1 - \theta)x_j^i + \theta G_{y^i}(x_j^i), \qquad (13)$$

with $\theta \in [0, 1]$.

3.4 Iterative Refinement of the Conditional Distribution

Matching the marginal distributions does not guarantee that the conditional distribution of the target can be approximated to that of the source. To our knowledge, most of the recent works related to this issue [7, 20–22] are Inductive TL methods and they have access to some labelled data in the target domain which in practice makes the posteriors' estimations easier.

Instead, our class-specific transformation method (TST), reduces the difference between the likelihoods $P(G_y^3(\mathbf{x}^{src})|y = c)$ and $P(\mathbf{x}|y = c)$ by using target posteriors estimated from a model trained on gradually modified source domain (Eq. 13). Hence, these likelihood approximations will not be reliable unless we iterate over the whole distribution adaptation process and retrain the classifier model using $G_y^3(\mathbf{x}^{src})$.

3.5 Stopping Criterion

In order to automatically control the number of the iterations in our pipeline, we introduce a domain dissimilarity measure inspired by sample selection bias corrections techniques [4, 23].

---

[2] Equations (10) and (11) rectify equations from [16], as we discussed in [17].

Many of the sample selection bias techniques are based on weighting samples $\mathbf{x}_i^{src}$ using the ratio $w(\mathbf{x}_i^{src}) = P(\mathbf{x}_i^{trg})/P(\mathbf{x}_i^{src})$. This ratio can be estimated using a classifier that is trained to distinguish between source and target domains, i.e., samples are labelled as either belonging to class src or trg. Based on this idea, we use this classification performance as a measure of dissimilarity between two domains, i.e., if it is easy to distinguish between source and target samples, it means they are dissimilar. The intuition is that if the domain dissimilarity is high, then more iterations are required for achieving a better match between the domains.

3.6   Algorithm and Computational Complexity

The proposed method is illustrated in Fig. 2 and Algorithm 1. Its computational cost is as follows, where n is the size of the dataset, f is its dimensionality and K is the number of GMM components:

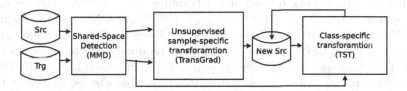

Fig. 2. The Transductive Transfer Machine (TTM).

1. MMD: $O(n^2)$ for constructing the MMD matrix, $O(nf^2)$ for covariance computation and $O(f^3)$ for eigendecomposition.
2. TransGrad: $O(nK)$ for Expectation step of GMM computation, $O(nKf)$ for the computation of diagonal covariance matrices and $O(K)$ for the Maximisation step of the GMM computation. Once the GMM is built, the Trans-Grad transformation itself is $O(nKf)$.
3. TST: $O(Kf)$ for class specific TST transformations.
4. NN classifier: zero for training and $O(n^2f)$ for reapplying the classifier.

Algorithm 1. TTM: Transductive Transfer Machine

Input: $\mathbf{X}^{src}, \mathbf{Y}^{src}, \mathbf{X}^{trg}$
Output: $\mathbf{Y}^{trg}$
1. MMD: search for the shared subspace between the two domains (Eq. 2)
2. TransGrad: adjust the marginal distribution mismatch between the two domains (Eq. 3)
while $(T < max\_iter)$ and $(\|D(G^t(\mathbf{X}^{src}), \mathbf{X}^{trg}\|) > threshold)$ **do**
    3. Find the feature-wise TST transformation (Eqs. 10, 12, 13)
    4. Transform the source domain clusters (Eq. 14)
    5. Retrain the classifier using the transformed source
end while

The max_iter parameter is set to 10 for all the experiments, though in the majority of cases, the iterations stop before that because of the criterion of Sect. 3.5. For each of the T iterations, the classifier is re-applied and TST is computed. Therefore, the overall complexity of our training algorithm is dominated by the cost of training a GMM (which is low by using diagonal covariances) and iteratively applying a classifier. The core transformations proposed in this paper, TransGrand and TST are $O(nKf)$ and $O(nf)$, respectively, i.e., much cheaper than most methods in the literature.

4   Experimental Evaluation

4.1   Datasets and Feature Extraction

USPS, MNIST, COIL20 and Caltech + office are four benchmark datasets widely adopted to evaluate computer vision and pattern recognition algorithms.

USPS dataset consists of 7,291 training images and 2,007 test images of size 16×16 [24]. *MNIST* dataset has a training set of 60,000 examples and a test set of 10,000 examples of size 28×28. USPS and MNIST datasets follow very different distributions but they share 10 classes of digits. We followed the settings of [12] for USPS→MNIST using their randomly selected samples composed of 1,800 images in USPS as the source data, and 2,000 images in MNIST to form the target data and also switch source-target pairs to get another dataset MNIST→USPS. The images were rescaled to 16×16 pixels, and each represented by a feature vector encoding the gray-scale pixel values. Hence the source and target data can share the same feature space.

COIL20 contains 20 objects classes with 1,440 images [25]. The images of each object were taken 5 degrees apart as the object is rotated on a turntable and each object has 72 images. Each image is 32×32 pixels with 256 gray levels. In our experiments, we followed the settings of [12] and partitioned the dataset into two subsets. *COIL1* and *COIL2:* COIL1 contains all images taken with objects in the orientations of $[0°, 85°] \cup [180°, 265°]$ (quadrants 1 and 3); COIL2 contains all images taken in the orientations of $[90°, 175°] \cup [270°, 355°]$ (quadrants 2 and 4). In this way, subsets COIL1 and COIL2 follow different distributions. One dataset, COIL1→COIL2, was constructed by selecting all 720 images in COIL1 to form the source data, and all 720 images in COIL2 to form the target data. Source-target pairs were switched to form another dataset COIL2→COIL1. Following Long et al. [12], we carried out a pre-processing l_2-normalisation on the raw features of MNIST, USPS, COIL1 and COIL2 datasets.

CALTECH + OFFICE [26,27] is composed of a 10-class sampling of four datasets; Amazon (images downloaded from online merchants), Webcam (low-resolution images by web camera), DSLR (high-resolution images by a digital SLR camera) and Caltech-256. For the settings we followed [26]: 10 common classes are extracted from all four datasets: Back-pack, Touring-bike, Calculator, Head-phones, Computer-keyboard, Laptop, Computer-monitor, Computer-mouse, Coffee-mug and Video-projector. Each dataset is assumed as a different domain and there are between 8 and 151 samples per category per domain, and

2533 images in total. We followed the feature extraction and experimental settings used in previous works [26,27]. Briefly, SURF features were extracted and the images encoded with 800-bins histograms with the codebook trained from a subset of Amazon images. The histograms were then normalised and z-scored to follow a normal distribution in each dimension. We further performed experiments on $CALTECH + OFFICE$ where DeCAF features are used as descriptors. DeCAF features are extracted by first training a deep conventional model in a fully supervised setting using a state-of-the-art method [28]. The outputs from the 6th Neural Network layer was used as the visual features, leading to 4096 dimensional DeCAF features.

The second column in Table 2 shows the baseline dissimilarity measure (Sect. 3.5) between the two transfer domains.

4.2 Experiments and Results

We coin the iterative version of all our proposed algorithms as Transductive Transfer Machine (TTM) where TTM0 refers to when we have an iterative version of TST, TTM1 is the combination of the MMD and TST and finally TTM2 is the TTM1 with a further intermediate sample-wise marginal adaptation (TransGrad). We have evaluated the performance of these three methods and compared the performance with two state-of-the-art approaches [12,26] using the same public datasets and the same settings as those of [12,26]. Further comparisons with other transductive transfer learning methods such as Transfer Component Analysis [29], Transfer Subspace Learning [30] and Sampling Geodesic Flow (SGF) using the Grassmann manifolds [31] are reported in [12,26].

Table 2 shows a comparison between our methods and the state-of-the-art methods. As one can note, all the transfer learning methods improve the accuracy over the baseline. Furthermore, our TTM methods generally outperform all the other methods. The main reason for that is that our methods combine three different adaptation techniques which jointly implement a complex transformation that would be difficult to determine in a single step. The order in which these transformations are applied, global (MDD) + sample-based (TransGrad) + conditional (TST), is important because neither MMD nor TransGrad take class labels into account. TST achieves better results if it is applied to data in which the difference between source and target domains is not too large, as it uses estimates of $P_{A_{src}}(y|\mathbf{x})$ based on classifiers learnt on the (adapted) source domain. If the marginals were far off the desired solution, the classifier could generate poor estimates of $P_{A_{src}}(y|\mathbf{x})$, leading to poor transfer. Similarly, the TransGrad transformation is less constrained than MMD, which is why it is important that it is applied after MMD. These three steps complement each other, as each applies transformations of a different nature.

Table 2 shows that in most of the tasks our methods give the best results. The average performance accuracy of TTM2 on 12 transfer tasks is **56.20 %**, which is an improvement of **1.32 %** over the best performing previous method JDA [12]. JDA also benefits from jointly adapting the marginal and conditional distributions but their approach has the global and class specific adaptations along each other at each iteration which in practice these two might cancel the effect of each other hence limiting the final model from being well fitted into the target clusters. While in JDA the number of iterations is fixed to 10, in our algorithm we based this number on a sensible measure of domain dissimilarity.

GFK [26] performs well on some of the Office + Caltech experiments but poorly on the others. The reason is that the subspace dimension should be small enough to ensure that different sub-spaces transit smoothly along the geodesic flow, which may not be an accurate representation of the input data. JDA and TTM perform much better by learning an accurate shared space.

For a comparison using state-of-the-art features, in Table 3 we present further results using Deep Convolutional Activation Features (DeCAF) features [32]. We followed the experimental setting in [26] for unsupervised domain adaptation for Caltech + office dataset, except that instead of using SURF, we used DeCAF. In this set of experiments we compared our TTM method with methods that adapt the classifiers hyperplanes or using auxiliary classifiers, namely; the Adaptive Support Vector Machines (SVM-A) [7], Domain Adaptation Machine (DAM) [33] and DA-M2S [34]. DAM was designed to make use of multiple source domains. For a single source domain scenario, the experiments were repeated 10 times by using randomly generated subsets of source and target domains and the mean performance is reported in Table 3.

Table 2. Recognition accuracies with Nearest Neighbour classifiers on target domains using TTL algorithms. The datasets are abbreviated as M: MNIST, U: USPS, C: Caltech, A: Amazon, W: Webcam, and D: DSLR.

TTL Experiment	Domain Dissimilarity	NN Baseline	GFK (PLS, PCA) [26]	JDA (1NN) [12]	TTM0 (TST + NN)	TTM1 (MMD + TTM0)	TTM2 (TransGrad + TTM1)
M→ U	0.984	65.94	67.22	67.28	75.94	76.61	**77.94**
U→ M	0.981	44.70	46.45	59.65	59.79	59.41	**61.15**
COIL1→ 2	0.627	83.61	72.50	89.31	88.89	88.75	**93.19**
COIL2→1	0.556	82.78	74.17	88.47	**88.89**	88.61	88.75
C→ A	0.548	23.70	41.4	44.78	39.87	44.25	**46.76**
C→ W	0.78	25.76	40.68	**41.69**	41.02	39.66	41.02
C→ D	0.786	25.48	41.1	45.22	50.31	44.58	**47.13**
A→ C	0.604	26.00	37.9	39.36	36.24	35.53	**39.62**
A→ W	0.743	29.83	35.7	37.97	37.63	**42.37**	39.32
A→ D	0.85	25.48	36.31	**39.49**	33.75	29.30	29.94
W→ C	0.752	19.86	29.3	**31.17**	26.99	29.83	30.36
W→ A	0.717	22.96	**35.5**	32.78	29.12	30.69	31.11
W→ D	0.51	59.24	80.89	89.17	85.98	89.17	**89.81**
D→ C	0.78	26.27	30.28	31.52	29.65	31.25	**32.06**
D→ A	0.790	28.50	**36.1**	33.09	31.21	29.75	30.27
D→ W	0.471	63.39	79.1	89.49	85.08	**90.84**	88.81

Table 3. Results on Caltech + office dataset using DeCAF features. The methods are abbreviated as: M0: Baseline (no transfer), M1: SVM-A [7], M2: DAM [33], M3: DA-M2S (w/o depth) [34], M4: JDA (1NN) [12] and M5: TTM (NN).

	C→A	C→W	C→D	A→C	A→W	A→D	W→C	W→A	W→D	D→C	D→A	D→W
M0	85.70	66.10	74.52	70.35	64.97	57.29	60.37	62.53	98.73	52.09	62.73	89.15
M1	83.54	81.72	74.58	74.36	70.58	96.56	85.37	96.71	78.14	91.00	76.61	83.89
M2	84.73	82.48	78.14	76.60	74.32	93.82	**87.88**	96.31	81.27	**91.75**	79.39	84.59
M3	84.27	82.87	75.83	78.11	71.04	**96.62**	86.38	**97.12**	77.60	91.37	78.14	83.31
M4	89.77	83.73	86.62	82.28	78.64	80.25	83.53	90.19	100	85.13	**91.44**	98.98
M5	**89.98**	**86.78**	**89.17**	**83.70**	**89.81**	81.36	80.41	88.52	100	82.90	90.81	**98.98**

Note that in Table 3 the baseline without any transformation using DeCAF features and NN classifier is significantly better than the results of Table 2, simply because DeCAF features are better than SURF. As one can see our TTM method outperforms the other state-of-the-art approaches in most of the cases, gaining on average 2.10 % over the best performing state-of-the-art method of M2S(w/o depth).

To validate that TTM can achieve an optimal performance under a wide range of parameter values, we conducted sensitivity analysis on MNIST→USPS, Caltech→Amazon and Webcam→Caltech. We ran TTM with varying values of the regulator γ of the TransGrad step, and the results are in Fig. 3(a). One can see that for all these datasets, the performance improves as γ grows but it plateaus when $\gamma = 5$. For this reason we used $\gamma = 5$ in all experiments in the remaining of this paper.

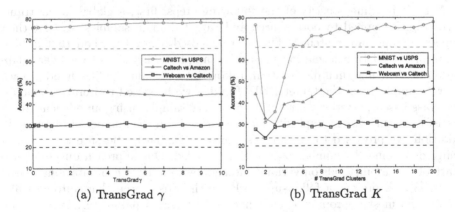

(a) TransGrad γ (b) TransGrad K

Fig. 3. Effect of different γ values and number of GMM clusters in the TransGrad step of our framework on the final performance of the pipeline for three cross-domain experiments. The dashed line shows the baseline accuracy for each experiment.

We also ran TTM with varying number Gaussians K in the TransGrad step for the target GMM. Theoretically as the number of GMM components increases the translations get more accurate and the performance becomes more stable. We plot the classification accuracy w.r.t. K in Fig. 3(b). Note that for $K = 1$, TransGrad contributes to an improvement over the baseline, as it induces a global shift towards the target set. But in general, for values of K smaller than the number of classes, we do not actually expect TransGrad to help, as it will shift samples from different classes towards the same clusters. This explains why the performance increases with K for $K > 2$. Based on this result, we adopted $K = 20$ in all other experiments of this paper.

We have also compared the time complexity of our TTM algorithm against JDA [12] in the transfer task from MNIST digits dataset to USPS digits dataset. Both algorithms were implemented in Matlab and were evaluated on a Intel Core2 64 bit, 3 GHz machine running Linux. We averaged time measurements of 5 experiments. The JDA algorithm took 21.38 ± 0.26 s and our full TTM framework took 4.42 ± 0.12 s, broken down as: 0.40 ± 0.01 s to find the appropriate shared space using the MMD, 1.90 ± 0.06 to perform the sample-wise marginal distribution adaptations using TransGrad and finally 2.42 ± 0.12 s to apply the iterative conditional distribution adaptations (TST). Therefore, the proposed TTM outperforms JDA in most of the cases requiring one fifth of its computational time.

5   Conclusions

In this paper, we introduced transductive transfer machine (TTM), which aims to adapt both the marginal and conditional distributions of the source samples so that they become more similar to those of target samples, leading to an improvement in the classification results in transfer learning scenarios.

TTM's pipeline consists of the following steps: first, a global linear transformation is applied to both source and target domain samples, so that their expected values are matched. Then we proposed a novel method that applies a sample-based transformation to source samples. This leads to a finer adaptation of their marginal distribution, taking into account the likelihood of each source sample given the target PDF. Finally, we proposed to iteratively adapt the class-based posterior distribution of source samples using an efficient linear transformation whose complexity mostly depends on the number of features. In addition, we proposed to use an unsupervised similarity measure to automatically determine the number of iterations needed. Our approach outperformed state-of-the-art methods on various datasets, with a lower computational cost.

In [3], we present a follow-up work which adds a step that automatically selects the most appropriated classifier and its kernel parameter, leading to a significant improvement of the results presented here.

It is worth pointing out that TTM is a general framework with applicability beyond object recognition and could be easily applied to other domains, even outside Computer Vision. For future work, we suggest studying combinations of TTM with semi-supervised learning methods and feature learning algorithms. Another exciting direction is to combine TTM with voting classification algorithms (c.f. [35]).

Acknowledgements. We are grateful for the support of EPSRC/dstl contract EP/ K014307/1 (Signal processing in a network battlespace) and EPSRC project S3A, EP/L000539/1. During part of the development of this work, TdC had been working in Neil Lawrence's group at the University of Sheffield.

References

1. Pan, S.J., Yang, Q.: A survey on transfer learning. IEEE Trans. Knowl. Data Eng. **22**, 1345–1359 (2010)
2. Torralba, A., Efros, A.A.: Unbiased look at dataset bias. In: Proceedings of the IEEE Conference on Computer Vision and Pattern Recognition, CVPR (2011)
3. FarajiDavar, N., deCampos, T., Kittler, J.: Adaptive transductive transfer machines. In: Proceedings of the British Machine Vision Conference (BMVC), Nottingham (2014)
4. Cortes, C., Mohri, M., Riley, M.D., Rostamizadeh, A.: Sample selection bias correction theory. In: Freund, Y., Györfi, L., Turán, G., Zeugmann, T. (eds.) ALT 2008. LNCS (LNAI), vol. 5254, pp. 38–53. Springer, Heidelberg (2008)
5. Gretton, A., Smola, A., Huang, J., Schmittfull, M., Borgwardt, K., Schölkopf, B.: Covariate shift by kernel mean matching. Dataset Shift Mach. Learn. **3**, 131–160 (2009)
6. Joachims, T.: Transductive inference for text classification using support vector machines. In: Proceedings of the International Conference Machine Learning, ICML, San Francisco, CA, USA, pp. 200–209 (1999)
7. Yang, J., Yan, R., Hauptmann, A.G.: Cross-domain video concept detection using adaptive. In: Proceedings of the 15th International Conference on Multimedia (2007). doi:10.1145/1291233.1291276
8. Gopalan, R., Li, R., Chellappa, R.: Unsupervised adaptation across domain shifts by generating intermediate data representations. IEEE Trans. Pattern Anal. Mach. Intell. PAMI **36**(11), 2288–2302 (2014). doi:10.1109/TPAMI.2013.249
9. Chu, W.S., De la Torre, F., Cohn, J.F.: Selective transfer machine for personalized facial action unit detection. In: Proceedings of the IEEE Conference on Computer Vision and Pattern Recognition, CVPR (2013)
10. Dai, W., Chen, Y., Xue, G., Yang, Q., Yu, Y.: Translated learning: transfer learning across different feature spaces. In: Neural Information Processing Systems, pp. 353–360 (2008)
11. Borgwardt, K.M., Gretton, A., Rasch, M.J., Kriegel, H., Schalkopf, B., Smola, A.J.: Integrating structured biological data by kernel maximum mean discrepancy. In: Proceedings of the International Conference Intelligent Systems for Molecular Biology (2006)
12. Long, M., Wang, J., Ding, G., Yu, P.: Transfer learning with joint distribution adaptation. In: Proceedings of the International Conference on Computer Vision, ICCV (2013)
13. Aytar, Y., Zisserman, A.: Tabula rasa: model transfer for object category detection. In: Proceedings of the International Conference on Computer Vision, ICCV (2011)
14. Gretton, A., Borgwardt, K., Rasch, M., Scholkopf, B., Smola, A.: A kernel method for the two sample problem. In: Proceedings of the Neural Information Processing Systems, NIPS, pp. 513–520. MIT Press (2007)
15. Sun, Q., Chattopadhyay, R., Panchanathan, S., Ye, J.: A two-stage weighting framework for multi-source domain adaptation. In: Proceedings of the Neural Information Processing Systems, NIPS, pp. 505–513 (2011)

16. Arnold, A., Nallapati, R., Cohen, W.W.: A comparative study of methods for transductive transfer learning. In: Proceedings of the Seventh IEEE International Conference on Data Mining Workshops, ICDMW, pp. 77–82. IEEE Computer Society, Washington (2007)

17. FarajiDavar, N., deCampos, T., Kittler, J., Yan, F.: Transductive transfer learning for action recognition in tennis games. In: VECTaR Workshop, in Conjunction with ICCV (2011)

18. Pan, S.J., Tsang, I.W., Kwok, J.T., Yang, Q.: Domain adaptation via transfer component analysis. In: Proceedings of the 21st International Joint Conference on Artificial Intelligence, pp. 1187–1192. Morgan Kaufmann Publishers Inc., San Francisco (2009)

19. Reynolds, D.A., Quatieri, T.F., Dunn, R.B.: Speaker verification using adapted gaussian mixture models. Digit. Sig. Process. **10**, 19–41 (2000)

20. Chen, M., Weinberger, K.Q., Blitzer, J.: Co-training for domain adaptation. In: Proceedings of the Neural Information Processing Systems, NIPS, pp. 2456–2464 (2011)

21. Quanz, B., Huan, J., Mishra, M.: Knowledge transfer with low-quality data: a feature extraction issue. In: Abiteboul, S., Bolhm, K., Koch, C., Tan, K. (eds.) Proceedings of the 27th International Conference on Data Engineering (ICDE), pp. 769–779. IEEE Computer Society, Hannover, Germany (2011)

22. Zhong, E., Fan, W., Peng, J., Zhang, K., Ren, J., Turaga, D.S., Verscheure, O.: Cross domain distribution adaptation via kernel mapping. In: International Conference on Knowledge Discovery and Data mining, KDD, pp. 1027–1036. ACM (2009)

23. Shimodaira, H.: Improving predictive inference under covariate shift by weighting the log-likelihood function. J. Stat. Plan. Infer. **90**, 227–244 (2000)

24. Cun, Y.L., Boser, B., Denker, J.S., Howard, R.E., Habbard, W., Jackel, L.D., Henderson, D.: Handwritten digit recognition with a back-propagation network. In: Touretzky, D.S. (ed.) Advances in Neural Information Processing Systems, vol. 2, pp. 396–404. Morgan Kaufmann Publishers Inc., San Francisco (1990)

25. Nene, S.A., Nayar, S.K., Murase, H.: Columbia university image library COIL-20 (1996). http://www.cs.columbia.edu/CAVE/software/softlib/coil-20.php (retrieved 30 June 2014)

26. Gong, B., Shi, Y., Sha, F., Grauman, K.: Geodesic flow kernel for unsupervised domain adaptation. In: Proceedings of the IEEE Conference on Computer Vision and Pattern Recognition, CVPR, pp. 2066–2073 (2012)

27. Bay, H., Ess, A., Tuytelaars, T., Van Gool, L.: Speeded-up robust features (SURF). Comput. Vis. Image Underst. **110**, 346–359 (2008)

28. Krizhevsky, A., Sutskever, I., Hinton, G.E.: Imagenet classification with deep convolutional neural networks. In: Proceedings of the Neural Information Processing Systems, NIPS, pp. 1106–1114 (2012)

29. Pan, S.J., Tsang, I.W., Kwok, J.T., Yang, Q.: Domain adaptation via transfer component analysis. IEEE Trans. Neural Netw. **22**, 199–210 (2011)

30. Si, S., Tao, D., Geng, B.: Bregman divergence-based regularization for transfer subspace learning. IEEE Trans. Knowl. Data Eng. **22**, 929–942 (2010)

31. Gopalan, R., Li, R., Chellappa, R.: Domain adaptation for object recognition: an unsupervised approach. In: Metaxas, D.N., Quan, L., Sanfeliu, A., Gool, L.J.V. (eds.) Proceedings of the International Conference on Computer Vision, ICCV, pp. 999–1006 (2011)

32. Donahue, J., Jia, Y., Vinyals, O., Hoffman, J., Zhang, N., Tzeng, E., Darrell, T.: DeCAF: A deep convolutional activation feature for generic visual recognition. Technical report CoRR arXiv:1310.1531, Cornell University Library (2013)
33. Duan, L., Tsang, I.W., Xu, D., Chua, T.: Domain adaptation from multiple sources via auxiliary classifiers. In: Proceedings of the 26th Annual International Conference on Machine Learning, ICML, pp. 289–296. ACM, New York (2009)
34. Chen, L., Li, W., Xu, D.: Recognizing RGB images by learning from RGB-D data. In: IEEE International Conference on Computer Vision and Pattern Recognition, CVPR (2014)
35. Gao, J., Fan, W., Jiang, J., Han, J.: Knowledge transfer via multiple model local structure mapping. In: Knowledge Discovery and Data Mining, pp. 283–291 (2008)

Fully Automatic Segmentation of Hip CT Images via Random Forest Regression-Based Atlas Selection and Optimal Graph Search-Based Surface Detection

Chengwen Chu[1], Junjie Bai[2], Li Liu[1], Xiaodong Wu[2], and Guoyan Zheng[1]($\boxtimes$)

[1] Institute for Surgical Technology and Biomechanics, University of Bern,
Bern, Switzerland
{chengwen.chu,li.liu}@istb.unibe.ch, guoyan.zheng@ieee.org
[2] Department of Electrical and Computer Engineering, The University of Iowa,
Iowa City, USA
{junjie-bai,xiaodong-wu}@uiowa.edu

Abstract. Automatic extraction of surface models of both pelvis and proximal femur of a hip joint from 3D CT images is an important and challenging task for computer assisted diagnosis and planning of peri-acetabular osteotomy (PAO). Due to the narrowness of hip joint space, the adjacent surfaces of the acetabulum and the femoral head are hardly distinguishable from each other in the target CT images. This paper presents a fully automatic method for segmenting hip CT images using random forest (RF) regression-based atlas selection and optimal graph search-based surface detection. The two fundamental contributions of our method are: (1) An efficient RF regression framework is developed for a fast and accurate landmark detection from the hip CT images. The detected landmarks allow for not only a robust and accurate initialization of the atlases within the target image space but also an effective selection of a subset of atlases for a fast atlas-based segmentation; and (2) 3-D graph theory-based optimal surface detection is used to refine the extraction of the surfaces of the acetabulum and the femoral head with the ultimate goal to preserve hip joint structure and to avoid penetration between the two extracted surfaces. Validation on 30 hip CT images shows that our method achieves high performance in segmenting pelvis, left proximal femur, and right proximal femur with an average accuracy of 0.56 mm, 0.61 mm, and 0.57 mm, respectively.

1 Introduction

Developmental dysplasia of hip (DDH) is a congenital defect that seriously affects young people nowadays. In many treatment procedures for patients with DDH, periacetabular osteotomy (PAO) recently becomes a common surgical intervention [1], aiming to improve ability of weight bearing and stability of the diseased hip joint. To reach this goal, knowing acetabular coverage, which is defined as a ratio between the femoral head surface covered by the acetabulum and the

© Springer International Publishing Switzerland 2015
D. Cremers et al. (Eds.): ACCV 2014, Part III, LNCS 9005, pp. 640–654, 2015.
DOI: 10.1007/978-3-319-16811-1_42

complete femoral head surface, is important for operative planning for PAO. For this purpose, we need to extract surface models of both the pelvis and the proximal femur from hip CT images.

Automatic extraction of the surface models of both the pelvis and the proximal femur from hip CT images comprises two key steps. Firstly, both anatomical structures have to be detected in the target volume data and secondly, both models need to be segmented. Furthermore, the fact that the two structures compose a hip joint should not be neglected. Otherwise, the resultant models may penetrate each other due to the narrowness of the hip joint and hence do not represent a true hip joint.

For detection, reported methods in literature address the problem either by assuming an user-supplied initialization [2,3] or by using Generalized Hough Transform (GHT) [4,5]. For segmentation, both multi-atlas-based segmentation methods [6–8] and statistical shape model (SSM)-based segmentation methods [2–5,9,10] are proposed. Here we define an atlas as a pair of data consisting of a CT volume and its corresponding segmentation. Given a set of atlases, atlas-based segmentation methods segment a target volume by registering the atlases to the volume first, followed by a label fusion process. Multi-atlas-based segmentation methods may be applicable for extraction of surface models of individual structures of the hip joint, but they cannot guarantee the preservation of the hip joint space and the prevention of the penetration of the extracted surface models. The other segmentation option is the SSM-based methods, which perform an adaption of the SSM to the target image data. Similar to atlas-based methods, conventional SSM-based methods are difficult, if not impossible, to guarantee the preservation of the hip joint structure [2–4,9]. This problem is recently addressed by introducing an articulated statistical shape model (aSSM) [5]. Another solution is to simultaneously detecting both surfaces of the adjacent structures based on graph optimization theory [10]. By incorporating prior knowledge about spatial relationship in the graph optimization, the adjacent surfaces can be segmented without penetration to each other.

In this paper, we propose a two-stage automatic hip CT segmentation method. In the first stage, we use a multi-atlas-based method to segment the regions of the pelvis and the bilateral proximal femurs. An efficient random forest (RF) regression-based landmark detection method is developed to detect landmarks from the target CT images. The detected landmarks allow for not only a robust and accurate initialization of the atlases within the target image space but also an effective selection of a subset of atlases for a fast atlas-based segmentation. In the second stage, we refine the segmentation of the hip joint area using graph optimization theory-based multi-surface detection [11,12], which guarantees the preservation of the hip joint space and the prevention of the penetration of the extracted surface models with a carefully constructed graph. Different from the method introduced in [10], where the optimal surfaces are detected in the original CT image space, here we propose to first unfold the hip joint area obtained from the multi-atlas-based segmentation stage using a spherical coordinate transform and then detect the surfaces of the acetabulum and the femoral head in the unfolded space. By unfolding the hip joint area using the spherical

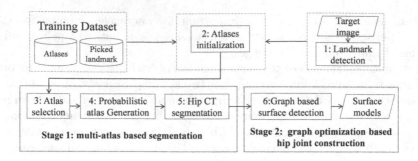

Fig. 1. The flowchart of our proposed segmentation method

coordinate transform, we convert the problem of detection of two half-spherically shaped surfaces of the acetabulum and the femoral head in the original image space to a problem of detection of two terrain-like surfaces in the unfolded space, which can be efficiently solved using the methods presented in [11,12]. Figure 1 presents a schematic overview of the complete workflow of our method.

2 Multi-atlas Based Hip CT Segmentation

2.1 Landmark Detection by Fast Random Forest Regression

Basic Algorithm. We have a separate RF landmark detector for each land-mark. During training, in each training image, we sample a set of image volumes around the ground-truth landmark position which is known. Each sampled volume is represented by its visual feature $\mathbf{f}_i \in \mathbb{R}^{d_f}$ and the displacement $\mathbf{d}_i \in \mathbb{R}^3$ from its center to the landmark (Fig. 2(a)). Let us denote all the sampled volumes in all training images as $\{P_i = (\mathbf{f}_i, \mathbf{d}_i)\}_{i=1...N}$ (Fig. 2(b)). The goal is then to learn a mapping function $\phi : \mathbb{R}^{d_f} \rightarrow \mathbb{R}^3$ from the feature space to the displacement space. Principally, any regression method can be used. In this paper, similar to [13,14], we utilize the random forest regressors [15].

Once the regressor is trained, given a new image (Fig. 2(c)), we randomly sample another set of volumes $\{P'_k = (\mathbf{f}'_k, \mathbf{c}'_k)\}_{k=1...N'}$ all over the image (or a region of interest if an initial guess of the landmark position is known), where $\mathbf{f}'_k$ and $\mathbf{c}'_k$ are the visual feature and center coordinate of the kth volume, respectively (Fig. 2(d)). Through the trained regressor ϕ, we can calculate the predicted displacement $\mathbf{d}'_k = \phi(\mathbf{f}'_k)$, and then $\mathbf{d}'_k + \mathbf{c}'_k$ becomes the prediction of the landmark position by a single volume P'_k (Fig. 2(e)). Note that each tree in the random forest will return a prediction. Therefore, supposing that there are t trees in the forest, we will get $N' \times t$ predictions. These individual predictions are very noisy, but when combined, they approach an accurate prediction. To this end, we consider each single vote as a small Gaussian distribution. We developed a fast probability aggregating algorithm as described below to add these distributions to get a soft probability map called *response volume* which gives, for every position of the CT volume, its probability of being the landmark (Fig. 2(f)).

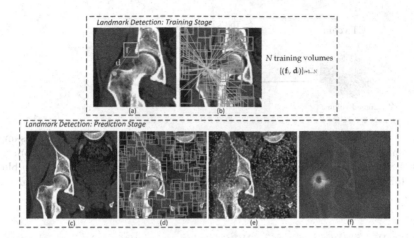

Fig. 2. The RF training and landmark detection. Illustration on coronal slice for easy understanding. (a) A volume sampled around the true landmark position. (b) Multiple sampled training volumes from one atlas. (c) A target image. (d) Multiple sampled test volumes over target image. (e) Each volume gives a single vote for landmark position. (f) Response volume calculated using improved fast Gaussian transform.

Fast Probability Aggregation. As described above, $N' \times t$ predictions are produced to detect each landmark. We consider each prediction a Gaussian model $\mathcal{N} \sim (\bar{\mathbf{d}}_k, \Sigma(\mathbf{d}_k))$, where $\bar{\mathbf{d}}_k$ and $\Sigma(\mathbf{d}_k) = diag(\sigma_{k,x}^2 \ \sigma_{k,y}^2 \ \sigma_{k,z}^2)$ are mean and covariance (which can be calculated from the displacements of the training samples that arrived at particular leaf node). All the $N' \times t$ predictions are accumulated to compute the likelihood of being a true landmark position for all M voxels in the image. This finally yields a response volume for each landmark. Once the response volume has been obtained for each landmark, the position mode is selected as the landmark position.

The computational time of landmark prediction is mainly on multivariate Gaussian accumulation which is usually computed using

$$G(\mathbf{y}_i) = \sum_k^{N' \times t} \frac{1}{\sqrt{(2\pi)^3 |\Sigma(\mathbf{d}_k)|}} exp(-\frac{1}{2}(\mathbf{d}_{\mathbf{y}_i} - \bar{\mathbf{d}}_k)^T \Sigma(\mathbf{d}_k)^{-1}(\mathbf{d}_{\mathbf{y}_i} - \bar{\mathbf{d}}_k)) \quad (1)$$

where $\mathbf{d}_{\mathbf{y}_i} = \mathbf{y}_i - \mathbf{x}_k$, $\mathbf{y}_i$ is a voxel in target image and $\mathbf{x}_k$ is the center of volume k. For all of the N_l landmarks, such calculation will result in prohibitively expensive computation time of $O(M \times N' \times t \times N_l)$ on a 3D CT image with M voxels. In this paper, we propose to approximate Eq. 1 by:

$$G(\mathbf{y}_i) = \sum_k^{N' \times t} W_k \cdot e^{(\|\mathbf{d}_{\mathbf{y}_i} - \bar{\mathbf{d}}_k\|^2 / h^2)} \quad (2)$$

Here we rewrite the Eq. 1 by introducing a constant kernel size of h, and moving the constrains of the variance out of the exponential part by introducing

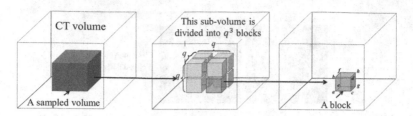

Fig. 3. A schematic view illustrating how to compute the visual feature of a sampled sub-volume for RF training and regression. Left: a sub-volume is sampled from a hip joint CT volume. Middle: we subdivide the sampled sub-volume into $q \times q \times q$ blocks. Right: for each block, we compute its mean and variance using the integral image technique

a weight $W_k = 1/\sigma_{k,x}\sigma_{k,y}\sigma_{k,z}$. With such an approximation, we develop an efficient probability aggregation strategy based on the Improved Fast Gaussian Transform (IFGT) [16] to calculate the response volumes with highly reduced time of $O((M + N' \times t) \times N_l)$.

Visual Feature. As for the visual feature over the sampled sub-volume, we use mean and variance of intensities in a small volume obtained by subdividing the sampled sub-volume. In this paper, we subdivide each sampled sub-volume into a grid of $q \times q \times q$ blocks (see Fig. 3 for details). To accelerate the feature extraction within each block, we use the well-known integral image technique as introduced in [17]. Details about how to compute the integral image of a quantity can be found in [17]. The quantity can be the voxel intensity value or any arithmetic computation on the intensity value. Advantage of using integral image lies in the fact that once we obtain an integral image of the quantity over the complete hip CT volume, the sum of the quantity in any sub-volume can be calculated quickly in constant time O(1) regardless of the size of the volume [17]. Here we assume that we already computed the integral image of the voxel intensity I and the integral image of the squared voxel intensity S of the complete hip CT volume using the technique introduced in [17]. We then compute the mean $E[X]$ and the variance $Var(X)$ of the intensity value of any block (Fig. 3, right) as:

$$
\begin{cases}
E[X] = (I(\mathbf{h}) - I(\mathbf{d}) - I(\mathbf{f}) - I(\mathbf{g}) + I(\mathbf{b}) + I(\mathbf{c}) + I(\mathbf{e}) - I(\mathbf{a}))/N \\
E[X^2] = (S(\mathbf{h}) - S(\mathbf{d}) - S(\mathbf{f}) - S(\mathbf{g}) + S(\mathbf{b}) + S(\mathbf{c}) + S(\mathbf{e}) - S(\mathbf{a}))/N \\
\qquad\qquad Var(X) = E[X^2] - (E[X])^2
\end{cases}
$$

where $\{\mathbf{a}, \ldots \mathbf{h}\} \in \mathcal{R}^3$ are the eight vertices of a block and N is the number of voxels within the block, as shown in Fig. 3, right.

2.2 Atlas Initialization and Atlas-Based Segmentation

Using the detected N_l anatomical landmarks, scaled rigid registrations are performed to align all the N_A atlases to the target image space. Then we select N_s most similar atlases for the given target image. This is achieved by comparing the sum of the distance of the landmarks for all the aligned atlases after the scaled rigid registration. The selected atlases are further registered to the target image with a Markov Random Field (MRF) based non-rigid registration [18]. We then use the selected atlases to generate probabilistic atlas (PA) for pelvis, bilateral proximal femurs and background following the idea introduced in [19]. The generated PAs are further incorporated to a Maximum-a-Posteriori (MAP) estimation which is then optimized by a graph cut method [20] to obtain segmentation results.

3 Graph Optimization Based Hip Joint Surface Detection

3.1 Problem Formulation

After we extract surface models of the pelvis and femur using multi-atlas based segmentation, we expect to refine the hip joint segmentation in the second stage by separating two surfaces of the adjacent structures, i.e., separating the surface of the acetabulum from the surface of the femoral head. In the CT image space, both the acetabulum and the femoral head are ball-like structures and their surfaces can be approximately represented as half-spherically shaped models. To separate these two surfaces, directly applying graph optimization-based surface detection in the CT image space as described in [10,12] would be an option. However, construction of a graph in the original CT image is not straightforward and requires finding correspondences between two adjacent surfaces obtained from a rough segmentation stage as done in [10,12], which is challenging.

In our method, instead of performing surface detection in the original CT image space, we first define a hip joint area in the CT image based on the multi-atlas-based segmentation results, and then unfold this area using a spherical coordinate transform as shown in Fig. 4. Since the spherical coordinate transform converts a half-spherically shaped surface to a planar surface, the surfaces of the acetabulum and the femoral head can therefore be unfolded to two terrain-like surfaces with a gap (joint space) between them as shown in Fig. 4. We reach this goal with following steps:

1. Detecting rim points of the acetabulum from segmented surface model of the pelvis using the method that we developed before [21] (Fig. 4: 1).
2. Fitting a circle to the detected rim points, determining radius R_c and center of the circle, as well as normal to the plane where the fitted circle is located (Fig. 4: 2).
3. Constructing a spherical coordinate system as shown in Fig. 4: 3, taking the center of the fitted circle as the origin, the normal to the fitted circle as the fixed zenith direction, and one randomly selected direction on the plane where the fitted circle is located as the reference direction on that plane. Now, the position of a point in this coordinate system is specified by three numbers: the radial distance R of that point from the origin, its polar angle Θ measured from the zenith direction and the azimuth angle Φ measured from the reference direction on the plane where the fitted circle is located.
4. Sampling points in the spherical coordinate system from the hip joint area (see Fig. 4: 4) using a radial resolution of 0.25 mm and angular resolutions of

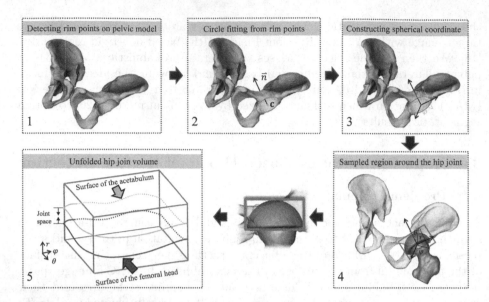

Fig. 4. A schematic illustration of defining and unfolding a hip joint. Please see text in Sect. 3.1 for a detailed explanation.

0.03 radians (for both polar and azimuth angles). Furthermore, we require the sampled points satisfying following conditions:

$$\begin{cases} R_c + 10 \leq R \leq R_c/2 \\ 0 \leq \Theta \leq \pi/2 \\ 0 \leq \Phi \leq 2\pi \end{cases} \tag{3}$$

5. Getting corresponding intensity values of the sampled points from the CT image, which finally forms an image volume $I(\theta, \varphi, r)$ (Fig. 4: 5), where $0 \leq r \leq \lceil (10 + \frac{R_c}{2})/0.25 \rceil$, $0 \leq \theta \leq \lceil \pi/0.06 \rceil$ and $0 \leq \varphi \leq \lceil 2\pi/0.03 \rceil$. The dimension of r depends on the radius of the fitted circle while the dimensions of θ and φ are fixed. To easy the description later, here we define the dimension of r as D_r.

Figure 5 shows an example of the unfolded volume $I(\theta, \varphi, r)$ of a hip joint. With such an unfolded volume, graph construction and optimal multiple-surface detection will be straightforward when the graph optimization-based multiple-surface detection strategy as introduced in [11,12] is used.

3.2   Graph Construction for Multi-surface Detection

For the generated volume $I(\theta, \varphi, r)$ as shown in Fig. 5, we assume that r is implicitly represented by a pair of (θ, φ), e.g. $r = p(\theta, \varphi)$. For a fixed (θ, φ) pair, the voxel subset $\{I(\theta, \varphi, r)|0 \leq r < D_r\}$ forms a column along the $r - axis$ and is defined as $Col(p)$. Each column has a set of neighbors and in this paper

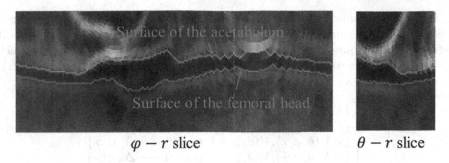

$\varphi - r$ slice $\theta - r$ slice

Fig. 5. An example of unfolded volume $I(\theta, \varphi, r)$ of a hip joint, visualized in 2D slices. **Left:** a 2-D φ-r slice. **Right:** a 2-D θ-r slice. In both slices, the green line indicates the surface of the femoral head and the red line indicates the surface of the acetabulum. The gap between these two surface corresponds to the joint space of the hip (Color figure online).

4-neighbor system is adopted. The problem is now to find k coupled surfaces such that each surface intersects each column exactly at one voxel. In our case, we expect to detect two adjacent surfaces of a hip joint, i.e., the surface of the acetabulum S_a and the surface of the femoral head S_f. To accurately detect these two surfaces using graph optimization-based approach, following geometric constraints need to be considered:

1. For each individual surface, the shape changes of this surface on two neighboring columns $Col(p)$ and $Col(q)$ are constrained by smoothness conditions. Specifically, if $Col(p)$ and $Col(q)$ are neighbored columns along the $\theta - axis$, for each surface S (either S_a or S_f), the shape change should satisfy the constraint of $|S(p) - S(q)| = |r_p - r_q| \leq \Delta_\theta$, where $r_p = p(\theta_1, \varphi)$ and $r_q = q(\theta_2, \varphi)$ are coordinate values of the surface S (either S_a or S_f) intersecting columns $Col(p)$ and $Col(q)$, respectively. The same constraint could also be applied along the $\varphi - axis$ with a smoothness parameter Δ_φ.
2. For the pair of surfaces S_a and S_f, their surface distance in the same column is constrained. For example, in column $Col(p)$, the distance between these two surface should be constrained in a specified range of $0 \leq \delta_p^l \leq (|S_a(p) - S_f(p)|) \leq \delta_p^u$. In addition, S_f requires to be located below the S_a (as shown in Fig. 5).

To enforce above geometric constraints, three types of arcs are constructed to define a directed graph $G = \{G_a \cup G_s\}$ (see Fig. 6 for details), where G_a and G_s are two subgraphs and each for detecting one surface of S_a and S_f, respectively. For each subgraph, we construct both *intra-* and *inter-* column arcs. We also construct *inter*-surface arcs between two subgraphs G_a and G_s, following the graph construction methods introduced in [11,12].

Intra-column arcs: This type of arcs is added to ensure that the target surface intersects each column at exactly one position. In our case, along each column $p(\theta, \varphi)$, every node $V(\theta, \varphi, r)$ has a directed arc to the node immediately below it $V(\theta, \varphi, r - 1)$ with $+\infty$ weight (Fig. 6 left).

Inter-column arcs: This type of arcs is added to constrain the shape changes of each individual surface S on neighboring columns under a 4-neighborhood system. With two pre-defined smoothness parameters Δ_θ and Δ_φ, we construct these arcs with $+\infty$ weight along both the $\theta - axis$ and the $\varphi - axis$ (Fig. 6 left). In summary, we have arcs:

$$E = \begin{cases} \{< V(\theta, \varphi, r), V(\theta + 1, \varphi, max(0, r - \Delta_\theta)) >\}\cup \\ \{< V(\theta, \varphi, r), V(\theta - 1, \varphi, max(0, r - \Delta_\theta)) >\}\cup \\ \{< V(\theta, \varphi, r), V(\theta, \varphi + 1, max(0, r - \Delta_\varphi)) >\}\cup \\ \{< V(\theta, \varphi, r), V(\theta, \varphi - 1, max(0, r - \Delta_\varphi)) >\} \end{cases} \quad (4)$$

To get a smooth segmentation, we further enforce soft smoothness shape compliance by adding another type of intra-column arcs (Fig. 6 left) [12]:

$$E = \begin{cases} \{< V(\theta, \varphi, r), V(\theta + 1, \varphi, r) > |r \geq 1\}\cup \\ \{< V(\theta, \varphi, r), V(\theta - 1, \varphi, r) > |r \geq 1\}\cup \\ \{< V(\theta, \varphi, r), V(\theta, \varphi + 1, r) > |r \geq 1\}\cup \\ \{< V(\theta, \varphi, r), V(\theta, \varphi - 1, r) > |r \geq 1\} \end{cases} \quad (5)$$

Again we construct these arcs along both the $\theta - axis$ and the $\varphi - axis$ using a 4-neighborhood system. The *a prior* shape compliance smoothness energy that assigned to these arcs are determined by a non-decreasing function $f_{p,q}(|S(p) - S(q)|)$, where $|S(p) - S(q)|$ represent the shape change (determined by the smoothness parameters Δ_θ and Δ_φ) for a surface S on neighbored columns $Col(p)$ and $Col(q)$. We select a linear function $f_{p,q}(|S(p) - S(q)|) = a(|S(p) - S(q)|) + b$, following the method introduced in [12]. Thus, along the $\theta - axis$, we assign a weight a to the arcs. Likewise, for the arcs along the $\varphi - axis$, we assign a similar weight for each arc.

Inter-surface arcs: This type of arcs is added to constrain surface distance between S_a and S_f in each column. In our case S_f is required to be below the S_a. Thus, assuming that distance in column p between surfaces S_a and S_f ranges from δ_p^l to δ_p^u, we add the following arcs (Fig. 6 right):

$$E_s = \begin{cases} \{< V_a(\theta, \varphi, r), V_f(\theta, \varphi, r - \delta_p^u) > |r \geq \delta_p^u\}\cup \\ \{< V_f(\theta, \varphi, r), V_a(\theta, \varphi, r + \delta_p^l) > |r < R - \delta_p^l\}\cup \\ \{< V_a(0, 0, \delta_p^l), V_f(0, 0, 0) >\} \end{cases} \quad (6)$$

where V_a and V_f denote the node in the corresponding column from each subgraph as shown in (Fig. 6 right). For each column p, we have a different distance range (δ_p^l, δ_p^u) that is statistically learned from a set of training data.

By adding all the arcs as described above, we establish a directed graph $G = (V, E)$, where $V = V_a \cup V_f$ and $E = E_a \cup E_f \cup E_s$. Here, V_a and V_f are node sets from each subgraph, E_a and E_f are intra- and inter-column arcs from each subgraph, and E_s is the inter-surface arcs between two subgraphs. In order to detect surfaces based on graph optimization, a new digraph $G_{st}(V \cup \{s, t\}, E \cup E_{st})$ is defined. This is achieved by adding a source node s and a sink node t as well as new edge set E_{st} which includes the edges between nodes in the graph G

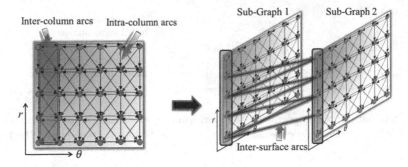

Fig. 6. Graph construction for detecting adjacent two surfaces of a hip joint. An example is presented in 2-D r-θ slice from the unfolded volume $I(\theta, \varphi, r)$. Left: intra-column (black arrows) and inter-column (red and blue) arcs for each subgraph; right: inter-surface arcs to connect two subgraphs. Please note that these two subgraphs share the same nodes as well as the same inter- and intra-column arcs. The inter-surface arcs are constructed between the corresponding two columns which have exactly the same column of voxels in the unfolded volume (Color figure online).

and the nodes of $\{s, t\}$. Then surface detection can be solved using the minimum s-t cuts established by Kolmogorov et al. [22]. We add new edges for the edge set E_{st} following the method introduced in [11]. The most important point here is to assign an appropriate penalty for each edge which is also called $t - link$. As described in [11], the penalty for each $t - link$ is determined by a pre-computed cost of each node. In our method, a carefully designed node cost function is calculated by considering both intensity information and a *prior* information. In the next section, we will introduce how such a cost function is calculated for each graph node.

3.3 Node Cost Function

Node cost function plays an important role for a successful surface detection. In our method, we first encode the boundary information to the cost function using the gradient information of each node following the method introduced in [11]. The negative magnitude of the gradient of the volume $I(\theta, \varphi, r)$ is computed at each voxel as $c_{edge}(\theta, \varphi, r) = -|\nabla I(\theta, \varphi, r)|$. We give each node a weight as:

$$w(\theta, \varphi, r) = \begin{cases} c_{edge}(\theta, \varphi, r) & if \quad z = 0 \\ c_{edge}(\theta, \varphi, r) - c_{edge}(\theta, \varphi, r - 1) & otherwise \end{cases} \quad (7)$$

These weights are then modified by adding three types of constraints from a *prior* information: (1) The generated PA of the pelvis and the femur in the multi-atlas based segmentation stage. (2) Intensity histograms of surface points which approximately indicate the intensity distribution of the points on each surface. They are statistically learned from a set of training data by extracting all the points on manually segmented surfaces from each training data. We learned

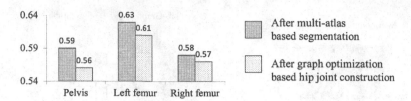

Fig. 7. Evaluation of the segmentation performance after each stage in the present method. The average surface distance (mm) on 10 test images are shown in the figure.

two histograms, one for the acetabulum surface and the other for the femoral head surface. (3) The orientation of the gradient along the $r - axis$, which is determined by a sign function $Sgn(I_i(\theta, \varphi, r) - I_i(\theta, \varphi, r - 1))$, where $I_i(\theta, \varphi, r)$ is the intensity of voxel $V(\theta, \varphi, r)$.

The PA gives the probability of each voxel belonging to a specified bone region (background, pelvis or bilateral proximal femurs). If any voxel have probability close or equal to 1 in the PA, it means that the atlases used for generating PA voted for this voxel, and thus this voxel is more likely to appear inside the bone region rather than on the surface of the bone. Considering that our purpose is to detect the surfaces of the bones, we decrease the weights for such nodes by:

$$w'(\theta, \varphi, r) = \begin{cases} w(\theta, \varphi, r) - h \cdot PA(\theta, \varphi, r), & if \ w(\theta, \varphi, r) > 0 \\ w(\theta, \varphi, r) + h \cdot PA(\theta, \varphi, r), & if \ w(\theta, \varphi, r) \leq 0 \end{cases} \quad (8)$$

where h is a constant value and $PA(\theta, \varphi, r)$ is the probability for a voxel $V(\theta, \varphi, r)$. For the nodes in the subgraph for detecting the surface of the acetabulum, we perform such a modification using the PA of the pelvis. Likewise, we encode information from the PA of the femur for the nodes in the other subgraph.

The intensity distribution of the bone surface points is limited in a specified range. For voxels whose intensity values are in this specified range, they are more likely to appear on the bone surfaces. We increase the weights for these nodes using the associated intensity histograms of surface points that are learned from a set of training data as described above.

$$w''(\theta, \varphi, r) = \begin{cases} w'(\theta, \varphi, r) + m \cdot Hist(I_i(\theta, \varphi, r)), & if \ w(\theta, \varphi, r) > 0 \\ w'(\theta, \varphi, r) - m \cdot Hist(I_i(\theta, \varphi, r)), & if \ w(\theta, \varphi, r) \leq 0 \end{cases} \quad (9)$$

where m is a constant value and $Hist(I_i(\theta, \varphi, r))$ is the corresponding value in the associated histogram for voxel $V(\theta, \varphi, r)$ which have intensity value of $I_i(\theta, \varphi, r)$. Please note that we have learned two intensity histograms, one for surface points of the acetabulum and the other for the surface points of the femoral head. When modifying the weights of nodes in each subgraph, the associated histogram is used.

As shown in Fig. 5, for voxels on the surface of the acetabulum, since the intensity at $V(\theta, \varphi, r)$ is bigger than $V(\theta, \varphi, r - 1))$, the value of the $Sgn(I_i(\theta, \varphi, r) - I_i(\theta, \varphi, r - 1))$ should be positive and we define the orientation of these voxels

Table 1. Surface distance (mm) between automatic and ground-truth segmentation of the bilateral hip joints from 10 CT data. Results after stage I (multi-atlas-based segmentation: MA) and after stage II (graph optimization-based surface detection: GO) are shown, where LA stands for the left acetabulum, LFH for the left femoral head, RA for the right acetabulum and RFH for the right femoral head.

Bone	Stage	CT 1	CT 2	CT 3	CT 4	CT 5	CT 6	CT 7	CT 8	CT 9	CT 10	Average
LA	MA	0.42	0.30	0.24	0.24	0.26	0.30	0.46	0.40	0.29	0.35	0.33
	GO	0.20	0.29	0.21	0.23	0.23	0.17	0.31	0.26	0.26	0.24	0.24
LFH	MA	0.40	0.56	0.41	0.34	0.51	0.36	0.51	0.81	0.38	0.49	0.48
	GO	0.30	0.25	0.24	0.37	0.33	0.32	0.41	0.64	0.31	0.27	0.34
RA	MA	0.43	0.36	0.22	0.33	0.24	0.30	0.48	0.31	0.25	0.32	0.32
	GO	0.23	0.23	0.18	0.30	0.17	0.22	0.22	0.21	0.22	0.30	0.23
RFH	MA	0.40	0.42	0.54	0.29	0.34	0.39	0.55	0.52	0.43	0.53	0.44
	GO	0.41	0.40	0.46	0.36	0.38	0.38	0.45	0.59	0.38	0.28	0.41

as positive too. Similarly, for voxels on the surface of the femoral head, we define their orientation in $r - axis$ as negative. Therefore, for a node in the subgraph for detecting the surface of the acetabulum, if its gradient orientation is not consistent with our definition, we set its weight to 0. For a node in the subgraph for detecting the surface of the femoral head, we perform a similar modification.

After we modify the weight for each node in the Graph G_{st}, we assign penalty for each t-link based on the modified weight using the method introduced in [11]. Our problem is then to optimally detect two surfaces from the constructed graph, which can be solved using the minimum s-t cuts algorithm [20,22].

4   Experiments and Results

We evaluated the present method on hip CT data of 30 patients after ethical approval. The intra-slice resolutions range from 0.576 mm to 0.744 mm while the inter-slice resolutions are 1.6 mm for all CT data. Manual segmentation of all 30 CT data were done by a trained rater. 20 of them were selected as the training data both for the RF regression-based landmark detection and the multi-atlas-based segmentation. The rest 10 datasets (20 hip joints) were used for evaluation.

As for performance evaluation, we computed two different metrics. First, surface distance (SD) between automatic segmentation and ground-truth segmentation are computed after each stage of the present method. Figure 7 shows the average SD which was computed on the entire pelvis and femur regions. More specifically, our method achieves high performance in segmenting pelvis, left proximal femur, and right proximal femur with an average accuracy of 0.56 mm, 0.61 mm, and 0.57 mm, respectively. Furthermore, we also looked at the segmentation accuracy around the hip joint local areas which are important for our target clinical applications. The local evaluation results are shown in Table 1. It is observed from Fig. 7 that the segmentation results of the two stages in the present method are quite close if we evaluate the performance in the entire

Table 2. Comparison of the results achieved by the present method with those reported in the literature.

Method	Preserving hip joint	Average SD (mm)	Average DOC (%)
Lamecker et al. [9]	No	1.80	-
Semi et al. [4]	No	0.70	-
Kainmueller et al. [5]	Yes	0.60	-
Yokota et al. [2]	No	1.10	92.7
Yokota et al. [3]	No	0.98	-
The present method	Yes	0.58	94.7

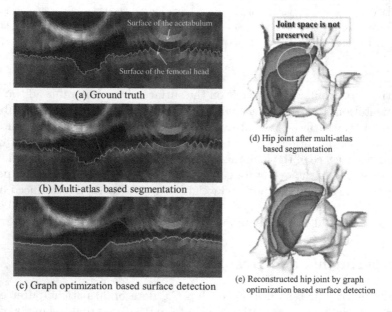

(a) Ground truth

(b) Multi-atlas based segmentation

(c) Graph optimization based surface detection

(d) Hip joint after multi-atlas based segmentation

(e) Reconstructed hip joint by graph optimization based surface detection

Fig. 8. An example of segmenting a hip joint with the present method. Both 2D and 3D visualizations of results from different stages of our method are presented.

regions of the pelvis and the femur. However, when we focus on the local hip joint area, one can find from Table 1 that the graph optimization-based surface detection improves the hip joint segmentation accuracy. Second, we also computed the Dice overlap coefficients (DOC) between automatic segmentation and ground-truth segmentation. The present method achieved a mean DOC of $93.3 \pm 1.1\%$, $95.2 \pm 1.3\%$, and $95.5 \pm 0.8\%$ for pelvis, left femur and right femur, respectively.

We checked whether the present method could preserve the hip joint space and prevent the penetration of the extracted surface models. For all the 20 hip joints that were segmented with the present method, we have consistently found that the hip joint spaces were preserved and that there was no penetration between the extracted adjacent surface models. Figure 8 shows a segmentation example. From this figure, we can clearly see that the graph optimization-based surface detection stage further improve the results from the multi-atlas-based segmentation.

5   Discussions and Conclusion

The goal of the present study is to develop and validate a fully automatic hip joint segmentation approach. Our experimental results showed that the present method not only achieved a good overall segmentation accuracy for both the pelvis and the proximal femur, but also had the advantages of preservation of hip joint space and prevention of the penetration of the extracted adjacent surface models, which are prerequisite conditions to use the segmented models for computer assisted diagnosis and planning of PAO surgery.

The performance of the present method is compared with those of the state-of-the-art hip CT segmentation methods [2–5,9]. The comparison results are summarized in Table 2. From this table, one can see that the performace of the present method is comparable to other state-of-the-art hip CT segmentation methods [2–5,9].

In conclusion, we presented a fully automatic and accurate method for segmenting CT images of a hip joint. The strength of the present method lies in the combination of a multi-atlas-based hip CT segmentation with a graph optimization-based multi-surface detection. The present method can be extended to segment CT data of other anatomical structures.

References

1. Ganz, R., Klaue, K., Vinh, T., Mast, J.: A new periacetabular osteotomy for the treatment of hip dysplasia: technique and preliminary results. Clin. Orthop. **232**, 26–36 (1988)
2. Yokota, F., Okada, T., Takao, M., Sugano, N., Tada, Y., Sato, Y.: Automated segmentation of the femur and pelvis from 3D CT data of diseased hip using hierarchical statistical shape model of joint structure. In: Yang, G.-Z., Hawkes, D., Rueckert, D., Noble, A., Taylor, C. (eds.) MICCAI 2009, Part II. LNCS, vol. 5762, pp. 811–818. Springer, Heidelberg (2009)
3. Yokota, F., Okada, T., Takao, M., Sugano, N., Tada, Y., Tomiyama, N., Sato, Y.: Automated CT segmentation of diseased hip using hierarchical and conditional statistical shape models. In: Mori, K., Sakuma, I., Sato, Y., Barillot, C., Navab, N. (eds.) MICCAI 2013, Part II. LNCS, vol. 8150, pp. 190–197. Springer, Heidelberg (2013)
4. Seim, H., Kainmueller, D., Heller, M., Lamecker, H., Zachow, S., Hege, H.C.: Automatic segmentation of the pelvic bones from CT data based on a statistical shape model. In: Eurographics Workshop on Visual Computing for Biomedicine, pp. 67–78 (2008)
5. Kainmueller, D., Lamecker, H., Zachow, S., Hege, H.C.: An articulated statistical shape model for accurate hip joint segmentation. In: IEEE EMBC 2009, pp. 6345–6351 (2009)

6. Ehrhardte, J., Handels, H., Plotz, W., Poppl, S.J.: Atlas-based recognition of anatomical structures and landmarks and the automatic computation of orthopedic parameters. Methods Inf. Med. **43**, 391–397 (2004)
7. Pettersson, J., Knutsson, H., Borga., M.: Automatic hip bone segmentation using non-rigid registration. In: ICPR 2006 (2006)
8. Ying, X., Jurgen, F., Shekhar, S., Raphael, S., Craig, E., Stuart, C.: Automated bone segmentation from large field of view 3D MR images of the hip joint. Phys. Med. Biol. **58**, 7375–7390 (2013)
9. Lamecker, H., Seeba, M., Hege, H.C., Deuflhard, P.: A 3D statistical shape model of the pelvic bone for segmentation. In: SPIE, vol. 5370, pp. 1341–1351 (2004)
10. Kainmueller, D., Lamecker, H., Zachow, S., Hege, H.-C.: coupling deformable models for multi-object segmentation. In: Bello, F., Edwards, E. (eds.) ISBMS 2008. LNCS, vol. 5104, pp. 69–78. Springer, Heidelberg (2008)
11. Li, K., Wu, X., Chen, D., Sonka, M.: Optimal surface segmentation in volumetric images - a graph-theoretic approach. IEEE Trans. Pattern Anal. Mach. Itell. **28**, 119–134 (2006)
12. Song, Q., Wu, X., Liu, Y., Smith, M., Buatti, J., Sonka, M.: Optimal graph search segmentation using arc-weighted graph for simultaneous surface detection of bladder and prostate. In: Yang, G.-Z., Hawkes, D., Rueckert, D., Noble, A., Taylor, C. (eds.) MICCAI 2009, Part II. LNCS, vol. 5762, pp. 827–835. Springer, Heidelberg (2009)
13. Criminisi, A., Shotton, J., Robertson, D., Konukoglu, E.: Regression forests for efficient anatomy detection and localization in CT studies. In: Menze, B., Langs, G., Tu, Z., Criminisi, A. (eds.) MICCAI 2010. LNCS, vol. 6533, pp. 106–117. Springer, Heidelberg (2011)
14. Lindner, C., Thiagarajah, S., Wilkinson, J.M., arcOGEN Consortium, Wallis, G., Cootes, T.F.: Fully automatic segmentation of the proximal femur using random forest regression voting. IEEE TMI 32, 1462–1472 (2013)
15. Breiman, L.: Random forests. Mach. Learn. **45**, 5–32 (2001)
16. Yang, C., Duraiswami, R., Davis, L.: Efficient kernel machines using the improved fast gauss transform. In: Advances in Neural Information Processing Systems, vol. 17, pp. 1561–1568 (2005)
17. Viola, P., Jones, M.: Rapid object detection using a boosted cascade of simple features. In: CVPR 2001, vol. I, pp. 511–518 (2001)
18. Glocker, B., Komodakis, M., Tziritas, G., Navab, N., Paragios, N.: Dense image registration through mrfs and efficient linear programming. Med. Image Anal. **12**, 731–741 (2008)
19. Chu, C., et al.: Multi-organ segmentation based on spatially-divided probabilistic atlas from 3D abdominal CT images. In: Mori, K., Sakuma, I., Sato, Y., Barillot, C., Navab, N. (eds.) MICCAI 2013, Part II. LNCS, vol. 8150, pp. 165–172. Springer, Heidelberg (2013)
20. Boykov, Y., Veksler, O., Zabih, R.: Fast approximate energy minimization via graph cuts. IEEE PAMI **23**, 1222–1239 (2001)
21. Liu, L., Ecker, T., Schumann, S., Siebenrock, K., Nolte, L., Zheng, G.: Computer assisted planning and navigation of periacetabular osteotomy with range of motion optimization. In: Golland, P., Hata, N., Barillot, C., Hornegger, J., Howe, R. (eds.) MICCAI 2014, Part II. LNCS, vol. 8674, pp. 643–650. Springer, Heidelberg (2014)
22. Kolmogorov, V., Zabih, R.: What energy functions can be minimized via graph cuts? IEEE Trans. PAMI **26**, 147–159 (2004)

Optimal Transportation for Example-Guided Color Transfer

Oriel Frigo[✉], Neus Sabater, Vincent Demoulin, and Pierre Hellier

Technicolor Research and Innovation, Avenue des Champs Blancs,
35570 Cesson-Sévigné, France
oriel.frigo@technicolor.com

Abstract. In this work, a novel and generic method for example-based color transfer is presented. The color transfer is formulated in two steps: first, an example-based Chromatic Adaptation Transform (CAT) has been designed to obtain an illuminant matching between input and example images. Second, the dominant colors of the input and example images are optimally mapped. The main strength of the method comes from using optimal transportation to map a pair of meaningful color palettes, and regularizing this mapping through thin plate splines. In addition, we show that additional visual or semantic constraints can be seamlessly incorporated to obtain a consistent color mapping. Experiments have shown that the proposed method outperforms state-of-the-art techniques for challenging images. In particular, color mapping artifacts have been objectively assessed by the Structural Similarity (SSIM) measure [26], showing that the proposed approach preserves structures while transferring color. Finally, results on video color transfer show the effectiveness of the method.

1 Introduction

Color transfer is the process to modify the color of an *input* image according to the color palette of an *example* image. The color changes could be more or less realistic (or artistic) depending on the choice of the *example* image and the final sought appearance. Image and video color transfer is useful for a variety of computer vision applications. For example, coloring gray scale images, picture contrast change acquired in bad climatic conditions or image denoising using flash/no flash pairs.

In the movie industry, to ensure that a movie has the appropriate color mood, color grading (changes in color, contrast, white balance and hues) is performed manually by the colorist, a highly qualified art professional, who could clearly benefit from automatic and consistent color transfer methods. Similarly, editing tools for large personal photo collections could be improved with example-based

Electronic supplementary material The online version of this chapter (doi:10. 1007/978-3-319-16811-1_43) contains supplementary material, which is available to authorized users.

D. Cremers et al. (Eds.): ACCV 2014, Part III, LNCS 9005, pp. 655–670, 2015.
DOI: 10.1007/978-3-319-16811-1_43

algorithms [8,11], specially considering the last trend of editing sets of multi-contributor images of a given event (party, wedding, *etc.*).

A common drawback of color transfer methods is the strong tendency to create undesired visual artifacts. For instance, existing noise or compression "block effects", that are initially barely noticeable, can become prominent. Hence, in order to achieve automatic color transfer, the considered method must achieve a visually-plausible and appropriate color transformation. Artifacts and unnatural colors should be avoided, while computational space and time complexity should be kept as low as possible. Considering these requirements, in this paper we propose an example-based method for automatic color transfer where the illuminant matching and the transfer of dominant colors of the images are treated separately. Moreover, our method carries out a final regularization of the color transform avoiding new parasite structures in the image. Thanks to this regularization, the color transformation can easily be applied to videos without any color flickering. Experimental video results are included on the supplementary material.

2   Related Work

Reinhard *et al.* [21] were pioneers in establishing the concept of color transfer, with an approach to modify the color distribution of one given original image based on the global color statistics (mean and variance) of an example image in the decorrelated color space $l\alpha\beta$. Other works have proposed global color transfer in terms of non-linear histogram matching [16,17,19] or N-Dimensional Probability Distribution Function (N-PDF) transfer [18]. Removing the inherent artifacts due to color modifications is the main goal of some other works. For example, in [20] a nonlocal filter is studied to remove spatial artifacts.

Related work also include [24] in which the color transfer is defined on color segments given by an Expectation-Maximization adapted algorithm. However their color mapping is essentially different from our color mapping which is based on the Monge-Kantorovitch optimal transportation problem. In [5,6] the color transfer problem is also presented in terms of optimal transportation. Other works adapted the flow-based color transfer representing the colors in the image by compact signatures given by Gaussian Mixture Models [15] or super-pixel segmentation [27].

Another class of methods such as [7,10,23] assumes that there are spatial correspondences to be found between the input and example image, these correspondences being used to derive a color transformation. The assumption of geometrical relationship drastically reduces the scope and genericity of the method.

Few works have introduced semantic constraints in the context of color transfer or color enhancement. In [3], a semantic annotation of input and example images is obtained by training a Support Vector Machines and classifying regions in the image according to a trained model. The method proposed by [13] performs semantic image enhancement based on correspondences between image characteristics and semantic concepts.

Despite the significant progress made since the Reinhard *et al.* seminal paper [21], color transfer remains a challenging problem. Indeed, we think that the current approaches are still limited in some situations (strongly dependent on the selected images) and are prone to create image artifacts. On the one hand, linear color transfer methods are robust and usually do not introduce noise. However, they do not perform well when there are several objects with different colors, since the linear transformation cannot account for the magnitude of color change that is expected. On the other hand, highly non-linear transformations seem to be more robust but at the cost of amplifying noise and introducing undesired structures when a local histogram stretching arises. Besides, all techniques may transform the image with unnatural results. For example, an object receiving non-plausible colors as a green face.

3   Our Approach

In this section, we present two contributions to color transfer: an example-based CAT for illuminant matching (Sect. 3.1) and a color transfer based on automatic color palette associations (Sect. 3.2). These two methods are independent and complementary, and achieve convincing results for challenging images when used together. Moreover, we show how our color transfer can optionally be constrained with semantic attributes like saliency or faces (Sect. 3.3).

In order to limit the aforementioned artifacts, we propose to process separately the luminance and chroma channels of the image. Basically, the luminance channel will be addressed using a novel example-based CAT, accounting for the illuminant change, while the chroma channels will be transformed using optimal transportation. In fact, we have observed a substantial improvement in our results with this approach compared to other color transfer techniques that treat jointly luminance and chroma.

3.1   Example-Based CAT

In [21], it is mentioned that one interesting application for color transfer is to remove undesirable color cast from an image, such as the yellowish colors in photos taken under incandescent illumination. Although this description reminds the color constancy problem, as far as we know, color constancy and chromatic adaptation has not been approached in the color transfer literature. In digital photography, adjusting the lighting is known as white-balance or color-balance and is modified with respect to a standard illuminant. In this work we propose to modify the illuminant of the input image with respect of the example image illuminant.

In most cases, no information is available about the spectral power distribution of the illuminant in the scene. Hence, the solution is to estimate the color of the illuminant (the white point in the scene) based on the digital image. A simple approach to address this problem is to consider a variant of the "grey world assumption" [9], which assumes that the mean value of a natural image tends to be a greyish color corresponding to the color of the illuminant. Formally, given an input image I and an example image E, the goal is to modify I so as to adapt its illuminant to the estimated illuminant of E. For that, we propose the following example-based CAT algorithm:

1. Estimate the white point (illuminant) of image E. *For a given value t (we set $t = 0.3$, more discussion on [9]), the white point of an image is defined as the mean color value of all pixels such that*

$$\frac{|a^*| + |b^*|}{L^*} < t , \tag{1}$$

   where a^*, b^* and L^* denote the pixel coordinates in the CIELAB color space.
2. Estimate similarly the white point of image I.
3. Perform the chromatic adaptation transform (CAT) on I to adapt its white point to the white point of E. This transformation is described below.
4. Repeat Steps 2 and 3 until (a) the maximum number of iterations has been reached or; (b) the I white point has not changed from the previous iteration.
5. Return image I' which has the same geometry of I but with colors adapted to the illuminant of E.

Now, let us describe the CAT transform (Step 3). Let (L_I, M_I, S_I) and (L_E, M_E, S_E) denote respectively the estimated white points in LMS color space. Then, the CAT linear transform is defined as:

$$M_A^{-1} \cdot \text{diag}\left(L_E/L_I, M_E/M_I, S_E/S_I\right) \cdot M_A , \tag{2}$$

where M_A is a CAT matrix[1] that transforms from XYZ to LMS cone space. This transformation rescales the color values of I based on the ratio of input and example white points so that the colors of I appear to have the same illuminant of E.

The algorithm is performed iteratively, hence the user can control the desired degree of adaptation to the example image according to the maximum number of iterations parameter. Experimentally, it was assessed that no more than 30 iterations are needed for an acceptable illuminant adaptation, limiting the risk of over-adaptation.

Figure 1 shows a result of the example-based CAT, where an input image (left) is corrected so as to match the warm cast of an example image (middle column) or the cold cast of another example (right column).

Notice that the example-based CAT depicted here can be used either as a pre-processing step before applying chroma color transfer, or as a standalone technique to perform a smooth color transfer accounting only for the illuminant of the example image.

---

[1] Many CAT matrices exist in literature, such as CAT02, Bradford, CMCCAT2000, Sharp, *etc.* The state-of-the-art CAT02 transformation matrix [14] is used in our work.

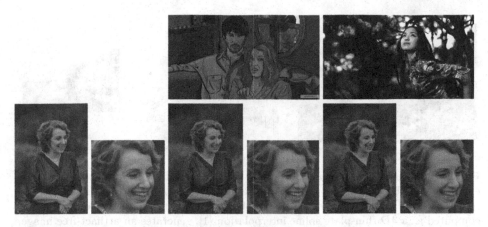

Fig. 1. Illustration of the example-guided chromatic adaptation transform (CAT), where the illuminant of an example image is estimated and transferred to another image. Left column: input image and cropped image around the face. Middle column: result of the example-guided CAT with a warm light estimated from the example drawing on the top. Right column: result of the example-guided CAT with a cold light estimated from the example image on the top. In both cases, the light cast has been estimated and transferred to the input image, specially visible on the face. Images are best viewed on the electronic version.

3.2 Color Chroma Transfer

The intuition of our color chroma transfer method is to use optimal transportation as an efficient tool to map two color distributions approximated by their palettes, regardless of the number of colors in each set. In order to define the color chroma transfer, we propose to use a compact and robust description of the image by its set of meaningful color modes. In particular, we rely on a nonparametric color segmentation known as ACoPa (Automatic Color Palette) [4]. This is a non-supervised technique, so the user does not need to specify the number of color modes in advance, as they are automatically extracted from the color histogram based on meaningful (*a contrario*) peaks. After extracting the set of modes from the input and example images, the color transfer based on the optimal mapping between these two sets of modes is performed (see Fig. 2).

More precisely, given an input image I and an example image E with its set of meaningful modes P (and Q respectively), the mode mapping function $f : P \to Q$ matches each input image mode with one or more example image modes. In practice, we propose a soft assignment method to compute many-to-many matches that minimizes the transportation cost between the set of modes P and Q. An effective solution for this problem comes from the Monge-Kantorovich theory of optimal transportation. Optimal transportation is a well-grounded and solid mathematical field that proves and characterizes the existence of optimal solutions for the transportation problem, minimizing the total displacement cost between two probability distributions. This displacement cost is also known as Wasserstein distance or Earth Mover's Distance (EMD) [22]. Let $P = \{\mathbf{p}_i\}_{i \in [1,m]}$

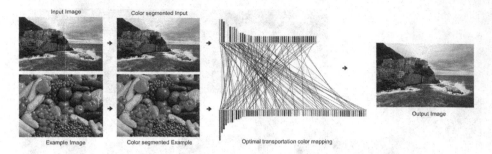

Fig. 2. Overview of the proposed example-guided color transfer methodology. After extraction of the meaningful color palettes [4], a color mapping is estimated as the solution of the optimal transportation problem. Finally, a smooth color transform, computed as a $3D$ thin plate spline interpolation [1], generates an artifact-free image.

and $Q = \{\mathbf{q}_j\}_{j\in[1,n]}$ be the input and example signatures with m and n modes respectively, where $\mathbf{p}_i$ and $\mathbf{q}_j$ are the mode representatives. Each mode representative is a six-dimensional vector $\mathbf{p}_i = (\mu_i^l, \mu_i^a, \mu_i^b, \sigma_i^l, \sigma_i^a, \sigma_i^b)$ composed of its mean and standard deviation (both defined as three-dimensional points in the CIELAB color space).

Let $\mathbf{D} = [d_{ij}]$ be the distance matrix where d_{ij} denotes the distance between modes i and j: $d_{ij} = \|\mu_i - \mu_j\|_2 + \|\sigma_i - \sigma_j\|_2$, where μ_i and μ_j (resp. σ_i and σ_j) are the mean (resp. standard deviation) color values of I and E over the modes i and j. Thus we aim to find $\mathbf{F} = [f_{ij}]$, with f_{ij} being the flow of the assignment between i and j minimizing the cost $\sum_{i=1}^{m}\sum_{j=1}^{n} f_{ij}d_{ij}$, subject to the four following constraints:

$$(1)\quad \forall j \in [1,n],\quad \sum_{i=1}^{m} f_{ij} \leqslant \frac{1}{n}; \qquad (2)\quad \forall i \in [1,m],\quad \sum_{j=1}^{n} f_{ij} \leqslant \frac{1}{m};$$

$$(3)\quad \forall i \in [1,m], \forall j \in [1,n],\quad f_{ij} \geqslant 0; \qquad (4)\quad \sum_{i=1}^{m}\sum_{j=1}^{n} f_{ij} = 1.$$

In practice, the soft assignment matrix $\mathbf{F} = [f_{ij}]$ is obtained using the Simplex linear programming algorithm [22]. After finding $\mathbf{F}$, for each input mode $i = 1, ..., m$, an averaged and weighted mean is computed

$$\widehat{\mu}_i^k = \frac{\sum_{j=1}^{n} f_{ij}\mu_j^k}{\sum_{j=1}^{n} f_{ij}}, \tag{3}$$

where $k = \{a, b\}$ stands for chroma channels in the CIELAB color space. Based on the fact that the human visual system is more sensitive to differences in luminance than in chroma, we only use chroma channels in the color transformation, avoiding artifacts that would occur if the luminance channel was also used. Then, the color transfer between E and I is encoded giving the set of color correspondences $\Upsilon = \left\{(L_i, \mu_i^a, \mu_i^b), (L_i, \widehat{\mu}_i^a, \widehat{\mu}_i^b)\right\}_i$. Now, we have seen in practice that using Υ to apply a piecewise linear color transform to image I would create an output image with new undesired color edges at the color segment borders. Instead, we apply a *smooth* color transform to image I, computed as a $3D$ thin plate splines interpolation [1] using the set of color correspondences Υ in the RGB color space. Hence, it is guaranteed that the color transform applied to I is the best color transform in terms of optimal transportation and smoothness. Thin plate splines interpolation is only used as a final regularization to reduce edge artifacts. Note that the described method could create new colors i.e. colors that are not present in the input nor in the example image. Indeed, color statistics values $\widehat{\mu}_i^k$ are computed based on the weighted average of associated color statistics from the example image (Eq. 3). So, these averaged values can be seen as the result of an additive color mixture which is likely to create new colors. The risk of such color mixture model is to modify the input image with false or non realistic colors. However, this risk is limited thanks to the matching between the I illuminant and the E illuminant (cf. Sect. 3.1). Furthermore, the mapping can be constrained with visual or semantic priors as described in the next section.

3.3   Semantic Constraints on Color Transfer

The color chroma transfer described above does not need any prior knowledge of the input and example images. Nonetheless the color mode mapping can be easily adapted to take into account some semantic information. The main idea is to constrain the color transfer in such a way that modes corresponding to the same semantic components of the input and example images are matched together. Given the two images I and E, let us assume that the color modes can be separated into two classes $P = \{\hat{P} \cup \tilde{P}\}$ (resp. $Q = \{\hat{Q} \cup \tilde{Q}\}$) based on a spatial knowledge as visual attention or object segmentation. Then, two different color mappings g and h are computed as solutions to the bipartite graph matching in terms of Earth Mover's distance such that:

$$g : \hat{P} \to \hat{Q}, \text{ and } h : \tilde{P} \to \tilde{Q}. \tag{4}$$

In order to satisfy these constraints, the optimization is split into two different transportation problems. In the following, we describe how semantic constraints as visual saliency and faces can be easily adapted to this framework.

Saliency. The saliency map is a two-dimensional representation of conspicuity (gaze points) for every pixel in an image. In this work we use the saliency map S deduced from a coherent psychovisual space proposed in [12]. Given the saliency map S of an image, each color mode i is considered as salient if

$$\frac{1}{\sharp R_i} \sum_{x,y \in R_i} S(x, y) > \rho,$$

where R_i is the list of pixel coordinates (x, y) belonging to the color mode i and $\sharp R_i$ is its cardinal. The parameter ρ is typically set to $\rho = 0.7$, meaning that at least 70 % of the pixels belonging to a color mode are salient. Finally, salient modes are mapped to salient modes (and non salient modes to non salient modes), as described in Eq. (4).

Faces. Face detection can be also easily incorporated in the color transfer method. The main objective is to ensure fidelity to skin tones and avoid unrealistic colors being assigned to faces and skin. Here, the popular face detector methodology[2] of Viola *et al.* [25] is used. The face detection is performed on both images I and E. Two cases of interest are considered:

- Faces are found in I and E. In this situation, we impose that the modes extracted from faces in I are mapped with the modes extracted from faces in E to ensure skin tones transfer.
- Faces are found in I, but not in E. In this case, colors corresponding to face and skin are not modified to ensure skin tones fidelity.

4   Results

In this section we present experimental results that illustrate the efficiency of our color transfer method. We strongly recommend the reader to look the figures on the digital version of the paper to appreciate the results. For all the experiments we use the example-based CAT followed by the color chroma transfer. We present four result sections. In Sect. 4.1, a comparison with five state-of-the-art color transfer methods is performed, and an objective assessment of the transformation consistency is proposed. Then, a comparison to a state-of-the-art local color transfer method is presented in Sect. 4.2. We also show the benefit of adding additional semantic constraints in specific situations in Sect. 4.4. Finally, results on video color transfer are presented in Sect. 4.3.

4.1   Evaluation of Image Color Transfer

First of all, we compare our results with five state-of-the-art global color transfer techniques from which authors have made their code available (see Figs. 3, 4 and 5): the seminal method of Reinhard [21], the N-PDF method from Pitié *et al.* followed by the regularization proposed by Rabin *et al.* [18,20]; the variational method from Papadakis *et al.* [17], the histogram reshaping method described in [19]; and the regularized transportation method from Ferradans *et al.* [5]. Note that for the experiment on Fig. 3 (Scotland landscape, firstly appeared on [18]), methods [17,19] produces a result with noise amplification artifacts, while the result of [5] has undesired edges on regions that were originally homogeneous on the input image. On the other hand, our method produces a result without artifacts, similarly to the result obtained by [18,20], with the advantage that we do not need to rely on post-processing image regularization that blurs the output image. For the challenging test pair of Fig. 4, only our

---

[2] Implementation available in the OpenCV library. http://opencv.org/.

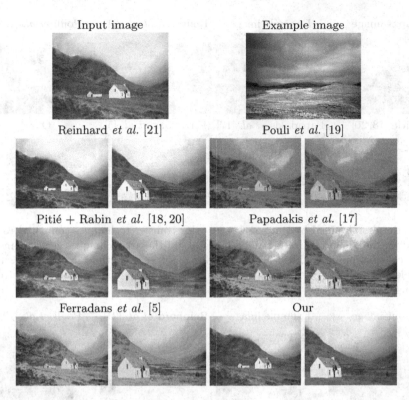

Fig. 3. Results obtained by state-of-the-art color transfer techniques compared to our method for the Scotland image. For this image pair, a zoom shows color mapping artifacts. For instance, the whitish appearance of the house should be preserved, and banding/noise artifacts are visible in the sky. On the contrary, our method generates a visually plausible and artifact-free result. Images are best viewed in color and on the electronic version.

method is able to adapt the low-saturated colors of the original image (Manarola, Italy on a cloudy day) to the colorful palette of the example image (fruits and vegetables) while keeping a natural and convincing result. Note that state-of-the-art methods produce results with lower color dynamics where all the houses and the rock are reddish. Finally, for Fig. 5, the state-of-the-art methods produce color aberrations on the sky and houses, leading to unnatural colors. Color transfer evaluation is not at all straightforward, since it depends on subjective aesthetic preferences. In addition, the purpose of color transfer can be diverse, for example content homogenization or artistic content colorization. However, we argue that color artifacts are not accepted as good results. In Fig. 3, the halos in the sky in [18,20], the uniform reddish color transfer for the fruits in Fig. 4 or the inconsistent and unnatural color transfer (e.g. Fig. 5) are examples of not tolerable color artifacts. We claim that non plausible results lead to the introduction of new structures in the images. Thus, the perceptual metric Structural

Input image   Example image   Reinhard *et al.* [21]   Pouli *et al.* [19]

Pitie [18, 20]   Papadakis *et al.* [17]   Ferradans *et al.* [5]   Our

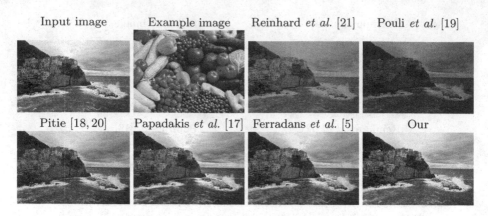

Fig. 4. Results obtained by state-of-the-art color transfer techniques compared to our method for the Manarola/fruits pair. While state-of-the-art techniques generate inconsistent color mapping (reddish houses and halo sky), our method leads to a visually plausible and artifact-free result. Images are best viewed in color and on the electronic version.

Input image   Example image   Reinhard *et al.* [21]   Pouli *et al.* [19]

Pitie [18, 20]   Papadakis *et al.* [17]   Ferradans *et al.* [5]   Our

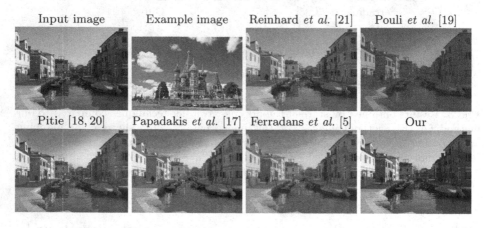

Fig. 5. Results obtained by state-of-the-art color transfer techniques compared to our method for the Burano/moscow pair. While state-of-the-art techniques generate inconsistent color mapping (sky halo, incoherent color on the water), our method leads to a visually plausible and artifact-free result. Images are best viewed in color and on the electronic version.

Similarity (SSIM) [26] is used to assess the artifacts of color transfer, as already proposed in [2,28] and more recently in [10]. Since SSIM was employed with the goal of evaluating the capability of the method to produce an artifact-free result, we computed the SSIM between the luminances of the input and the output images, not taking the color into account. In Table 1, we compare our method with state-of-the-art in terms of artifact generation. Results show that in all cases, our method was able to transfer the color palette while preserving the geometric structure of the image.

Table 1. Comparison of the SSIM measure [26] between input and output images for different color transfer methods, corresponding to Figs. 3, 4 and 5. A SSIM value of 1 denotes that no artifacts have been generated after color transfer. Our method creates no artifacts compared to other techniques.

	Reinhard [21]	Pouli [19]	Pitié+Rabin [18, 20]	Papadakis [17]	Ferradans [5]	Our
Figure 3	0.98	0.87	0.96	0.86	0.68	**0.99**
Figure 4	0.84	0.56	0.94	0.91	0.87	**0.98**
Figure 5	0.83	0.76	0.91	0.78	0.80	**0.98**

4.2 Comparison to Local Patch-Based Color Transfer

In Fig. 6, we compare our results with the method of HaCohen *et al.* [7], which performs color transfer with a transformation based on non-rigid patch correspondences between the input and the example images. Both methods lead to reasonable results, and the objective comparison of methods is difficult. Although [7] has better recovered the specularity of the dress, our result is less saturated (arguably more natural) on the skin, on the hair and on the background. The methods were compared on a larger set of images (results are visible in the supplementary material) and both methods produce comparable results. However, while [7] assumes that the scenes are visually similar which is a very restrictive

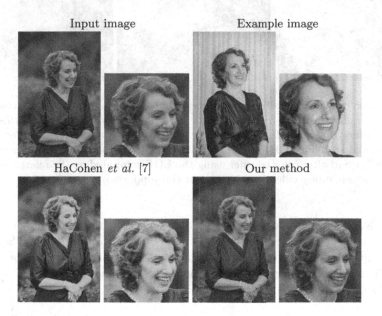

Fig. 6. Results obtained with the color transfer technique of [7] compared to our method. Although [7] uses the restrictive hypothesis of spatial correspondences, we obtain a visually plausible result with a highly generic method.

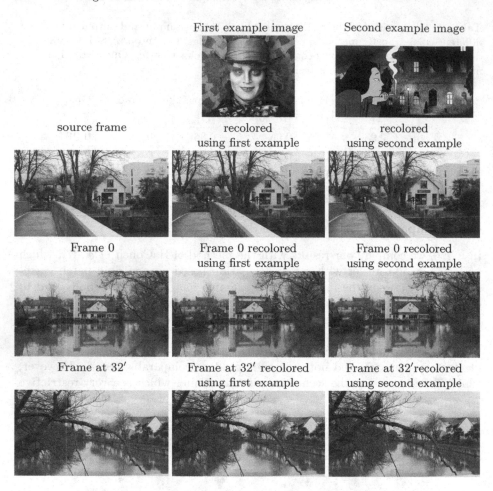

Fig. 7. Video color transfer. Top row shows two possible example images. Second row, from left to right: the input frame chosen to perform the color transfer, and this frame recolored using the example images. For each example, the color transformation is computed and stored as a $3D$ Look-up Table (LUT). Bottoms rows show some video frames before and after color transfer using the LUT computed on the reference frame. The two corresponding videos can be seen in the supplementary material.

hypothesis, our framework is generic and can be used without any *a priori* of the scene. In particular, the method in [7] is ineffective with the images of Sect. 4.1. To sum up, our method is suitable for all types of images and in the case in which the images are very similar, our method is as good as the state-of-the-art method specifically tailored for this specific case.

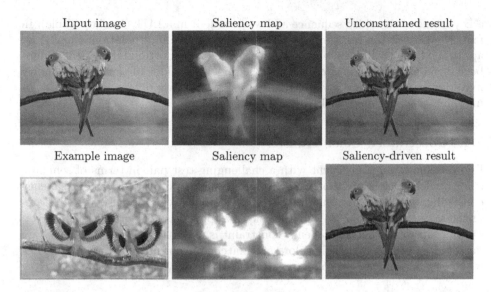

Fig. 8. Illustration of saliency constraint: without the saliency constraint, the colors of the birds are not correctly transferred; while in the saliency-driven color transfer both the birds and the background are assigned to the expected colors.

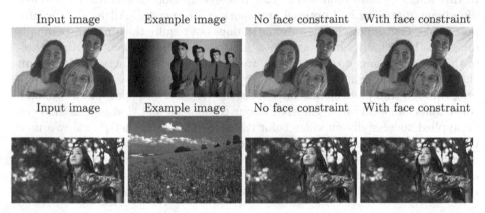

Fig. 9. Top part: Skin tones mapping. From left to right: input and example images containing faces. The result without incorporating face constraint leads to undesirable reddish skin tones, while the result with the face constraint has mapped efficiently the skin tones. **Bottom part: Skin tones fidelity.** From left to right: input and example images. The result without incorporating face constraint leads to non plausible reddish skin tones, while the result with the face constraint has ensured skin tones fidelity (Color figure online).

4.3 Video Color Transfer

The color transfer method presented in this paper can also be used for example-guided video color transfer. The extension of our technique to video is straight-forward. We estimate the color transformation between the example image and a key frame of the video sequence and we encode it in a LUT (Lookup Table). In fact, the LUT is the result of the 3D thin plate spline interpolation. Finally, we apply the LUT to all frames in the video sequence. Unfortunately, videos cannot be shown on this version and we invite the reviewer to look at the supplementary material where videos are visible. Results show that we obtain consistent color mappings without color flickering (Fig. 7).

4.4   Constrained Color Transfer

Figure 8 shows an experiment with a challenging test pair in terms of semantic color associations. Note that when color transfer is performed without saliency constraint, the result is semantically inconsistent. We have also tested state-of-the-art methods [5,17–20] and the color mapping was not semantically correct. On the contrary, when the saliency constraint is used, the birds in the images are detected as salient and their colors are matched accordingly. Finally, in Fig. 9, we illustrate two cases of color transfer constrained by face detection.

5   Conclusion

In this work, we have proposed a color transfer method that is based on global illuminant matching and optimal transport color transfer. All in all, the proposed color transfer method is automatic, does not require the input and example images to be visually similar and does not create visual artifacts as other state-of-the-art algorithms do. Our results present no visible artifacts since we limit changes in the luminance channel and regularize discontinuities in the color mapping through thin plate splines interpolation. We have also shown how semantic constraints can easily be considered in our framework and that our method can be applied successfully on video color transfer. The SSIM metric [26] was used to objectively assess our method compared to other techniques. Since SSIM is a metric limited to the evaluation of artifacts, future work will comprehend on one hand an extensive subjective evaluation of our method and on the other hand the assessment of color transfer quality through objective evaluation criteria.

References

1. Bookstein, F.: Principal warps: thin-plate splines and the decomposition of deformations. IEEE Trans. Pattern Anal. Mach. Intell. **11**, 567–585 (1989)
2. Chiou, W.C., Chen, Y.L., Hsu, C.T.: Color transfer for complex content images based on intrinsic component. In: IEEE Multimedia Signal Processing, pp. 156–161 (2010)
3. Cusano, C., Gasparini, F., Schettini, R.: Color transfer using semantic image annotation. In: IS&T/SPIE Electronic Imaging, International Society for Optics and Photonics, pp. 82990U–82990U-8 (2012)
4. Delon, J., Desolneux, A., Lisani, J.L., Petro, A.: A nonparametric approach for histogram segmentation. IEEE Trans. Image Process. **16**, 253–261 (2007)

5. Ferradans, S., Papadakis, N., Rabin, J., Peyré, G., Aujol, J.-F.: Regularized discrete optimal transport. In: Pack, T. (ed.) SSVM 2013. LNCS, vol. 7893, pp. 428–439. Springer, Heidelberg (2013)

6. Freedman, D., Kisilev, P.: Object-to-object color transfer: optimal flows and smsp transformations. In: Proceedings of the IEEE Conference on Computer Vision and Pattern Recognition (CVPR), pp. 287–294 (2010)

7. HaCohen, Y., Shechtman, E., Goldman, D.B., Lischinski, D.: Non-rigid dense correspondence with applications for image enhancement. ACM Trans. Graph. **30**, 70:1–70:10 (2011)

8. HaCohen, Y., Shechtman, E., Goldman, D.B., Lischinski, D.: Optimizing color consistency in photo collections. ACM Trans. Graph. **32**, 1–10 (2013)

9. Huo, J.y., Chang, Y.l., Wang, J., Wei, X.x.: Robust automatic white balance algorithm using gray color points in images. IEEE Trans. Consum. Electron. **52**, 541–546 (2006)

10. Hwang, Y., Lee, J.Y., So Kweon, I., Joo Kim, S.: Color transfer using probabilistic moving least squares. In: Proceedings of the IEEE Computer Society Conference on Computer Vision and Pattern Recognition (CVPR), pp. 3342–3349 (2014)

11. Jiang, J., Gu, J.: An exemplar-based method for automatic visual editing and retouching of fine art reproduction. In: Color and Imaging Conference, pp. 85–91 (2013)

12. Le Meur, O., Le Callet, P., Barba, D., Thoreau, D.: A coherent computational approach to model bottom-up visual attention. IEEE Pattern Anal. Mach. Intell. **28**, 802–817 (2006)

13. Lindner, A., Shaji, A., Bonnier, N., Süsstrunk, S.: Joint statistical analysis of images and keywords with applications in semantic image enhancement. In: Proceedings of the 20th ACM International Conference on Multimedia, pp. 489–498 (2012)

14. Moroney, N., Fairchild, M.D., Hunt, R.W.G., Li, C., Luo, M.R., Newman, T.: The CIECAM02 color appearance model. In: Color and Imaging Conference, pp. 23–27 (2002)

15. Murray, N., Skaff, S., Marchesotti, L., Perronnin, F.: Toward automatic and flexible concept transfer. Comput. Graph. **36**, 622–634 (2012)

16. Neumann, L., Neumann, A.: Color style transfer techniques using hue, lightness and saturation histogram matching. In: Computational Aesthetics in Graphics, Visualization and Imaging, pp. 111–122 (2005)

17. Papadakis, N., Provenzi, E., Caselles, V.: A variational model for histogram transfer of color images. IEEE Trans. Image Process. **20**, 1682–1695 (2011)

18. Pitié, F., Kokaram, A.C., Dahyot, R.: Automated colour grading using colour distribution transfer. Comput. Vis. Image Underst. **107**, 123–137 (2007)

19. Pouli, T., Reinhard, E.: Progressive color transfer for images of arbitrary dynamic range. Comput. Graph. **35**, 67–80 (2011)

20. Rabin, J., Delon, J., Gousseau, Y.: Removing artefacts from color and contrast modifications. IEEE Trans. Image Process. **20**, 3073–3085 (2011)

21. Reinhard, E., Adhikhmin, M., Gooch, B., Shirley, P.: Color transfer between images. IEEE Comput. Graph. Appl. **21**, 34–41 (2001)

22. Rubner, Y., Tomasi, C., Guibas, L.J.: The earth mover's distance as a metric for image retrieval. Int. J. Comput. Vision **40**, 99–121 (2000)

23. Sheikh Faridul, H., Stauder, J., Kervec, J., Tremeau, A.: Approximate cross channel color mapping from sparse color correspondences. In: The IEEE International Conference on Computer Vision (ICCV) Workshops (2013)

24. Tai, Y.W., Jia, J., Tang, C.K.: Local color transfer via probabilistic segmentation by expectation-maximization. In: Proceedings of the IEEE Conference on Computer Vision and Pattern Recognition (CVPR), pp. 747–754 (2005)
25. Viola, P., Jones, M.J.: Robust real-time face detection. Int. J. Comput. Vision **57**, 137–154 (2004)
26. Wang, Z., Bovik, A.C., Sheikh, H.R., Simoncelli, E.P.: Image quality assessment: from error visibility to structural similarity. IEEE Trans. Image Process. **13**, 600–612 (2004)
27. Wu, F., Dong, W., Kong, Y., Mei, X., Paul, J.C., Zhang, X.: Content-based colour transfer. Comput. Graph. Forum **32**, 190–203 (2013)
28. Xu, W., Mulligan, J.: Performance evaluation of color correction approaches for automatic multi-view image and video stitching. In: Proceedings of the IEEE Conference on Computer Vision and Pattern Recognition (CVPR), pp. 263–270 (2010)

Evaluation of Discriminative Models for the Reconstruction of Hand-Torn Documents

Fabian Richter[✉], Christian X. Ries, and Rainer Lienhart

Multimedia Computing and Computer Vision Lab, University of Augsburg,
Augsburg, Germany
richter@informatik.uni-augsburg.de

Abstract. This work deals with the reconstruction of hand-torn documents from pairs of aligned fragments. In the first step we use a recent approach to estimate hypotheses for aligning pieces from a set of magazine pages. We then train a structural support vector machine to determine the compatibility of previously aligned pieces along their adjacent contour regions. Based on the output of this discriminative model we induce a ranking among all pairs of pieces, as high compatibility scores often correlate with spatial configurations found in the original document. To evaluate our system's performance we provide a new baseline on a publicly available benchmark dataset in terms of mean average precision (mAP). With the (mean) average precision being widely recognized as de facto standard for evaluation of object detection and retrieval methods, our work is devoted to establish this performance measure for document reconstruction to enable a rigorous comparison of different methods.

1 Introduction

Efficient and robust matching of hand-torn document pieces is of great interest in many scientific disciplines, for instance in the fields of forensics, archaeology, and criminal investigation. Successfully aligned pieces can be used in many different scenarios, be it for guiding human users by suggesting partial solutions or for fully automatic reconstruction. For example, according to [1], the winning team of the 2011 DARPA Shredder Challenge partly relied on automatically generated piece-pair recommendations that had to be reviewed by team members for final decision making. While this challenge was focused around extracting information from shredded documents, there is also a famous example for investigators being faced with hand-torn documents: The majority of documents abandoned by the East German secret police in 1989 were simply destroyed by hand, and large efforts have been made to recover their valuable confidential content.

This paper specifically deals with the problem of reconstructing hand-torn documents as a two-stage procedure: In the first part (Sect. 4) we align pairs of pieces based on their outer contours. To do so we extend a recent approach [2] that builds on MSAC [3] (M-estimator SAmple Consensus). We explain how to determine orientation estimates for pieces from the Fourier transform and

© Springer International Publishing Switzerland 2015
D. Cremers et al. (Eds.): ACCV 2014, Part III, LNCS 9005, pp. 671–686, 2015.
DOI: 10.1007/978-3-319-16811-1_44

show how to make use of this prior knowledge in computing alignments. In the second part (Sect. 5) we then focus on the verification of contour regions that become adjacent through alignments. To validate the compatibility of these regions, we compare their local visual characteristics in terms of shape, color, and texture. Our system therefore uses structured output prediction and dynamic programming to infer optimal sequences of matched contour points.

Our main contributions can be summarized as follows:

- Since our approach employs supervised learning, it provides a well-founded way to enrich geometric contour representations by content-based features. Unlike in unsupervised approaches, we can for example integrate color- and texture information without having to adjust thresholds manually.
- We provide two new baselines on a public dataset [4] in terms of overlap-recall curves for the a priori alignment step, and mean average precision (mAP) for the ranking of piece-pairs induced by our structural model. Using these standard performance measures enables an easily comprehensible evaluation and may facilitate comparison of different methods.

2   Related Work

A large number of recent work deals with the reconstruction of two-dimensional objects, for a wide range of applications, e.g., reassembling of jigsaw puzzles [5,6], hand-torn documents and photos [4,7–12], or archaeological findings [13,14].

At the core of most approaches is the feature extraction from polygonal curves that approximate the pieces' outer contours. One popular approach used in many works, e.g., [8,10,11], is the turning function [15] proposed by Wolfson. It allows to represent curves by shape signature strings, which are invariant against rotation and translation. Because of that, this signature is well suited for sub-string matching techniques. For partial contour matching in particular, many approaches [6,10,13,16] use variants of the Smith-Waterman algorithm [17] or similar dynamic programming methods. However, effectively matching contours often requires a priori corner detection [10], as this limits the procedure to sub-segments between two consecutive points with high curvature. Since corners can be difficult to identify [13] in some settings, our approach relies on a different partial contour matching approach [2] based on MSAC [3].

To reassemble the intact document layout, pairs of aligned pieces are commonly ranked before being merged. In the approach of da Gama Leitão et al. [13], the authors compare curvature-encoded fragment outlines by dynamic programming. Since their approach uses progressively increasing scales of resolution, the overall computational complexity can be reduced. For each discrete pairing between two matched outline segments, the authors compute a discriminant value to discard likely incorrect candidates. A quite different route is taken by Zhu et al. [11], who aim to find a globally consistent solution to the reconstruction task. After identifying initial candidate matches based on the turning function, the authors disambiguate these candidates by considering the spatial compatibility of neighboring matches. To obtain a consistent solution, they use an iterative procedure that alternates between gradient projection and merging steps. Another approach closely related to our work is that of Stieber et al. [10]. The authors also apply the Smith-Waterman algorithm to align contour points. However, their reliance on fixed costs for sequence operations seems to be a weak point. In contrast, our system employs supervised learning to obtain the cost model, which also allows to incorporate shape- and content-based local features seamlessly.

3 Dataset of Hand-Torn Documents

Preprocessing. In this work we use the *bdw082010* dataset [4], which consists of 96 hand-torn document pages that show either pictures, text, or both. Our preprocessing closely follows [4] to obtain an approximation of each fragment's contour: From a binary segmentation mask that identifies the foreground region of each piece we determine the set of outer contour points P using the algorithm of Suzuki et al. [18]. Afterwards we apply the Douglas-Peucker algorithm [19] to find a small subset of *support points* $\hat{P} = \{\hat{p}_1, \ldots, \hat{p}_n\} \subseteq P$ that constitutes a less complex description of the piece's contour. By connecting consecutive pairs of support points through line segments one finally obtains a polygon that approximates the exact contour up to a predefined precision.

Ground Truth. As explained in [4] the dataset is partitioned into three disjoint sets: {train}, {val}, and {test}. After the data preprocessing step, each page has been put together manually. Hence the layout of each page as well as the upright orientation of each piece is known. Based on this manual reconstruction, we call two fragments s and t *connected* iff four or more support points have an adjacent counterpart on the other piece. Each such pair of support points is called an *inlier*. We found that examples with less than four inliers are only loosely connected and tend to be negligible for document reconstruction – hence these examples were left out in our experiments.

Throughout the rest of this work, adjacent contour regions are represented by intervals of support points, which are denoted by $R(s)$ and $R(t)$. Each of these intervals contains its inliers as well as all intermediate support points from its respective polygon. Thus each interval defines a polyline that approximates a subsegment of the piece's exact outer contour P. For example, Fig. 5 gives a schematic illustration how inliers and intermediate points between ground truth intervals $R(s) = \{i, \ldots, i+5\}$ and $R(t) = \{j, \ldots, j+4\}$ are used for the extraction of a training example.

4 Partial Contour Matching for Document Pieces

We define partial contour matching between pieces s and t as the task of identifying contour regions $R(s)$ and $R(t)$ along which those pieces were once adjacent

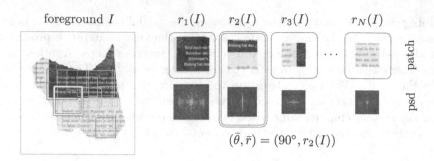

Fig. 1. Left: Patches of different sizes are positioned greedily to cover foreground region I. **Right:** Below a few highlighted patches we show their power spectral density (psd). Estimate $\bar{\theta}$ for the piece's orientation always stems from a single patch $\bar{r}$, which is chosen according to Eq. (2).

in the original document. Our method builds on recent work [2] that introduces a variant of MSAC for aligning pairs of fragments. To determine boundary segments where pieces complement each other, the authors create an initial set of hypotheses (Euclidean transformations) from pairs of candidate inliers. All hypotheses are then verified in a two-step procedure, to identify the one alignment that best recovers the pieces' spatial relationship. The authors show experimentally that incorporating prior knowledge about the pieces' orientations helps to improve alignment results. Besides, discarding inconsistent hypotheses effectively reduces the search space and hence speeds up alignment.

Since the studies in [2] are limited to a simulated text detector for orientation assignment, our first contribution is to introduce a method for estimating orientations in practice. For this purpose we implement the recent approach of Hollitt and Deeb [20], who estimate an image's orientation from its Fourier transform. In Sect. 4.1 we first adapt their method for arbitrarily shaped document pieces. Although this approach gives robust estimates in many cases, it is likely to fail when document pieces convey little or no information about their dominant orientation. As discussed in Sect. 4.2 we overcome this issue by using a discriminative model that identifies incorrect estimates. Finally, we explain in Sect. 4.3 how this classifier is integrated into the alignment procedure.

4.1   Orientation Estimate from Fourier Transform

We briefly recap the technique of Hollitt and Deeb [20] to estimate the dominant orientation of an image. The idea is to find the direction along which the image shows the greatest variation in intensity values, because usually, its *upright direction* is either equivalent or perpendicular to that direction. Instead of working in the spatial domain, the authors apply a Fourier transform on the image to find its dominant orientation in the frequency domain. Therefore let $I(x,y) \in \mathbb{N}^{n \times n}$ denote an image, and let $(\mathcal{F}I)(\xi_x, \xi_y) \in \mathbb{C}^{n \times n}$ be its Fourier transform. Instead of ξ_x, ξ_y, which are conjugate to axes x and y, one can equivalently consider the

Fourier transform to be a function of polar coordinates ξ_ρ, ξ_θ. To find the direction of strongest spatial variation we sum over the *power spectral density (psd)* along θ:

$$g(\theta; I) = \sum_{\xi_\rho} |(\mathcal{F}I)_m(\xi_\rho, \xi_\theta)|^2 \tag{1}$$

The subscript in $(\mathcal{F}I)_m$ refers to a masked output after applying a bandpass filter. By filtering high frequencies we avoid a bias for diagonal orientations. On the other hand, ignoring very low frequencies eliminates the impact of illumination changes.

Aside from bandpass filtering we also need to account for the fact that we are dealing with arbitarily shaped pieces. First of all, we need to ignore strong gradients at the piece's outer contour, which are uninformative for its true upright orientation. On the other hand, some foreground regions may be detrimental for orientation estimation, e.g., if the foreground region partially covers a natural image. To choose an optimal foreground subregion we hence use a sliding window approach to position patches of varying size. As shown in Fig. 1, each patch covers a square region of interest on foreground I. We greedily position patches $[r_i(I)]_{i=1...N}$ one by one, from large to small. Before a new patch is placed, we verify that its mutual overlap with any of the previously positioned patches is not too high. Finally we compute the Fourier transform, separately for each patch, and choose the orientation that shows the strongest spatial variation among all orientations and patches:

$$(\bar{\theta}, \bar{r}) = \underset{\theta, r_i(I)}{\mathrm{argmax}} \left\{ g(\theta; r_i(I))/B_i \right\} \tag{2}$$

In the above equation, bandwidth B_i of the bandpass filter for the i-th patch is used for normalization to avoid a systematic bias for larger patches.

4.2 A Discriminative Model for Orientation Estimates

Since the method discussed so far always yields an orientation estimate, we now turn to learn a discriminative model (SVM) to decide whether an estimate should be trusted or needs to be invalidated.

We found that a strong peak $g(\bar{\theta}; \bar{r})$ is indicative for a robust estimate and hence should not be discarded. In contrast, we need to reject ambiguous orientation estimates in cases where multiple peaks occur (e.g., for textured image regions). We formalize this idea by sampling sums of spectral densities along different directions $\theta \in [\bar{\theta} - 45°, \bar{\theta} + 45°]$ in steps of $\omega = 0.5°$, using Eq. (1). This yields a 181-dimensional descriptor:

$$\boldsymbol{\vartheta}_{ori}[90 \pm i] = g(\bar{\theta} \pm i\omega; \bar{r}) \, / \, g(\bar{\theta}; \bar{r}), \; \forall i \in \{0, \ldots, 90\} \tag{3}$$

By centering the descriptor around $\bar{\theta}$ we make it comparable with descriptors of other patches, because they all have their peak at the same position. Furthermore, we normalize it by $g(\bar{\theta}; \bar{r})$ to obtain a characterization of the relative strength of the peak. To gain partial invariance against shifts we further aggregate descriptor values into blocks of 5°, 15°, and 45°, respectively. For each

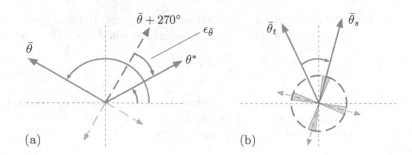

Fig. 2. Left: The minimal relative error $\epsilon_{\bar{\theta}}$ (see Eq. (4)) is computed from orientation estimate $\bar{\theta}$ (modulo 90°) and true orientation θ^*. **Right:** Orientation estimates for two fragments s and t. If both estimates $\bar{\theta}_s$ and $\bar{\theta}_t$ were approximately correct, one could restrict the orientation domain to only four intervals during alignment.

of these $2 \times (9 + 3 + 1)$ blocks we compute its mean and standard deviation and append these values to ϑ_{ori}. Note that all the information needed is readily available from the spectral densities computed in Eq. (2). Finally, to complement this representation from the frequency domain, we extract four Haralick texture features [21] (*angular second moment, contrast, correlation,* and *entropy*) on patch $\bar{r}$ and add them to our final descriptor of $(181 + 26 + 4)$ values.

To distinguish correct from incorrect orientation estimates, we then train a linear support vector machine using SVMLight [22]. For this purpose we categorize patches into positive and negative training examples. Therefore we compute orientations $\bar{\theta}$ of randomly oriented pieces, according to Eq. (2), and keep track of the error regarding their ideal upright directions θ^* that are known from the ground truth. Since our approach works in the frequency domain, $\bar{\theta}$ often fails to give a piece's upright direction; however, it may still identify its correct orientation. We note that in some cases, straight lines in vertical direction can also cause the estimate to be correct modulo 90°. For this reason we categorize training examples based on their *minimal relative error*, which we define by:

$$\epsilon_{\bar{\theta}} = \min_{k} \left\{ \theta^* - (\bar{\theta} + k \cdot 90°) \right\} \in [0°, 45°] \tag{4}$$

It becomes clear from Fig. 2a that this relative error is zero only if orientation estimate $\bar{\theta}$ is correct modulo 90°. We found that our orientation estimates are very precise for the majority of examples. Hence if $\epsilon_{\bar{\theta}}$ is less than 2° we consider the descriptor of patch $\bar{r}$ to be a positive example – otherwise it yields a negative example. Next we discuss different strategies how to incorporate our orientation estimates during alignment, and explain how to adjust the decision threshold of our SVM by performing cross-validation on pairwise examples.

4.3   Experiments

Given two pieces s and t that were digitized with unknown orientation, we first estimate their orientations $(\bar{\theta}_s, \bar{\theta}_t)$ to bring them in presumably upright direction. We denote these rotated fragments by $\bar{s}$ and $\bar{t}$. To actually align the rectified

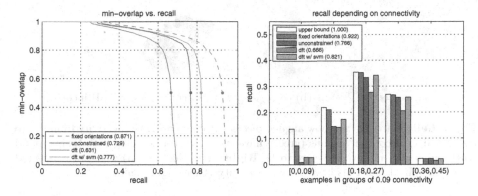

Fig. 3. Left: Evaluation in terms of min-overlap vs. recall. Reducing the search space selectively (dft w/ svm) gives the overall best performance. **Right:** Recall evaluated for different levels of connectivity, at a fixed min-overlap of 0.5. The white bar represents all examples within each connectivity group and hence upper bounds the recall to 1.0.

fragments according to [2], we hold $\bar{s}$ fixed, while computing an Euclidean transformation h that aligns the second piece onto the first. This aligned version of $\bar{t}$ is in the following referred to by $h(\bar{t})$. We now want to discuss different strategies for computing hypothesis h:

Baseline (Fixed Orientations). As baseline for our experiments we compute the best possible hypothesis by treating the upright orientation of both pieces as known and fixed. Since we use the true orientations from ground truth we only have to determine an optimal translation for h.

Unconstrained. As illustrated by the broken circle in Fig. 2b, not using any orientation estimate comes down to considering all relative orientations between pieces. While this approach ensures that the correct hypothesis can not be falsely discarded, it is also computationally very expensive.

Use Estimates from DFT. To accelerate the computation of h, the key idea put forward in [2] is to discard transformations for which the relative orientation between $\bar{s}$ and $h(\bar{t})$ is inconsistent with their estimate. Applying this simple rule speeds up the alignment process significantly due to the limited number of hypotheses that need to be evaluated. As illustrated in Fig. 2b, trusting the estimates (mod. 90°) narrows the search range to only four small intervals. Obviously, this inevitably yields an incorrect result if either estimate is incorrect.

Conditionally Use Estimates from DFT. To get the best of both worlds, we reduce the search space selectively, e.g., when clear lines or text are present on both pieces. Whenever the estimates for both pieces are predicted to be correct by our SVM model, we can safely shrink the hypothesis space as explained above. Otherwise, if either of the two estimates is presumably incorrect (e.g., for pieces showing natural images), we perform an unconstrained search instead.

To optimize prediction performance, we perform cross-validation on all pairwise examples from {train}+{val}. If we encounter pieces with correct estimates,

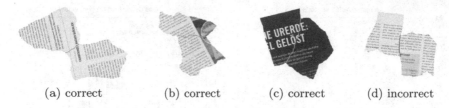

(a) correct	(b) correct	(c) correct	(d) incorrect

Fig. 4. Left: In (a)–(c) we show aligned pieces with increasing connectivity from left to right. Adjacent contour regions (green) have strong mutual overlap with their ground truth segments (min-overlap close to 1). **Right:** The pieces in (d) were not connected in the document and thus have 0 % connectivity (Color figure online).

we want the SVM to give a positive prediction for both. We call this a *joint true positive* example. A *joint false positive* on the other hand is if any of the two examples is assigned an incorrect estimate, but the SVM still classifies both as positive. Based on these outcomes we tune the model threshold to optimize the F_β score, which is a weighted average of precision and recall. While $\beta = 1$ is the harmonic mean of the two, we use $\beta = 0.5$ to attach a higher importance to precision than recall. We feel that precision is more important, because joint false positives likely yield incorrect alignments. After adjusting the threshold, we retrain the model on the full {train}+{val} datasplit and report performances on {test}: There we achieve a $F_{0.5}$ score of 0.9155, which corresponds to a precision of 92.0 % and recall of 89.7 %. Using the so chosen threshold effectively narrows the search from examining all relative orientations (unconstrained) to only four intervals (dft) for 66.9 % of all pairwise examples.

Conclusions and Results. To assess the quality of alignments we follow the methodology in [2] and report performances in terms of min-overlap vs. recall. The *min-overlap* for two aligned pieces takes on values from $[0, 1]$ that reflect how accurately two regions $R(\bar{s})$ and $R(h(\bar{t}))$ match with their ground truth segments. Formally, the min-overlap is defined as

$$min\text{-}overlap(\hat{l}_s, \hat{l}_t) = \left\lfloor \frac{\hat{l}_s \cap l_s}{\hat{l}_s \cup l_s}, \frac{\hat{l}_t \cap l_t}{\hat{l}_t \cup l_t} \right\rfloor, \tag{5}$$

where l_s and l_t are the pieces' adjacent line segments stemming from ground truth intervals $R(s)$ and $R(t)$, and $\hat{l}_s$ and $\hat{l}_t$ are the polylines associated with predictions $R(\bar{s})$ and $R(h(\bar{t}))$, respectively. As illustrated in Fig. 4(a)–(c), correctly aligned pieces yield adjacent contour regions (green) having high mutual overlap with the annotated segments. On the other hand, Fig. 4(d) shows that originally disconnected pieces always score min-overlap 0, because $l_s = l_t = \emptyset$.

In Fig. 3a we finally plot overlap-recall curves for our different search strategies. We note that an unconstrained search gives better results than blindly relying on estimates from the Fourier transform (dft). However, using conditional estimates (dft w/ svm) improves the area under curve from 72.9 % to 77.7 %, at a maximum recall of 82.9 %. We achieve comparable results to those reported in [2], despite not relying on a simulated text detector. Since the dataset contains a substantial number of pieces that lack text and straight lines, assuming reliable orientation estimates for those pieces would be an overly idealized assumption. In these situations our SVM proves to be very reliable in deciding whether or not to shrink the search space, depending on the pieces at hand.

In our second experiment we evaluate recall for different levels of connectivity. In [2] the *connectivity* of two pieces is defined as the length of their adjacent boundary segments relative to their overall contour lengths. As common sense suggests, correctly aligning pieces with low connectivity (Fig. 4a) is inherently more difficult than others sharing large parts of their boundaries (Fig. 4c). This claim is substantiated by the plot in Fig. 3b, which shows that our alignment mostly fails when facing low-connectivity examples (0 %–18 %). In this scenario, using the SVM clearly improves the recall over an unconstrained search. For high-connectivity examples (18 %–45 %), the SVM still performs on a par, despite being much faster due to the inherently smaller hypothesis space.

5   Ranking Sequences by Structured Output Prediction

To quantify the compatibility of adjacent contour regions we learn a stuctured prediction model that incorporates contour information as well as content-based local features. In Sects. 5.1 and 5.2 we formulate our prediction problem and give details about the model. Afterwards in Sect. 5.3 we briefly introduce the dynamic programming algorithm used for solving the inference task at training- and test time. Finally in Sect. 5.4 we discuss how to train the structural support vector machine, before concluding the paper with an evaluation in Sect. 5.5.

5.1   Structured Output Prediction

As introduced before, we denote by $\bar{s}$, $h(\bar{t})$ two aligned fragments that become adjacent along intervals $R(\bar{s})$ and $R(h(\bar{t}))$. Motivated by the protein alignment model of Yu et al. [23], let us first define a *sequence* $y \in \mathcal{Y}$ between two contour regions as list of subsequent operations $y = (y^1, \ldots, y^{|y|})$. Each of these elements corresponds to exactly one *operation* between the two pieces. In the ideal case, a sequence is only composed of *matches* between support points, i.e., a point from the first polygon becomes associated with one from the second polygon. To score any sequence defined over output space $\mathcal{Y}$ we next define a linear function

$$\Omega_w(y; R(\bar{s}), R(h(\bar{t}))) = w \cdot \Psi(y; R(\bar{s}), R(h(\bar{t}))) , \qquad (6)$$

in which $[\cdot]$ denotes the dot product, w is the cost model that is to be learned, and $\Psi(y; R(\bar{s}), R(h(\bar{t})))$ is a joint feature vector of fixed size that describes the structured output y on intervals $R(\bar{s})$, $R(h(\bar{t}))$. To rank hypothesis h that aligns piece t onto s, we aim to find the most promising sequence y^* among all possible sequences along the contour regions:

$$y^* = \underset{\hat{y} \in \mathcal{Y}}{\operatorname{argmax}} \left\{ \Omega_w(\hat{y}; R(\bar{s}), R(h(\bar{t}))) \right\} \qquad (7)$$

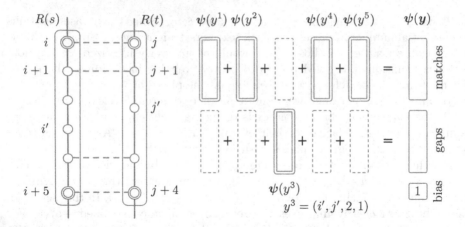

Fig. 5. Left: Schematic illustration of a ground truth sequence of length five, with four match operations (green). In between, gap y^3 (red) spans over two support points on $R(s)$ and one point on $R(t)$, respectively. According to Eq. (8), descriptors for individual operations sum up to the sequence's descriptor, as illustrated on the righthand side (Color figure online).

As we will see shortly in Sect. 5.3, we are able to find this optimal sequence regarding model w by dynamic programming.

5.2 Decomposition of Sequences into Operations

We begin by motivating the *match* operation, which associates one support point from piece s with another on piece t. For instance, we write $y^k = (i', j', 0, 0)$ to associate support point $i' \in R(s)$ with $j' \in R(t)$. The latter two 0's indicate that a match operation does not affect any points other than i' and j'. Intuitively, we only want to create a match if i' has been adjacent to j' in the original document (i.e., an inlier). When dealing with real-world documents however, pieces do not always have well aligned support points.

To account for this we complement matches with *gap* operations, which allow to skip (possibly multiple) support points on either of the two fragments. A gap is denoted by $y^k = (i', j', \delta_s, \delta_t)$ to indicate that immediately before i' and j', δ_s and δ_t many points are omitted, respectively. Following [23] we define a joint feature descriptor that is linear in its operations. The descriptor for the entire sequence is decomposed into the sum over descriptors $\psi(y^k)$ for individual operations:

$$\Psi(y) = \left[\sum_{k=1}^{|y|} \psi(y^k), 1 \right] \qquad (8)$$

A constant 1 is appended for learning a global bias in our model. For notational simplicity we omit contour ranges, e.g., by writing $\Psi(y) \equiv \Psi(y; R(s), R(t))$ in short. An example for a sequence that is decomposed into its individual operations is given in Fig. 5. Since one operation can either be a match or a gap, it is possible to split the descriptor from Eq. (8) into blocks. Using our simplified notation we write $\psi(y^k) = [\psi_M(y^k), \psi_G(y^k)]$, where subscripts in ψ_M and ψ_G refer to match and gap, respectively. Note that depending on the operation, only one descriptor is set, while the other one is initialized to $\mathbf{0}$. Each descriptor reflects the compatibility of only those parts of $R(s)$ and $R(t)$ that are affected by the respective operation. Analogous to the descriptor, our model decomposes into $w = [w_M, w_G, w_B]$. Due to space limitations we keep the discussion about implementation details short:

Match Operation. The descriptor for a match operation $y^k = (i', j', 0, 0)$ describes the compatibility of support point i' on $R(s)$ to j' on $R(t)$. In Eq. (9) the first two elements introduce an absolute- and a relative offset. The latter is set to the reciprocal of the minimum over contour lengths $R_s = |R(s)|$ and $R_t = |R(t)|$. This effectively rewards matches between short contour intervals stronger than for long ones.

The remaining component $d_M(y^k)$ introduces a set of dissimilarities computed from a multimodal feature representation. These values can be interpreted as the inherent cost imposed on matching support points. From a geometric perspective, we determine the points' dissimilarity in terms of their local polygonal approximation (line length and enclosed angle), as well as their spatial proximity after alignment through hypothesis h. In addition we use three content-based features, introduced in [4], to represent shape, color and texture within the vicinity around each point. For each feature channel we compute a dissimilarity value from the feature descriptors. All dissimilarities[1] are stacked into vector $d_M(y^k)$, which is finally appended to the offsets to give our *match descriptor*:

$$\psi_M(y^k) = [1, 1/\lfloor R_s, R_t \rfloor, -d_M(y^k)] \tag{9}$$

Gap Operation. Gaps allow us to deal with noise in the contour approximation. The principle idea is that each gap operation $y^k = (i', j', \delta_s, \delta_t)$ is delimited by two matches. For example, the gap y^3 in Fig. 5 is immediately followed by a match $y^{k+1} = (i' + 1, j' + 1, 0, 0)$, and it is preceded by a second match $y^{k-1} = (i' - \delta_s, j' - \delta_t, 0, 0)$. Analogous to a match, the first two values in Eq. (10) introduce offsets to learn a flat penalty. Since gaps should always have a negative contribution to the sequence score, those offsets have a negative sign.

In the second component we want to penalize long gaps and those that are uneven in size (in terms of δ_s and δ_t). Therefore we introduce two dissimilarity values $\delta_s + \delta_t$ and $\lceil \delta_s, \delta_t \rceil - \lfloor \delta_s, \delta_t \rfloor$. Furthermore, we add dissimilarities to encode the divergence of the pieces' polygon approximations along the gap regions. Once again, all dissimilarities[1] are combined into a vector $d_G(y^k)$. Our *gap descriptor* is obtained by stacking the dissimilarity vector onto the gap penalty offsets:

$$\psi_G(y^k) = [-1, -1/\lfloor R_s, R_t \rfloor, -d_G(y^k)] \tag{10}$$

---

[1] Dissimilarities are computed from feature-dependent kernel functions that yield positive real numbers within comparable value ranges.

5.3   Inference via Dynamic Programming

Assuming two adjacent contour regions $R(s)$ and $R(t)$ we now introduce a modified variant of the Smith-Waterman algorithm [17] to determine the best sequence along these intervals. We found those regions $R(s) = \{i, \ldots, i + R_s - 1\}$ and $R(t) = \{j, \ldots, j + R_t - 1\}$ to provide very reliable estimates for delimiting sequences – hence we restrict each sequence to start with a match in (i, j) and end with a match in $(i + R_s - 1, j + R_t - 1)$.

Since each sequence is decomposable into individual operations, one can incrementally extend sequence prefixes into longer sequences. Therefore we append only one operation at a time to an existing prefix. By $p[i', j']$ we refer to the score of the prefix that starts in (i, j) and ends in (i', j'). To compute this score one has to choose the operation that yields the overall highest score for $p[i', j']$. That is, we either append a match operation with score

$$p[i', j'] = p[i' - 1, j' - 1] + \boldsymbol{w}_M \cdot \boldsymbol{\psi}_M((i', j', 0, 0)), \tag{11}$$

or else introduce a gap if

$$p[i', j'] = \max_{\delta_s, \delta_t} \left\{ p[i' - \delta_s, j' - \delta_t] + \boldsymbol{w}_G \cdot \boldsymbol{\psi}_G((i', j', \delta_s, \delta_t)) \right\} \tag{12}$$

is a higher score. By performing a traceback from the last to the first match we get a sequence that fully extends over intervals $R(s)$ and $R(t)$. Note that the global bias w_B has to be added only once for the first match in (i, j) as each prefix builds upon this initial operation.

5.4   Learning Problem

Learning cost model $\boldsymbol{w}$ is treated as regularized empirical risk minimization problem. Our training set $\{(\boldsymbol{x}_1, \boldsymbol{z}_1), \ldots, (\boldsymbol{x}_N, \boldsymbol{z}_N)\}$ consists of pairs of fragments $\boldsymbol{x}_i = (s_i, t_i)$ and annotations $\boldsymbol{z}_i = (l_i, \boldsymbol{y}_i)$. Labels $l_i \in \{-1, +1\}$ are needed to distinguish positive from negative examples. For positive (connected) examples, their correct sequences $\boldsymbol{y}_i$ are part of ground truth data. Pieces from negative examples on the other hand do not share a common border in the original document – thus we align them once in advance to also infer non-empty sequences. Using the hinge loss we obtain the following optimization problem:

$$\operatorname*{argmin}_{\boldsymbol{w}, \xi_i \geq 0} \left\{ \frac{1}{2} \|\boldsymbol{w}\|^2 + C \sum_i \xi_i \right\} \tag{13}$$

$$\text{s.t.} \quad \forall \boldsymbol{x}_i \in P_{pos} : \boldsymbol{w} \cdot \boldsymbol{\Psi}(\boldsymbol{y}_i; R(s_i), R(t_i)) \geq +1 - \xi_i$$

$$\forall \boldsymbol{x}_i \in P_{neg}, \forall \hat{\boldsymbol{y}}_i : \boldsymbol{w} \cdot \boldsymbol{\Psi}(\hat{\boldsymbol{y}}_i; R(\bar{s}_i), R(h(\bar{t}_i))) \leq -1 + \xi_i$$

$$\boldsymbol{w}_M, \boldsymbol{w}_G \geq \boldsymbol{0}$$

This formulation establishes one margin constraint on each example, whose violation yields a positive slack value ξ_i that is penalized in the objective function. Parameter C balances these training errors versus the model's capability of generalizing beyond training examples.

Table 1. Left: Performance evaluation for different feature combinations. **Right:** Evaluation of the ranking capabilities of our structural SVM in terms of (i) mean average precision (mAP), and (ii) mean accumulated cost (mAC) from [4]. See text for details.

Feature evaluation	16 pieces	Ranking performance	16 pieces	24 pieces[a]	32 pieces[a]
mAP (all features)	**0.7906**	mAP	**0.7906**	**0.6626**	**0.5835**
mAP (base)	0.7252	mAP (w/ pruning)	0.9903	0.8962	0.8740
mAP (base w/ shape)	0.7258	mAP (w/ pruning + overlap)	0.9917	0.9601	0.9462
mAP (base w/ color)	0.7754	mAC (w/ pruning)	0.0113	0.1193	0.1092
mAP (base w/ texture)	0.7895	mAC (w/ pruning + overlap)	0.0113	0.0493	0.0350
		mAP [4]	**0.7341**	**0.5932**	**0.5374**
		mAC [4]	0.0109	0.0380	0.0378

[a]For 24 and 32 pieces the bdw082010 test set contains only 12 pages.

To train our model we use the stochastic gradient descent solver from [24]. After obtaining an initial model from a moderate number of examples, we iteratively infer new hard negative examples using the dynamic programming method introduced in Sect. 5.3. We continue to re-train the model from a cache of hard examples until either (i) a fixed number of iterations is reached, or (ii) no new hard negative examples can be found.

5.5 Experiments

Despite the interest of researchers on this topic, related work reporting quantitative results on a standardized dataset is sparse. Thus we provide a reproducible baseline on the publically available bdw082010 dataset (see Sect. 3). The test set of this dataset consists of $M = 48$ magazine pages, which have been torn into N pieces each. Since each page contributes $(N^2 - N)/2$ unique piece pairs, the test set consists of $M \cdot (N^2 - N)/2$ examples in total. We first align each pair of pieces and then assign a compatibility score (see Eq. (6)) according to the predicted optimal sequence. An example is positive if its pieces were connected in the original document, and only aligned pieces with min-overlap 0.5 or higher are considered to be true positives. For our experiments we treat each individual page as "*query*", and examples from that very page are ranked according to their scores. From the resulting ranked lists we compute the average precision (AP) for each page, and finally the mean average precision (mAP) over the entire test set with 48 queries in total. We argue that the mAP is indicative for the performance of many approaches [4,10–12], as they all rely on successively merging the most compatible pieces.

In our first set of experiments we evaluate the importance of content-based features. Using only information from the pieces' polygons in our match descriptor (Eq. (9)) yields 72.5 % mAP. Next we augment this basic representation with either shape-, color-, or texture information. As can be seen in Table 1 (left), we do not gain much by adding shape information. This is because alignments are very accurate and hence shape dissimilarities add only little discriminativeness. However, using color or texture information results in substantial performance

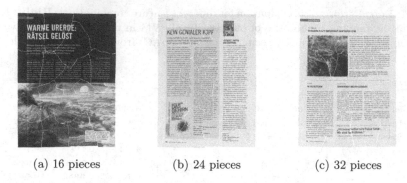

(a) 16 pieces   (b) 24 pieces   (c) 32 pieces

Fig. 6. Examples for pages that are reconstructed only from pairwise alignments.

improvements to 77.5 % and 78.9 %, respectively. A combination of all local features gives the overall best performance with 79.1 % mAP. As can also be seen from the table, the mAP declines with an increasing number of pieces per page. This comes at no surprise, as the number of negative (disconnected) examples grows quadratically, while the number of positive examples only increases approximately linearly with N. As summarized in Table 1, we outperform previous work [4] on this dataset in terms of mAP, for all degrees of fragmentation.

In the second set of experiments we analyze how mAP relates to the quality of individually reconstructed pages. As explained in [4], the layout of each page can be recovered by constructing a spanning tree from alignments (edges) between pairs of pieces (nodes). Using our compatibility score for the edge weights we create a maximum spanning tree using Kruskal's algorithm [25]. To reconstruct the document we retain only those alignments that correspond to spanning tree edges. This effectively prunes all but $N-1$ alignments, hence why the results are named mAP (w /pruning) in Table 1. Again we compute the AP, separately for each page, and report the mAP over all 48 pages. Using all features combined we achieve 99.0 % for $N = 16$, which means that only very few alignments were false positives. In Fig. 6 we give examples for pages that were reconstructed very accurately just from local alignments between pairs of pieces. To further improve our reconstruction results (mAP w/ pruning + overlap), we augment our spanning tree algorithm with a geometric verification that invalidates alignments resulting in overlapping pieces. While its effect is less pronounced for 16 pieces per page, we note that for $N = 32$ the mAP increases from 87.4 % to 94.6 %.

Finally, we report results regarding a complementary performance measure that was put forward with the release of the dataset [4]. The mAC in Table 1 corresponds to the median over the mean accumulated costs per page. Intuitively, this value is an indicator for the effort of repositioning pieces within an existing solution, according to the ground truth page layout. Despite that our preliminary postprocessing does not yet account for evidence from previous alignments, our approach gives competitive results compared to those obtained with a revised implementation of [4]. Although differences in terms of mAC are seemingly insignificant, a comparison by mAP clearly proves the superiority of our method.

We conclude that mAP makes for a rigorous and transparent comparison of results, because prediction outcomes (true positives and false positives) have an immediate interpretation, just as for object detection and retrieval methods.

References

1. Geller, T.: Darpa shredder challenge solved. Commun. ACM **55**, 16–17 (2012)
2. Richter, F., Ries, C.X., Romberg, S., Lienhart, R.: Partial contour matching for document pieces with content-based prior. In: IEEE International Conference on Multimedia and Expo (2014)
3. Torr, P.H.S., Zisserman, A.: Mlesac: a new robust estimator with application to estimating image geometry. Comput. Vis. Image Underst. **78**, 138–156 (2000)
4. Richter, F., Ries, C.X., Cebron, N., Lienhart, R.: Learning to reassemble shredded documents. IEEE Trans. Multimedia **15**, 582–593 (2012)
5. Yao, F., Shao, G.: A shape and image merging technique to solve jigsaw puzzles. Pattern Recogn. Lett. **24**, 1819–1835 (2003)
6. Bunke, H., Bühler, U.: Applications of approximate string matching to 2D shape recognition. Pattern Recogn. **26**, 1797–1812 (1993)
7. Biswas, A., Bhowmick, P., Bhattacharya, B.B.: Reconstruction of torn documents using contour maps. In: IEEE International Conference on Image Processing, vol. 3, pp. 517–520 (2005)
8. Zhu, L., Zhou, Z., Zhang, J., Hu, D.: A partial curve matching method for automatic reassembly of 2d fragments. In: Huang, D.-S., Li, K., Irwin, G.W. (eds.) ICIC 2006. LNCIS, vol. 345, pp. 645–650. Springer, Heidelberg (2006)
9. Justino, E., Oliveira, L.S., Freitas, C.: Reconstructing shredded documents through feature matching. Forensic Sci. Int. **160**, 140–147 (2006)
10. Stieber, A., Schneider, J., Nickolay, B., Krüger, J.: A contour matching algorithm to reconstruct ruptured documents. In: Goesele, M., Roth, S., Kuijper, A., Schiele, B., Schindler, K. (eds.) Pattern Recognition. DAGM, vol. 6376, pp. 121–130. Springer, Heidelberg (2010)
11. Zhu, L., Zhou, T., Hu, D.: Globally consistent reconstruction of ripped-up documents. IEEE Trans. Pattern Anal. Mach. Intell. **30**, 1–13 (2008)
12. Cao, S., Liu, H., Yan, S.: Automated assembly of shredded pieces from multiple photos. In: IEEE International Conference on Multimedia and Expo, pp. 358–363 (2010)
13. da Gama Leitão, H.C., Stolfi, J.: A multiscale method for the reassembly of two-dimensional fragmented objects. IEEE Trans. Pattern Anal. Mach. Intell. **24**, 1239–1251 (2002)
14. Papaodysseus, C., Panagopoulos, T., Exarhos, M., Triantafillou, C., Fragoulis, D., Doumas, C.: Contour-shape based reconstruction of fragmented, 1600 BC wall paintings. IEEE Trans. Sig. Process. **50**, 1277–1288 (2002)
15. Wolfson, H.J.: On curve matching. IEEE Trans. Pattern Anal. Mach. Intell. **12**, 483–489 (1990)
16. Chen, L., Feris, R., Turk, M.: Efficient partial shape matching using smith-waterman algorithm. In: CVPR Workshop (2008)
17. Smith, T.F., Waterman, M.S.: Identification of common molecular subsequences. J. Mol. Biol. **147**, 195–197 (1981)

18. Suzuki, S., Abe, K.: Topological structural analysis of digital binary images by border following. Comput. Vis. Graph. Image Process. **30**, 32–46 (1985)
19. Douglas, D., Peucker, T.: Algorithms for the reduction of the number of points required to represent a digitized line or its caricature. Can. Cartographer **10**, 112–122 (1973)
20. Hollitt, C., Deeb, A.S.: Determining image orientation using the hough and fourier transforms. In: Proceedings of the 27th Conference on Image and Vision Computing, pp. 346–351 (2012)
21. Haralick, R.M., Shanmugam, K., Dinstein, I.: Textural features for image classification. IEEE Trans. Syst. Man Cybern. **SMC–3**, 610–621 (1973)
22. Joachims, T.: Advances in Kernel Methods - Support Vector Learning. MIT Press, Cambridge (1999)
23. Yu, C.J., Joachims, T., Elber, R., Pillardy, J.: Support vector training of protein alignment models. J. Comput. Biol. **15**, 867–880 (2008)
24. Felzenszwalb, P.F., Girshick, R.B., McAllester, D., Ramanan, D.: Object detection with discriminatively trained part based models. IEEE Trans. Pattern Anal. Mach. Intell. **32**, 1627–1645 (2010)
25. Kruskal, J.: On the shortest spanning subtree and the traveling salesman problem. Proc. Am. Math. Soc. **7**, 48–50 (1956)

Hand Segmentation with Structured Convolutional Learning

Natalia Neverova[1,2]($\boxtimes$), Christian Wolf[1,2], Graham W. Taylor[3],
and Florian Nebout[4]

[1] CNRS, Université de Lyon, Lyon, France
[2] INSA-Lyon, LIRIS, UMR5205, 69621 Lyon, France
{natalia.neverova,Christian.Wolf}@liris.cnrs.fr
[3] University of Guelph, Guelph, Canada
gwtaylor@uoguelph.ca
[4] Awabot, Lyon, France
florian.nebout@awabot.com

Abstract. The availability of cheap and effective depth sensors has resulted in recent advances in human pose estimation and tracking. Detailed estimation of hand pose, however, remains a challenge since fingers are often occluded and may only represent just a few pixels. Moreover, labelled data is difficult to obtain. We propose a deep learning based-approach for hand pose estimation, targeting gesture recognition, that requires very little labelled data. It leverages both unlabeled data and synthetic data from renderings. The key to making it work is to integrate structural information not into the model architecture, which would slow down inference, but into the training objective. We show that adding unlabelled real-world samples significantly improves results compared to a purely supervised setting.

1 Introduction

We present a new method for hand pose estimation from depth images targeting gesture recognition. We focus on *intentional* gestures, bearing *communicative function*, with an emphasis on the recognition of fine-grained and smooth gestures. In particular, our aim is to go beyond classification and estimate hand motion with great accuracy, allowing for richer human-computer interactions. From an application perspective, this ensures a tight coupling between users and objects of interest, for instance a cursor, or a manipulated virtual object.

Most existing methods are based on the estimation of articulated pose of the body or the hands. Made possible by the introduction of cheap and reliable consumer depth sensors, these representations have revolutionized the field, effectively putting visual recognition into the hands of non-specialists in vision. While the robust estimation of body joints is now possible in real time, at least in controlled settings [1], most systems provide coarse body joints and do not give the positions of individual joints of the hand. This restricts applications to full body motion, whereas fine-grained interaction requires hand pose estimation.

© Springer International Publishing Switzerland 2015
D. Cremers et al. (Eds.): ACCV 2014, Part III, LNCS 9005, pp. 687–702, 2015.
DOI: 10.1007/978-3-319-16811-1_45

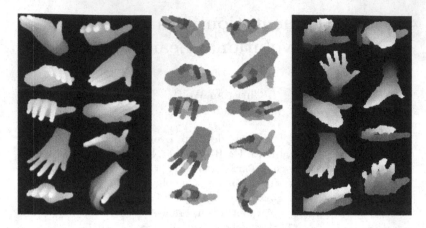

Fig. 1. Our model learns from labeled synthetic data and unlabeled real data. Left: Synthetic depth input images. Middle: Ground truth for synthetic input. Right: Real depth data.

Estimating hand pose is inherently more difficult than full body pose. Given the low resolution of current sensors and the strong noise they produce, fingers usually are composed of only a few pixels. To make matters worse, individual fingers frequently are not discernible. Existing work is mostly applicable in situations where the hands are close to the sensor, which is suited to applications where the user interacts with a computer he or she is close to or sitting in front of. However, applications in domotics, mobile robotics and games, to cite a few, do not fall into this category.

One way to address these issues is to add strong spatial and structural priors or hard constraints, for instance by fitting an articulated model to the data [2]. The computational complexity of the underlying optimization is a disadvantage of this solution. Machine learning has a preponderant role, where most solutions estimate joint positions through an intermediate representation based on hand part segmentation [3–5], or direct regression of finger joint positions [6], or both [5]. However, methods based on learning are hungry for labelled training data, which is difficult to come by. This is especially true for hand pose estimation, where manual annotation of both joint positions and finger parts is difficult.

Existing work deals with this issue by including priors, for instance by including structural information combining the learned predictions with graphical models [7]. Transductive learning is an alternative, where a few labelled samples are combined with a large amount of unlabelled samples, and a transfer function between both sets is learned [5].

In this work we tackle this problem in a structured machine learning setting by segmenting hands into parts. In a semi-supervised context, a deep convolutional network is trained on a large dataset of labelled synthetic hand gestures rendered as depth images, as well as unlabelled real depth images acquired with a consumer depth sensor (Fig. 1). The main contribution of this paper is the way in which structural information is treated in the learning process. Instead of combining a learned prediction model with a structured model, for instance a graphical model, we integrate structural information directly into the learning algorithm aiming to improve the prediction model. As as consequence, at test time, pixels are classified independently, keeping the advantages of low computational complexity and retaining the ability to parallelize.

The information integrated into the training procedure is related to prior information which can be assumed on a segmented image. Our method is based on two contributions. Firstly, contextual information is extracted from local context in unlabelled samples through a model trained on synthetic labelled examples. Secondly, similar to body part maps, ground truth hand part segmentation maps are assumed to feature a single connected region per part, which commonly holds ignoring rare exceptions due to severe self occlusion. We show that this information can be formalized and leveraged to integrate unlabelled samples into the training set in a semi-supervised setting.

Although we focus on the application of hand pose estimation, the proposed method is also applicable to other problems involving segmentation of entities, for example, objects, people, and scenes into parts.

2   Related Work

Hand Pose Estimation — the majority of approaches to pose estimation are conventionally assigned to one of two groups: 3D model or appearance-based methods. One of the most notable recent works in the spirit of 3D modeling and inverse rendering [8] is based on pixelwise comparison of rendered and observed depth maps. Liang et al. [2] apply the iterative closest point (ICP) algorithm to hand pose reconstruction and 3D fingertip localization under spatial and temporal constraints. Qian et al. [9] proposed a hybrid method for realtime hand tracking using a simple hand model consisting of a number of spheres. Appearance-based methods typically include global matching of observed visual inputs with pose instances from training data. Athitsos et al. [10], for example, use a synthetic dataset featuring a great number of hand shape prototypes and viewpoints and perform matching by calculating approximate directed Chamfer distances between observed and synthetic edge images.

A seminal paper on pixel-based body segmentation with random decision forests [1] gave birth to a whole group of follow-up works including several adaptations for hand segmentation [3–5]. Deep learning of representations has been applied to body part or hand part segmentation [7,11,12]. In [13], hand part segmentation using random forests is combined with deep convolutional networks for gesture recognition.

A great amount of ad-hoc methods have been proposed specifically for hand-gesture recognition in narrow contexts. Most of them rely on hand detection, tracking, and gesture recognition based on global hand shape descriptors such as contours, silhouettes, fingertip positions, palm centers, number of visible fingers, etc. [14,15]. Similar descriptors have been proposed for depth and RGBD data [16]. Sridhar et al. [17] proposed a hybrid model for hand tracking using a multi-view RGB camera setup combined with a depth sensor.

Segmentation, Structural Information and Context Models — there has been renewed interest lately in semantic segmentation or semantic labelling methods. In these tasks, taking into account structural (contextual) information in addition to local appearance information is primordial. Contextual information often allows the model to disambiguate decisions where local information is not discriminative enough. In principle, increasing the support region of a learning machine can increase the amount of context taken into account for the decision. In practice, this places all of the burden on the classifier, which needs to learn a highly complex prediction model from a limited amount of training data, most frequently leading to poor performance. An elegant alternative is to apply multi-scale approaches. Farabet et al. [18] propose a multi-scale convolutional net for scene parsing which naturally integrates local and global context.

Structural information can be directly modeled through spatial relationships, which are frequently formulated as probabilistic graphical models like Markov Random Fields, Conditional Random Fields [19] or Bayesian networks. Inference in these models amounts to solving combinatorial problems, which in the case of high-level contextual information are often intractable in the general case. In comparison, classical feed forward networks are causal models, which allow fast inference but which are inherently ill-suited to deal with cyclic dependencies. Architectures which permit feedback connections such as Deep Boltzmann Machines [20] are difficult to train and do not scale to high-resolution images.

An alternative way to approximate cyclic dependencies with causal models has recently gained attention in computer vision. In *auto-context models* [21], cascades of classifiers are trained, where each classifier takes as input the output of the preceding classifier and eventual intermediate representations. Follow-up work recast this task as a graphical model in which inference is performed through message passing [22,23]. In [24], a sequential schema is proposed using randomized decision forests to incorporate semantic context to guide the classifier. In [25], auto-context is integrated into a single random forest, where pixels are classified breadth first, and each level can use decisions of previous levels of neighboring pixels. In [11], spatial neighborhood relationships between labels, as they are available in body part and part segmentation problems, are integrated into convolutional networks as prior knowledge.

Our proposed method is similar to auto-context in that the output of a first classifier is fed into a second classifier, which is learned to integrate the context of the pixel to predict. However, whereas auto-context models aim at repairing the errors of individual classifiers, our model uses contextual information to extract structural information from unlabelled images in a semi-supervised setting. The ability to seamlessly combine unlabeled examples and labeled examples is an important motivation behind the field of deep learning of representations [26,27]. Also relevant to our work are paradigms in which the test task is similar but different than the training task – transfer learning and domain adaptation [28]. Although we do not explicitly treat domain adaptation, in our task we exploit synthetic data at training time but not at test time.

3   Semi-Supervised Structured Learning

The pixelwise hand segmentation in this work is performed with a classifier which we call a *direct learner*. It operates frame-by-frame, ignoring inter-frame temporal dependencies. Given the constraint of real-time performance typical for this class of applications, we keep the test architecture as simple as possible and focus mainly on developing an effective training procedure to learn meaningful data representations that are robust to noise typical of real-world data.

The training data consists of input depth maps: $X = \{X^{(i)}\}$, $i = 1 \ldots |X|$. From this whole set of maps, L maps are synthetic and annotated, denoted as $X_L = \{X^{(i)}\}$, where $i = 1 \ldots L$, $L < |X|$. The subset of unlabeled real images is denoted as $X_U = \{X^{(i)}\}$, where $i > L$. The set of ground truth segmentation maps corresponding to the labelled set is denoted as $G = \{G^{(i)}\}$, where $i = 1 \ldots L$, $L \leq |X|$. No ground truth is available for $X^{(i)}$, $i > L$. Pixels in the different maps are indexed using a linear index j: $X^{(i,j)}$ denotes the jth pixel of the ith depth map.

The synthetic frames are rendered using a deformable 3D hand model. A large variety of viewpoints and hand poses (typical for interactive interfaces) is obtained under manually defined physical and physiological constraints. For the sake of generalization, and also keeping in mind that manually labeling data is tedious and impractical, we do not assume that ground-truth segmentation of real data is available in any amount. Instead, in parallel with supervised learning on annotated synthetic images, we use unlabeled frames for global optimization during training time.

Optimization criteria are based on, first, consistency of each predicted pixel class with its local neighborhood on the output segmentation map and, second, global compactness and homogeneity of the predicted hand segments.

For the first task, at training time we introduce an additional classification path, called the *context learner* [29], which is trained to predict each pixel's

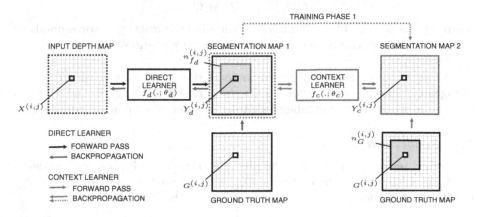

Fig. 2. The two learning pathways involving a direct learner f_d and a context learner f_d. The context learner operates on punctured neighborhood maps $n^{(i,j)}$, where the (to be predicted) middle pixel is missing.

class given labels of its local neighborhood. Both the direct and context learners are first pre-trained simultaneously in a purely supervised way on the synthetic images (see Fig. 2). The pre-training of the context learner is divided into two steps. First, ground truth label maps are used as the training input. After convergence of the direct learner, its output is used instead for input to the context learner, and the context learner is fine-tuned to cope with realistic output segmentation maps.

Let us introduce notation that will be used to formalize the training algorithm: $f_d(\theta_d)\colon X^{(i,j)} \to Y_d^{(i,j)}$ denotes a *direct learner* with parameters θ_d mapping each pixel $j = 1 \ldots M$ in a depth map i (having depth value $X^{(i,j)}$) into a corresponding pixel of an output segmentation map Y_d with elements $Y_d^{(i,j)}$, having one of possible $k = 1 \ldots K$ values corresponding to hand segments.

$f_c(\theta_c)\colon N^{(i,j)} \to Y_c^{(i,j)}$ denotes a *context learner* predicting the pixel label $Y_c^{(i,j)}$ from its neighborhood $N^{(i,j)}$ on the same segmentation map. The neighborhood is *punctured*, i.e. the center pixel to be predicted, j, is missing. As we have already mentioned, this classifier is first pre-trained on the ground truth images $G^{(i)}$ followed by fine-tuning on the segmentation maps produced by the direct learner f_d.

The probabilistic setting of our training algorithm makes it convient to introduce a difference between a random variable and its realization. In the following and as usual, uppercase letters denote random variables or fields of random variables and lower case letters denote realizations of values of random variables or of fields of random values. Realizations of random fields X, Y_c, Y_d and G defined above are thus denoted as x, y_c, y_d and g. Furthermore, $P(X = x)$ will be abbreviated as $P(x)$ when it is convenient. Figure 2 illustrates the configuration of the two learners f_d and f_c and the corresponding notation.

The loss function used for training the direct learner f_d in conjunction with the context learner f_c is composed of three terms whose activation depends on whether or not ground truth labels for the given training image are available:

$$Q = Q_{sd} + Q_{sc} + Q_u, \tag{1}$$

where Q_{sd} is responsible for training of the direct learner, Q_{sc} corresponds to the context learner (both) and Q_u is an unsupervised term serving as a natural regularizer.

During training, annotated and unannotated examples are considered interchangeably, starting with labeled data (supervised learning) followed by an increase in the amount of unlabeled samples (unsupervised domain adaptation).

3.1   Supervised Terms

Supervised terms classically link the predicted class of each pixel to the ground truth hand part label. The first term Q_{sd} is formulated as vanilla negative log-likelihood (NLL) for pixel-wise classification with the direct learner f_d.

$$Q_{sd}(\theta_d \,|\, X_L) = -\sum_{i=0}^{L} \sum_{j=0}^{M} \log P\left(Y_d^{(i,j)} = g^{(i,j)} \,\middle|\, x^{(i,j)}; \theta_d\right) \tag{2}$$

Recall here, that $Y_d^{(i,j)}$ is the output of the direct learner and $g^{(i,j)}$ is a ground truth label.

The second term Q_{sc} is also a negative log-likelihood loss for pixelwise classification, this time using the context learner f_c. Learning of θ_c proceeds in two steps. First, ground truth segmentation maps are fed to the learner, denoted as $n_G^{(i,j)}$, minimizing NLL:

$$Q_{sc}^{(1)}(\theta_c \,|\, G) = - \sum_{i=0}^{L} \sum_{j=0}^{M} \log P \left(Y_c^{(i,j)} = g^{(i,j)} \,\Big|\, N^{(i,j)} = n_G^{(i,j)}; \theta_c \right) \qquad (3)$$

After convergence, in a second phase, segmentation maps produced by the direct learner are fed into the context learner, denoted as $n_{f_d}^{(i,j)}$.

$$Q_{sc}^{(2)}(\theta_c \,|\, f_d(X_L)) = - \sum_{i=0}^{L} \sum_{j=0}^{M} \log P \left(Y_c^{(i,j)} = g^{(i,j)} \,\Big|\, N^{(i,j)} = n_{f_d}^{(i,j)}; \theta_c \right) \qquad (4)$$

Parameters θ_d are kept fixed during this step, and depth maps are not used during both steps.

3.2   Unsupervised Terms

In the unsupervised case, ground truth labels are not available. Instead, the loss function measures structural properties of the predicted segmentation at two different scales, either on context (at a neighborhood level), or globally on the full image. The estimated properties are then related to individual pixelwise loss.

$$Q_u = f(Q_{loc}, Q_{glb}) \qquad (5)$$

Local Structure. Q_{loc} is a term capturing local structure. It favors predictions which are consistent with other predictions in a local neighborhood. In particular, it favors predictions where the direct learner agrees with the context learner (recall that the context learner is not learned in this phase).

This term is formulated as a conditional negative likelihood loss. For each given pixel, if both classifiers f_d and f_c (the latter one operates on the output of the former one) agree on the same label, this pixel is used to update parameters θ_d of the direct learner and the error is minimized using the classical NLL scenario treating the predicted label as corresponding to the ground truth:

$$Q_{loc}(\theta_d \,|\, X_U) = - \sum_{j=0}^{M} \mathbb{I}_{y_d^{(i,j)} = y_c^{(i,j)}} \log P \left(Y_d = y_c^{(i,j)} \,\Big|\, x^{(i,j)}; \theta_d, \theta_c \right), \qquad (6)$$

where $\mathbb{I}_\omega = 1$ if ω holds and 0 else. In this case the parameters θ_c of the context learner remain unchanged. The indicator function is non-smooth with respect to the parameters. For backpropagation, we treat it as a constant once both segmentation maps are computed.

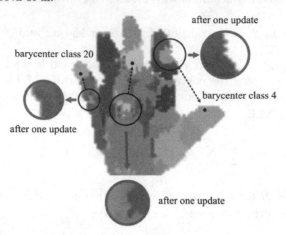

Fig. 3. Global structural information which can be extracted from a segmented image even if ground truth labels are **not** available. Small circles with thin black borders contain segmented pixels which are far away from the principal pixel mass of the given hand part, indicated by the barycenter of the hand part. The global unsupervised loss term Q_{glb} punishes these results. Large circles with thick blue borders show the same content after a single network parameter update using Q_{glb} (Colour figure online).

Global Structure. Q_{glb} is a term capturing global structure. It favors predictions which fit into global image statistics and penalizes the ones which do not by changing parameters in the direction of a more probable class. Technically, this term aims on minimizing variance (in terms of pixel coordinates) of each hand segment. Figure 3 illustrates the intuitive understanding of this terms. Ground truth labels are **not** available for the real images dealt with in this part, but there is intrinsic structural information which can be extracted from a segmented image, and which is related to strong priors we can impose on the segmentation map. In particular, unlike general segmentation problems, body and hand part segmentation maps contain a single connected region per hand part label (ignoring cases of strong partial self-occlusion, which are extremely rare). In Fig. 3, small circles with thin black borders contain segmented pixels which are not connected to the principal region of the given hand part, indicated by the barycenter of the pixels of this hand part. The global unsupervised loss term Q_{glb} punishes these results. Large circles with thick blue borders show the same content after a single network parameter update using Q_{glb}.

We formalize this concept as follows. For each class k present in the output map Y_d, barycentric coordinates of the corresponding segment are calculated:

$$\mathbf{R}_k = \frac{\displaystyle\sum_{j:Y_d^{(i,j)}=k} P(y_d^{(i,j)}|x^{(i,j)})\mathbf{r}^{(i,j)}}{\displaystyle\sum_{j:Y_d^{(i,j)}=k} P(y_d^{(i,j)}|x^{(i,j)})}, \tag{7}$$

where pixel coordinates, in vector form, are denoted as $\mathbf{r}^{(i,j)}$.

If $\left|\mathbf{r}^{(i,j)} - \mathbf{R}_k\right| > \tau$, i.e. the pixel (i,j) is close enough to its barycenter (τ is estimated from the labelled synthetic data), then the pixel is considered as correctly classified and used to update parameters of the direct learner θ_d. The loss function term for one pixel (i,j) is given as follows:

$$Q_{glb}^{+}(\theta_d \left| y_d^{(i,j)} \right.) = -F_{y_d}^{(i)} \log P \left(Y_d = y_d^{(i,j)} \left| x^{(i,j)}, \theta_d, \theta_c \right. \right), \tag{8}$$

where $F_k^{(i)}$ is a weight related to the size of class components:

$$F_k^{(i)} = |\{j : Y_d^{(i,j)} = k\}|^{-\alpha} \tag{9}$$

and $\alpha > 0$ is a gain parameter. In the opposite case, when $\left|\mathbf{r}^{(i,j)} - \mathbf{R}_k\right| \leq \tau$, the current prediction is penalized and the class γ corresponding to the closest segment in the given distance τ is promoted:

$$Q_{glb}^{-}(\theta_d \left| y_d^{(i,j)} \right.) = -F_{\gamma}^{(i)} \log P \left(Y_d = \gamma \left| x^{(i,j)}, \theta_d, \theta_c \right. \right), \tag{10}$$

where

$$\gamma = \operatorname{argmin}\left(|\mathbf{r}^{(i,j)} - \mathbf{R}_k|\right). \tag{11}$$

This formulation is related to the k-means algorithm. However, data points in our setting are embedded in two spaces: the space spanned by the network outputs (or, alternatively, feature space), and the 2D geometric space of the part positions. Assigning cluster centers requires therefore optimizing multiple criteria and distances in heterogeneous spaces. Other clustering costs could be also adopted.

Integrating Local and Global Structure. Local structure and global structure are fused emphasizing agreement between both terms. In particular, activation of the penalizing global term (which favors parameters pushing a pixel away from currently predicted class) is confirmed by a similar structural information captured by the local term ($Q_{loc} = 0$):

$$Q_u = \beta_{loc} Q_{loc} + \beta_{glb} \begin{cases} Q_{glb}^{+} & \text{if } \left|\mathbf{r}^{(i,j)} - \mathbf{R}_k\right| \leq \tau, \\ Q_{glb}^{-} & \text{if } \left|\mathbf{r}^{(i,j)} - \mathbf{R}_k\right| > \tau \text{ and } Q_{loc} = 0, \\ 0 & \text{else} \end{cases} \tag{12}$$

where β_{loc} and β_{glb} are weights.

Combining the two terms, Q_{loc} and Q_{glb}, is essential as they are acting in an adversarial way. The local term alone leads to convergence to a trivial solution when all pixels in the image are assigned to the same class by both classifiers. The global term favors multi-segment structure composed of homogeneous regions, while exact shapes of the segments may be distorted as to not satisfy the desirability of of compactness. The two terms acting together, as well as mixing the labeled and unlabeled data, allow the classifier to find a balanced solution.

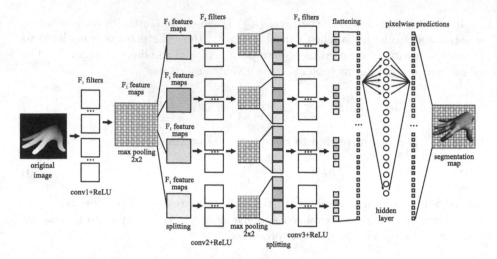

Fig. 4. The proposed deep convolutional architecture of a single learner.

4   Architecture

The direct and context learners are based on a convolutional network architecture and have the same general structure (see Fig. 4) including three consecutive convolutional layers F_1, F_2 and F_3 with rectified linear activation units (ReLU). Layers F_1 and F_2 are followed by 2×2 max pooling and reduction.

As opposed to most existing methods for scene labeling, instead of randomly sampling pixels (or patches), training is performed image-wise, i.e. all pixels from the given image are provided to the classifier at once and each pixel gets assigned with an output class label based on information extracted from its neighborhood.

Applying of the convolutional classifier with pooling/reduction layers to an image in the traditional way would lead to loss in resolution by a factor of 4 (in the given configuration). On the other hand, simply not reducing the image resolution will prevent higher layers from learning higher level features, as the size of the filter support does not grow with respect to the image content. To avoid this dilemma, we employ specifically designed splitting functions originally proposed for image scanning in [30] and further exploited in *Over Feat* networks [31]. Intuitively speaking, each map at a given resolution is reduced to four different maps of lower resolution using max pooling. The amount of elements is preserved, but the resolution of each map is lower compared to the maps of previous layers.

In more detail, let us consider the output of the first convolutional layer F_1 of the network. Once the output feature maps are obtained, 4 virtual extended copies of them are created by zero padding with (1) one column on the left, (2) one column on the right, (3) one row on top, (4) one row in the bottom. Therefore, each copy will contain the original feature map but shifted in 4 different directions. On the next step, we apply max pooling (2×2 with stride 2×2) to each of the extended maps producing 4 low-resolution maps. By introducing the shifts, pixels from all extended maps combined together can reconstruct the original feature map as if max pooling with stride 1×1 had been applied. This operation allows the network to preserve results of all computations for each pixel on each step and, at the same time, perform the necessary reduction, resulting in a significantly speed up during training and testing.

After pooling, convolutions of the following layer F_2 are applied to all 4 low-resolution maps separately (but in parallel). The same procedure is repeated after the second convolutional layer F_2, where each of 4 branches is split again into 4, producing 16 parallel pathways overall. If necessary, the algorithm can be extended to an arbitrary number of layers and employed each time when reduction is required.

All outputs of the third convolutional layer F_3 are flattened and classified with an MLP, producing a label for each pixel. Finally, the labels are rearranged to form the output segmentation map corresponding to the original image.

The direct and the context learners have the same architecture with the only difference that the middle parts of the first layer filters of the context learner are removed. It helps to prevent the network from converging to a trivial solution where a pixel label is produced by directly reproducing its input. This is especially important on the initial training stage, when the context learner is trained on ground truth segmentation maps.

5   Experiments

For this project, we have created a vast collection of about 60,000 synthetic training samples, including both normalized 8 bit depth maps and ground truth segmentations with resolution 640×640 pixels. Hand shapes, proportions, poses and orientations are generated with a random set of parameters. Each pose is captured from 5 different camera view points sampled randomly for each frame. An additional set of 6000 images is used for validation and testing.

The unlabeled part of the training set consists of 3000 images captured with a depth sensor. To evaluate the algorithm performance on the real-world data, we have manually annotated 50 test samples. An example of a ground truth segmentation map is shown in Fig. 5, where the hand is divided into 20 segment classes. Background pixels are set to 0 and assigned a class label of 0.

For training, synthetic depth maps are downsampled by a factor of 4 (to imitate real world conditions), and cropped. As a result, the network input is of size 80×80 pixels.

Both direct and context learners have 3 convolutional layers F_1, F_2 and F_3 with 16, 32, 48 filters respectively, where each filter is of size 7×7. Max pooling 2×2 is performed after the first two convolutional layers. The hidden layer is composed of 150 units. Thus, each pixel is classified based on its receptive field of size 46×46. In the context learner, the middle parts of size 3×3 of the first layer filters are removed. The learning rate is initially set to 0.1. Unsupervised learning parameters are set to $\beta_{loc} = 0.1$, $\beta_{glb} = 1.2$, and $\alpha = 0.5$.

The current pure CPU implementation of the entire pipeline runs at 436 ms per frame (with a potential speed-up by a factor of 20–30 [13] on GPU).

Table 1. Performance of networks trained with different objective functions.

Loss function	Training data	Test data	Accuracy (%)	Average per class (%)
Q_{sd} (supervised baseline)	synth.	synth.	85.90	78.50
		real	47.15	34.98
$Q_{sd} + Q_{loc} + Q_{glb}$ (semi-supervised, ours)	all	synth.	85.49	78.31
		real	**50.50**	**43.25**

Table 2. Perf. improvement on a real image after updating parameters using different supervised and unsupervised terms, estimated as an average over 50 real images.

Terms	Q_{loc}	Q_{glb}^{+}	$Q_{glb}^{+} + Q_{glb}^{-}$	$Q_{loc} + Q_{glb}^{+} + Q_{glb}^{-}$	Q_{sd}
Requires labels	No	No	No	No	Yes
Gain in % points	+0.60	+0.36	+0.41	**+0.82**	+16.05

The training procedure is started with purely supervised learning by backpropagation which proceeds until 50 % of the synthetic training data is seen by the network. From this moment on, we replace 10 % of the training set with unlabeled real world samples. A single training image consisting of $80 \times 80 = 6400$ pixel samples is used for each step of gradient descent.

Comparative performance of classifiers trained by including and excluding different unsupervised terms of the loss function is summarized in Table 1. Exploiting unlabeled real data for unsupervised training and network regularization has proven to be generally beneficial, especially for reconstruction of small segments (such as finger parts), which leads to a significant increase of average per-class accuracy. The bar plot on the Fig. 5 demonstrates significant improvement of recognition rates for almost all classes except for the first, base "palm" class which can be seen as a background for a hand image against which finger segments are usually detected. Therefore, this reflects the fact that more confident detection in the case of semi-supervised training comes together with a certain increase in the amount of false positives.

Table 2 illustrates the impact of one update of the network parameters for different loss functions on the performance on a given image which was used for computing the gradients. We note that a combination of two competitive unsupervised terms (local and global) produces a more balanced solution than the same terms separately.

The local term alone forces the network to favor the most statistically probable class (i.e. the "palm" in our settings), while the global one on its own tends to shift boundaries between regions producing segmentation maps similar to a Voronoi diagram. In the latter case, the number of cells is typically defined by an initial guess of the network on the given image and is unlikely to be changed by global unsupervised learning alone.

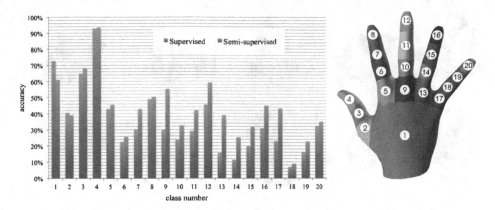

Fig. 5. Left: average accuracy per class obtained with the supervised method (in blue) and with semi-supervised structured learning (in red); Right: labeling of hand segments (Colour figure online).

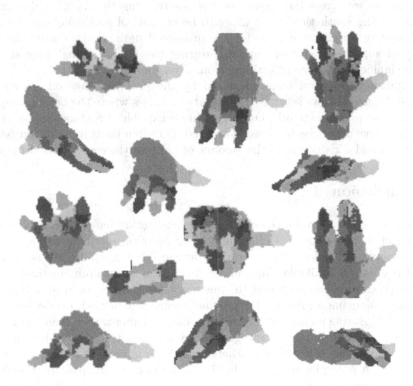

Fig. 6. Output segmentation maps produced by the semi-supervised network for real-world images.

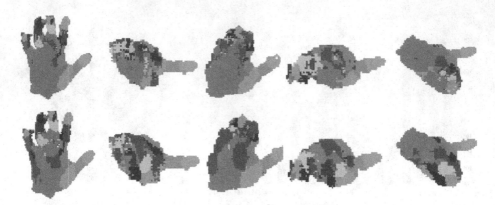

Fig. 7. Challenging examples. Top row: examples where the baseline method has difficulty in segmentation. Bottom row: the results of our proposed algorithm on the same examples.

Therefore we stress the importance of pre-training the direct and context learners on the synthetic data in order to be capable of producing structurally representative initial predictions for the unlabeled data. Furthermore, the frequency of supervised gradient updates during the final training stage should remain significant to prevent training from diverging.

Output segmentation maps produced by the proposed method are shown in Fig. 6. Figure 7 shows several "problematic" images where the baseline supervised network performs poorly. Our algorithm is capable of finding regions which would not have otherwise been reconstructed and often leads to more consistent predictions and a reduction in the amount of noise in the segmentation maps.

6   Conclusion

We have proposed a novel method for part segmentation based on convolutional learning of representations. Unlike most deep learning methods which require large amounts of labeled data, we do not assume that ground-truth segmentation of real data is available. Our main contribution is a training method which exploits (i) context learning; and (ii) unsupervised learning of local and global structure, balancing a prior for large homogenous regions with pixel-wise accuracy. By integrating structural information into learning rather than the model architecture, we retain the advantages of very fast test-time processing and the ability to parallelize. The use of synthetic data is an important part of our training strategy. A potential area of further improvement is domain adaptation from synthetic to real images.

Acknowledgements. This work was partially funded by French grants **Interabot**, call *Investissements d'Avenir*, and **SoLStiCe** (ANR-13-BS02-0002-01), call *ANR blanc*.

References

1. Shotton, J., Fitzgibbon, A., Cook, M., Sharp, T., Finocchio, M., Moore, R., Kipman, A., Blake, A.: Real-time human pose recognition in parts from single depth images. In: CVPR, pp. 1297–1304 (2011)
2. Liang, H., Yuan, J., Thalmann, D., Zhang, Z.: Model-based hand pose estimation via spatial-temporal hand parsing and 3D fingertip localization. Vis. Comput. **29**, 837–848 (2013)
3. Keskin, C., Kiraç, F., Kara, Y., Akarun, L.: Real time hand pose estimation using depth sensors. In: ICCV Workshop on Consumer Depth Cameras. IEEE (2011)
4. Półrola, M., Wojciechowski, A.: Real-time hand pose estimation using classifiers. In: Bolc, L., Tadeusiewicz, R., Chmielewski, L.J., Wojciechowski, K. (eds.) ICCVG 2012. LNCS, vol. 7594, pp. 573–580. Springer, Heidelberg (2012)
5. Tang, D., Yu, T., Kim, T.K.: Real-time articulated hand pose estimation using semi-supervised transductive regression forests. In: ICCV (2013)
6. Shotton, J.: Conditional regression forests for human pose estimation. In: CVPR, pp. 3394–3401 (2012)
7. Jain, A., Tompson, J., Andriluka, M., Taylor, G., Bregler, C.: Learning human pose estimation features with convolutional networks. In: ICLR (2014)
8. Oikonomidis, I., Kyriazis, N., Argyros, A.: Efficient model-based 3D tracking of hand articulations using kinect. In: BMVC, pp. 101.1–101.11 (2011)
9. Qian, C., Sun, X., Wei, Y., Tang, X., Sun, J.: Realtime and robust hand tracking from depth. In: CVPR (2014)
10. Athitsos, V., Liu, Z., Wu, Y., Yuan, J.: Estimating 3D hand pose from a cluttered image. In: CVPR. IEEE (2003)
11. Jiu, M., Wolf, C., Taylor, G., Baskurt, A.: Human body part estimation from depth images via spatially-constrained deep learning. Pattern Recogn. Lett. **50**(1), 122–129 (2014)
12. Toshev, A., Szegedy, C.: DeepPose: human pose estimation via deep neural networks. In: CVPR (2014)
13. Tompson, J., Stein, M., LeCun, Y., Perlin, K.: Real time continuous pose recovery of human hands using convolutional networks. In: SIGGRAPH/ACM-ToG (2014)
14. Stergiopoulou, E., Papamarkos, N.: Hand gesture recognition using a neural network shape fitting technique. Eng. Appl. Artif. Intell. **22**, 1141–1158 (2009)
15. Malima, A., Özgür, E., Çetin, M.: A fast algorithm for vision-based hand gesture recognition for robot control. In: IEEE 14th Conference on Signal Processing and Communications Applications (2006)
16. Mateo, C.M., Gil, P., Corrales, J.A., Puente, S.T., Torres, F.: RGBD human-hand recognition for the interaction with robot-hand. In: IROS (2012)
17. Sridhar, S., Oulasvirta, A., Theobalt, C.: Interactive markerless articulated hand motion tracking using RGB and depth data. In: ICCV (2013)
18. Farabet, C., Couprie, C., Najman, L., LeCun, Y.: Scene parsing with multiscale feature learning, purity trees, and optimal covers. In: ICML (2012)
19. Tighe, J., Lazebnik, S.: Superparsing: scalable nonparametric image parsing with superpixels. In: Daniilidis, K., Maragos, P., Paragios, N. (eds.) ECCV 2010, Part V. LNCS, vol. 6315, pp. 352–365. Springer, Heidelberg (2010)
20. Salakhutdinov, R., Hinton, G.E.: Deep boltzmann machines. In: International Conference on Artificial Intelligence and Statistics, pp. 448–455 (2009)
21. Tu, Z.: Auto-context and its application to high-level vision tasks. In: CVPR (2008)

22. Ross, S., Munoz, D., Hebert, M., Bagnell, J.A.: Learningmessage-passing inference machines for structured prediction. In: CVPR, pp. 2737–2744 (2011)
23. Shapovalov, R., Vetrov, D., Kohli, P.: Spatial inference machines. In: CVPR, pp. 2985–2992 (2013)
24. Shotton, J., Johnson, M., Cipolla, R.: Semantic texton forests for image categorization and segmentation. In: CVPR, pp. 1–8 (2008)
25. Montillo, A., Shotton, J., Winn, J., Iglesias, J.E., Metaxas, D., Criminisi, A.: Entangled decision forests and their application for semantic segmentation of CT images. In: Székely, G., Hahn, H.K. (eds.) IPMI 2011. LNCS, vol. 6801, pp. 184–196. Springer, Heidelberg (2011)
26. Bengio, Y., Courville, A., Vincent, P.: Representation learning: A review and new perspectives. IEEE Trans. Pattern Anal. Mach. Intell. **35**, 1798–1828 (2013)
27. Weston, J., Ratle, F., Mobahi, H., Collobert, R.: Deep learning via semi-supervised embedding. In: Montavon, G., Orr, G.B., Müller, K.-R. (eds.) Neural Networks: Tricks of the Trade, 2nd edn. LNCS, vol. 7700, 2nd edn, pp. 639–655. Springer, Heidelberg (2012)
28. Bengio, Y.: Deep learning of representations for unsupervised and transfer learning. Unsupervised Transf. Learn. Challenges Mach. Learn. **7**, 19 (2012)
29. Fromont, E., Emonet, R., Kekeç, T., Trémeau, A., Wolf, C.: Contextually constrained deep networks for scene labeling. In: BMVC (2014)
30. Giusti, A., Ciresan, D.C., Masci, J., Gambardella, L.M., Schmidhuber, J.: Fast image scanning with deep max-pooling convolutional neural networks. In: ICIP (2013)
31. Sermanet, P., Eigen, D., Zhang, X., Mathieu, M., Fergus, R., LeCun, Y.: Overfeat: Integrated recognition, localization and detection using convolutional networks. In: ICLR (2014)

Topic-Aware Deep Auto-Encoders (TDA) for Face Alignment

Jie Zhang[1,2], Meina Kan[1], Shiguang Shan[1(✉)], Xiaowei Zhao[3], and Xilin Chen[1]

[1] Key Lab of Intelligent Information Processing of Chinese Academy of Sciences (CAS), Institute of Computing Technology, CAS, Beijing 100190, China
shiguang.shan@vipl.ict.ac.cn
[2] University of Chinese Academy of Sciences, Beijing 100049, China
[3] Imperial College London, London, UK

Abstract. Facial landmark localization plays an important role for many computer vision tasks, e.g., face recognition, face parsing, facial expression analysis, face animation, etc. However, it remains a challenging problem due to the diverse variations, such as head poses, facial expressions, occlusions and so on. In this work, we propose a topic-aware face alignment method to divide the difficult task of estimating the target shape into several much easier subtasks according to the topics. Specifically, topics are determined automatically by clustering according to the target shapes or shape deviations which are more compatible with the task of alignment. Then, within each topic, a deep auto-encoder network is employed to regress from the shape-indexed feature to the target shape. Deep model specific to each topic can capture more subtle variations in shape and appearance, and thus leading to better alignment results. This process is conducted in a cascade structure to further improve the performance. Experiments on three challenging databases demonstrate that our method significantly outperforms the state-of-the-art methods and performs in real-time.

1 Introduction

Face alignment or facial landmark localization is a vital problem in computer vision since many vision tasks depend on accurate face alignment results, including face recognition, facial expression analysis, face animation, etc. Although it has been studied for many years, facial landmark detection on the wild face images is still a challenging problem due to large shape variations, such as extreme head poses and facial expressions.

Typical *parametric methods*, such as Active Shape Model (ASM) [1,2] and Active Appearance Model (AAM) [3,4], employ the statistical model such as Principal Component Analysis (PCA) to capture the shape and appearance variations respectively. They perform well for face images with little pose variation, normal facial expression and good light conditions. However, they fail to get accurate shapes for those images with large head pose and exaggerated facial expressions since single linear model can hardly well capture the complex non-linear variations in the wild data. To handle the large texture variations, van

© Springer International Publishing Switzerland 2015
D. Cremers et al. (Eds.): ACCV 2014, Part III, LNCS 9005, pp. 703–718, 2015.
DOI: 10.1007/978-3-319-16811-1_46

et al. [5] extend the traditional AAM to MPPCA-AAM by using a mixture of probabilistic PCA [6] to model the complex appearance variations resulting in better performance. However, it is still sensitive to shape initializations as the traditional AAM.

Recently, *regression based methods* have achieved impressive results on both controlled and uncontrolled face images [7–10]. Instead of explicitly representing the shape or appearance variations with parametric models, these methods attempt to directly learn a mapping from appearance to face shape. As one of the most promising regression based method, SDM [9] employs a linear regression to estimate the shape deviation based on shape-indexed feature [7] under a cascade framework, and it achieves the state-of-the-art performance for facial landmark detection and tracking on the wild databases, e.g., LFPW [11], LFW-A&C [12], RU-FACS [13] and Youtube Celebrities [14]. To some extent, SDM is more robust to inaccurate shape initialization, but it may still get stuck on the images with extreme pose and exaggerated facial expressions when the initialization shape is far from the ground truth [15].

To relieve the influence of inaccurate initializations, [7,8] use multiple initializations for testing and take the median result of all random fern regressors as the final estimation. Burgos-Artizzu et al. [16] propose a Robust Cascaded Pose Regression (RCPR) method to further improve the performance of CPR [7] under a novel restart scheme. Specifically, given an image, 10 % of the cascade is applied for different initializations and then the variance of their predictions are checked. If the variance is low enough, the left 90 % of the cascade is applied, otherwise restart with a different set of initializations.

Different from [7,8,16], Dantone et al. [17] employ a regression forest to estimate the head pose and then individually model the shape and appearance variations of facial landmarks for each head pose by using conditional regression forest. They argue that the exploiting of head pose provides a good shape prior for face alignment and conditional regression forests are easier to learn since the trees have no need to capture all shape and appearance variations. A good shape prior can provide better shape initialization even under extreme pose. Furthermore, Zhao et al. [18] propose an iterative Multi-Output Random Forests (IMOFR) algorithm to jointly estimate head pose, facial expressions and facial landmarks, which divides facial landmark detection into subtasks based on both head poses and facial expressions. It further achieves more accurate face alignment results than [17]. Zhu et al. [19] employ a mixture-of-trees model to capture the diverse variations of each viewpoint and partially address the initialization problem by evaluating the models of all viewpoints, which is thus accompanied by a high computation problem. Yu et al. [20] propose a group sparse learning method to select optimized salient facial landmarks for mixture-of-trees models and further refine the detection result by using two-step cascaded deformable shape model. This method can perform faster than [19]. However, it still cannot meet the real-time requirement and the performance degenerates when it fails to get accurate estimation of salient facial landmarks. In another interesting work [15], an exemplar-based approach is proposed to model the correlations between landmarks and their surrounding information and then a feature voting-based face alignment method is employed with non-parametric shape regularization. This method does not require initial face shape based on face detection result. Impressive results are achieved on two challenging data sets, i.e., AFW [19] and IBUG [21], but it is extremely time-consuming.

Auto-encoders and other deep models are widely applied for computer vision problem and achieve great success for image denoising, image classification, face analysis, etc [22–26]. Inspired by the success of deep network, some researches propose to employ it to solve the facial landmark detection problem. Sun et al. [24] design a deep convolutional neural network (DCNN) for facial landmark detection and achieve impressive results on two public datasets. However, the performance under extreme pose and exaggerated facial expressions may degenerates since it is hard to train a robust deep model to capture all facial variations without any prior knowledge. In [26], Wu et al. propose a deep model based on the Restricted Boltzmann Machines (RBM) for facial landmark tracking with shape prior in consideration of face pose and expressions. Specifically, deep belief network is employed to capture the shape variations due to facial expressions and a 3-way RBM is further used for modeling pose variations. Yet, it is still hard to handle the extreme variations of face poses and facial expressions simultaneously.

To deal with the facial landmark detection with large shape variations, we propose a topic-aware face alignment method to divide the difficult task of estimating the target shape into several much easier subtasks according to the topics, and an overview of the proposed method is shown in Fig. 1. Different from [17,18], in which the topics are manually defined based on the appearance variations of head poses or facial expressions, we define the topics by automatically clustering the target shapes or shape deviations which are more compatible with the task of alignment. Then, within each topic, a deep auto-encoder network is exploited to detect the facial landmarks. Deep models specific to each topic can well capture the variations in shape and appearance even under extreme poses and facial expressions. This process is further conducted in a cascade structure to improve the performance. It is important to note that topic definitions in each cascaded stage are updated based on target shapes or shape deviations rather than the fixed manual definitions used in [17,18]. As a result, the topics are closely related to the task, i.e., predicting the target shape.

The main contributions of this work are summarized as bellow:

1. By automatically discovering topics according to the target shapes/target shape deviations, the difficult face alignment task is divided into several much easier subtasks. As the defined topic is related to the shape, more compact subtasks can be achieved leading to better alignment results.
2. Deep model is employed as the alignment model for each topic. Benefited the great ability of modeling nonlinearity, deep model can well capture the diverse variations in shape and appearance leading to more accurate alignment results.
3. Our method outperforms the state-of-the-arts methods on three public data sets, i.e., XM2VTS, LFPW, IBUG, and performs in real time.

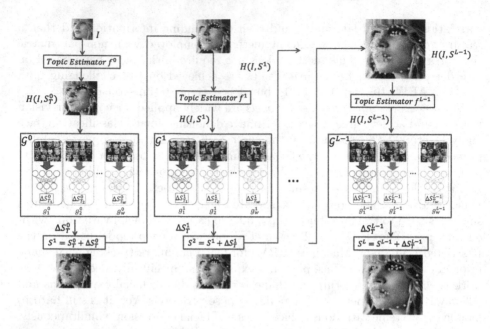

Fig. 1. Overview of our Topic-aware Face Alignment Algorithm with Deep Auto-encoders. f denotes a topic prediction function and $\mathcal{G}$ is the topic-specific deep models for face alignment. $H(I,S)$ is the joint shape-indexed features extracted around the landmarks of face shape S. ΔS is the shape difference between the ground truth and the current shape.

2 Topic-Aware Deep Auto-Encoder for Face Alignment

In this section, we will first give an overview of our topic-aware deep auto-encoder (TDA) method for face alignment. Then we will describe the technical details about each component of our approach.

2.1 Method Overview

Facial landmark detection on the wild face images is quite challenging mainly due to the large shape variations. To tackle this problem, we propose a topic-aware deep auto-encoders for the wild face alignment, which divides the difficult task of predicting the target shape into several much easier subtasks according to the topics, as illustrated in Fig. 1. To make the division of subtasks more compatible with the whole task, the topics are defined according to the target shape (or shape deviations). Furthermore, considering the great ability of capturing the nonlinearity, the deep auto-encoder is employed to solve the subtask within each topic to achieve better prediction.

Given an image I, the problem of facial landmark detection is generally formulated as learning a non-linear function D to predict the shape from the image:

$$D : S \leftarrow I, \tag{1}$$

where S is the face shape of input image I, i.e., the location of each landmark. In the wild condition, D is quite difficult to learn due to the large variations of shape and appearance. Therefore, we propose to divide D into several easier ones $\{D_1, D_2, \cdots, D_w\}$ according to the topics $T = \{T_1, T_2, ..., T_w\}$. In this work, the topics T are defined by clustering the face images according to the shape (or shape deviation if the output of D_i is the deviation rather than the shape). To predict the topic of any input image, a deep auto-encoder f is used to model the regression from the input image to the topics:

$$T = f(I), T \in \mathcal{T}. \tag{2}$$

Within each topic, the variations are more compact than the overall topics, and a better shape prior S_T, i.e., the mean shape specific to each topic, can be achieved.

Then, for each topic $T \in \mathcal{T}$, we design another deep auto-encoder network, denoted as g_T, which attempts to infer the shape deviation $\Delta S = S_g - S_T$ as follows:

$$g_T : \Delta S \leftarrow H(I, S_T), \tag{3}$$

where S_g is the ground truth face shape (i.e., the target shape), H is the feature extraction function, and S_T is the shape prior of topic T or the shape from the previous stage.

After learning all topic-specific face alignment models $\mathcal{G} = \{g_{T_1}, g_{T_2}, ..., g_{T_w}\}$, the mapping function D from image I to face shape S can be reformulated as:

$$S = D(I) = S_T + \mathcal{G}(I, T), \tag{4}$$

with $\mathcal{G}(I, T) = g_T$.

The above process is further conducted in a cascade procedure to improve the performance.

2.2   Topic Definition and Prediction

Topic Definition. In our method, the topics are defined by clustering the target shapes or shape deviations via k-means in each cascade stage. For the first stage, the topics are achieved by clustering according to the target shape, i.e., the ground truth shape S_g. As shown in Fig. 2(a), five topics are exploited by clustering which are roughly consistent with head pose variations since the head pose variations dominate the shape distribution of that dataset. A good shape prior can be easily achieved by taking mean face shape specific to each obtained topic.

For the successive stages, the topics are achieved by clustering according to the shape deviations, i.e., the difference between the ground truth shape and the shape from previous stage $\Delta S^{j-1} = S_g - S^{j-1}$, because the alignment model in the jth ($j \geqslant 2$) stage attempts to predict the shape deviations rather than the shape directly. In other words, the topics are defined according to the face shape deviations(i.e., the target of the task) rather than appearance. Finally,

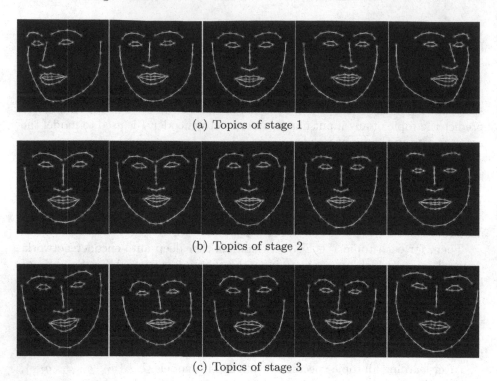

(a) Topics of stage 1

(b) Topics of stage 2

(c) Topics of stage 3

Fig. 2. Topic discovery at each stage. Five topics are exploited by clustering the target shapes or shape deviations for each stage. For stage 1, we directly show the cluster centers of each topic, i.e., the mean shape of each topic. For stage 2 and 3, the cluster centers, i.e., the mean shape deviation, is added to the frontal face shape for better exhibitions.

as shown in Fig. 2(b) and (c), the topics in each stage are different since the tasks, i.e., the deviations are different in each stage. Compared with the existing methods [17,18] which also divide the overall tasks into several subtasks, our method is different in two-folds: (1) [17,18] define the topics according to five head pose (profile left, left, front, right, profile right) or together with three facial expressions (neutral, happy and others), i.e., the characteristic of input image, while our method defines the topics according to the target shapes or shape deviations, i.e., the output of alignment task; (2) In [18], the topics are kept the same in all stages since characteristic of the input image is the same across all stages, while in our method, the topics in each stage are different since the task, i.e., the shape deviation, in each stage is different. Overall, the definition of topics in our methods can make division of topics more compatible with the overall task, leading to better results.

Topic Prediction. After topics $\mathcal{T}$ are defined based on face shapes, a nonlinear function, i.e., f in Eq. (2), is designed to predict the topic $T \in \mathcal{T}$ of any input image I. Deep models like deep auto-encoder networks [22] is a good choice for its favorable ability of modeling the nonlinearity. Specifically, a deep network with $m - 1$ hidden layers is designed. The prediction function f can be formulated as the following optimization problem:

$$f^* = \arg\min_f ||T - \psi_m(\psi_{m-1}(...\psi_1(I)))||_2^2 + \lambda \sum_{i=1}^m ||W_i||_F^2, \tag{5}$$

$$\psi_i(a_{i-1}) = \sigma(W_i a_{i-1} + b_i) \triangleq a_i, \ i = 1, ..., m - 1, \tag{6}$$

$$\psi_m(a_{m-1}) = W_m a_{m-1} + b_m \triangleq a_m, \ a_m \in \mathcal{T}, \tag{7}$$

where ψ_i is the nonlinear mapping of ith layer of deep auto-encoder networks parameterized with W_i and b_i, $\sum_{i=1}^m ||W_i||_F^2$ is a weight decay term to prevent over-fitting, σ is a sigmoid function which characterizes the nonlinearity mapping for feature representations $\{a_1, a_2, ..., a_{m-1}\}$ at the first $m - 1$ layers. At the last layer, linear regression is employed to get the topic prediction T. Equation (5) is iteratively optimized by L-BFGS [27]. After obtaining the solution f^*, the topic T of given image I can be achieved as $T = f^*(I) = \psi_m(\psi_{m-1}(...\psi_1(I)))$.

2.3 Topic-Specific Deep Auto-encoder for Face Alignment

For a topic T, the face alignment task can be formulated as learning a regression function to predict the shape deviations ΔS between current shape S_T and the ground truth S_g. Considering that the regression function is a complex nonlinear mapping, a deep auto-encoder network denoted as g_T, $T \in \mathcal{T}$ is designed to infer the shape deviations, as shown in Fig. 1.

Specifically, within each topic T ($T \in \mathcal{T}$), the shape-indexed SIFT [28] features denoted as $H(I, S_T)$ are extracted around all facial points and further concatenated as the input for the deep network g_T. The deep network is optimized as follows:

$$g_T^* = \arg\min_{g_T} ||\Delta S_T - \phi_{T,n}(\phi_{T,(n-1)}(...\phi_{T,1}(H(I, S_T))))||_2^2 + \eta \sum_{i=1}^n ||W_{T,i}||_F^2. \tag{8}$$

$$\phi_{T,i}(a_{T,(i-1)}) = \sigma(W_{T,i} a_{T,(i-1)} + b_{T,i}) \triangleq a_{T,i}, i = 1, ..., n - 1, \tag{9}$$

$$\phi_{T,n}(a_{T,(n-1)}) = W_{T,n} a_{T,(n-1)} + b_{T,n} \triangleq \Delta S_T, \tag{10}$$

where $\phi_{T,i}$ is the nonlinear mapping of ith layer of g_T parameterized with $W_{T,i}$ and $b_{T,i}$. n is the number of layers in the deep network and $\sum_{i=1}^n ||W_{T,i}||_F^2$ is a weight decay term. After obtaining the solution g_T^*, the shape deviations can be achieved as $\Delta S_T = g_T^*(I) = \phi_{T,n}(\phi_{T,(n-1)}(...\phi_{T,1}(H(I, S_T))))$.

The deep network g_T with n layers has many parameters and is easier to get stuck in local minimum. To relieve this, we initialize the first $n - 1$ layers through an unsupervised pre-train process. The objective function of the pre-train process for ith layer is:

$$\{\phi_{T,i}{}^*, \varphi_{T,i}{}^*\} = \arg\min_{\phi_{T,i}, \varphi_{T,i}} ||a_{T,(i-1)} - \varphi_{T,i}(\phi_{T,i}(a_{T,(i-1)}))||^2$$
$$+ \alpha(||W_{T,i}||_F^2 + ||W_{T,i}'||_F^2), \tag{11}$$

where $\phi_{T,i}(x) = \sigma(W_{T,i}x + b_{T,i})$ and $\varphi_{T,i}(x) = \sigma(W'_{T,i}x + b'_{T,i})$. For the first layer, we take the shape-indexed SIFT feature as input, e.g., $a_0 = H(I, S_T)$ and the output of this hidden layer is treated as the input of following layer. With the pretrained parameters of the first $n-1$ layers and randomly initialized parameters of the last layer, the whole network is fine-tuned according to Eq. (8).

After learning all topic-specific face alignment models $\mathcal{G} = \{g_{T_1}, g_{T_2}, ..., g_{T_w}\}$, the face shape S of any image can be achieved by adding the predicted shape deviation ΔS_T from the corresponding model g_T to the shape prior $S_T : S = S_T + \Delta S_T$, where T is predicted topic from deep model f. The topic-specific deep models for face alignment can well capture the detailed variations in shape and appearance of each topic, which show favorable ability for handling extreme head pose and facial expression variations.

2.4   Cascade Topic-Aware Face Alignment

Given an image I, we can get a shape prediction S from topic estimation model f and topic specific face alignment models $\mathcal{G}$. However, it is hardly to achieve accurate face alignment result with only one stage process as demonstrated above. So we perform topic-aware face alignment algorithm in a cascade structure.

After obtaining the shape estimation S^1 from the first stage, we further cascade $L-1$ stages to refine the face alignment result, where the jth stage attempts to predict the shape deviation $\Delta S^{j-1} = S_g - S^{j-1}$ based on shape-indexed feature $H(I, S^{j-1})$, $j = 2, 3, ..., L$. It is worth noting that topics T^j at each stage j is redefined by clustering with current target shape deviation ΔS^{j-1}. After defining the topics, we employ a deep auto-encoder network to predict the topic $T \in T^j$ based on shape-indexed feature $H(I, S^{j-1})$. For each stage j, the objective function of topic estimation model f^j is formulated as follows:

$$f^{j*} = \arg\min_{f^j} ||T^j - \psi^j_m(\psi^j_{m-1}(...\psi^j_1(H(I, S^{j-1}))))||_2^2 + \lambda \sum_{i=1}^m ||W_i^j||_F^2, \quad (12)$$

After getting the topic estimation at stage j, we divide the whole training set into several subset based on the topic estimation result. Then a deep face alignment model g_T^j specific to each topic $T \in T^j$ are trained with face images of the corresponding topic. The objective function of deep model g_T^j is shown below:

$$g_T^{j*} = \arg\min_{g_T^j} ||\Delta S_T^{j-1} - \phi^j_{T,n}(\phi^j_{T,(n-1)}(...\phi^j_{T,1}(H(I, S^{j-1}))))||_2^2 + \eta \sum_{i=1}^n ||W_{T,i}^j||_F^2.$$

$$(13)$$

Finally, the overall model $\mathcal{G}^j = \{g_{T_1}^j, g_{T_2}^j, ..., g_{T_w}^j\}$ for the jth stage consists of the face alignment models specific to each topic.

After cascading L stages, the overall topic-aware face alignment model D can be represented as: $D = \{f^1, f^2, ..., f^L; \mathcal{G}^1, \mathcal{G}^2, ..., \mathcal{G}^L\}$. As a result, the face alignment performance is gradually improved stage by stage as shown in Sect. 3.2. Our algorithm converged with 3 or 4 stages.

3   Experiments

In this section, the proposed topic-aware deep auto-encoder (TDA) method is evaluated on three public datasets. Firstly, the performance of each stage of TDA is investigated, and then the overall method is compared with the state-of-the-art methods.

3.1   Datasets and Methods for Comparison

To evaluate the effectiveness of the proposed TDA method, five public datasets are used, i.e., **XM2VTS** [29], **LFPW** [11], **HELEN** [30], **AFW** [19] and **IBUG** [31], among which three ones, i.e., IBUG, XM2VTS and LFPW test set, are used for testing, while the others are used for training. XM2VTS dataset contains 2360 face images of 295 individuals collected under laboratory conditions and the other datasets are collected from the internet, which contain more challenging images in the wild. LFPW contains 1432 images, including 1132 images for training and 300 images for testing. It is firstly published with 29 landmarks annotations by [11]. HELEN consists of 2330 high resolution images from *Flickr* with 194 annotated landmarks, which contains large variations such as head pose, facial expression, partially occlusion, etc. In AFW, 205 images with 468 faces are also collected from *Flickr*, containing complex backgrounds with large variations in head pose and facial expressions. However, only 6 landmarks(the center of eyes, tip of nose, the two corners and center of mouth) are released for this dataset [19]. Recently, the four datasets, i.e., XM2VTS, LFPW, HELEN and AFW, mentioned above, are relabeled with 68 landmarks and published in website [21]. Figure 3(a) shows the definitions of 68 landmarks. The face detection results are also provided in website [21]. Besides these datasets, another 135 images with extreme head pose and facial expressions are released in website [21], denoted as IBUG dataset.

The proposed TDA model is trained with the images from LFPW training set, HELEN and AFW. For testing, the XM2VTS, LFPW test set and IBUG dataset are employed. XM2VTS dataset formulates a laboratory scenario, while LFPW test set and IBUG formulate the uncontrolled scenario which means much more challenging. Especially, IBUG dataset is even more challenging than LFPW due to the extreme head pose and exaggerated facial expressions. For all experiments, the number of stages is 3 and the number of topics is 3 for each stage.

The proposed TDA method is compared with a few state-of-the-art methods, e.g., Dantone et al. [17], Zhu et al. [19], Yu et al. [20], DRMF [10] and SDM [9]. For Dantone et al.'s method, the model released by authors can only detect 10 landmarks, we retrain it to detect 68 landmarks with the same training set for fair comparison. For Zhu et al.'s method, we use the model provided by Asthana et al., which shows better performance in [10]. The public code of SDM only predict 49 inner landmarks (as shown in Fig. 3(b)), so we retrain the SDM method to detect the 68 landmarks with the same training set as ours. Following the CMU 68 points mark-up, the methods, i.e., Dantone et al., Zhu et al., and SDM, are trained to detect 68 landmarks, while the original implementations

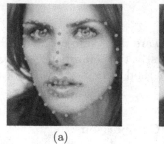 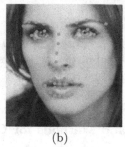

(a)   (b)

Fig. 3. Definition of facial landmarks: (a) 68 points mark-up. (b) 49 points mark-up.

of Yu et al.'s method and DRMF are directly used and they can only estimate 66 facial landmarks (as shown in Fig. 3(a) except two inner mouth corners). Therefore, in order to conduct a fair comparison, all methods are evaluated with the common 66 facial points.

Since all methods are initialized from face detection result, our TDA, SDM [9] and Dantone et al. [17] are conducted with face detection results from [21] and the face detectors for other methods [10,19,20] are kept the same as their papers.

To measure the performance of face alignment, the normalized root-mean-squared error (NRMSE) is employed. On XM2VTS and LFPW datasets, the NRMSE is normalized by the inter-ocular distance, while on IBUG, it is normalized by the face size for clear exhibition since this dataset is extremely difficult. Besides, the cumulative function (CDF) of NRMSE is used for performance evaluation.

3.2   Experimental Results

Performance of Each Stage. The proposed TDA is designed in a cascade structure, and thus we investigate the performance of facial landmark detection at each stage. The experiments are conducted on the most challenging IBUG dataset in terms of average detection accuracy of 66 facial landmarks. The experiment results are shown in Fig. 4. The "Mean Shape" denotes the alignment result by fitting a mean face shape to the face detection window. The "Top-aware Shape Prior" also takes the mean shape as the fitting results, but the mean shape is from the corresponding topic at the first stage rather than the overall mean shape. "Stage 1, 2, 3" represent the facial detection result from the topic-aware deep face alignment model at each stage respectively.

As seen from Fig. 4, shape priors provided by topic discovery is more accurate than simply taking the mean shape as initialization, which demonstrates the effectiveness of topic-aware strategy for face alignment, especially under extreme head poses and facial expressions. Moreover, the deep auto-encoder network specific to each topic significantly improve the detection accuracy at stage 1. This improvement comes from two aspects, better shape prior from topic discovery and better capture of the detailed variations in shape and appearance from the

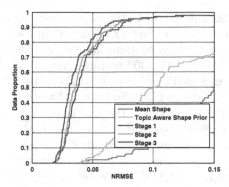
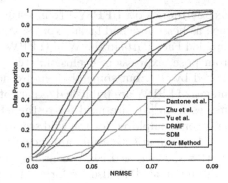

Fig. 4. Performance of each stage on IBUG.

Fig. 5. Experiment on XM2VTS.

deep model. Stage 1 handles the large variations and achieves a much better shape, but it is not accurate enough. To further handle the small shape variations and ensure a better shape, stage 2 and 3 are cascaded. As expected, the performance is improved progressively. It should be noted that, in order to well capture the subtle variations, a higher resolution image containing more subtle information is used in stage 3.

The experiments are conducted on a desktop (Intel i7-3770 3.4 GHz CPU) with MATLAB implementation. The overall run time of TDA is about 150 ms for one image, which means TDA is less time-consuming and can run in real-time.

Experiments on XM2VTS. We firstly compare the proposed TDA with the existing methods on the XM2VTS dataset. In XM2VTS, 2360 face images are collected over 4 sessions under the laboratory environment. It contains variations in shape and appearance due to identity, glasses, beard and so on. In DRMF [10], two face detectors are attached, and we choose the Viola-Jones face detector since all face images in this dataset are almost near frontal. For fair comparison, only the common face images returned by all face detectors are used for evaluation.

Figure 5 shows the comparison results in terms of cumulative error distribution curves. Although Dantone et al. [17] divide the face alignment task as ours, it performs the worst as seen from Fig. 5, mainly due to the limitations of *manual* division of variations and its limited ability of capturing complex nonlinearity. Zhu et al. [19] performs a little better followed by Yu et al. [20], however both are worse than DRMF [10] and SDM [9], possibly because Zhu et al. does not model the correlation of nonadjacent nodes in the mixture-of-trees model, and Yu et al. suffer from the local minimum problem caused by Gauss-Newton optimization. Benefitted from the regression based framework, DRMF and SDM perform much better, and SDM performs even better than DRMF with finer shape-indexed feature. Moreover, our TDA method outperforms SDM, with an improvement up to 5 % when NRMSE is 0.05, by taking the advantages of the topic-aware strategy and the deep models in a cascade structure.

Experiments on LFPW. To investigate the robustness to the large variations such as head pose and facial expression, all methods are further evaluated on the Labeled Face Parts in the Wild (LFPW) dataset, which contains large variations from pose, expression, occlusion, etc. The URLs of the 300 testing images are shared by [11], but some of them are no longer available. Recently, 224 testing images of LFPW are published as part of 300-W dataset [31]. So these 224 testing images from [31] are used for testing. For DRMF method, the tree-based face detector is employed for the wild scenario to achieve better face detection result.

The comparison results are shown in Fig. 6. As seen, all methods degenerate on this dataset as LFPW contains larger shape variations. On this dataset, Dantone et al. [17] also performs the worst as on XM2VTS. Yu et al. [20] is comparable to Zhu et al. [19] since Yu et al. degenerates a little due to inaccurate initializations from optimized part mixture models, especially in case of large variations. Similarly as on XM2VTS, DRMF and SDM perform better, and our TDA outperform all of them. Compared with the best performer SDM, the improvement of our TDA is even up to 10 % when NRMSE is 0.05. Moreover, TDA achieves nearly perfect result, i.e., 100 %, when NRMSE is 0.1. These comparisons demonstrate that our TDA is more robust to the large variations. On one hand, the improvement comes from the better shape prior from the topic-aware strategy, and on the other hand, the deep auto-encoder network can well model the nonlinear mapping from the shape-indexed feature to shape, leading to further improvements.

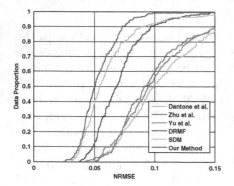 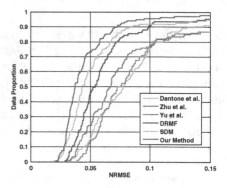

Fig. 6. Experiment on LFPW.   **Fig. 7.** Experiment on IBUG.

Experiments on IBUG. IBUG, as another wild dataset, is more challenging than LFPW due to the extreme head poses and exaggerated facial expressions. The evaluation results of all methods are presented in Fig. 7. Considering the extreme challenges on this dataset, NRMSE is normalized by the face size rather than inter-ocular distance for clear exhibition.

As seen from Fig. 7, the similar conclusions can be obtained that SDM performs the best among the existing methods and our TDA method outperforms

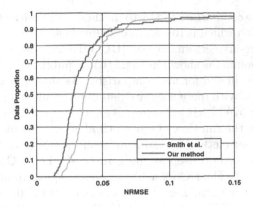

Fig. 8. Comparison with [15] on IBUG.

SDM. Even under the extreme shape variations, our algorithm outperforms all the other methods, demonstrating the effectiveness of our TDA, especially under the large variations.

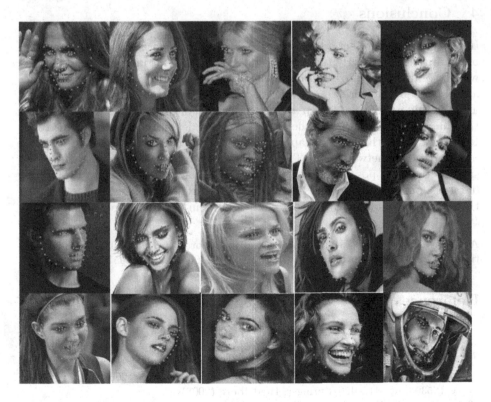

Fig. 9. Exemplar results from IBUG dataset.

Furthermore, we compare our TDA to method [15]. Smith et al. [15] propose a data-driven approach which is robust to extreme head pose and expressions and achieves state-of-the-art performance on IBUG dataset. Since only the detection result of 49 facial points (as shown in Fig. 3(b)) is published in [15], the common 49 landmarks are evaluated for fair comparison. As shown in Fig. 8, our method also outperforms [15] with more accurate detection result when NRMSE is below 0.07. Moreover, the MATLAB implementation of [15] requires 25.5 s for processing one image while the run time of our method is only 150 ms per image, which demonstrates that our method performs more efficiently than [15]. We also compare our TDA with several deep learning methods, i.e., DCNN [24] and Zhou et al. [32] on IBUG: (1) The DCNN achieves an average error of 0.1052, while our TDA achieves better performance with an average error of 0.0848 in terms of five common landmarks. (2) The mean error of Zhou et al. is 0.1455, and our TDA achieves a much lower mean error as 0.1156 in terms of 19 common points. From these comparisons, our TDA also outperforms DCNN [24] and Zhou et al. [32] on the extremely challenging dataset benefited from automatic topic discovery. Figure 9 shows the detection results of our TDA on some challenging images with simultaneous extreme poses, facial expressions and partial occlusions.

4   Conclusions

In this paper, we present a topic-aware deep auto-encoder network for face alignment. Instead of directly tackling the difficult alignment under large variations, we firstly divide it into several easier subtasks according to the topics, which are defined by clustering according to the target shapes or shape deviations. Then within each topic, a deep auto-encoder network is designed to regress from the shape-indexed feature to the shape or shape deviation specific to this topic. Benefitted from the better shape prior from the topic-aware strategy and the non-linear deep networks, our TDA method is robust to large shape variations, such as the head pose and facial expression. As evaluated on three challenging datasets, our method achieves the state-of-the-art performance, demonstrating the effectiveness of TDA. Moreover, our TDA can perform in real-time.

Acknowledgements. This work is partially supported by Natural Science Foundation of China under contracts Nos. 61025010, 61173065, and 61390511.

References

1. Cootes, T.F., Taylor, C.J., Cooper, D.H., Graham, J.: Active shape models-their training and application. Comput. Vis. Image Underst. (CVIU) **61**, 38–59 (1995)
2. Gu, L., Kanade, T.: A generative shape regularization model for robust face alignment. In: Forsyth, D., Torr, P., Zisserman, A. (eds.) ECCV 2008, Part I. LNCS, vol. 5302, pp. 413–426. Springer, Heidelberg (2008)
3. Cootes, T.F., Edwards, G.J., Taylor, C.J.: Active appearance models. IEEE Trans. Pattern Anal. Mach. Intell. (TPAMI) **23**, 681–685 (2001)

4. Matthews, I., Baker, S.: Active appearance models revisited. Int. J. Comput. Vis. (IJCV) **60**, 135–164 (2004)
5. van der Maaten, L., Hendriks, E.: Capturing appearance variation in active appearance models. In: IEEE Conference on Computer Vision and Pattern Recognition Workshops (CVPRW), pp. 34–41 (2010)
6. Tipping, M.E., Bishop, C.M.: Mixtures of probabilistic principal component analyzers. Neural Comput. **11**, 443–482 (1999)
7. Dollár, P., Welinder, P., Perona, P.: Cascaded pose regression. In: IEEE Conference on Computer Vision and Pattern Recognition (CVPR), pp. 1078–1085 (2010)
8. Cao, X., Wei, Y., Wen, F., Sun, J.: Face alignment by explicit shape regression. In: IEEE Conference on Computer Vision and Pattern Recognition (CVPR), pp. 2887–2894 (2012)
9. Xiong, X., De la Torre, F.: Supervised descent method and its applications to face alignment. In: IEEE Conference on Computer Vision and Pattern Recognition (CVPR) (2013)
10. Asthana, A., Zafeiriou, S., Cheng, S., Pantic, M.: Robust discriminative response map fitting with constrained local models. In: IEEE Conference on Computer Vision and Pattern Recognition (CVPR), pp. 3444–3451 (2013)
11. Belhumeur, P.N., Jacobs, D.W., Kriegman, D.J., Kumar, N.: Localizing parts of faces using a consensus of exemplars. In: IEEE Conference on Computer Vision and Pattern Recognition (CVPR), pp. 545–552 (2011)
12. Saragih, J.: Principal regression analysis. In: IEEE Conference on Computer Vision and Pattern Recognition (CVPR), pp. 2881–2888 (2011)
13. Bartlett, M.S., Littlewort, G.C., Frank, M.G., Lainscsek, C., Fasel, I.R., Movellan, J.R.: Automatic recognition of facial actions in spontaneous expressions. J. Multimedia **1**, 22–35 (2006)
14. Kim, M., Kumar, S., Pavlovic, V., Rowley, H.: Face tracking and recognition with visual constraints in real-world videos. In: IEEE Conference on Computer Vision and Pattern Recognition (CVPR), pp. 1–8 (2008)
15. Smith, B.M., Brandt, J., Lin, Z., Zhang, L.: Nonparametric context modeling of local appearance for pose-and expression-robust facial landmark localization. In: IEEE Conference on Computer Vision and Pattern Recognition (CVPR) (2014)
16. Burgos-Artizzu, X.P., Perona, P., Dollár, P.: Robust face landmark estimation under occlusion. In: IEEE International Conference on Computer Vision (ICCV) (2013)
17. Dantone, M., Gall, J., Fanelli, G., Van Gool, L.: Real-time facial feature detection using conditional regression forests. In: IEEE Conference on Computer Vision and Pattern Recognition (CVPR), pp. 2578–2585 (2012)
18. Zhao, X., Kim, T.K., Luo, W.: Unified face analysis by iterative multi-output random forests. In: IEEE Conference on Computer Vision and Pattern Recognition (CVPR) (2014)
19. Zhu, X., Ramanan, D.: Face detection, pose estimation, and landmark localization in the wild. In: IEEE Conference on Computer Vision and Pattern Recognition (CVPR), pp. 2879–2886 (2012)
20. Yu, X., Huang, J., Zhang, S., Yan, W., Metaxas, D.N.: Pose-free facial landmark fitting via optimized part mixtures and cascaded deformable shape model. In: IEEE International Conference on Computer Vision (ICCV) (2013)
21. 300 faces in-the-wild challenge. (http://ibug.doc.ic.ac.uk/resources/300-W/)
22. Bengio, Y.: Learning deep architectures for AI. Found. Trends Mach. Learn. **2**, 1–127 (2009)

23. Krizhevsky, A., Sutskever, I., Hinton, G.: Imagenet classification with deep convolutional neural networks. In: Advances in Neural Information Processing Systems (NIPS), pp. 1106–1114 (2012)
24. Sun, Y., Wang, X., Tang, X.: Deep convolutional network cascade for facial point detection. In: IEEE Conference on Computer Vision and Pattern Recognition (CVPR), pp. 3476–3483 (2013)
25. Luo, P., Wang, X., Tang, X.: Hierarchical face parsing via deep learning. In: IEEE Conference on Computer Vision and Pattern Recognition (CVPR), pp. 2480–2487 (2012)
26. Wu, Y., Wang, Z., Ji, Q.: Facial feature tracking under varying facial expressions and face poses based on restricted boltzmann machines. In: IEEE Conference on Computer Vision and Pattern Recognition (CVPR), pp. 3452–3459 (2013)
27. Le, Q.V., Coates, A., Prochnow, B., Ng, A.Y.: On optimization methods for deep learning. In: International Conference on Machine Learning (ICML), pp. 265–272 (2011)
28. Lowe, D.G.: Distinctive image features from scale-invariant keypoints. Int. J. Comput. Vis. (IJCV) **60**, 91–110 (2004)
29. Messer, K., Matas, J., Kittler, J., Luettin, J., Maitre, G.: Xm2vtsdb: the extended m2vts database. In: Second International Conference on Audio and Video-Based Biometric Person Authentication (AVBPA), vol. 964, pp. 965–966 (1999)
30. Le, V., Brandt, J., Lin, Z., Bourdev, L., Huang, T.S.: Interactive facial feature localization. In: Fitzgibbon, A., Lazebnik, S., Perona, P., Sato, Y., Schmid, C. (eds.) ECCV 2012, Part III. LNCS, vol. 7574, pp. 679–692. Springer, Heidelberg (2012)
31. Sagonas, C., Tzimiropoulos, G., Zafeiriou, S., Pantic, M.: 300 faces in-the-wild challenge: the first facial landmark localization challenge. In: The IEEE International Conference on Computer Vision Workshops (ICCVW) (2013)
32. Zhou, E., Fan, H., Cao, Z., Jiang, Y., Yin, Q.: Extensive facial landmark localization with coarse-to-fine convolutional network cascade. In: The IEEE International Conference on Computer Vision Workshops (ICCVW) (2013)

Author Index

Printed in the United States
By Bookmasters